NURSING IN THE COMMUNITY

NURSING IN THE COMMUNITY

Bonnie Bullough, RNC, PhD, FAAN
Professor, School of Nursing
State University of New York at Buffalo
Buffalo, New York

Vern Bullough, RN, PhD, FAAN
SUNY Distinguished Professor
State University of New York College at Buffalo
Buffalo, New York

with 95 *illustrations*

THE C.V. MOSBY COMPANY
ST. LOUIS • BALTIMORE • PHILADELPHIA • TORONTO 1990

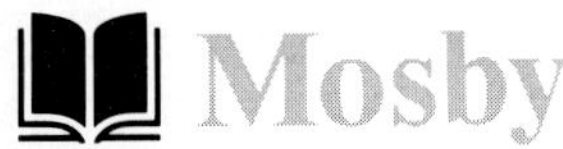

Editor N. Darlene Como
Developmental Editor Laurie Sparks
Project Manager Patricia Tannian
Production Editor Tim Sainz
Design Candace Conner

Printed in the United States of America

The C.V. Mosby Company
11830 Westline Industrial Drive, St. Louis, Missouri 63146

Library of Congress Cataloging in Publication Data

Nursing in the community
[edited by] Bonnie Bullough, Vern Bullough.
p. cm.
Includes bibliographical references.
ISBN 0-8016-6065-3
1. Community health nursing. I. Bullough, Bonnie. II. Bullough, Vern L.
[DNLM: 1. Community Health Nursing. WY 106 N97553]
RT98.N88 1990
610.73'43—dc20
DNLM/DLC 89-13540
for Library of Congress CIP
ISBN 0-8016-6065-3

GW/VH/VH 9 8 7 6 5 4 3 2 1

Contributors

Sherrie H. Bernat, RNC, MS
Women's Health Care Nurse Practitioner and Doctoral Student
School of Nursing
State University of New York at Buffalo
Buffalo, New York

Jeri Bigbee, RNC, PhD, FNP
Associate Professor
School of Nursing
University of Wyoming
Laramie, Wyoming

Constance D. Blair, RN, MS, MPH
Certified Family Nurse Practitioner
Arroyo Vista Family Health Center
Los Angeles, California

Alma J. Blake, PhD, RD
Associate Professor, Nutrition Program
State University of New York at Buffalo
Buffalo, New York

G. Lorain Brault, MS, RN
President, Hospital Home Health Agency of California
Torrance, California

Gwen M. Felton, PhD, RNC
Associate Professor, Community Health Nursing
Department of Nursing Systems
University of South Carolina
Columbia, South Carolina

Cathleen I. Getty, RN, MS
Associate Professor
School of Nursing
State University of New York at Buffalo
Buffalo, New York

Althea M. Glenister, RN, PhD, MPH
Associate Professor
School of Nursing
State University of New York at Buffalo
Buffalo, New York

G. Winnifred Humphreys, MSW
Clinical Associate Professor
School of Nursing
State University of New York at Buffalo
Buffalo, New York

Matthew Leopard, MA
Executive Officer
New York State National Guard
Buffalo, New York

Mary Ann Ludwig, RN, PhD
Clinical Assistant Professor
School of Nursing
State University of New York at Buffalo
Buffalo, New York

Lucy N. Marion, RNC, MN
Doctoral Student
University of Illinois
Chicago, Illinois

Lisa A. Monagle, RN, CNM, PhD
Adjunct Clinical Assistant Professor
School of Nursing
State University of New York at Buffalo
Buffalo, New York

Mary Anne Neary, MSN, RN
Clinical Assistant Professor
School of Nursing
State University of New York at Buffalo
Buffalo, New York

Mary Anne Noble, RN, DNSc
Clinical Associate Professor
School of Nursing
State University of New York at Buffalo
Buffalo, New York

Mary Ann Parsons, PhD, RNC
Professor, Community Health Nursing
Department of Nursing Systems
University of South Carolina
Columbia, South Carolina

Stephen Pendleton, DA
Assistant Professor, Political Science
State University of New York at Buffalo
Buffalo, New York

Janice Roes Salter, MN, MA
In-Service Education Coordinator
Erie County Home and Infirmary
Alden, New York

Anne Herrstrom Skelly, RN, MS, ANP-C
Director, Undergraduate Nursing Program
School of Nursing
State University of New York at Buffalo
Buffalo, New York

Linda H. Snell, RNC, MS
Women's Health Care Nurse Practitioner and Doctoral Student
School of Nursing
State University of New York at Buffalo
Buffalo, New York

Marietta P. Stanton, PhD, RN
Director, Continuing Nurse Education
School of Nursing
State University of New York at Buffalo
Buffalo, New York

Preface

Nursing in the Community can be summarized briefly as a comprehensive text for all nurses who work in the community and all students who are preparing for community nursing roles. But the text does more, since it recognizes that the traditional community health nursing role is changing. For much of its history community health nursing focused on preventive health care. Although this still remains the primary nursing role in the community, other nursing positions are developing in response to trends in society and the health care system. Some of the changes have been forced by federal legislation such as the 1983 federal action that changed the reimbursement system for Medicare from a primary emphasis on hospitalization to one that encouraged early discharge of most hospitalized clients. This in effect both changed and expanded the work of home health care nurses, case managers, and discharge planning nurses. Other changes have occurred in the roles of nurse practitioners, nurse-midwives, school nurses, and occupational health nurses. The result has been a change from the traditional role of nurses in the community delivering only preventive care to a varied role demanding more skills and ability as nurses are called on to fill a variety of nursing jobs in the community.

To tie these changes together the nursing process is used as the organizing framework for a discussion of these roles. The nursing process can be applied to a variety of community settings with a variety of clients. Since these changes did not occur in a vacuum, we have attempted to put them in their historical and sociologic perspective, more so than most other community health texts. It is hoped that by understanding where nurses came from and where we are now, readers can plan more effectively for the future.

We clustered the content of the book into seven units that help focus topics. Chapter outlines and objectives are presented at the beginning of each chapter to highlight and organize the material, and each chapter concludes with a summary and some questions for discussion. It is hoped that any discussion will move away from the material in the text and allow readers to use their own knowledge and experience in the discussion. For those interested in further reading or even further research into special topics, references and bibliographies are included at the end of each chapter.

Community nursing has always been demanding of nurses, but it seems to be more demanding now than ever before. This demand places a responsibility on nurses to obtain the most advanced knowledge and skills possible for their practice. This book provides the beginning framework and basic knowledge of community nursing, but community health nursing encompasses more than any single book can include. Additional reading and observation in the field are needed to meet the challenge of work in the community.

This book represents a collaborative effort, not only between the two editors, nurses who happen to be married to each other and longtime collaborators, but also between all the contributors. Our contributors were picked because of their expertise and their ability to communicate ideas. They represent all sections of the United States and have a wide variety of backgrounds and experiences. We believe they are an outstanding group, and we hope that you will agree.

A book, however, requires much more than an author sitting down at a word processor and typing. It requires the collaborative effort of a whole array of workers from editors and copyeditors to secretaries and reference checkers. Many people helped put this book together, not the least of whom are Mary Boldt and Ann Marie Bindert, secretaries in the dean's office at the State University of New York at Buffalo School of Nursing. Although these two are mentioned by name, the secretaries of all the contributors, some of whose names we do not know, are equally important. Ruth Heintz deserves special thanks for her prizewinning photographs. Special acknowledgement is due to the Hospital Home Health Care Agency of California, which also furnished some of the photographs. Janet Roes Salter wrote the instructor's manual for *Nursing in the Community*, which professors of community health nursing will find useful. Last but not least, thanks are due to those at Mosby who did the final work on the manuscript, particularly Darlene Como, Laurie Sparks, and Tim Sainz. Obviously there are many others who contributed whom we have not mentioned, and we hope they accept our love and appreciation. We think *Nursing in the Community* is an outstanding book, and we hope you will agree.

Bonnie Bullough
Vern Bullough

Contents

NURSING IN THE COMMUNITY

NURSES have filled a variety of community-based roles since the nineteenth century, although their titles and job descriptions have changed over time. The nineteenth century district nurse became the public health nurse of the early twentieth century and the community health nurse of the current era. The visiting nurse of the past is now the home health care nurse, and the industrial nurse of the 1940s is today's occupational health care nurse. School nurses have retained their title, but in many settings they are facing expanded role expectations. In addition, some new community nursing roles are developing, including those of case manager, nurse practitioner, and hospital discharge planning nurse.

The two chapters in the first section trace the history of these changes and describe the current array of community nursing positions. This broader focus departs somewhat from the tradition in community texts, which in the past emphasized the preventive care–oriented community health nurse. This book includes that focus but adds material about the new developments in the community. The decision to include the new and changing roles is based primarily on recent developments in the health care delivery system. Clients are being discharged from hospitals, mental institutions, and skilled nursing homes earlier in the illness cycle. The result is an increased demand for nursing care in the community and new challenges for the community-oriented nursing work force.

Nursing in the Community: the Context

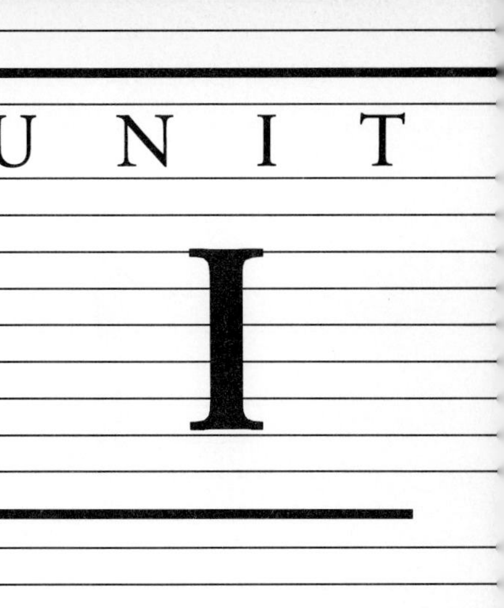

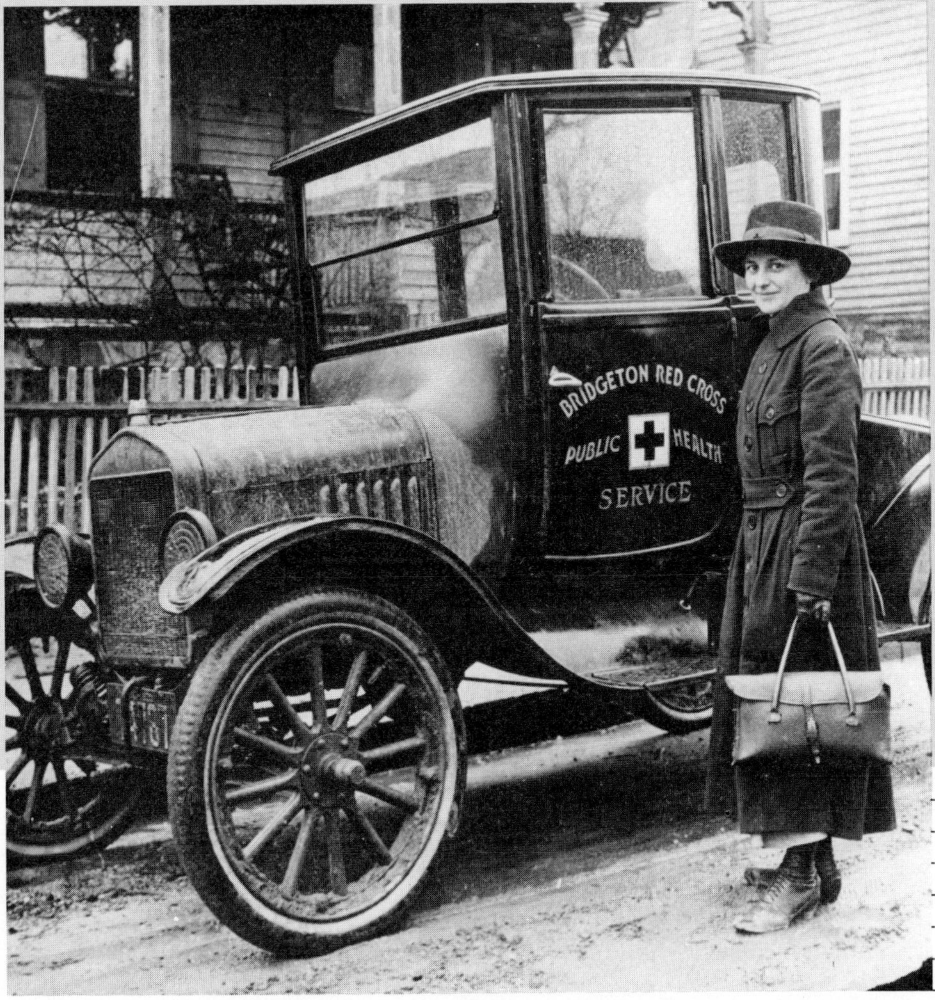

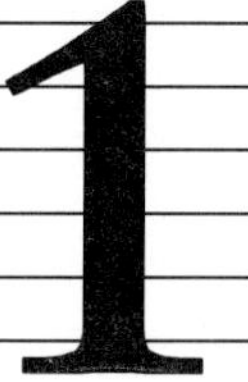

CHAPTER 1

Dynamic Nature of Community Nursing: Early Historical Background

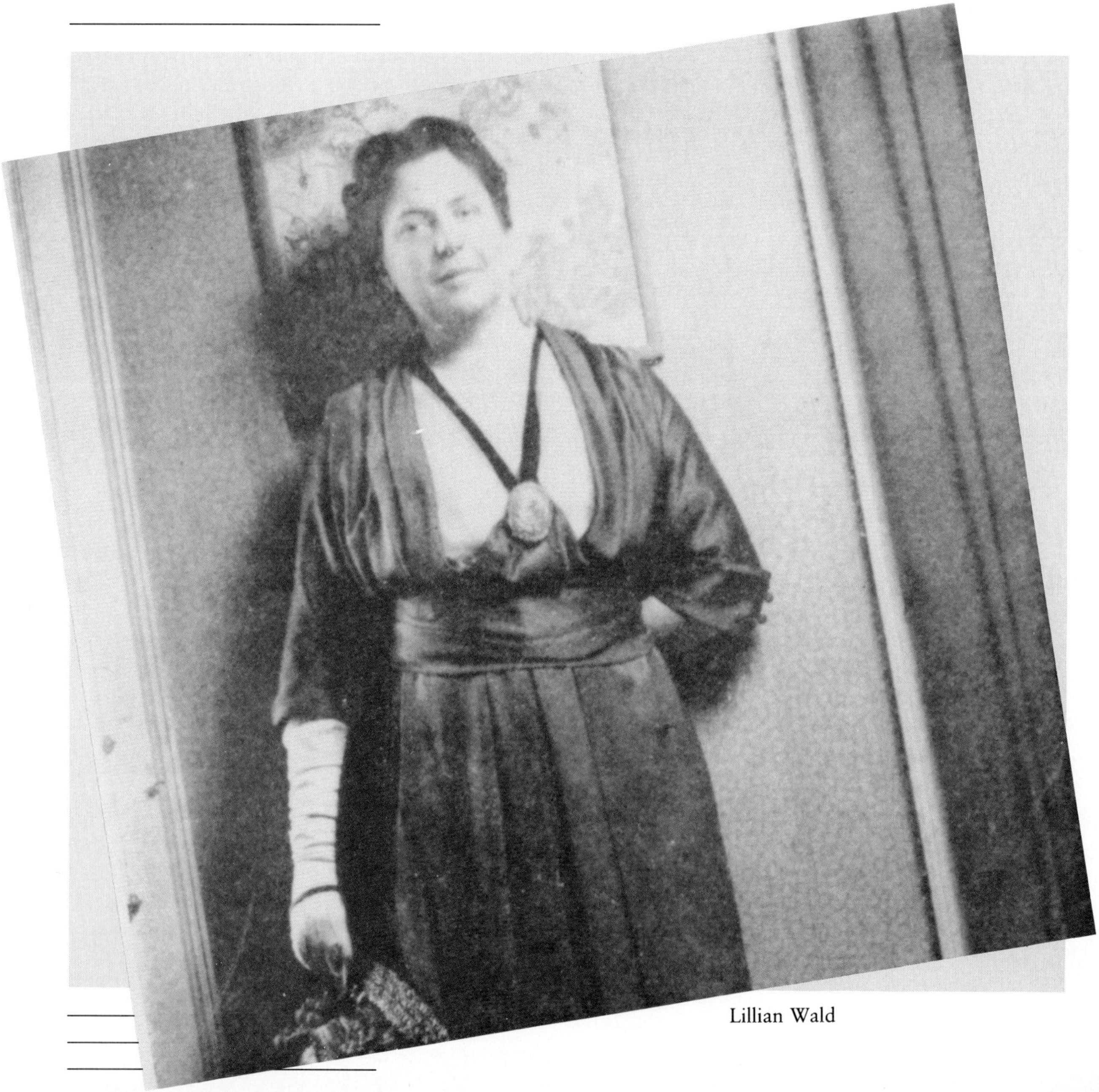

Lillian Wald

CHAPTER OUTLINE

Beginnings of public health
Development of modern public health
Melting pot
Early public health efforts
District nursing
Visiting nurses
Lillian Wald and the settlement houses
Public health nursing
Rural public health nursing
Increasing government support
Summary

OBJECTIVES

After completing this chapter, the reader should be able to:

1. Trace the highlights of the history of the interdisciplinary public health movement.
2. Understand the impact of immigration on the public health needs of Americans.
3. Describe the accomplishments of Lillian Wald.
4. Trace the development of the community nursing role from its origins in district nursing to the present.

NURSES who work in the community fill a variety of roles. Although some of these roles are new, others have their roots in community-focused roles that developed in the nineteenth and early twentieth centuries as a part of an interdisciplinary public health movement. C.E.A. Winslow, a leading figure in the movement, described public health in 1920 as the science and art of preventing disease, prolonging life, and promoting health through organized community efforts. These efforts included sanitation of the environment, control of communicable diseases, personal hygiene education, organization of medical and nursing services to establish an early diagnosis and to give preventive treatment of disease, and the development of social machinery to ensure a standard of living adequate for health maintenance (Winslow, 1920).

These nursing tasks remain part of the public health field even though their nature has changed and new tasks have emerged, including a growing concern with environmental issues and different communicable diseases, delivering medical care differently, and dealing with the rising standards of health maintenance along with the changing definition of what constitutes an adequate standard of living. In the process, Winslow's concepts of the role of the nurse have been extended to include all nursing activities in the community—even many functions that go far beyond duties he envisioned a public health nurse carrying out. Modern community health practice also reflects an orientation toward wellness, and although the preventive aspect of Winslow's definition still exists, its meaning has been broadened to include primary, secondary, and even tertiary preventive action. Primary prevention is aimed at the healthy population and takes place before symptoms appear. It entails providing the necessary information and support for decision making to maintain maximal functioning. Secondary prevention occurs with early diagnosis and treatment of illness or disability and is aimed at helping the patient recover as soon as possible. Tertiary prevention involves restoring people either to health or to the most functional condition possible after disease or disability occurs. Thus community health nursing encompasses public health, but it goes beyond traditional public health and in fact is a new frontier of nursing care.

BEGINNINGS OF PUBLIC HEALTH

Preventive nursing efforts predate the twentieth century movement. Public health policies can be traced from the beginning of recorded history. Papyri from ancient Egypt and clay tablets from the civilizations in the Tigris-Euphrates valley emphasize the importance of maintaining good health. These records include incantations, recipes, and advice on how to remain well or recover from illness. The legal tradition of Judaism has always emphasized preventive health measures. Judaic scriptures encouraged the disposal of garbage and excrement outside the city or camp, provided for quarantine of certain diseased persons, outlawed spitting, and emphasized body cleanliness. Many of these ideas came from Egypt and Babylon but became part of the ancient Hebrews' religious tradition and as such have come down to us. Other civilizations, such as that of China, gave similar emphasis to public health. Much of the Chinese medical advice was concerned with keeping yin and yang in harmony. This involved diet, exercises, and abstinence from certain activities and foods.

Preventive measures were in fact the most effective way for early people to deal with potential problems of sickness, disease, and deformity even though they did not know what actually caused such anomalies. Without knowledge of microorganisms or insect and animal vectors, people still learned from experience that certain areas were more unhealthy or dangerous than others, that certain times of the year seemed more likely to bring sickness, and that certain foods and practices should be avoided. Often what ancient peoples did for religious reasons or as part of a tradition now can be seen to have public health implications. For example, in south China, the people created fish ponds where they later planned to establish settlements, and although this apparently was done for esthetic and dietary reasons, it also seems clear from today's knowledge that the creation of such ponds cut down the mosquitoes that carried malaria because the fish ate the mosquito larva. A different example, this time in Europe, was the isolation of lepers and their removal from contact with society. Often their banishment was due to the belief that only sinners contract leprosy. Although this seems a particularly cruel way to deal with leprosy, researchers today believe the resulting isolation was one of the major factors that eliminated the disease in Europe during the late medieval period.

Many effective techniques associated with public health developed during the great bubonic pandemic of 1347-1351, which killed about one third of the people of Europe. The plague, known as black death, became endemic to Europe for the next three centuries, flaring up periodically and killing many people. It was during the first pandemic that various governments in Italy developed health boards. These boards were widely adopted elsewhere. In Venice on March 30, 1348, the Maggior Consiglio (Great Council), confronted with the frightening spread of plague, hurriedly resolved to appoint a committee of three wise men chosen among the Council members to consider "diligently all possible ways to preserve public health and avoid the corruption of the environment." It was not until a century later that such boards were made permanent. They were called Provveditori di Sanita' (literally Commissioners of Public Health), and their purpose was to seek "remedies" to prevent the outbreak and spread of contagion. Cities were organized by districts, and health officials were elected from each district. Their duty was to report outbreaks of plague or disease so that immediate steps could be taken. As late as 1721, the Public Health Board of Venice was regarded as unequaled elsewhere in Europe. In that year the Consul of Holland requested detailed information on its organization and functioning for his government in the Netherlands (Cipolla, 1976).

Once the power of public health officials was established, it expanded. Among duties assumed by various boards in Europe were supervision of the quality of the meat, fish, and wine sold in local markets, control of beggars and prostitutes, regulation of burials, cemeteries, and pesthouses, supervision of physicians, surgeons, and apothecaries, including the sale and preparation of drugs, and many additional duties assigned to them from time to time by government officials. Since it was clear that the health boards could hurt many interests, including powerful and entrenched ones, they were protected, at least during outbreaks of disease, by having them answerable only to the ruling bodies of the state.

England and America were slower to develop such boards, but the urbanization brought on by the Industrial Revolution ultimately resulted in more effective public health legislation. Nevertheless, developments were slower in Great Britain and areas settled by the British. Even as late as the beginning of the nineteenth century, a German writer noted that the British attached little importance to the regulation of public health and that Americans did almost nothing at all to regulate public health (Mohl, 1833).

This meant that what action did take place often resulted from the efforts of dedicated individual advocates or action by volunteer groups. The famous New England minister Cotton Mather (1663-1728) was a vocal advocate of smallpox inoculation. He learned about the inoculation from slaves brought from Africa, and after observing its effectiveness, he began advocating it. Mather was supported by some English publications that commented on the Turkish experience with inoculation. Unfortunately, inoculation was risky, and even though it had great value in preventing smallpox, some patients who were inoculated with the live virus contracted the disease and died. Vaccination with cowpox, a method developed by the English physician Edward Jenner (1749-1823), was more effective in the long run and eliminated smallpox from the world.

Also important in helping improve public health were popular manuals designed to teach health measures. This movement has gone under various names from the "personal hygiene movement" at the turn of the century to the "wellness movement" of today. The ancient Greeks had a number of manuals that gave advice on diet, child care, and personal life-styles. Similar manuals existed in medieval and early modern Europe. Much of the advice in the past is helpful even today, but some of it was doubtful when it was first offered and over the years has proved unhelpful or even harmful. Many people still subscribe to outmoded ideas that have been passed down through families or entire cultures. Some of this advice can be traced to the ancient Greeks who held that good health was maintained in a balance between four humors (phlegm, blood, black bile, and yellow bile). Some of these humors were thought to be disproportionately hot, whereas others were thought to be cold; an imbalance between the various humors caused illness that needed treatment. Greek physicians prescribed things that were cold for illnesses resulting from heat. Whether a remedy was hot or cold, however, was not necessarily related to its actual temperature; for example, ice was considered hot because it "burned" the mouth.

In some of the immigrant cultures in the United States, particularly those that come from Spanish-speaking areas of the Americas, there is still a widespread belief that infants are particularly susceptible to "cold stomach." Infants diagnosed as suffering from this do not receive cold foods such as citrus fruits even though the nurse might recommend such foods. Expectant mothers in such cultural groups are often cautious about eating too many foods that are classified as hot because it is believed this causes their babies to have diaper rashes when they are born.

DEVELOPMENT OF MODERN PUBLIC HEALTH

Although some of these ideas of the past seem quaint and others seem harmful, it must be remembered that they date from a period before the cause of disease was known. Knowledge of causality for disease dates primarily from the last part of the nineteenth century. A key figure was Louis Pasteur (1822-1895), who demonstrated a correlation between microorganisms and disease—a correlation that was developed further by individuals such as Ferdinand Cohn (1828-1898), who classified a number of bacteria, Joseph Schroeter (1835-1894), who developed a technique for growing pure colonies of bacteria, and most notably Robert Koch (1843-1910). It was Koch in 1876 who demonstrated in a public trial that lasted 3 days that anthrax is caused by the anthrax bacillus. Once this was demonstrated, other disease-causing organisms were quickly identified (Table 1-1).

Once the causal microorganism was found, the next stage was to trace the development of the disease, develop vaccines, control insect or animal vectors, and mount effective preventive campaigns. Public health had come of age. Most of the continental countries could quickly develop effective disease prevention programs because there was a tradition of government support of public health measures. But in the United States, and to a certain extent in England, there was a reluctance to intervene as directly or as drastically because of differing concepts about the nature of the state. The economic beliefs of the day held that individuals were supposed to fend for themselves. Those unable to do so would be helped by private charitable action. Undoubtedly this lack of intervention was acceptable to the majority of Americans who lived on farms and villages and small towns, but it proved totally inadequate in urbanized settings that developed with the industrialization of the United States during the last part of the nineteenth century. The shift in population that occurred with industrialization in the

TABLE 1-1 Discovery of Pathogenic Organisms

Year	Disease organism	Investigator
1876	Anthrax (bacillus)	Koch
1879	Gonorrhea (gonococcus)	Neisser
1880	Typhoid (bacillus found in tissues)	Ebert
	Leprosy	Hansen
	Malaria	Laveran
1882	Tuberculosis	Koch
	Glanders	Loeffler and Schutz
1883	Cholera	Koch
	Streptococcus (erysipelas)	Fehleisen
1884	Diphtheria	Klebs and Loeffler
	Typhoid (bacillus isolated)	Gaffky
	Staphylococcus	Rosenbach
	Streptococcus	Rosenbach
	Tetanus	Nicolaier
1885	*Escherichia coli*	Escherich
1886	Pneumococcus	Fraenkel
1887	Malta fever	Bruce
	Soft chancre	Ducrey
1892	Gas gangrene	Welch and Nuttal
1894	Plague	Yersin and Kitasato
	Botulism	van Ermengem
1898	Dysentery bacillus	Shiga

United States, coupled with the growing realization that diseases and epidemics common among the poor could easily spread to the upper and middle classes, resulted in public health activities receiving far more attention than they had before the Industrial Revolution.

MELTING POT

In addition to urbanization, America was literally besieged by immigrants in the nineteenth century. All Americans who cannot trace their descent to Native Americans are either immigrants or descendants of immigrants or slaves. The trickle of immigrants in the colonial period grew to flood tides in the nineteenth century. The first big wave followed in the aftermath of the Napoleonic Wars, which ended in 1815, and there were increases during each successive decade until the 1850s when more than 2 million Europeans migrated to this country. The reasons for coming to America varied from individual to individual, but there were some general motivations. There had been a rapid expansion of European population during the nineteenth century that put a premium on land, which was plentiful in America. Political discontent played a role, as evidenced by the German migration following the failed Revolution of 1848, and so did religion (witness the converts to the Mormon Church and their westward trek), but the most important motives were economic. Immigrants sought land, jobs, and a better life. National tragedies that led to displacement of populations should not be overlooked. The potato blight hit Ireland's main food crop between 1845 and 1849, caused widespread famine, and forced the survivors to seek new homes and opportunities in America. Later in the century pogroms in Russia encouraged a mass migration of Jews from that country (Gordon, 1964; Jones, 1960).

Most eighteenth century immigrants settled on the undeveloped frontier land close to the eastern seaboard, and although many nineteenth century immigrants headed for the western frontier, disproportionate numbers ended up in the rapidly growing eastern cities. Here they were crowded into slums that were usually located in and around the business or factory district of the city. The wealthier inhabitants of the city moved farther out, but commuter railroads and ultimately streetcars made it possible for them to continue working in the city. Adjustment to the New World and to new conditions has never been easy. Affluent or successful people were less likely to emigrate to America. Consequently many of those who did come to the United States were poor. What little money they had was used on transportation to the new land. In fact, this was one of the reasons these people often settled in the city rather than in the countryside in the nineteenth and twentieth centuries; many of them lacked the resources to go much farther (Handlin, 1952). A second wave of immigration after the Civil War added to the growth of the cities, but new immigrants and American city dwellers also took advantage of the offer of unsettled land made by the developing railroads. This land was given to settlers free so that the railroads would have a better chance of succeeding.

The immigrants were strangers to the immediate world around them. They fought the loneliness of their condition and created a variety of formal and informal institutions to help them adjust. Usually immigrants settled in the same neighborhood as their former countrymen. In the process, they created Germantowns, New Irelands, and Little Polands. Eventually, as these settlers became successful, some of them were able to move from the ethnic communities into more comfortable neighborhoods. The abandoned ethnic neighborhood was taken over by new immigrants who, like their predecessors, were attracted by the cheap rents and central location. As the changeover took place, the new arrivals filtered into the district, occupying house after house as they became vacant, until the whole character of a Germantown had changed into a Little Italy or an Irish enclave had given way to a Russian Jewish ghetto. This challenge to the old settled groups by the new immigrants was often associated with hostility and conflict, and the poverty of the new was accentuated by the poor quality of their housing, which was constantly deteriorating, since the landlords were generally reluctant to improve the tenements or apartments that the new immigrants crowded.

The immigrants were also exploited. Sometimes this exploitation was by individuals of the same ethnic group whose experience or knowledge of English enabled them to deal with the more established Americans. However, outsiders who had little sympathy for or understanding of the new immigrants were often the manipulators. The outsiders could use the immigrants' naivete, poverty, and lack of English language skills to exploit them. Unfortunately, the tendency of the immigrants to "ghettoize" themselves made them more exploitable. The land near the center of the city, not the existing structures, might eventually have great value. Inevitably the housing became dilapidated, and essential repairs were neglected as the absentee owners waited for their land to appreciate while milking it for all it was worth. The newcomers lacked the economic or political power to demand improvements. Moreover, their segregation made it possible for the cities to neglect essential services in their areas without inconveniencing richer and more politically powerful citizens. Municipal services provided for the immigrants ranging from garbage collection to police protection were inferior to those supplied to the residents of the newer sections of the city (Burgess, 1929).

For newcomers trapped in the city, life was hard and death rates were high. New York City and the other major Atlantic ports where the immigrant concentration was great allowed newcomers to be crowded into multistory tenements. In the interior of the country, smaller units were more the norm, but it was not unusual to crowd six families into units built for one. This overcrowding helped spread disease; tuberculosis rates were particularly high among the foreign-born population. The newest immigrants were also pushed into the least desirable places to live. In Chicago, a transportation center, they were forced to live in areas next to the slaughterhouses; in Boston they were hemmed in by the docks and markets of the North End, and in other cities and towns they were forced to live near railroad switching yards. A great problem in tenements was sanitation. Many of the early buildings had been built without privies. Although after the middle of the nineteenth century most tenements were built with privies or water closets, which washed away the sewage, these were located outside in the backyards and the alleys. For people who lived on the sixth floor, an outside toilet was inconvenient to say the least. Later, as the modern flush toilet was developed, the newer tenements were built with inside toilets, usually two on each floor. However, these were open to all comers, but charged to the care of none and left to the neglect of all. In the winter the pipes overflowed, and weeks might go by before the landlord set matters right. Some of the most neglected tenements retained the odor of human excrement until they were torn down.

Filth was inescapable. Open drainage ditches were common, and even in a city as large as Chicago it was not until well into the twentieth century that all the sewers were covered, so flyborne diseases were prevalent until then. Since an adequate water supply was difficult to obtain, it was often necessary to carry tubs and jugs from taps in the alley. Contamination of this water supply led to epidemics. Illness was rampant, drunkenness was common, and behavioral disorders and neuroses—all classified as insanity then—were ever present. The American people however, were slow to deal with these problems (Burgess, 1929). The New York State Senate appointed a committee to look into the need for municipal health measures in 1858. The committee attributed the high rate of mortality in New York City at the time to the

> overcrowded condition of tenement houses, the want of practical knowledge of the proper mode of constructing such houses, deficiency of light, imperfect ventilation, impurities in domestic economy, unwholesome food and beverages, insufficient sewage (i.e., sewers), want of cleanliness in the streets and at the wharves and piers, to a general disregard of sanitary precautions, and finally, to the imperfect execution of existing ordinance, and the total absence of a regularly organized sanitary police (Rosen, 1958).

One of the great motivators for action was the possibility that the various epidemics, most of which started in the slum areas, could spread into wealthier areas. Cholera epidemics hit in 1832, 1848, 1866, and 1873. Yellow fever and smallpox were more or less endemic during much of the nineteenth century. Diphtheria and scarlet fever were major causes of death among children, and during the 40 years from 1840 to 1880 scarlet fever was particularly virulent.

EARLY PUBLIC HEALTH EFFORTS

Communities were slow to do anything about sickness in an organized way except to rely on charity. Probably the most important health care institutions for the poor in the nineteenth century were the dispensaries that appeared in England in the late eighteenth century and were imported to Philadelphia in 1786. Growth of the movement escalated after the Civil War, and by 1874 there were 29 dispensaries in New York City alone, which treated 213,000 patients per year. By 1900 some 876,000 patients were being treated per year. Most dispensaries had a resident physician who performed minor surgery, pulled teeth, and treated minor medical complications. The primary task of the physician was to issue prescriptions, and it was the routine and exclusive dependence on drug therapy that distinguished the medicine of the poor from that of the middle class. As dispensaries grew in size, their staffs increased, but almost all dispensaries operated on shoestring budgets of no more than $4000 to $5000 per year. Financial backing was mostly through private charities; only in New York City did the dispensaries receive any city or state money.

Reforms in health care began with individual calls for action, often joined by groups of individuals who were usually located in the rapidly growing eastern seaport cities that were the focus of much of the early immigration. John C. Griscom, a New York City inspector for the Board of Health (a position dating back to 1804), appended a brief report of the sanitary conditions of the city to his formal report in 1845. Lemuel Shattuck of Boston issued a *Census of Boston* in 1845 and in the process established a solid foundation for the accurate reporting of vital statistics.

LEMUEL SHATTUCK

Lemuel Shattuck believed that sickness and death could be repelled by adherence to a moral code emphasizing godliness and cleanliness. Although his *Report to the Committee of the City Council Appointed to Obtain the Census of Boston for the Year 1845* (Shattuck, 1846) emphasized the importance and obligation of municipal government to assume supervision over the necessities of life, which in an earlier age and in more rural areas could be properly left to the individual, he was also a great advocate of private and corporate responsibility. Much of his life in fact was spent trying to restrain the functions of the city and state government from expanding into private areas. Thus, although Shattuck believed that pure water should be piped into every dwelling, he initially argued against municipal control and against the expansion of the public water supply. He believed that any extension of municipal responsibility would lead both to private negligence and to political corruption.

By 1850 when Shattuck made his report to the Massachusetts State Lesiglature in the *Report of the Sanitary Commission,* he had begun to recognize that only municipal or state intervention could solve many of the problems with which he was concerned. Still his proposals were primarily a call for moral reform and went on the assumption that, if filth could be eliminated, vice would also be eliminated. Cleansing the body in his mind was much more than a physical act, it was a means and condition to obtain inward purity.

Shattuck thus emphasizes how strong a hold the belief that disease and poverty was a retribution for sin had on the American mind. It was not until after the Civil War that these beliefs began to change (Rosenkrantz, 1972).

The newly formed American Medical Association joined with the medical department of the National Institute, a scientific body based in Washington, D.C., in 1848 to collect sanitary surveys from the various areas of the country. In that same year Griscom published *The Sanitary Condition of the Laboring Population of New York,* which was similar to studies being published in England at that same time. Lemuel Shattuck followed with another *Report* in 1850 recommending that a Massachusetts state board of health be established.

It was not until after the Civil War, however, that the states began to take action. Massachusetts in 1869 was the first state to establish a state health department, followed the next year by California and soon after by other states. By the end of the nineteenth century there were 38 state boards. The organization of the American Public Health Association in 1872 indicated health professionals' and other citizens' concern with health. The federal government in 1878 passed the National Quarantine Act, creating a short-lived National Board of Health that went out of existence in 1883. When the federal government finally became involved again, it did so more gradually and on a smaller scale.

Most of the frontline action took place in the cities, where the problems remained the greatest. In 1859 the New York Infirmary for Women and Children appointed a "sanitary visitor" to give simple practical instruction to "poor mothers on the management of infants, and the preservation of health of families." Unfortunately, this effort lost out in the crisis brought on by the Civil War. During the Panic of 1873, a period of economic depression, the New York Diet Kitchen set up food stations to feed the poor, and as economic conditions improved, the food station became a milk station for babies. Adding impetus to the movement was the effort of Nathan Strauss, a private philanthropist who supported the establishment of milk stations throughout New York City beginning in 1893. By 1902 the milk stations were distributing 250,000 bottles monthly. Milk stations replaced wet nurses as the invention of the rubber nipple allowed alternatives to breast milk.

Some farsighted reformers saw the milk stations as a foundation for a maternal and child care center. Leading efforts for this were the husband and wife team of Wilbur and Elsie Cole Phillips, who started their work in Milwaukee and carried it to fruition in Cincinnati. Ultimately the projects in both Milwaukee and Cincinnati were terminated because the Phillipses, as well as many of those working with them, were socialists. The Phillipses' ideology encouraged opposition from the medical and political establishment (Rosen, 1971).

DISTRICT NURSING

Nursing involvement in the community started in England. The leader of this effort was William Rathbone (1819-1902), a Liverpool merchant-shipowner and a member of a family with strong philanthropic and liberal traditions. In 1859 Rathbone was concerned with home nursing in Liverpool, so he hired a nurse to practice among the poor and in their homes. A single nurse soon proved so insufficient that Rathbone decided to establish a corps of nurses at his own expense to nurse the sick poor in their own homes. This raised the problem of where such nurses were to come from, and Rathbone turned to Florence Nightingale for advice. On her recommendation Rathbone opened the Training School and Home for Nurses in cooperation with the Royal Liverpool Infirmary. In 1867 Rathbone divided Liverpool into 18 districts, with a nurse and "lady visitor" in each district. This Liverpool idea of districts was copied and spread in England and to the United States (Bullough and Bullough, 1978). Soon after the founding of the first three Nightingale training schools in the United States in 1873, nurses were hired for district nursing. Mary Gardner, one of the first American authors of a major public health text, estimated that there were 200 district health nurses by 1900 and 3000 by 1912 (Gardner, 1936).

The first district nursing in the United States was established in New York City in 1877 when the Women's Board of the New York Mission hired Frances Root, a graduate of Bellevue Hospital's first nursing class, to visit among the sick poor. Root's primary duty was nursing, but she was also cautioned not to "forget the soul's interest" and to use every opportunity to give godly advice and Christian comfort. Somewhat less religious was the program begun a year later by the Society for Ethical Culture, a secular religious group pledged to promoting the highest ethical conduct in all phases of life. Since its nurses worked out of dispensaries, they had the advantage of medical advice from dispensary physicians. The women of the Society also made certain that the nurses had supplies of linen, food, and clothes for patients who might need them. Since district nursing was emerging almost simultaneously with social work (social workers were originally called friendly visitors), early visiting nurses often combined both functions.

VISITING NURSES

The term "visiting nursing" was first used when a Buffalo group, now known as the Buffalo Visiting Nurses' Association, started an outreach program from a Sunday school class in 1885. It was quickly followed in 1886 by a Boston program, which was organized by the Women's Education Association, and by the Philadelphia Visiting Nurse Society. The fact that almost all the original visiting nurses were graduates of the hospital training schools helped establish the principle that visiting nurses should be trained nurses; this gave the American district nurses a decided advantage over their European counterparts who were often not so well trained (Brainard, 1922).

These early visiting nurse associations usually began as small undertakings with a few wealthy "lady managers" financing and supervising the work of one or two nurses. Thus, even though the nursing aspect was emphasized, control was not in the hands of the nurses, most of whom worked six days a week, eight to 10 hours a day, and visited eight to 12 patients each day. The nurses were expected not only to do nursing care but to raise the "household existence" with their "delicate instruction and firm convictions" in physical and moral hygiene. "The image of the visiting nurse climbing the tenement stairs to save the indigent from illness and bad habits struck the fancy of a wide variety of social reformers" (Buhler-Wilkerson, 1985).

Although there was some tension between private dispensaries and physicians who went to care for the sick poor in their homes, the visiting nurse was rapidly accepted by both the medical establishment and the community. It has been hypothesized that one reason for this was that the visiting nurse reduced the number of charity patients seeking hospitalization and thereby helped lessen the burden of the rising cost of hospital care (Rosner, 1982). This is because the solution to what some contemporaries claimed was excessive and indiscriminate charity was to provide the poor with more care in their homes while simultaneously teaching them to stay healthy (Rosner, 1980).

Nurses for their part were attracted to community work because they had greater independence. They were no longer the handmaidens of physicians, but their associates or co-workers. By making their own diagnoses, they could set priorities for those in the home they thought needed more intensive care. Patients often went for months without seeing physicians, since the nurse was in charge of the patient's care.

As the idea caught on, visiting nurses were soon working for department stores, factories, insurance companies, boards of health and education, hospitals, settlement houses, milk and baby clinics, playgrounds, and hotels, as well as for visiting nurse associations. Some of the visiting nurse associations were government agencies, and some were voluntary agencies. This led to growing confusion and competition for resources and credit for accomplishments.

Conflicts concerning the sponsorship of visiting nurses were accentuated by the traditional attitude of American medicine, which regarded medical care as a private affair that might well be supplemented by charitable enterprises such as visiting nurse associations, but not by paid government employees. Inevitably most tax-supported public health departments were forced to abandon any claims to curative activities that might threaten the economic well-being of private physicians. Instead they turned to a hygienic, rather than a therapeutic, focus and left the care of the sick to the privately financed visiting nurse associations. Nurses generally opposed such a separation, but in spite of this, they lost ground as both health departments and school health services became increasingly preventive instead of curative (Buhler-Wilkerson, 1985). These issues, which were first raised at the turn of the century, still concern nurses. The setting is different, but the issues remain the same.

Probably the most influential community nursing figure in the United States during the late nineteenth and early twentieth centuries was Lillian D. Wald, a New York Hospital Training School graduate. Wald began teaching home nursing classes on New York's Lower East Side, a neighborhood of recent immigrants and grinding poverty. One day a small child asked Wald to visit her sick mother, whom Wald found confined to the family's only bed, which was badly soiled by two days of hemorrhaging. For Wald, all of "the maladjustments of our social and economic relations seemed epitomized in this brief journey."

Determined to do something about the lack of adequate health care in the neighborhood and filled with enthusiasm to serve humanity, Wald convinced two well-to-do friends, Mrs. Solomon Loeb and Jacob Schiff, to finance an effort to help such people. Wald and Mary Brewster, another nurse, moved into a top floor walk-up apartment and offered their services to the neighborhood. To lessen the stigma of charity, they asked their patients to pay for services whenever and however possible. At the end of two years they moved to more permanent quarters—the famous house on Henry Street in New York City that Schiff paid for. Other nurses and social workers joined them and made the Henry Street Settlement second only to Jane Addams' Hull House in Chicago as a focus for welfare activities. Wald thus became one of the best-known women in the country.

LILLIAN WALD AND THE SETTLEMENT HOUSES

Settlement houses were formed in a number of other communities with nurses often in influential roles. Settlement houses differed from the other developing social agencies of the time in that they were concerned with the neighborhood as a whole. They differed from the dispensaries and health centers in that the physician was not the controlling influence. In fact, the settlement house originally sought to develop relationships among the culturally, religiously, and socially different community groups to bring people together so that they could improve their living conditions and environments. Wald summed up these aims as "fusing these people who come to us from the Old World Civilization into . . . a real brotherhood among men" (Addams, 1912; Wald, 1915).

Settlement houses across the country emphasized health care and education and did much to develop both social work and public health nursing. Wald and others emphasized that poor health and physical disability were the "most constant attendants of poverty." It has been estimated that a serious disabling condition existed in about three fourths of the families needing charity. Although the settlement house movement, and particularly Hull House and the Henry Street Settlement, are now looked on with universal favor and even reverence, in their own days they were considered quite radical. They helped develop autonomous neighborhood organizations, and the leaders of the movement, including a large number of nurses, saw the poverty of their day as something that could be corrected.

In 1908 Lillian Wald's efforts led to the establishment of a New York City Division of Child Hygiene, which staffed nurse visits to mothers of every newborn in a densely populated section of New York City's Lower East Side. In keeping with the growing distinction between private and public health nursing, this was more preventive and educational than therapeutic. In 1909 Wald managed to extend the realm of the visiting nurse even further when she suggested to officials of the Metropolitan Life Insurance Company that a nurse on its staff could actually save money by reducing mortality. The company followed her suggestion, and administrators were so impressed with the results that they set up a visiting nurse for their policyholders, a service that was continued for some 44 years by which time government intervention into health care was so well established and the nature of health care had changed so much that the service was no longer necessary. It was also Wald who first used the term "public health nursing," which soon replaced the other names, such as district nurse, by which these nurses had been designated. The term "visiting nurse" did, however, remain in use to signify a nurse who gave hands-on care in the community.

Another of Wald's great achievements was the United States Children's Bureau, which was created by federal legislation in 1912, and whose

LILLIAN WALD

Despite her many great accomplishments, Lillian Wald was a controversial figure in her lifetime. She supported the Russian Revolution, and although she did not approve of the Bolsheviks' methods, she remained receptive to their efforts to modernize Russia. Her opinions cost her some influential support in the United States, but she never hesitated to speak her mind. Like most people who were passionately involved in social reform causes, Wald had more than one cause that she advocated. One of these was Prohibition. When her friends pointed out that Prohibition led to bootlegging and a rise in crime, she argued that the bootleggers harmed only the idle rich, and she considered herself "a member of the 4,000,000, not the 400."

DISTRICT NURSING: LILLIAN D. WALD, HEADWORKER, NURSES SETTLEMENT

The possibilities of caring for the sick poor and for those of small means in their own homes have not been developed proportionately with the development of hospitals. Perhaps the rapid growth of the hospitals has overshadowed or retarded the other.

I have long felt that home nursing deserved to be considered by communities in a large way, as a legitimate branch of the whole care of the public health and as a logical correlation with the work of the hospitals. Moreover, I am convinced that a systematic extension of this service would considerably relieve the pressure now put on hospitals for free or low-priced bed space, thus diminishing the problem of overcrowding with its attendant increasing budgets.

In New York City, where land and buildings are so costly, it would be worthwhile to extend the work of visiting nurses just as a matter of convenience, even if the actual cost of the service were not greatly less than that of institutions.

If on the other hand the results were not as good for the patient, if he did not recover as well, or if his comfort and happiness were less, home nursing ought not to be advocated on grounds of expediency or economy.

But the experience of all visiting nursing work proves that such is not the case, but that many classes of cases do as well, from the medical standpoint, in the home as in the hospital, while the peace of mind and contentment of the patient are often much greater.

There are of course many cases, which from the medical as well as the social viewpoint, demand hospital treatment, where conditions impossible of attainment in the private house are indicated, and these the public have been so long familiar with that they probably do not need more than reference in this article.

It is legitimate to regard the nurse as a social factor of large opportunities, opportunities of which she has availed herself in many communities. The nurse has the supreme advantage of having her services understood, and the demand for her as soon as she is known in her neighborhood frequently becomes a tax to the limit of her strength.

She is an educator, carrying education to a large number of people who from stress of circumstances cannot go out to obtain this education; hard-worked women, overwhelmed with difficult housing and domestic conditions; people house-ridden on account of illness; and those who have not come in contact with the city and whose social experiences are limited to the little group that perhaps has come from their own small continental town.

It seems obvious to those of us who have watched the district nurse's activity that much is demanded of her; technical skills, physical endurance, and the social training which will include a knowledge of and interest in the conditions that make up her neighborhood. This seems only possible of attainment if she lives in the neighborhood in which she works, in a settlement where all matters affecting the neighborhood of her patients are of concern.

Without entering into the wide outlook that is suggested by the social servant I would like to draw attention to one or two results directly in her profession that have followed the nurse's experience; the school nurse, concerning which another paper will report, the nurses in the tuberculosis campaign, and their participation in other prophylactic measures relating to the physical welfare of the community; better housing, parks and playgrounds, convalescent homes.

The nurses would make a plea to have the community, that concerns itself with social matters, make high demands upon them, and ask that the *adequate* care of the sick in their homes be made a matter of serious consideration. (Wald Papers)

purpose was to investigate and report matters pertaining to the welfare of children among all classes of people. Wald together with Florence Kelly, another remarkable woman leader at the turn of the century, conceived the idea of the bureau and based their arguments for its existence on their belief that infant health depends on the protection of mothers.

Once nursing in the community was established, it expanded rapidly. Most of the large urban areas soon had visiting nurse services of some kind, and governments were following the example of Los Angeles, which had put a nurse on the city payroll in 1897, and hiring increasing numbers of nurses in many public health roles. After Koch's discovery of the cause of tuberculosis, Reba Thelin was hired by Johns Hopkins Hospital in 1903 to work in the homes of tuberculosis patients. Her job was to make certain that the patients received the fresh air, rest, and regular meals that were then part of the regimen for the disease; she was also to keep the danger of infection to a minimum (Sachs, 1908). In Cleveland by 1904, largely through the efforts of John and Isabel Lowman, the Visiting Nurses' Association began visiting homes of tuberculosis patients being treated by tuberculosis dispensaries (Bower, 1932).

PUBLIC HEALTH NURSING

By 1912 the community focus in nursing had become so important and its practitioners so numerous that a separate organization seemed necessary to set standards and guide its further expansion. The result was the formation of the National Organization for Public Health Nursing (NOPHN), the first nursing organization to admit nonnurses. It included both public health nurses and interested lay persons and agencies. Wald's term "public health nursing" was chosen because it reflected a hope that the visiting nurse and the newly emerging field of public health and preventive medicine could be linked together. The Cleveland Visiting Nurse Association contributed its quarterly journal to the organization. *Public Health Nursing* was published until 1952 when a nursing reorganization amalgamated it with *Nursing Outlook* (Roberts, 1961). A new journal with the same name, but no connection, began publishing in 1984.

The most obvious field in which public health nurses demonstrated their usefulness and effectiveness was in infant and child care. High infant mortality rates had always been accepted as more or less inevitable, but by 1900 there was an increasing belief that they could be diminished. Milk distribution programs remained the only operative infant welfare program until 1906 when the Cleveland Visiting Nurse Association and the Cleveland Milk Fund Association jointly opened the Babies' Dispensary, which offered medical and nursing supervision of both healthy and ill children. The service was copied in other cities, and with the formation of the Division of Child Hygiene in the New York City Department of Health in 1908, municipal government became a major factor in public health nursing (Brainard, 1922; Fulmer, 1902; Rosen 1958; Waters, 1909; Winslow, 1911).

Part of the approach in reducing infant mortality rates was to raise the educational standards of midwives, a group who had no particular legal standards to meet. Often they were neighborhood women who had had children or who had observed several births and then had started delivering babies themselves. A New York City survey published in 1913 indicated that more than 40% of infants were delivered by untrained attendants, some 3000 of whom were practicing in the city. Many reformers felt that training and supervision of midwives were absolutely essential before maternal and neonatal death rates could be cut. Any such suggestions were, however, opposed by organized medicine, which thought that midwives should be abolished and the whole field of obstetrics should be turned over to physicians.

Not all nurses agreed with this. One of the more famous American nurse-midwives was Emma Goldman (1869-1940), whose public career as an anarchist soon took precedence over her role both in nursing and in midwifery.

In general nurses, or at least that segment of nursing that was the most influential in the nursing organizations, were ambivalent about midwifery. Shortly after NOPHN was founded, the training of nurse-midwives was discussed, but no positive action was taken even though in Europe nurse-midwives were becoming common. With the establishment of the federal Children's Bureau in 1912, systematic study of the mortality and morbidity rates for infants and mothers was begun. These studies and the publicity they received

EMMA GOLDMAN

Emma Goldman had become interested in nursing while in prison where she was serving a sentence for inciting a riot in 1893. The prison physician asked her to help him, and she finished up her training while still in jail. After her release she continued her studies in Vienna where she received diplomas in both nursing and midwifery and attended lectures by Freud. When she returned to the United States, she set up practice as a nurse-midwife but soon left to campaign for birth control and more effective social change. However, she never entirely lost her interest in nursing or her ability as a nurse.

emphasized the need for better obstetric care, particularly for low-income mothers. Nurses as a group were unwilling to antagonize organized medicine and reluctant to establish programs to train nurse-midwives. A compromise was reached with the passage of the Sheppard-Towner Act of 1921, which provided among other things that public health nurses were to instruct local midwives. To supplement this act, various states began regulating the education, licensing, and practice of midwives; more important, the states also enacted legislation to use the funds available under the Sheppard-Towner Act for public health nursing care of infants and mothers.

RURAL PUBLIC HEALTH NURSING

Most of the early American development of public health nursing took place in the larger cities. Although Great Britain, Canada, and Germany had begun to organize rural district nursing around the turn of the century, little was done in the United States. Wald as early as 1908, recognizing this deficiency, proposed that the Red Cross undertake rural nursing. Wald believed that the Red Cross could do for rural nursing what the visiting nurse associations were doing for the cities and at the same time broaden its own activities beyond disaster relief. The Red Cross initially ignored her suggestion, but when Jacob H. Schiff, a New York philanthropist, offered $100,000 for rural nursing, the Red Cross became interested. Approval was given in December 1911, and by 1912 the Rural Nursing Service was officially under way. Fannie F. Clement, a nurse and trained social worker, was appointed director of the project, which soon changed its name to the Town and Country Nursing Service.

Progress was slow, mainly because the Red Cross saw itself not as an employer of nurses, but rather as an agency to secure and train qualified nurses, advise interested communities, and lobby for the expansion of rural nursing. Getting local communities to pay salaries, however, was difficult.

It was mainly the Metropolitan Life Insurance Company's decision to use the existing rural nurses for the service of their policyholders that enabled rural nursing to continue. By 1916, 31 associations were cooperating with both the Metropolitan Life Insurance Company and the Red Cross, but most of the nursing salaries came through the insurance company's payment of 50 cents per call for its policyholders.

World War I temporarily interrupted the expansion of rural nursing, but a rapid expansion occurred at the end of the war. Such expansion, however, only exacerbated the tensions between nurses and the local Red Cross chapters. Much of the difficulty came because few local chapters really understood the programs, and some of those that did were openly opposed. There was also conflict with community officials about how much control the Red Cross should have. Despite this, between January 1919 and June 1930 nearly 3000 services were started, although not more than one third this number existed at any one time. With the entry of federal and state governments into the field in the 1930s the Red Cross began to withdraw, until by 1947 the whole rural health nursing program was discontin-

MRS. WHITELAW REID

Mrs. Whitelaw Reid originally contributed some financial support of rural nurses, but it was soon withdrawn under circumstances that revealed the exclusive social attitude that periodically plagued the Red Cross, as well as other charitable organizations at this time. Reid simply refused to contribute more money because she felt that the nurses selected for rural nursing were not ladies, although she added in the letter in which she withdrew her support that "to get on with the village people their not being ladies does not matter—I suppose the ladies would not like the work."

ed (Clement, 1913; Dock and Clement, 1922; Dubline and Lotka, 1937; Fox, 1922; Kernodle, 1949).

INCREASING GOVERNMENT SUPPORT

The first tentative steps toward a national health policy in the United States took place in 1878 when Congress passed the National Quarantine Act, which empowered the surgeon general of the Marine Hospital Service to enforce port quarantine as long as he did not interfere with the laws and procedures of the states. This was followed in 1879 by the creation of a National Board of Health comprising seven physicians who were representatives from the Army, Navy, and Marine Hospital Service, as well as the Justice Department. Its charge was modest: to collect information on public health matters, to advise the federal government departments, as well as state governments, and to report to Congress a plan for a national health organization. The Board failed to receive an appropriation from Congress in 1883, and its work was terminated. Only in 1912 when the director of the Marine Hospital had his title changed to surgeon general of the United States Public Health Service (USPHS) was there an official agency dedicated to public health. In 1917 the National Leprosarium was established, and in 1918 the USPHS assumed the responsibility for providing health examinations for all immigrants. The Division of Venereal Diseases was established during World War I, and in 1929 the Narcotics Division was added to the USPHS.

With the advent of Franklin D. Roosevelt's New Deal in 1933, public health in the United States came of age. Under regulations of the Federal Emergency Relief Act of 1933, passed to deal with the crisis of the Great Depression, bedside care for indigent patients was considered a legitimate use of public funds. Although only a few nurses were hired under this provision, the precedent had been set for federal government support of nursing and other public health services (Fitzpatrick, 1975).

The Works Progress Administration (WPA), created in 1935 to give work to unemployed workers, allowed nurses to be employed in public health organizations on a wider scale than ever before. New programs for crippled children were set up, and widespread immunization programs were started. By 1936 more than 2000 professional nurses were employed by the WPA in various public health programs (Woodward, 1937, 1938). More important in the long run was the Social Security Act of 1935. This initially provided pensions to the needy aged, old age insurance, unemployment insurance, benefit payments to the blind, dependent mothers and children, and crippled children, and expanded health programs. Title VI of the act provided for federal assistance to states and their subdivision in the establishment and maintenance of adequate community health service, including the training of personnel. Most of the health programs were administered either through the federal Children's Bureau or through the USPHS. Nurses were influential in the planning, since one of the leaders was Pearl McIver, who had been initially hired by the government in 1933 to encourage and assist local health agencies to use unemployed nurses. When the Social Security Act was passed, McIver became the public health nursing consultant for the USPHS, and she and the service drew heavily on the National Organization of Public Health Nurses for ideas and standards in public health nursing. Dorothy Deming, who had been editor of *Public Health Nursing,* also became a consultant.

Other programs also involved direct government intervention in public health–related measures, always on the assumption that improvements in nursing education or greater use of nurses would improve the health care delivery system and raise the standards of American health. Federal funds made available, particularly after 1935, allowed the states to allocate funds for community-focused programs aimed at providing preventive nursing care to selected groups including women, children, persons with infectious diseases, those needing immunizations, and those needing health education. Public health nurses provided these services in conjunction with other members of the health care team.

As nursing education improved in the last three decades, all nursing roles expanded and the role of the public health nurse was broadened to include additional activities such as primary health care. With this change the term "community health nurse" gained favor. It is the term used in this book. The role of the modern community health nurse is further defined in the next chapter.

There are still many agencies that are called visiting nursing services. However, their work is changing rapidly as modern health care technology is developed for homes. Additionally, recent changes in health care financing have moved clients out of the hospital sooner, so home nursing is becoming more complex. The broader descriptive term that is now being used to describe this type of nursing role is "home health nursing care.[22]

SUMMARY

Efforts to control the environment and prevent the spread of disease have been carried out throughout recorded history. However, modern public health measures could not exist had nineteenth century researchers not identified microorganisms as the cause of infectious disease. This discovery was significant in the development of an interdisciplinary public health movement that sought to prevent illness by improving isolation techniques, immunizing, carrying out client teaching campaigns, and other measures. Modern community health nurses are a part of that interdisciplinary public health movement.

American cities were greatly influenced by successive waves of poor immigrants. The needs of this population motivated many of the public health reformers, including Lillian Wald, a nurse who established the Henry Street Settlement.

The terms that have been used to describe the nurses who work in the community and participate in that movement have changed several times in the last century. The community nursing service established by William Rathbone in 1876 was called the "District Nursing Service." District nursing agencies were also established in the United States, but the term was soon replaced by "Visiting Nursing Services."

During the first part of the twentieth century the role of the nurse who worked in the community was divided into two different roles. The private philanthropic groups who sponsored visiting nursing services retained the term "visiting nurses" for their nursing work force, and their primary focus was on the provision of direct care with health teaching only a secondary responsibility. As the government bodies appropriated funds to establish community nursing programs, the term "public health nurses" developed. The programs' focus was on preventive activities including client teaching, immunizations, and work with other members of the public health team.

With further evolution and some expansion of these two roles, two new terms have appeared. "Community health nursing" is now the preferred term for the preventive role, and "home health nursing care" is the term most often used to describe the work of the nurses who provide direct care to clients in their homes.

QUESTIONS FOR DISCUSSION

1. What steps were taken by the Venetian Great Council in the fourteenth century to prevent the spread of bubonic plague?
2. Why was the research of Robert Koch extremely important to the development of the modern public health movement?
3. Compare the experiences of an immigrant family known to you with those described in the text.
4. What were the contributions made by Lilian Wald to the development of nursing in the community?

REFERENCES

Addams J: Twenty years at Hull House, New York, 1912, Macmillan Publishing Co.

Bower I: Public health nursing in Cleveland 1895-1928, Cleveland, 1932, Western Reserve University.

Brainard AM: The evolution of public health nursing, Philadelphia, 1922, WB Saunders Co.

Buhler-Wilkerson K: Public health nursing: in sickness or in health, Am J Nurs 75:1155, 1985.

Bullough V and Bullough B: The-care-of-the-sick: the emergence of modern nursing, New York, 1978, Prodist.

Burgess EW: Urban areas. In Smith TV and White L, editors: An experiment in social science research, Chicago, 1929, University of Chicago Press.

Cipolla CM: Public health and the medical profession in the Renaissance, Cambridge, England, 1976, Cambridge University Press.

Clement FF: Prospective Red Cross rural nursing in the Kentucky Mountains, Am J Nurs 13:768, 1913.

Dock LL and Clement FF: From rural nursing to the public health service. In Dock LL and others, editors: History of American Red Cross nursing, New York, 1922, Macmillan Publishing Co.

Dubline LI and Lotka AJ: Twenty-five years of health progress, New York, 1937, Metropolitan Life Insurance Co.

Fitzpatrick ML: Nurses in American history: nursing and the Great Depression, Am J Nurs 75:2188, 1975.

Fox EG: Red Cross public health nursing after the war. In Dock LL and others, editors: History-of-American Red-Cross-nursing, New York, 1922, Macmillan Publishing Co.

Fulmer H: History of visiting nurse work in America, Am J Nurs 2:411, 1902.

Gardner MS: Public health nursing, ed 3, New York, 1936, Macmillan Publishing Co.

Gordon M: Assimilation in American life: the role of race, religion and national origin, New York, 1964, Oxford University Press.

Handlin O: The uprooted, Boston, 1952, Atlantic Little Brown.

Jones MA: American immigration, Chicago, 1960, University of Chicago Press.

Kernodle PB: The Red-Cross nurse in action 1822-1946, New York, 1949, Harper & Brothers.

Mohl RV: Die Polizei-Wissenschaft nach den Grundsatzen der recht Staates, Tubingen, 1833, H Laup.

Roberts M: American nursing: history and interpretation, New York, 1961, Macmillan Publishing Co.

Rosen G: A history of public health, New York, 1958, MD Publications.

Rosen G: The first neighborhood health center movement—its rise and fall, Am J Public Health 61:1620, 1971.

Rosenkrantz BG: Public health and the state, Cambridge, Mass, 1972, Harvard University Press.

Rosner D: A once charitable enterprise: hospitals and health care in Brooklyn and New York, 1885-1915, Chicago, 1980, University of Chicago Press.

Rosner D: Health care for the "truly needy:" nineteenth century origins of the concept, Milbank Q 60:355, 1982.

Sachs TB: The tuberculosis nurse, Am J Nurs 8:597, 1908.

Shattuck L: Report to the committee of the city council appointed to obtain the census of Boston for the year 1845, Boston, 1846, JH Eastburn.

Wald L: The house on Henry Street, New York, 1915, Henry Holt.

Wald Papers, Reel 24, New York Public Library.

Waters Y: Visiting nursing in the United States, New York, 1909, Charities Publication Committee.

Winslow CE: The role of the visiting nurse in the campaign for public health, Am J Nurs 11:909, 1911.

Winslow CEA: The untitled field of public health, Mod Med 2:183, 1920.

Woodward ES: The WPA and nursing, Am J Nurs 37:994, 1937.

Woodward ES: WPA nursing, Am J Nurs 38:733, 1938.

BIBLIOGRAPHY

Bannister LA: A new field: the nurse's opportunity in factory work. In Fourteenth annual report of the American Society of Superintendents of Training Schools for Nurses, New York, 1908, American Society of Superintendents.

Buhler-Wilkerson K: Public health nursing: in sickness or in health, Am J Nurs 75:1155, 1985.

Buhler-Wilkerson K and Reverby S: Can a time honored model solve the dilemma of public health nursing? Am J Nurs 74:1081, 1985.

Charley I: The birth of industrial nursing: its history and development in Great Britain, London, 1954, Baillière Tindall.

Duffus RL: Lillian Wald, neighbor and crusader, New York, 1939, Macmillan Publishing Co.

Markolf AS: A study of industrial nursing service, Public Health Nurs 32:631, 1944.

Markolf AS: Industrial nursing begins in Vermont, Public Health Nurs 37:125, 1945.

McGrath BJ: Nursing in commerce and industry, New York, 1946, Commonwealth Fund.

CHAPTER

2

Nursing Roles in the Community

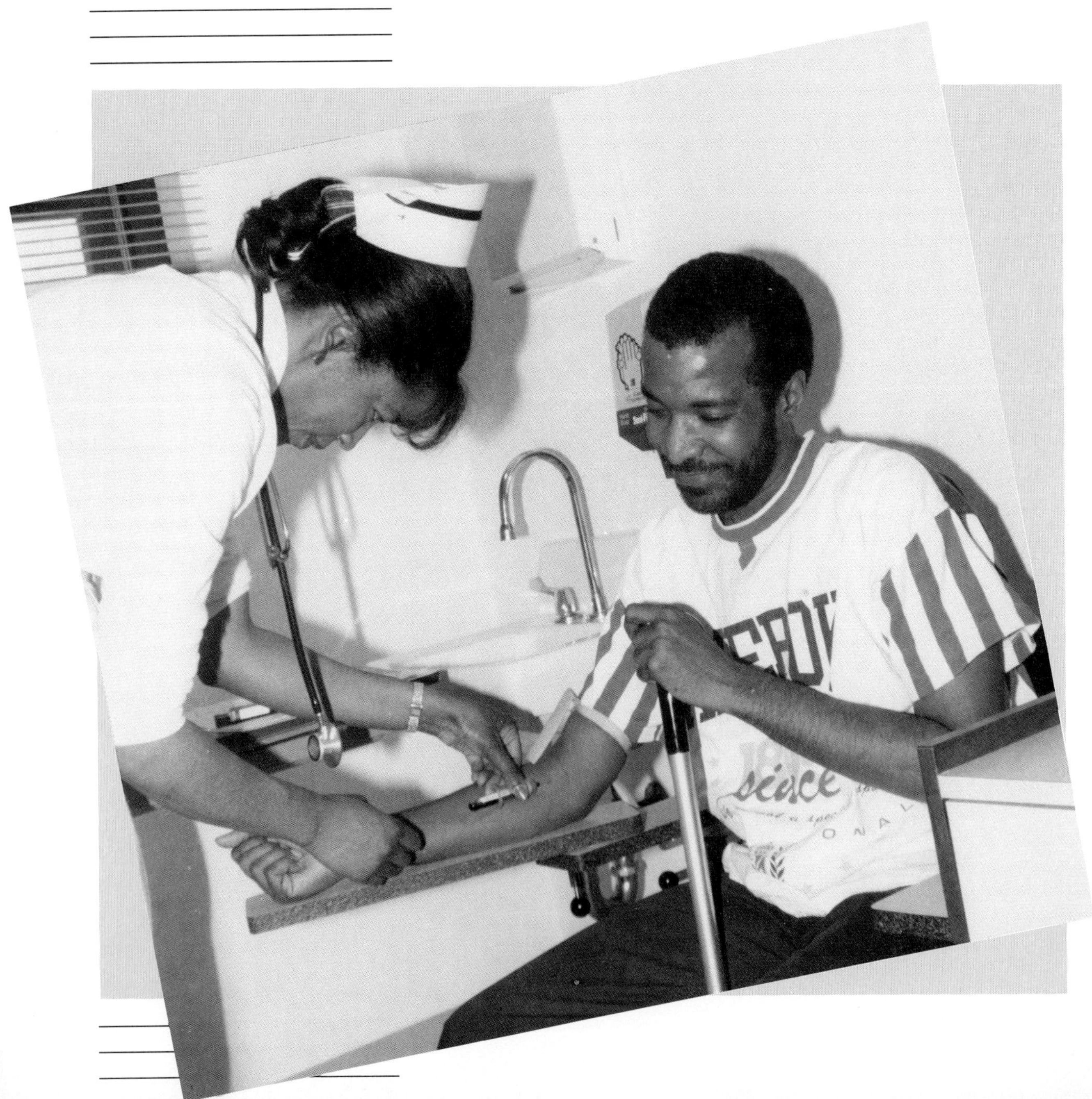

CHAPTER OUTLINE

- Community health nursing
  - High-risk populations
  - Concept of community
  - Preventive health care
- Home health care nursing
- Case manager
- Role of the hospital discharge planning nurse
  - Assessment of needs and resources
  - Nursing diagnosis
  - Planning
  - Implementation
  - Evaluation
- Case manager in the home health care agency
- School nursing
  - Current components of the school health program
  - School nurse practitioners
- Occupational health nursing
  - Role of the occupational health nurse
- Nurse practitioners
  - Role of the nurse practitioner
  - Nurse practitioner education
  - Nurse practitioner specialties
  - Certification
- Nurse-midwifery
- Clinical nurse specialists and nurse clinicians
  - Nurse Practice Acts
- Malpractice insurance crisis
- Summary

OBJECTIVES

After completing this chapter, the reader should be able to:

1. Describe the major community nursing roles, including:
   a. Community health nurse
   b. Home health care nurse
   c. Case manager
   d. Occupational health nurse
   e. Nurse practitioner
   f. Nurse-midwife
   g. Clinical nurse specialist and other specialists
2. Discuss the factors that led to the development of these roles.
3. Describe the changes in nursing practice law that have occurred in response to the development of advanced nursing specialties.

NURSES who want to work in the community have many varied and interesting roles to choose from. In addition to the major nursing roles of community health nurse and home health care nurse, nurses can choose several other related positions that fall under the umbrella of community nursing. The history of the two major roles is presented in Chapter 1. The more recent roles developed because of recent changes in the health care delivery system, the changing consumer demands for care, and the growing maturity of nursing as a learned profession.

COMMUNITY NURSING ROLES

1. Community health nurse (public health nurse)
2. Home health care nurse (visiting nurse)
3. Case manager
    a. Hospital discharge planning nurse
    b. Other case managers
4. Occupational health nurse
5. School health nurse
    a. School health nurse practitioner
6. Nurse practitioners
    a. Pediatric nurse practitioner
    b. Adult nurse practitioner
    c. Geriatric nurse practitioner
    d. Obstetric-gynecologic nurse practitioner
    e. Family nurse practitioner
7. Nurse-midwife
8. Clinical nurse specialist and other specialists

COMMUNITY HEALTH NURSING

The major ambulatory nursing role is filled by the community health nurse. Because of its importance to society, special graduate educational programs were developed in the 1920s and 1930s to prepare hospital diploma nurses for community work. When the integrated baccalaureate programs were developed after 1945, the community health content became a component of the basic programs, so graduates of American and Canadian university nursing programs are now prepared to function as beginning community health nurses (Bullough and Bullough, 1978).

Community health nursing focuses primarily on disease prevention and health promotion. To carry out this goal, community health nurses deliver care to the community as a whole—to populations within the community, to families, and to individuals. Although the actual services of the nurse are often given to families and individuals, the goal of community health nursing is to improve the health of the entire community by identifying every susceptible subgroup and delivering care to the aggregate of people who are at high risk of illness, disability, or death. Clients who are cared for by community health nurses are selected on the basis of programmatic policies that reflect the prioritized needs of the community and society. Usually these priorities are established using data collected in epidemiologic studies, although political forces also figure into the setting of priorities (ANA, 1985; APHA, 1980).

Community health nursing is defined by the American Nurses' Association Council of Community Nurses as a

> synthesis of nursing practice and public health practice applied to promoting and preserving the health of populations. . . . Health promotion, health maintenance, health education, and management, coordination, and continuity of care are utilized in a holistic approach to the management of the health care of individuals, families, and groups in a community (ANA, 1980).

As indicated in this definition, the work of the community health nurse is closely tied to the work of the interdisciplinary public health team, which includes physicians, sanitarians, nutritionists, and health educators. The community health nurse is responsible for the nursing component of the work of the team. Although the focus on community needs remains the cornerstone of the role, the tasks carried out change over time because public health needs and priorities change. For example, during the first part of the twentieth century the control of communicable diseases was the primary mission of all public health workers. Although the nurses on the public health team sometimes gave direct, hands-on care to the victims of these diseases, they primarily used public education, immunizations, and isolation techniques to control the spread of disease. As these diseases were controlled, community health nurses focused on other areas such as prenatal care, substance abuse, or accident prevention. These areas involved less hands-on care and more health teaching and counseling (Buhler-Wilkerson, 1985).

More recently the spread of acquired immunodeficiency syndrome (AIDS) has once again made communicable diseases a high-priority public health focus. However, actual care of the infected is carried out by home health care and hospital nurses with community health nurses carrying the responsibilities of the emotional support for clients and health teaching aimed at prevention (U.S. Department of Health and Human Services, 1986).

High-Risk Populations

As indicated above, community health nursing focuses on populations that are at a high risk for illness. The term "at risk" means that members of a population are susceptible to a disorder. For example, if the nurse were to study the population at risk for prostate cancer, only men would be included in the study. If the term "high risk" were used, the population would be narrowed to elderly men. The group at risk for rubella includes those persons without immunity to the disease. Within the context of the science of epidemiology, risk factors are the variables that are related to a given disease. For example, smoking is a risk factor for lung cancer. Its link was discovered through not just one study but a whole series of studies spanning many years.

High-risk populations are groups of people who have particularly high rates of a given health disorder (Higgs and Gustafson, 1985). Epidemiologic studies are carried out to identify the risk factors for the disorder. Thus it is necessary for community health nurses to understand the epidemiologic approach to research and to read the epidemiologic literature so that they understand the risk factors for conditions found in the communities they serve.

Concept of Community

Although the risk factors related to a specific illness, disability, or cause of death can be studied at the national or state level, the community health nurse is ordinarily concerned with the risk factors that have an impact on the daily lives of local people. Thus the focus is often on trying to identify the risk factors at the community level.

The term "community" is one of those words with a variety of meanings. It is possible to speak of a small town, a portion of a large city, a group of scholars, or the members of an occupational group as a community. Community health nurses tend to use the term in one of two ways. Nurses can refer to the community as the structure made up of a group of inhabitants who share contiguous living space and a common political structure. This community is ordinarily served by a formal political organization, such as a city government, agents of social control, such as the police and courts, and safety nets, such as fire departments.

The other use of the term refers to the community as an aggregate of people who relate to one another, share a common identity, or have common interests. These people do not necessarily live next to one another. Thus it is possible to relate public health programs to an occupational community or a minority community.

Preventive Health Care

Since the primary goal of community health nursing is to improve the health of the commu-

TABLE 2-1 Examples of the Three Levels of Preventive Health Care

Level	Activities	Goal
Primary	Providing immunizations	Prevention of communicable diseases such as diphtheria, pertussis, and rubella
	Smoking cessation programs	Prevention of lung cancer and cardiovascular disorders
	Sex education stressing the use of condoms with sexual contact	Prevention of AIDS and gonorrhea
Secondary	Programs to teach and motivate women to do breast self-examination	Early identification of breast cancer
	Blood pressure screening	Early identification of hypertension
	Throat cultures for people with pharyngitis	Prevention of rheumatic fever and other complications from streptococcal infections
Tertiary	Teaching exercises after first phase of treatment of an injured limb	Restored use of injured limb
	Counseling, low-salt diet, exercise, and management of stress for hypertensive clients	Limited or lessened hypertension
	Exercises and speech therapy after cerebrovascular accident or other neurologic insult	Restored function and limited disability

nity, a preventive focus is also a key element in the definition of the role. Preventive health care includes all activities aimed at promoting health, preventing illness, prolonging life, and improving the functioning of individuals. These activities can be divided into primary, secondary, and tertiary preventive care depending on the stage of the disease process (Shamansky and Clausen, 1980). The three levels of preventive care are listed and explained below with examples in Table 2-1.

1. Primary prevention takes place before the disease process occurs. Preventive activities include generalized health promotion, as well as specific activities aimed at blocking exposure to the causes of disease or disability.
2. Secondary prevention takes place early in the disease process. It is aimed at early diagnosis and treatment to prevent death or limit disability.
3. Tertiary prevention usually occurs when the disease process is clearly present but at a stable state. It is aimed at rehabilitation. The goal is to limit further deterioration or restore the individual to the best possible condition within the constraints of the disease process (ANA, 1980; Clemen-Stone and others, 1987; Pender, 1982).

HOME HEALTH CARE NURSING

The home health care nursing team delivers both preventive and sick care to clients in their home. Traditionally this type of care was called visiting nursing; "home health care" is now the preferred term. The work role is in many ways similar to that of institutional nurses except that home health care workers must function without the on-site support services of the hospital, including x-ray examinations, laboratories, and medical staff. Although home nursing agencies ordinarily use physicians' written orders for guidance, physicians are usually less accessible than they are in an institution, and equipment is also ordinarily more limited. This means that the home health care team members must be able to make client care decisions with minimum outside support, and they must be flexible and innovative.

Home nursing is in a period of rapid growth partly because the mechanisms for Medicare and Medicaid reimbursement have changed to encourage early discharge of clients from hospitals. (See Chapter 13.) However, since funds for home nursing are still limited, registered nurses are used sparingly. It is hoped that political activity by all community-based nurses will improve this situation, but until that happens the number of registered nurses deployed to give bedside care to patients with complex illnesses will remain limited. Most of the actual nursing care in the home is delivered by nursing aides, practical nurses, and patients' family members. Registered nurses, particularly those with collegiate preparation, are usually employed as supervisors or directors of community agencies or case managers.

The supervisors and directors of home health care agencies plan for large groups of clients, work out staffing patterns, implement government regulations, budget funds, and provide in-service education for other nursing personnel unless the agency is large enough to employ a separate in-service educator. That these nurses are moving up in the administrative structure has some advantages. They are better able to assess the community and to make major decisions about services in these positions than in the first-level nursing positions (Anderson, 1983).

The technology of home health care has changed radically in the last few years with a wide variety of complex machines and equipment being placed in clients' homes. Items such as home dialysis units, oxygen equipment, and apparatuses for delivering chemotherapy and hyperalimentation are now common. These developments are discussed in Chapter 14. The technology makes the work role more complex because home health care nurses not only must be able to use the equipment themselves, but must instruct clients, families, and other workers in its use. Mechanical training or a course in physics comes in handy.

CASE MANAGER

The health care delivery system is in the process of becoming more specialized, more technically oriented, and more bureaucratized. Although these changes have modernized the treatment of illness and made some improvements in the delivery of preventive services, the growing complexity of the system is having some negative consequences. Probably the major social cost of such a complex system that involves so many specialties is the loss of continuity in client care. Horror stories have appeared in the media and professional literature about people who receive double doses of medications from two specialists, people who suffer and die because they do not receive much-needed care because of bureaucratic technicalities or a lack of funds, and the common plight of people who are sent home from the hospital without adequate planning. These are everyday examples of the lack of coordination that the growth and increased complexity of the system has created. Nurses as a group are distressed by these developments and have whenever possible taken on the task of organizing the management of care to provide continuity for a wide vareity of clients. Coordination of care is defined as a process whereby clients' needs are assessed, planned for, and provided as they move from one level of care to another or from one provider to another.

Providing continuity of care is an important aspect of all community nursing roles, but it is the primary focus of the case manager. The concept of the case manager was borrowed from the field of social work. Social workers oversee many facets of their clients' lives, and they often speak of managing a "caseload"; hence the term "case management" came into existence. Case managers are now being used in a variety of health care settings. For example, private insurance companies, including the Blue Cross/Blue Shield groups and the health maintenance organizations (HMOs), have found that case managers who help clients find their way through the maze of health providers and secure second opinions related to costly procedures can save the company money, as well as provide better service (Colosi, 1986).

Case managers are also becoming important in the field of mental health. At one time most chronically ill persons were hospitalized in large state mental hospitals. The quality of life in these institutions was rightfully questioned, and starting approximately 20 years ago, a large-scale movement to deinstitutionalize this population occurred. Unfortunately, however, people were often sent into communities that had no facilities or plans to help them, so they migrated to skid-row neighborhoods or became the bag persons who sleep on the streets and exist on what they can pull from garbage cans (Arnhoff, 1975; Skelly and others, in press).

There is now a movement to hire case managers to work with the mentally ill population, to secure needed funds for their survival, to help them search for housing, to identify sheltered employment opportunities, and to arrange for needed health care. In areas where it has been tried, case managers have been able to improve the quality of life of this population significantly (Franklin and others, 1987).

In both of these examples the case manager need not necessarily be a nurse. The discharged mental patients can be and are managed by social workers, nurses, or psychologists. Insurance companies are hiring nurses and some nonnurses on the basis of the individual candidate's knowledge of the local health care situation and other attributes. However, there are several case manager positions that are more likely to be filled by nurses. These include the position of the hospital discharge planning nurse, the clinical nurse specialist who works with children dependent on high technology for survival at home or with groups of elderly clients or the case manager in the home health agency (Feeg, 1987; Jamieson, 1987). In these situations a nursing background is highly valued. The work of the hospital discharge planning nurse provides a good example of the case manager role.

ROLE OF THE HOSPITAL DISCHARGE PLANNING NURSE

Hospitals started hiring discharge planners about 20 years ago to help clients deal with complex transfers to facilities with skilled nurses or to their homes. The Social Security amendments of 1972 contributed to the growth of the concept. The amendments marked the first efforts of the federal government to improve the quality of the care given to Medicare and Medicaid recipients and to control the cost of the program. Professional Standards Review Organizations (PSROs) were established at the local level. As these organizations assessed the quality of care, they became advocates for discharge planning, particularly in light of the other provisions of the amendments, which mandated a review of the length of hospital stays and earlier discharges when it was feasible (Bullough, 1973). Nurses were often hired to carry out the reviews for the PSROs and to do the discharge planning. Sometimes one nurse did both, although as these roles have evolved, the Quality Assurance Nurse and the Discharge Planning Nurse have been separated. In 1977 discharge planning was recognized by the Joint Planning Committee on the Accreditation of Hospitals (JPCAH) as a criterion for accreditation of hospitals. The need for hospital discharge planning nurses escalated sharply after 1983 when further revisions of the Social Security Act drastically cut the hospital stays for Medicare and Medicaid recipients. These changes are sending many clients to skilled nursing facilities, nursing homes, or their own homes long before they are well enough to care for themselves.

The goal of hospital discharge planning is to provide continuity of care for clients who are leaving the hospital (Chisholm, 1983; Stone, 1979). Sometimes the planning task is carried out by the hospital discharge planning nurse alone, and sometimes the planning is done by a team that includes social workers, physical therapists, pharmacists, and others, as well as the nurse. An early model of high-quality, team discharge planning was developed by the Rancho Los Amigos Hospital near Los Angeles. The hospital focused on patients with complex needs for rehabilitation, including those with poliomyelitis, cerebral palsy, and spinal cord injuries. The team added engineers to the traditional group of health care workers. Members of the group were encouraged to brainstorm about new ways to help clients live outside institutional settings and manage as much of their own lives as possible. Special grasping tools or lifts that were designed for one client often proved helpful for others. Innovative social support systems that used traditional agencies, as well as nontraditional resources, helped team members think of other avenues of support for the next client.

Although this model may well be outside the reach of the financial resources of most hospitals, the hospital discharge planning nurse or the discharge planning team that has a spark of creativity does better planning. The nursing process is used to guide the day-to-day planning activities. The process starts with an assessment of both client needs and resources. The diagnostic statement is a summary of both facets of the assessment. The planning phase of the process is aimed at finding resources to fit the needs. Implementation usually includes both referrals and health teaching. The plan must be evaluated to see if it works so that a secondary plan can be used if necessary. These steps as they apply to the hospital discharge planning nurse are described in more detail later in this chapter.

Assessment of Needs and Resources

To carry out the two-pronged assessment process, the discharge planning nurse first reads the client chart, which includes demographic data, the nursing and medical diagnoses, and progress notes. Sometimes a list of the needs for care is prepared by a physician or a member of the nursing staff. The client's needs and resources are assessed using the chart data and a personal interview.

If the hospital discharge planning nurse sees everyone who is scheduled for discharge, the assessment step may sometimes be the only step in the nursing process that is needed. This is because some clients' needs for posthospital self-care or care by health care providers are minimal and the resources are adequate. These clients can be taught the necessary self-care and discharged without further services. However, in most settings these easy-to-discharge patients are assessed by the nursing staff in the hospital units. Only those clients with more complex needs or fewer available resources are referred to the hospital discharge planning nurse. Fig. 2-2 suggests a format that can be used to structure the data needed for discharge planning.

Nursing Diagnosis

The diagnostic statement that summarizes the assessment phase should include a statement about the level of care needed (for example, skilled nursing, nursing home, home care with support, or self-care). Nursing care needs and needs for other referrals should be listed in the diagnostic statement.

Planning

Overworked hospital discharge planning nurses are sometimes tempted simply to do the planning and inform clients of the plan. This strategy wastes time in the long run because it creates fear and uncertainty on the part of the clients. The

Client Name ______________________________

ASSESSMENT OF NEEDS

Date of admission ______________________ Anticipated discharge date ______________________

Discharge diagnosis ______________________________

Nursing service needs (Check needed services on left, explain on right)

___ 1. Medications: ______________________________

___ 2. Treatments:

___ IV therapy ______________________________

___ Dressings, casts ______________________________

___ Stitch removal ______________________________

___ Oxygen ______________________________

___ Bed care ______________________________

___ Passive exercises ______________________________

___ Other ______________________________

___ 3. Nutritional needs:

___ Special diet ______________________________

___ Assistance with eating ______________________________

___ 4. Activity:

___ Limitations ______________________________

___ Exercises ______________________________

___ Help needed ______________________________

___ 5. Health teaching needed ______________________________

Other services needed:

___ 1. Physical therapy ______________________________

___ 2. Social work ______________________________

___ 3. Occupational therapy ______________________________

___ 4. Dietition ______________________________

___ 5. Pharmacist ______________________________

___ Other ______________________________

General level of care needed:

___ 1. Skilled nursing ______________________________

___ 2. Custodial care ______________________________

___ 3. Home care with referrals ______________________________

___ 4. Home care ______________________________

EVALUATION OF RESOURCES

Assessment of client strengths and capabilities (Check as applicable on left, explain on right)

___ 1. Capabilities for self-care ____________________

___ 2. Knowledge deficits ____________________

___ 3. Other ____________________

Assessment of family support or support from significant others: ____________________

SUMMARY OF NEEDS TO BE ADDRESSED IN THE DISCHARGE PLAN

Discharge plan (Check as applicable on left, explain on right)

___ 1. Plan for teaching ____________________

___ 2. Plan for referrals and arrangements ____________________

___ 3. Other ____________________

IMPLEMENTATION

Teaching done (summary and date) ____________________

Referrals made (list and date) ____________________

EVALUATION

Teaching deficits ____________________

Referral outcomes ____________________

FIG. 2-1. Format for hospital discharge planning.

key to effective discharge planning with good compliance is joint planning. Clients should be fully informed of the nurse's perception of needs and should be given time to think and see if they agree with that perception. Then both parties can develop a plan that matches resources with needs. The nurse brings knowledge of the needs and referral possibilities to this discussion but must avoid using this knowledge base to take advantage of the client. Families should also be involved if they are to provide support services. When no family member is available, sometimes a friend or group of friends may be willing to serve as a source of support. If friends take on the role of surrogate family members, they should also be involved in the planning process. Identifying and encouraging nonfamily support persons is often a crucial step in planning for clients with AIDS, since social stigma sometimes motivates families to abandon these persons.

Implementation

The implementation phase of the process includes both the client teaching component and referrals. For example, a client who is recovering after a myocardial infarction needs instructions about medications, diet, and activity levels. In addition, a referral to the local cardiac rehabilitation project might be helpful if such a resource exists. A list of local agencies should be kept in the nurse's office. Sometimes nurses use a list published by the United Way or another local agency and augment it as they evaluate local resources and find new agencies that can assist clients in the community.

The referral process varies. Some clients need only be told about the available resources, and they make their own appointments. Others may not be capable of this activity. Some agencies demand an official referral form, so in these cases the nurse must write or telephone the referral even if the client is competent. Sometimes a visit to the agency by the nurse or a delegate of the nurse smooths the client's pathway. Flexibility is called for in the referral process (Brown and Trimberger, 1983).

Evaluation

After the discharge, a telephone call or even a visit is useful to make sure that the referrals were implemented and that teaching was comprehensive enough. Sometimes a change of plans is called for.

CASE MANAGER IN THE HOME HEALTH CARE AGENCY

The case manager who works for a home health care agency uses the basic nursing process as it was outlined for the discharge planning nurse, but the situation creates some demands for additional tasks. Discharge planning is usually a one-time event with possible adjustments when the plan is evaluated. Home health care case managers usually reevaluate a group of clients many times over the span of their illnesses, so the nursing process is repeated starting each time managers visit their clients. The cycle starts again with the evaluation phase from the current cycle merging with the assessment phase for the next cycle.

A more important difference in the roles of the case manager and the discharge planning nurse stems from the fact that the home health care case manager is often also the line supervisor for ancillary nursing personnel, including nursing aides and licensed practical nurses. This means that the case manager needs to develop a communication system for working with staff and methods of evaluating their work to make sure appropriate and essential nursing care is delivered. Sometimes the role includes a staff teaching role as well. The task of supervision in a home is further complicated by the fact that third party reimbursement levels are so low that stringent economies are necessary. Consequently two people are seldom sent to the home at the same time, so supervision must take place by telephone and through correspondence.

The system can be as follows: At the first client visit the case manager assesses the client's health status and resources. This may include taking a history, doing a brief physical examination, checking written documents, and interviewing family members. From these data a nursing diagnosis and plans for care are made, client teaching and referrals are negotiated with the client and family, and the hands-on nursing care for the day is done by the case manager. The next day, the nursing aide assesses the patient, reads the written care plan drawn up by the case manager, and gives the hands-on care. Nursing aides can call the case manager if they have problems. Some days later the case manager again visits the client, carries out the nursing process, and alters the written care plan if a new situation exists. Referrals to nonnurses (social workers, nutritionists, physicians, or physical therapists) are a part of the case manager's duties, although the nursing aide may well be the person who notified the case manager of the need for a referral. Thus good communication patterns between the staff members are crucial for high-quality care.

SCHOOL NURSING

Although there were nurses working in schools during the nineteenth century in Europe, American school nursing had its beginning in 1902 when Lillian Wald placed a Henry Street Settlement staff nurse in four New York City schools on an experimental basis. She wanted to see if the nurse, Linda Rogers, could reduce the absenteeism caused by communicable diseases. Rogers accomplished this goal by examining the children for early exclusion of the sick and thus reduced the spread of contagious diseases. She then visited selected children in their homes to teach their families how to care for them. The experiment was successful, and the idea of the school nurse spread (Wald, 1933; Wold and Dagg, 1981).

Inspection of children by the school nurse was the crucial element in the role of the school nurse during the early part of this century. A 1918 text advised the nurse to carry out the inspection without touching the child. Children were told to open their mouths, pull down their eyelids, and show their wrists. When examining the hair for pediculi or scabies, the nurse was advised to use two toothpicks "or if she is economically inclined one toothpick, broken in two, lifting and shaping the hair so as to expose the skin" (Wold and Dagg, 1981).

As epidemics of contagious diseases diminished and the medical profession became more powerful, inspections by nurses were replaced with examinations by physicians. The school nurse was reduced to an assistant to the physician. Interventions by school nurses were limited to those that did not compete with the private medical practitioners (Igoe, 1980; Wold and Dagg, 1981). However, on the positive side, the redirected efforts of school nurses were then focused on preventive care and health teaching of students and teachers. Since hospital training did not prepare nurses adequately for this role, it became apparent that at least some nurses needed more education. Eventually the need for nurses to fill this role was an important force in the development of baccalaureate nursing education (Gardner, 1926; Wold and Dagg, 1981).

Current Components of the School Health Program

The goal of the school health program is to support the educational process by helping keep children healthy and by teaching students and teachers preventive health measures (Newman and others, 1981). The role of the school nurse includes the following components (Wold and Dagg, 1981):

1. The identification and exclusion of students and staff with communicable diseases

2. The enforcement of laws and policies related to immunizations
3. Limiting disability of students with early diagnosis and prompt treatment or referral of children with chronic health problems
4. Maintaining a healthy, safe environment
5. Maintaining a workable system for providing first aid
6. Developing, implementing, and evaluating a comprehensive health education curriculum

Ordinarily the school nurse carries out this program in conjunction with a team that includes teachers, physicians, social workers, psychologists, school health aides, and parents. This means that the school nurse not only delivers direct services but also is involved in coordinating care, making referrals, supervising care, and working through others (Griffith and Whicker, 1981). The clientele of the school nurse is broad, ranging in age from 5 to 17 years. This means that a wide variety of problems must be understood. These problems are discussed in Chapter 16, which focuses on the school-aged child.

School Nurse Practitioners

Recently one group of school nurses, the school nurse practitioners, reclaimed the original territory of the early twentieth century school nurses. They have again made the physical examination of children a nursing function (Synoground, 1984). School districts started employing school nurse practitioners in the 1970s and found that money was saved by having them do examinations mandated by the 1972 amendments to the Social Security Act (Sobolewski, 1981).

Starting in 1978 the Robert Wood Johnson Foundation sponsored a school health demonstration project at 18 sites in Colorado, New York, North Dakota, and Utah. The goal was to see if the health of school-aged children could be improved by using school nurse practitioners with physician support. The projects were placed in areas where most of the children had no regular contact with physicians. School nurse practitioners took over routine care of most episodic illnesses of the children and also filled the traditional school nurse role of health teaching, observation of children, immunizations, and referrals. In a report published in 1985 the foundation indicated that the programs were a success. Large numbers of medically underserved children were reached, a significant amount of untreated illness was found, and the proportion of children who were immunized increased (R.W. Johnson, 1985). Currently only a minority of the school nurses are nurse practitioners, but they may well be the wave of the future, particularly if American political forces move again in the direction of concern for the welfare of all children regardless of their economic backgrounds.

Although the Robert Wood Johnson projects demonstrated that school nurse practitioners could improve the health of children from disadvantaged families, the foundation cannot finance the program on a national basis. Long-range financing of such a program would have to come out of public coffers. School nurses should watch and participate in these decisions as the politics evolve.

OCCUPATIONAL HEALTH NURSING

Probably the first occupational health nurse was Philippa Flowerday, an English nurse who was hired by J. and J. Colman in Norwich, England, in 1878.

The honor of being the first U.S. company to employ a nurse is usually given to the Vermont Marble Company, which started a nursing program in 1895 (Marlkolf, 1945). Ada Mayo Steward was hired to visit the workers and their families in their homes. She concentrated on the control of communicable diseases and the improvement of the health of the women and children in the families (Felton, 1986).

The growth of the concept was slow. By 1910

FIRST INDUSTRIAL NURSE

Probably the first industrial nurse was Philippa Flowerday (later Mrs. William Reid), who was employed by J. and J. Colman in Norwich, England, in 1878. The employees of the company had organized the Self-Help Medical Club to which they contributed a small monthly amount that entitled them to medical attention. It was part of Flowerday's duties to assist the physician hired by the club, after which she visited the sick employees or their families in their homes.

only 66 American firms employed graduate nurses. The number increased during World War I when various government agencies encouraged industries to hire nurses to cut down worker absenteeism. Many large companies realized the importance of first aid on the job, and although there was some cutback after the war, the concept of the industrial nurse was well established in some of the larger plants (Bullough and Bullough, 1978; Charley, 1954; Marlkolf, 1945).

Broader expansion of the role was dependent on a change in attitude toward workers. The Industrial Revolution, which started in England in the eighteenth century and reached the United States in the nineteenth century, brought a higher standard of living to the two nations. However, it also brought disequilibrium to the workforce as people moved from the farms to the cities, it brought seasonal unemployment, and it brought industries that were often dangerous for workers. Many great new captains of industry believed that none of these conditions was their concern, so growth of occupational nursing had to wait for union activities and legislation that made work a more humane place that included an occupational nurse.

Probably the first step in this process was the passage of child labor laws in the nineteenth century. These were followed by the first Workman's Compensation Act, which was passed in New Jersey in 1911. As other states followed this lead, more workers who were injured on the job could receive hospital and medical care. In the long run this legislation probably helped motivate employers to be more safety conscious to keep compensation rates down. The 1935 Social Security Act provided unemployment insurance, which helped workers cope with economic cycles, as well as seasonal characteristics of many jobs. The Federal Fair Labor Standards Act of 1938 set 16 years as the minimum age for most jobs and 18 years as the minimum age for hazardous work.

The key legislation in the field was the 1970 Occupational Safety and Health Act. This act established the Occupational Safety and Health Administration (OSHA), which enforces safety standards outlined in the act, and the National Institute for Occupational Safety and Health (NIOSH), which sponsors research and makes recommendations to the government regarding occupational health and safety. These acts and their subsequent revisions are discussed in Chapter 17. The problems faced by occupational health nurses are dealt with in more detail there. The 1970 legislation has served as a major impetus for industry to hire occupational health nurses who helped monitor the safety of the workplace, to prepare the reports called for in the legislation, and to deal with illness and injury in a timely manner (Babbitz, 1984; Clemen-Stone and others, 1987).

Role of the Occupational Health Nurse

The goals of occupational health nursing are to prevent occupational injuries and illness and to facilitate good health among workers. The role of the occupational nurse in meeting these goals is summarized in Table 2-2.

There are now an estimated 25,000 occupational health nurses. A professional society was organized in 1942 as the American Association of Industrial Health Nurses. The name was changed in 1977 to the American Association of Occupational Health Nurses (AAOHN). This

TABLE 2-2 Summary of the Role of the Occupational Health Nurse

Nursing process	Activities
1. Assessment	Assess health of individual workers Assess risks and hazards in the workplace Keep accurate and complete records
2. Diagnosis	List problems for individual employees Note risks and hazards in the workplace
3. Planning	Confer with management regarding all aspects of the program Counsel employees for better individual health Cooperate with employees to set up a wellness program Work with unions to ensure cooperation Use specialists such as industrial hygienists and safety engineers to lessen hazards
4. Implementation	Implement programs to increase safety and lessen hazards Teach workers good health and safety behaviors Enforce laws related to health and safety Carry out appropriate and timely first aid and see that workers get needed additional care Make referrals to other health workers
5. Research and evaluation	Monitor hazards Evaluate programs Conduct research to identify potential health problems

change reflects the broader focus of the specialty on other workplaces besides industry. AAOHN now has more than 10,000 members. A recent membership survey indicated that most members are diploma graduates, or nurses who received their training from hospital programs. However, the educational level of the group is escalating and a baccalaureate degree will probably be required in the future (Dees, 1984). Manufacturing plants employ the most occupational health nurses, followed in order by the chemical industry and the health care industry (Cox, 1987).

Nearly 2000 AAOHN members are certified. This certification represents additional education earned in degree or continuing education programs. Formal organized specialty training is available in only a few universities, but AAOHN offers an active, focused continuing education program. There is also a small group of occupational health nurse practitioners or adult health nurse practitioners in the field, particularly where employee wellness programs are instituted.

The wellness programs are a recent development. As the worst industrial hazards were dealt with, it has become apparent that the challenge of the future is to encourage employees to take charge of their own health risks. Thus occupational health nurses are now supporting drug and alcohol programs, obesity clinics, smoking cessation programs, and exercise programs (Richard, 1984). Some of these wellness programs use the nursing theory popularized by Orem, which stresses the importance of self-help activities in improving health and well-being (Dees, 1984).

The changing job market has also brought new challenges to the occupational health nurses. Medical centers bring clients who face such hazards as needle sticks, anesthesia dangers (particularly to pregnant workers), and back injuries (de Carteret, 1987; Kwapien and others, 1987). Teaching good health habits in a medical center is challenging, since many workers are also experts in the field. Unfortunately, some of the experts think the rules do not apply to them.

NURSE PRACTITIONERS

The nurse practitioner movement as a separate entity started in 1965. Trends in medicine were basic to its development. Starting with the 1910

Flexner report on medical education, medical education was upgraded and many substandard medical schools were closed. Although these reforms did not actually decrease the supply of physicians, they caused the physican ratio of 150: 100,000 standard population to stay the same for 50 years. At the same time medical science and technology developed, so the demand for services grew. This created a shortage of physicians that became acute in the 1960s (Fein, 1967).

Scientific development also helped stimulate a specialty orientation in medicine, so by the end of the 1960s medical specialists outnumbered generalists by more than three to one (National Center for Health Statistics, 1973). This meant that the supply of physicians who were available for primary care declined sharply during the century. The fees charged by these specialists also escalated, so available medical services became costly.

For a time a physician's assistant seemed to many people to be the most likely answer to the shortage of primary care services. The physician's assistant movement expanded so rapidly that by 1977 there were 56 educational programs operating in 30 states and physician assistant practice was legal in all states (Fisher and Horowitz, 1977).

However, the role of the nurse had already started expanding into territory that overlapped with medicine. There were public health nurses functioning in an expanded role in northern California as early as 1962 and probably in informal types of primary care situations much earlier (Siegel and Bryson, 1963). Starting also in 1962, outpatient nurses at Massachusetts General Hospital were responsible for the long-term management of patients with chronic illnesses (Noonan, 1972). The University of Colorado program to train pediatric nurse practitioners was started in 1965, the same year the Duke University physician assistant program began (Silver, 1967).

Organized medicine was supportive of the nurse practitioner movement in this era. The American Academy of Pediatrics furnished leadership by sponsoring conferences, research, and statements supporting practitioners whom they termed "nurse associates" (American Nurses' Association, 1971). The American Medical Association followed the academy's lead and in 1970 issued an official statement supporting the expansion of the nurse's role (American Medical Association, 1970).

Role expansion for registered nurses was also facilitated by trends in nursing education. Education reform in nursing was slow because of the virtual monopoly of the hospital apprenticeship–type programs. However, the struggle to move nursing education into the mainstream of higher education was finally succeeding (Bullough, 1976). In the 1965 academic year, when the first formal educational programs for nurse practitioners were started, 13.7% of the new nurse graduates were from baccalaureate programs and 2.6% were from associate degree programs (ANA, 1967). Even the 83.7% of the new graduates who finished with diplomas came from programs that were strengthened because of competition from the collegiate schools. By 1984 the pool of collegiate graduates had grown significantly with 29.5% of the new graduates finishing with baccalaureate degrees and 55.3% finishing with associate of arts degrees, whereas only 15% were finishing with hospital diplomas (Rosenfeld, 1985). Thus the upgrading of the nursing educational system has supported the development of the advanced nursing specialities, including nurse practitioners.

However, even with stronger educational background nurses faced some psychologic barriers to role expansion. Traditionally the physician-nurse relationship had been one of extreme superordination-subordination. Many physicians simply did not think nurses were capable of independent or even cooperative decision making. An even more important barrier was the image nurses held of themselves. Some nurses could not imagine themselves making diagnostic decisions. They had of course been making them for years but had disguised their decision making with elaborate games that left physicians sure they were the only decision makers (Bullough, 1975; Stein, 1967). Some nurses enjoyed these feminine games; others feared formal responsibility.

However, the women's liberation movement occurred simultaneously with the development of nurse practitioners, and it helped some nurses broaden their horizons and accept the expanded role of nurse practitioner.

Role of the Nurse Practitioner

The Council of Primary Health Care Nurse Practitioners has drawn up this description of the scope of practice:

> Nurse practitioners provide primary health care services to clients—individuals, families and groups—emphasizing the promotion of health and the prevention of disease. They manage actual and potential health problems, which include common diseases and human responses to disease. Consultation and referral occur as needed. Self-care is promoted as appropriate. Nurse practitioners provide holistic care, taking into account the needs and strengths of the whole person. Nurse practitioners collaborate with clients to establish realistic goals and activities to guide both the client and the provider in implementing the care plan. Nurse practitioners are accountable for the outcome of their practice.
>
> Nurse practitioners have expanded nursing practice boundaries by creating an additional model for delivery of nursing care directly to the public. They have also incorporated selected medical services into professional nursing practice and have helped to change the relationship between nurses and physicians from dependent to interdependent and independent with mutual referral and consultation. The role of nurse practitioner continues to evolve as changes in society and health care occur (ANA, 1987a).

The description of the obstetric-gynecologic nurse practitioner drawn up by the Nurses' Association of the American College of Obstetricians and Gynecologists is in many ways similar:

> The obstetric-gynecologic nurse practitioner is a registered nurse who has satisfactorily completed a formal obstetric-gynecologic nurse practitioner educational program. Thereby, the obstetric-gynecologic nurse practitioner will have acquired special knowledge and skills in health promotion and maintenance, disease prevention, psychosocial and physical assessment, and management of health-illness needs in the primary care of women. This care is provided predominantly in an ambulatory setting. The obstetric-gynecologic nurse practitioner will provide such care with the physician as well as with other members of the health-care team (Nurses' Association of the American College of Obstetricians and Gynecologists, 1984).

A key element in both of these official descriptions of the nurse practitioner role is the focus on primary health care. Nurse practitioners use a broad definition of the concept, including not only the care given to the client at the first contact with the health care delivery system, but also all services that prevent illness, promote health, and detect illness early.

An example of how the nurse practitioner role is implemented using the nursing process is furnished by the National Association of Pediatric Nurse Associates and Practitioners (NAPNAP, 1983).

Assessment:

1. Secure a health and developmental history.
2. Perform and record a health appraisal including physical assessment from the newborn period through adolescence.
3. Differentiate between normal findings and those that require consultation and/or referral.
4. Assess the child's and family's psychosocial, emotional, spiritual, physiologic and environmental needs and priorities.
5. Diagnose children with common acute conditions, illnesses, or minor trauma within legally accepted protocols or Nurse Practice Acts.

Plan:

6. Formulate a health plan emphasizing self-care responsibility through the participation of the child, family, physician and other health professionals.

7. Determine those cases that require consultation and/or referral with the pediatrician or other professional of the health care team.

Intervention:

8. Encourage health and provide preventive health care that includes immunizations, anticipatory guidance, health education, and counseling.
9. Treat children with common acute conditions, illnesses or minor trauma within legally accepted protocols or Nurse Practice Acts or in collaboration with the physician.
10. Collaborate with the pediatrician or other health professionals in the health care of children with chronic illnesses.
11. Counsel children and families as needed.
12. Identify resources and coordinate referrals for children and families requiring further evaluation or services.
13. Interact with appropriate community agencies to facilitate implementation of the health care plan.

Evaluation:

14. Analyze the results of the health care plan.
15. Modify the health care plan as indicated.
16. Implement and participate in appropriate follow-up.

Nurse Practitioner Education

The first formal training program for nurse practitioners was established in 1965 in Colorado. Henry Silver and Loretta Ford designed the program as a short-term (four-month) certificate course. There were several reasons that the early programs were not established as an integral part of regular nursing programs—they were experimental, many of the teachers were physicians who had no close ties with nursing schools, and there were nurse educators who questioned the validity of the new role.

These educators perceived the health care team as divided into workers who focused on care and workers whose job it was to cure. Nursing was thought of as the caring profession, so it followed that nurses should be interested only in the social and psychologic problems that accompany illness rather than in treating the actual illness. Nurses were described as maternal, expressive, supportive, and feminine, whereas physicians were described as paternal, instrumental, masculine, and cure oriented (ANA, 1965; Johnson, 1974; Kreuter, 1957; Rogers, 1964). The nurse practitioner role combined the care and cure elements, so it did not fit the format. Probably the most outspoken of the educators who did not favor nurse practitioners was Martha Rogers. She perceived the development of the nurse practitioner role as a ploy by physicians to lead nurses into "paying obeisance to an obsolete hierarchy." Rogers wanted nursing to be an independent profession and thought the nurse practitioner movement was a step backward. She argued that those who became nurse practitioners left the nursing profession (Rogers, 1972).

Educators who accepted this thinking were naturally unwilling to accept nurse practitioner programs in their schools; consequently this was a powerful barrier to the early institutionalization of the educational programs within mainstream nursing education. Nevertheless, there were a few university nursing schools willing to set up nurse practitioner programs at the graduate level. Gradually the fears and hostility lessened, and the educational pattern was upgraded and switched from the certificate to the graduate level. Women's health is now the only field with any appreciable number of certificate programs. The obstetric-gynecologic nurse practitioner is usually prepared in a 10-month certificate program, and there are a group of specialists in family planning who have even shorter programs (Geolot, 1987; Sultz and others, 1983, part I and part II).

The nurse practitioner movement is now almost 25 years old, and there are more than 15,000

TABLE 2-3 Nurse Practitioner Specialties

Specialty	Clients	Education	Certification by
Pediatric nurse practitioner	Infants Children Teenagers	Master's degree	NAPNAP* or ANA†
Adult nurse practitioner	Adults	Master's degree	ANA
Geriatric nurse practitioner	Older adults	Master's degree	ANA
Obstetric-gynecologic nurse practitioner	Women of all ages, including teenage women	Certificate or master's degree	NAACOG‡
Family nurse practitioner	Families and individuals	Master's degree	ANA

*National Association of Pediatric Nurse Associates and Practitioners.
†American Nurses' Association
‡Nurses' Association of the American College of Obstetricians and Gynecologists.

nurse practitioners in practice. Repeated studies have shown that nurse practitioners give safe, effective care that is well received by clients and other providers (Henry, 1986; U.S. Congress, Office of Technology Assessment, 1986; Ventura and others,1985).

Nurse Practitioner Specialties

The nurse practitioner movement started with many specialties, but five major divisions have now emerged. Three of the specialties, pediatrics, adult care, and geriatrics, use age as a developmental organizing framework. Women, including obstetrics and gynecology, are separated out as a fourth specialty, whereas family nursing, which focuses on individuals and family members of all ages, is the fifth specialty. All of the specialties, including occupational and school nurse practitioners and other smaller subspecialties, are important in the community, but the family focus of the family nurse practitioner makes the role most popular with community health nurses.

Certification

Certification varies by specialty. The American Nurses' Association (ANA) certifies family nurse practitioners, adult nurse practitioners, geriatric nurse practitioners, and pediatric nurse practitioners. However, most pediatric nurse practitioners are certified by a separate organization, the National Association of Pediatric Nurse Associates and Practitioners (NAPNAP). Obstetric-gynecologic nurse practitioners are certified only by the Nurses' Association of the American College of Obstetricians and Gynecologists (NAACOG). Each of these certifying bodies requires registered nurse licensure, graduation from a recognized nurse practitioner program, and successful completion of a certifying examination. Most states require certification for nurse practitioner practice, and even in states that do not require it, many employers look for the credential when they hire. Table 2-3 summarizes the specialties and their certifying organizations.

NURSE-MIDWIFERY

Traditionally, assisting with the birth process was considered a field for women only, and midwifery was a time-honored profession learned by apprenticeship (Leavett, 1986). Obstetrics developed into a medical specialty in the nineteenth century, and other physicians added deliveries to their functions, often moving the deliveries to hospitals, where analgesics and anesthesia were used and promises of "painless childbirth" were made. Physicians also promised safer childbirth, although this was not necessarily true until the twentieth century when the development of trained nurses made hospital clients safer from infections and nurses monitored the clients.

With the advent of the trained nurse, most European countries developed nurse-midwifery as a specialty. Often a collaborative agreement was made whereby nurse-midwives handled the normal deliveries and obstetricians took the problem cases. Nurse-midwifery was much slower to develop in the United States, and the specialty has had to struggle for its existence (Litoff, 1978).

The first American nurse-midwifery training program was established in connection with the Maternity Center of New York City in 1932 (Tom, 1982). It was at this school that most early American nurse-midwives received their training. Many of the graduates, however, were prevented from practicing as midwives and had to content themselves with serving as teachers or working in hospital maternity units. Nevertheless, many did practice, particularly in the New York City area and in certain economically deprived rural areas of the country. Nurse-midwives encountered the least opposition in the latter areas, and their best-known trailblazer was Mary Breckenridge of Kentucky.

Early in her nursing career Breckenridge surveyed the health problems of the people of rural Kentucky and decided that a crucial health care problem was the poor maternal care residents were receiving. Since there were no American training schools for midwifery at that time, Breckenridge went to England to study. On her return to Kentucky in 1925, she established a service for mothers and children that eventually came to be called the Frontier Nursing Service. Most of the nurse-midwives who worked in the project during its early years were British, although eventually the service established its own training program. Adopting the principle that if a husband could reach the nurse at the center, the nurse could make it back to the mother, nurses traveled on horseback and foot to the isolated hill residences (Breckenridge, 1952; Dammann, 1982).

Although the Frontier Nursing Service became a recognized outpost of expanded nursing function, nurse-midwives continued to be much less welcome in areas where there were more physicians. Such exclusion continued despite research evidence that indicated lives could be saved by nurse-midwives. A landmark study carried out from 1960 to 1963 proved this claim. The demonstration project employed two nurse-midwives to manage normal deliveries at the Madera County Hospital in rural California. They gave prenatal care, attended labor and delivery, and cared for mothers and infants in the postpartum period. The nurse-midwives were successful in breaking down cultural barriers between the patients and providers. The number of women seeking prenatal care and other preventive services increased significantly. Even more important was that, during the span of the project, prematurity and neonatal mortality rates among the patient population fell significantly. Yet when the project sponsors sought to institutionalize the practice and secure a change in California state law that would have allowed nurse-midwives to continue practicing, they were unsuccessful because of opposition from the California Medical Association (CMA). When CMA opposition forced the cancellation of the project, the neonatal mortality went from the project rate of 10.3:1000 to 32.1:1000 live births (Levy and others, 1971).

Other outcome studies have supported these positive findings (American Nurses' Association, 1987a; Institute of Medicine, 1985). In one recent study a comparison was done between team care (including medicine, nursing, nurse-midwifery, social work, and nutrition) and ordinary clinical care. The group cared for by the team showed significantly lower incidence of low birth weight. The findings were particularly dramatic among mothers younger than 15 years of age. This group, which was cared for by the team, had only half the incidence of low–birth weight infants as the control group (Institute of Medicine, 1985; Piechnic and Corbett, 1985).

The success of nurse-midwives stems partly from their interest in preventive health measures and their support of client participation in care (Philosophy, 1984). Nurse-midwives also spend more time with each client than do physicians. A 1981 study analyzed the content and process of prenatal care provided by certified nurse-midwives and found that the mean length of their prenatal visits was 23.7 minutes (Lehrman, 1981). An ambulatory medical care survey found that prenatal visits with office-based physicians did not include counseling and tended to last only about 10 minutes (National Center for Health Statistics, 1980).

Because nurse-midwives and nurse practitioners have a positive record of caring for women from all social strata including the socially and economically high-risk population, the Institute of Medicine recommended the following:

> More reliance should be placed on nurse-midwives and nurse practitioners to increase access to prenatal care for hard-to-reach, often high-risk groups. Maternity programs designed to serve socioeconomically high-risk mothers should increase their use of such providers; and state laws should be supportive of nurse-midwifery practice and of collaborations between physicians and nurse-midwives/nurse practitioners (Institute of Medicine, 1985).

The record of safe client care helped popularize nurse-midwifery. However, there were other factors that helped the movement grow. The organization that is now called the American College of Nurse-Midwives was established in 1955. It furnished a support system for its members (ACNM, 1984a). The women's movement has also been an important factor in the growth of the concept. Many women were distressed by the physician-dominated delivery process. Nurse-midwives were willing to play an important role in the decision making related to the birthing process. Consequently the popularity of the specialty grew.

There are now 32 educational programs accredited by the American College of Nurse-Midwifery. Of this group 16 are at the masters's degree level, 15 are certificate programs, and one awards a Doctor of Nursing Science (ACNM, 1984a).

CLINICAL NURSE SPECIALISTS AND NURSE CLINICIANS

The clinical nurse specialist is a specialist in nursing who has a master's degree. The nurse clinician is a more general term that describes a specialist who may or may not have a master's degree. These nursing roles developed during the same period as those of the nurse practitioner, and they constitute an alternative approach to an expanded role for nurses. The movement was facilitated by the Nurse Training Act, which was enacted in 1964 under Title VIII of the Public Health Service Act. This legislation was aimed at strengthening nursing education. In response to this opportunity, many schools of nursing established master's degree programs or expanded existing programs and made clinical specialization the focus of the new curriculums (Kalisch and Kalisch, 1987).

The early emphasis of the specialists was to improve client education and give social and psychologic support to clients (Reiter, 1966). Most of the specialists worked in hospitals where they attempted to improve nursing care by giving expert care to patients, serving as role models and carrying out formal or informal educational programs to upgrade nursing staff performance. In the last few years, some of the nursing specialists have moved the focus of their activity to the community. Alternatively some specialists work with

TABLE 2-4 Certification of Specialists by American Nurses' Association

Nurse	Generalist level registered nurse certified (R.N.C.)	Clinical specialty level registered nurse certified specialist (R.N.C.S.)
Medical surgical	X	X
Gerontologic	X	
Psychiatric mental health	X	
Maternal and child	X	
Child and adolescent	X	X
High-risk perinatal	X	
Community health	X	
Adult psychiatric mental health		X
Child and adolescent psychiatric mental health		X

groups of clients who are in and out of the hospital, so a significant portion of the work of the specialist is in the community.

The American Nurses' Association tests and certifies six types of specialists or clinicians at the generalist level and four types of clinical nurse specialists (Table 2-4) (ANA, 1987b). The master's degree is required for the specialist certification.

There are also several independent specialty nursing organizations that certify nurses who work in the community. These organizations include the Association of Rehabilitation Nurses and the International Association of Enterostomal Therapy.

Nurse Practice Acts

The development of the advanced nursing specialties has had a significant impact on nursing practice law. Some historical background is needed to put these recent changes in perspective. Nurse practice acts were developed at the beginning of the twentieth century to protect both nurses and the public. These acts were state laws rather than federal statutes because the U.S. Constitution includes no mechanism for national licensure. The early nurse practice acts recognized nurses who had gone through a formal nursing educational program and differentiated them from untrained nurses. Starting in 1938 the laws were revised to divide the nursing role into a registered and practical nursing level. During this same era, nurses were seeking mandatory licensure to make it illegal for untrained persons to practice nursing. To achieve this goal it was necessary to spell out the nursing role, so scope-of-function statements were written into the law. To avoid controversy with the medical establishment, nurses in many states suggested to legislators that a disclaimer be written into the nurse practice act indicating that nurses would not diagnose diseases or treat clients (Bullough, 1980; Bullough, 1984).

Consequently when the first nurse practitioner programs were started in 1965, the graduates were being prepared for a role that was outside the legal scope of practice in most states. Midwifery was recognized in New Mexico and New York City, although exemptions in some of the state laws written to cover lay midwives allowed nurse-midwives to practice. An important political task for nurses and their friends has been to update the practice acts to accommodate the expanded nursing role.

The first state to change its practice act was Idaho. In 1971 the following clause was inserted after the prohibition against diagnosis and treatment:

> except as may be authorized by rules and regulations jointly promulgated by the Idaho State Board of Medicine and the Idaho Board of Nursing which shall be implemented by the Idaho Board of Nursing (Idaho, 1971).

After the passage of this amendment, the combined boards met and adopted regulations that called for agencies employing nurse practitioners to draw up policies and procedures to guide their practice. Thus the Idaho legislature and boards established two precedents: to use the power of the boards to draw up regulations to facilitate the expanded role of the nurse and to use agency-generated protocols to guide the practice of the individual nurse.

A third approach to the accommodation of the nurse practitioner role was to expand the basic definition of the registered professional nurse by omitting or limiting the disclaimer against diagnosis and treatment by nurses or by rewriting the definition of the registered nurse using broader language. New York, in 1972, was the first state to use this approach (New York, 1972). Table 2-5 shows the mechanisms used for legal coverage of the advanced nursing specialties in each of the states. Most states have now expanded their basic definition of the functions of the registered nurse, removing the old prohibitions against nurses diagnosing. Although this facilitates an expanded role for all registered nurses, it does not cover such nurse practitioner activities as writing prescriptions for medications or ordering laboratory tests. This creates a problem because most medical practice acts forbid these practices by anyone except physicians, dentists, osteopaths, and veterinarians. Thus a statutory change is usually needed to allow nurses to carry out these responsibilities. As indicated in the table, a system of state certification has evolved allowing such activities for nurse practitioners in 36 states and for nurse-midwives in 40 states.

A second approach to coverage is laws or regulations that say that nurses can prescribe or carry out other medical functions when they are working under standing orders or protocols. The protocol approach has become more popular in recent years because of a 1983 Missouri Supreme Court decision supporting the use of standing orders or protocols. Missouri is one of the states that does not certify nurse practitioners or other specialists. A case was brought by the Missouri Medical Board against five physicians who were working with two nurse practitioners in a family planning clinic. The board argued that the two nurse practitioners were functioning illegally, so their physician supervisors were charged with aiding and abetting the illegal practice of medicine. The board won its case at the circuit court level, but the case was appealed to the Missouri State Supreme Court where the decision was reversed. The court ruled that the practice of the two nurses was legal. Although the 1975 Missouri Nurse Practice Act did not mention nurse practitioner activities, it was a broad general act and the legitimization of the expanded functions came from the use of standing orders and protocols (Greenlaw, 1984; Wolff, 1984).

The issue as to which is the best approach to coverage is controversial among nurses. The American Nurses' Association supports the Missouri model of a broad umbrella practice act with no mention of the specialties in the nurse practice acts (ANA, 1981). Most nurse-midwives, nurse practitioners, and the legal advisors who support them would prefer certification by the states (Bullough, 1984; Greenlaw, 1984).

MALPRACTICE INSURANCE CRISIS

As the roles of these ambulatory specialists have expanded into territory that was formerly considered part of the medical field, the possibility of

TABLE 2-5 Legal Coverage of Nurse Practitioners and Nurse-Midwives

	Expanded definition RN	State certification for nurse practitioner	State certification for nurse-midwife	Protocol	Other
Alabama	X	X	X	X	
Alaska	X	X			Nurse-midwife covered by nurse practitioner statute
Arizona	X	X	X		
Arkansas	X	X	X	X	
California	X	X	X	X	
Colorado	X				Nurse-midwife–medical practice act
Connecticut	X	X	X	X	
Delaware	X		X	X	
Washington, D.C.				X	Hospital licensing act
Florida	X	X	X	X	
Georgia	X	X	X	X	
Hawaii	X	X	X		
Idaho	X	X	X		
Illinois					
Indiana	X				Nurse-midwife–medical practice act
Iowa	X	X	X		
Kansas	X	X	X		
Kentucky	X	X	X		Nurse-midwife covered by nurse practitioner statute
Louisiana	X	X	X		
Maine	X	X	X		Physician delegation
Maryland	X	X	X		
Massachusetts	X	X	X		
Michigan	X	X	X		
Minnesota	X				
Mississippi	X	X	X	X	
Missouri	X			X	1983 Supreme Court Decision
Montana			X		
Nebraska	X	X	X	X	
Nevada	X	X		X	Nurse-midwife covered by nurse practitioner statute
New Hampshire	X	X	X	X	
New Jersey	X				Nurse-midwife board of medical examiners
New Mexico	X	X	X		
New York	X	X		X	Public health laws and regulations
North Carolina	X	X	X		
North Dakota	X	X			Nurse-midwife covered by nurse practitioner statute
Ohio			X		Nurse-midwife medical practice act
Oklahoma	X	X	X		
Oregon	X	X	X		
Pennsylvania	X	X	X	X	Nurse-midwife regulated by board of medicine

Continued

TABLE 2-5 Legal Coverage of Nurse Practitioners and Nurse-Midwives—cont'd.

	Expanded definition RN	State certification for nurse practitioner	State certification for nurse-midwife	Protocol	Other
Puerto Rico					
Rhode Island					Nurse-midwife department of health rules
South Carolina	X		X	X	Regulations by board of nursing and medicine
South Dakota	X	X	X		
Tennessee	X	X	X		
Texas	X	X	X		
Utah	X	X	X	X	
Vermont	X	X	X	X	
Virgin Islands			X		
Virginia	X	X	X		
Washington	X	X	X	X	
West Virginia	X		X		
Wisconsin			X		
Wyoming	X	X	X		

liability suits increased. Not unexpectedly the cost of malpractice insurance went up. However, the 1400 nurse-midwives who carried insurance through the American College of Nurse Midwives (ACNM) were shocked in 1985 when they lost their insurance completely and were quoted annual fees of between $25,000 and $80,000, which was much more than the annual salaries of most members of ACNM. The group turned to the U.S. Congress for help and with assistance from other nursing organizations was able to get the Risk Retention Amendments of 1986 passed. These amendments allow an insurance company to be licensed in one state and yet do business in all the states. This removed one barrier to ACNM starting its own insurance company. In the meantime the National Association of Insurance Carriers Commission took pity on the group and found coverage for its members (Bullough, 1987a).

In 1987 nurse practitioners faced a similar scenario. They first lost their ANA-sponsored insurance and then were reinstated with rate increases from $50 to $1500 anually. Nurse practitioners have found other carriers, but the price increase remains. Any long-range solution of the problem will undoubtedly involve more federal regulation of the insurance industry, which has even been exempt from federal antitrust regulations (Jonides and McGuire, 1987). It is now proposed that the industry be made subject to these laws so that the public can scrutinize it and some of the collusion between companies will be reduced (Bullough, 1987). Passage of this legislation or any similar efforts will involve heavy political activity by nurse practitioners and their colleagues. This development, along with the changes that have taken place in the state nurse practice acts, underscores a point that has been implied several times in this book. Increasingly, community nurses are called on for political activity and political sophistication. This marks a significant change from past practices when most nurses avoided politics.

SUMMARY

A broad array of choices is now available for nurses who choose to work in the community. Community health nursing, which evolved out of the earlier public health nursing role, is the major traditional community nursing position. However, the position of visiting nurse has also existed for more than a century. That position is now being filled by home health care nurses, and their job market is expanding rapidly. In addition, there is a varity of other developing community nursing roles, including those of case manager, school nurse, occupational health nurse, nurse practitioner, nurse-midwife, and clinical specialist.

Educational preparations for most of these positions is at the baccalaureate level, although requirements for nurse practitioner, nurse midwife, and clinical nurse specialist roles have moved to the graduate level.

The advanced specialists created pressure on the state nurse practice acts, which are being changed to accommodate a more autonomous nursing role. Unfortunately, however, the new specialists are at risk for rising malpractice insurance rates.

QUESTIONS FOR DISCUSSION

1. Define the term "preventive health care."
2. Differentiate between primary, secondary, and tertiary prevention. Give examples of each of these levels of preventive health care.
3. Do you think the hospital discharge planning nurse is an appropriate role for inclusion in a text that is focused on the community nursing role?
4. A variety of community nursing roles are described in this chapter. Select one of these roles, and examine it carefully. What do nurses who fill this role do, and who are the clients they serve? Is it a role you would like to fill?

REFERENCES

American College of Nurse-Midwives, Research and Statistics Committee, C Adams, Project Director: Nurse-midwifery in the United States: 1982, Washington DC, 1984a, The College.

American College of Nurse-Midwives: Education programs accredited by the division of accreditation, ACNM, Appendix V, J Nurse Midwifery 29(2):173, 1984b.

American Medical Association, Committee on Nursing: Medicine and nursing in the 1970s: a position statement, JAMA 213:1881, 1970.

American Nurses' Association, Education Committee: First position paper on education for nursing, Am J Nurs 65:106, 1965.

American Nurses' Association: Facts about nursing: a statistical summary, New York, 1967, The Association.

American Nurses' Association, Maternal Child Health Nursing Practice Division and American Academy of Pediatrics: Guidelines on short-term continuing education programs for pediatric nursing associates, Am J Nurs 71:509, 1971.

American Nurses' Association: A conceptual model of community health nursing, Kansas City, Mo, 1980, The Association.

American Nurses' Association: The nursing practice act: suggested state legislation, Kansas City, Mo, 1981, The Association.

American Nurses' Association, Council of Community Health Nurses: A guide for community based nursing services, Kansas City, Mo, 1985, The Association.

American Nurses' Association: Standards of practice for primary health care nurse practitioner, Kansas City, Mo, 1987a, The Association.

American Nurses' Association: The career credential: professional certification, the 1987 catalog of certification requirements, Kansas City, Mo, 1987b, The Association.

American Public Health Association: The definition and role of public health nursing in the delivery of health care, Washington DC, 1980, The Association.

American Public Health Association, Public Health Nursing Section: Operational definition of public health nursing. In ANA Council of Community Health Nurses: A guide for community based nursing services, Appendix B, Kansas City, Mo, 1985, American Nurses' Association.

Anderson ET: Community focus in public health nursing, Nurs Outlook 31:44, 1983.

Arnhoff F: Social consequences of policy toward mental illness, Science 188:1277, 1975.

Babbitz M: Occupational health nursing: influence on policy making, Occup Health Nurs 32:21, 1984.

Breckenridge M: Wide neighborhood: a study of frontier nursing service, New York, 1952, Harper & Row, Publishers Inc.

Brown S and Trimberger L: Discharge referrals, J Emerg Nurs 9:44, 1983.

Buhler-Wilkerson K: Public health nursing: in sickness or in health? Am J Public Health 75:1155, 1985.

Bullough B: The Medicare-Medicaid amendments, Am J Nurs 73:1926, 1973.

Bullough B: Barriers to the nurse practitioner movement: problems of women in a woman's field, Int J Health Serv 2(suppl):225, 1975.

Bullough B: Influences on role expansion, Am J Nurs 76:1476, 1976.

Bullough B, editor: The law and the expanding nursing role, ed 2, New York, 1980, Appleton-Century-Crofts.

Bullough B: The current phase in the development of nurse practice acts, Saint Louis University Law Journal 28(2):365, 1984.

Bullough B: The malpractice insurance crisis, J Pediatr Health Care 1(1):2, 1987a.

Bullough B: Nurse practitioners: the new victims of the malpractice crisis, J Pediatr Health Care 1(5):231, 1987b.

Bullough V and Bullough B: The care of the sick: the emergence of modern nursing, New York, 1978, Prodist.

de Carteret CJ: Needle stick injuries: occupational health hazard for nurses, AAOHN J 35(1):19, 1987.

Charley I: The birth of industrial nursing: its history and development in Great Britain, London, 1954, Baillière, Tindall & Cox.

Chisholm MM: Promises and pitfalls of discharge planning, Nurs Management 14:26, 1983.

Clemen-Stone S, Eigsti DG, and McGuire S: Comprehensive community health nursing, ed 2, New York, 1987, McGraw-Hill Inc.

Colosi E: Laser view of managed care, Case Management Perspective 1:4, 1986.

Cox AR: AAOHN membership profile, AAOHN J 35(7):324, 1987.

Dammann N: A social history of the Frontier Nursing Service, Sun City, Ariz, 1982, Social Change Press.

Dees J: Conceptual model for nursing practice in occupational health nursing, Occup Health Nurs 32:137, 1984.

Feeg VD: From the editor, Pediatr Nurs 13(4):226, 1987.

Fein R: The doctor shortage: an economic diagnosis (Studies in Social Economics), Washington, DC, 1967, The Brookings Institute.

Felton JS: The genesis of American occupational health nursing, part II, AAOHN J 34:31, 1986.

Fisher DW and Horowitz SM: The physician's assistant: profile of a new health profession. In Bliss AA and Cohen ED, editors: New health professionals, Germantown, Md, 1977, Aspen Systems.

Franklin JL and others: An evaluation of case management, Am J Public Health 77:674, 1987.

Gardner MS: Public health nursing, ed 2, New York, 1926, Macmillan Publishing Co.

Geolot DH: NP education: observations from a national perspective, Nurs Outlook 35:132, 1987.

Greenlaw J: Commentary: Sermchief v. Gonzales and the debate over advanced nursing practice legislation, Law Med Health Care 12(1):30, 1984.

Griffith BB and Whicker PH: Teacher observer of student health problems, J Sch Health 51(6):428, 1981.

Henry OM: How many nurse practitioners are enough? Am J Public Health 76:493, 1986.

Higgs ZR and Gustafson DD: Community as a client: assessment and diagnosis, Philadelphia, 1985, FA Davis Co.

Idaho Code: Section 54-1413(e), 1971 Revision.

Igoe JB: Changing patterns in school health and school nursing, Nurs Outlook 28(8):486, 1980.

Institute of Medicine, Committee to Study the Prevention of Low Birthweight, Division of Health Promotion and Disease Prevention: Preventing low birthweight, Washington, DC, 1985, National Academy Press.

Jamieson M: The St. Anthony park block nurse program: notes from the field, Am J Public Health 77(9):1227, 1987.

Johnson DE: Development of a theory: a requisite for nursing as a primary health profession, Nurs Res 23:372, 1974.

Jonides L and McGuire M: Malpractice insurance update, J Pediatr Health Care 1(4):228, 1987.

Kalisch PA and Kalisch BJ: The advance of American Nursing, Boston, 1987, Little, Brown & Co Inc.

Kreuter FR: What is good nursing care? Nurs Outlook 5:302, 1957.

Kwapien CA, Phillips DA, and Anderson L: Hepatitis B program for health personnel, AAOHN J 35(1):19, 1987.

Leavitt JW: Brought to bed—childbearing in America, 1750 to 1950, New York, 1986, Oxford University Press.

Lehrman E: Nurse-midwifery practice: a descriptive study of prenatal care, J Nurse Midwifery 26:27, 1981.

Levy BS, Wilkinson FS, and Marine WM: Reducing neonatal mortality rate with nurse-midwives, Am J Obstet Gynecol 109:50, 1971.

Litoff JB: American midwives: 1860 to present, Westport, Conn, 1978, Greenwood Press.

Maine Revised Statutes, Title 32, Chapter 31, Section 2102.

Marlkolf AS: Industrial nursing begins in Vermont, Public Health Nurs 37:125, 1945.

National Association of Pediatric Nurse Associates and Practitioners: Scope of practice, Pelman, NJ, 1983, The Association.

National Center for Health Statistics, Health Manpower and Health Facilities, US Public Health Service Publication No HSM 73-1509, Washington, DC, 1973, US Government Printing Office.

National Center for Health Statistics: Office visits by women: the national ambulatory medical care survey. Prepared by Cypress BK. Vital and Health Statistics, Series 13, No 45, DHHA No (PHS) 80-1976, Public Health Service, Washington, DC, 1980, US Government Printing Office.

Newman IM, Newman E, and Martin GL: School health services, what costs/what benefits? J Sch Health 51:423, 1981.

New York State Education Law, Op Title 8, Article 130, Section 6901, 1972 Revision.

Noonan BR: Eight years in a medical nurse clinic, Am J Nurs 72:1128, 1972.

Nurses' Association of the American College of Obstetricians and Gynecologists, The obstetric-gynecologic nurse practitioner, Washington, DC, 1984, The Association.

Pender NJ: Health promotion in nursing practice, Norwalk, Conn, 1982, Appleton-Century-Crofts.

Philosophy—American College of Nurse-Midwives, Appendix 1, J Nurse Midwifery 29:169, 1984.

Piechnik SL and Corbett MA: Reducing low birth weight among socioeconomically high-risk adolescent pregnancies, J Nurse Midwifery 30(2):88, 1985.

Reiter F: The nurse clinician, Am J Nurs 67:274, 1966.

Richard E: A rationale for incorporating wellness programs into existing occupational health programs, Occup Health Nurs 32:412, 1984.

Robert Wood Johnson Foundation: Special Report 1:1, 1985.

Rogers ME: Reveille in nursing, Philadelphia, 1964, FA Davis Co.

Rogers ME: Nursing: to be or not to be, Nurs Outlook 20:42, 1972.

Rosenfeld P: Nursing student census with policy implications, 1985, New York, 1985, National League for Nursing, Division of Policy and Research Pub. No. 19-2156.

Shamansky SL and Clausen C: Levels of prevention: examination of the concept, Nurs Outlook 28:104, 1980.

Siegel E and Bryson SC: Redefinition of the role of the public health nurse in child health supervision, Am J Public Health 53:1015, 1963.

Silver HK, Ford LC, and Day LR: The pediatric nurse practitioner program, JAMA 204:298, 1968.

Silver HK and others: A program to increase health care for children: the pediatric nurse practitioner program, Pediatrics 39:756, 1967.

Skelly A and others: A survey of the health perceptions of the homeless, J NY State Nurses Assoc, in press.

Sobolewski SD: Cost effective school nurse practitioner services, J Sch Health 50(1):585, 1981.

Stein LI: The doctor-nurse game, Arch Gen Psychiatry 16:699, 1967.

Stone M: Discharge planning guide, Am J Nurs 79:1446, 1979.

Sultz HA and others: A decade of change for nurse practitioners, Nurs Outlook 31(3):138, 1983.

Sultz HA and others: Part II. Nurse practitioners: a decade of change, Nurs Outlook 31(4):216, 1983.

Synoground G: A program to prepare prospective school nurses, J Sch Health 54:295, 1984.

Tom S: Nurse-midwifery: a developing profession, Law Med Health Care 10:262, 1982.

US Congress, Office of Technology Assessment: Nurse practitioners, physician assistants and certified nurse-midwives: a policy analysis, Health Technology Case Study 37, Washington, DC, US Government Printing Office, OTA-HCS-37, 1986.

US Department of Health and Human Services: Coping with AIDS: psychological and social considerations in helping people with HTLV-III infection, Washington, DC, 1986, US Department of HHS, National Institute of Mental Health, DDHS Publication No ADM 85-1432.

Ventura MR, Feldman MJ, and Crosby F: Information synthesis: effectiveness of nurse practitioners, Buffalo, NY, 1985, Veterans Administration Medical Center.

Wald LD: The house on Henry Street, ed 2, Boston, 1933, Little, Brown & Co Inc.

Wold SJ and Dagg NV: School nursing: a passing experiment? In Wold SJ, editor: School nursing: a framework for practice, St Louis, 1981, CV Mosby Co.

Wolff MA: NLE rounds: court upholds expanded practice role for nurses, Law Med Health Care 12(1):27, 1984.

BIBLIOGRAPHY

American Nurses' Association, Health Nursing Practice Division and American Academy of Pediatrics: Guidelines on short-term continuing education programs for pediatric nursing associates, Am J Nurs 71:509, 1971.

American Nurses' Association: A conceptual model of community health nursing, Kansas City, Mo, 1980, The Association.

American Nurses' Association: Standards of practice for primary health care nurse practitioner, Kansas City, Mo, 1987, The Association.

American Public Health Association: The definition and role of public health nursing in the delivery of health care, Washington DC, 1980, The Association.

Maine Revised Statutes, Title 32, Chapter 31, Section 2102.

Silver HK, Ford LC, and Day LR: The pediatric nurse practitioner program, JAMA 204:298, 1960.

Steinberg PM and Carter GW: Case management and the elderly, Lexington, Mass, 1983, Lexington Books.

NURSES who work in the community frequently interact with clients in one-to-one relationships without the support of teachers, peers, or supervisors. Consequently they need to call on a broad knowledge base as they carry out the nursing process. In this section the nursing process is reviewed and applied to the community setting. Then epidemiology, health teaching, environmental issues, and nutrition, four major elements of the knowledge base, are summarized. These chapters do not cover everything that is needed for a lifetime of practice, but rather they provide an effective starting point. Courses covering each of these topics alone would be even more useful.

Epidemiology is the key science and research method used in all five steps of the community nursing process—assessement, diagnosis, planning, intervention, and evaluation. Familarity with the theories of learning and methods of teaching clients is a crucial element in the intervention process. Environmental issues have become significant elements in the assessment and diagnostic process, as well as the intervention phase in the community, and a knowledge of nutrition is essential in the diagnosis and intervention of a variety of problems. Chapters in subsequent sections add to this knowledge base.

At one time nurses who went out into the community carried a black bag full of supplies and instruments. A few home health care nurses still carry such a bag. Today, however, the black bag has grown to a figurative suitcase filled with the nurse's knowledge base. This suitcase is expandable, and nurses must keep stuffing it with new knowledge to deal with new problems and techniques. In fact, almost everything a person learns can be useful for the community nursing role, and this is why the community is such an interesting and challenging work site.

Knowledge Base for Community Nursing

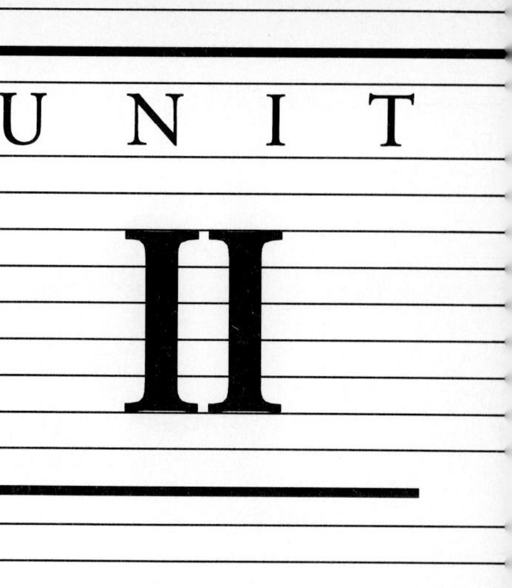

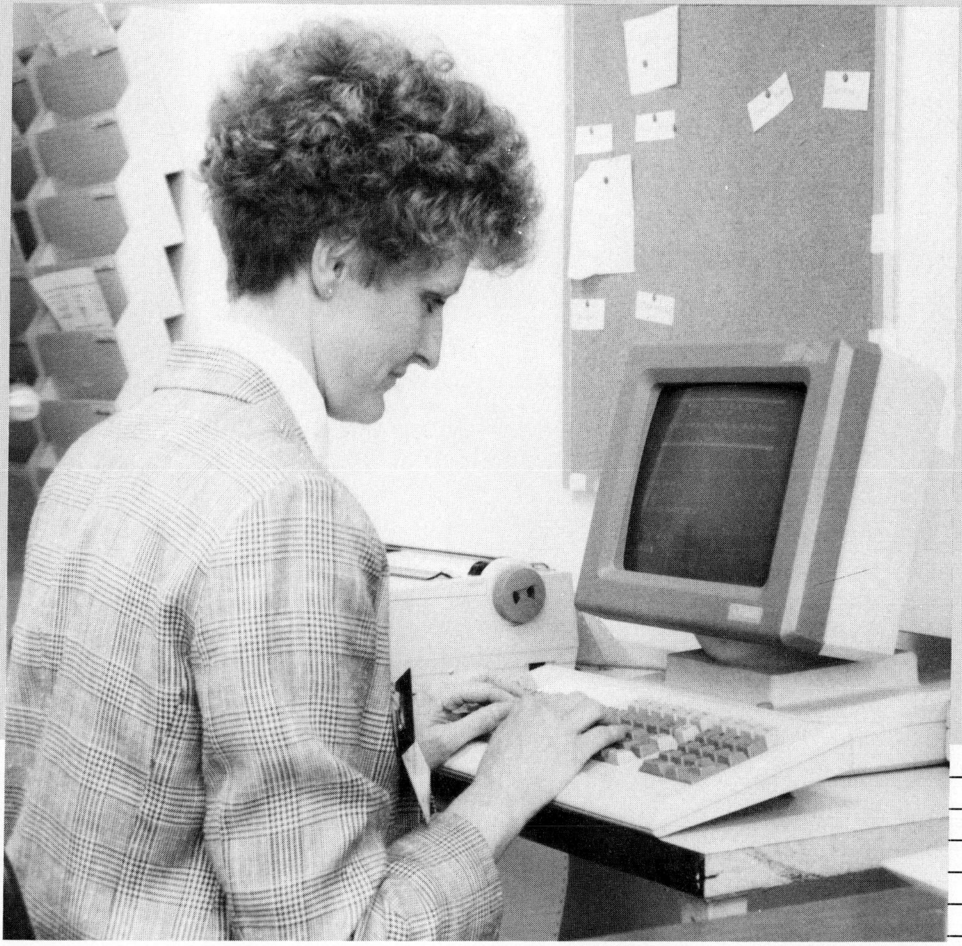

CHAPTER 3

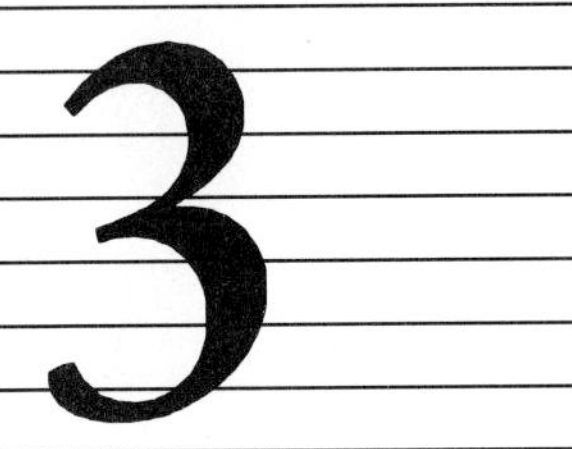

Nursing Process in the Community Setting

Janice Roes Salter

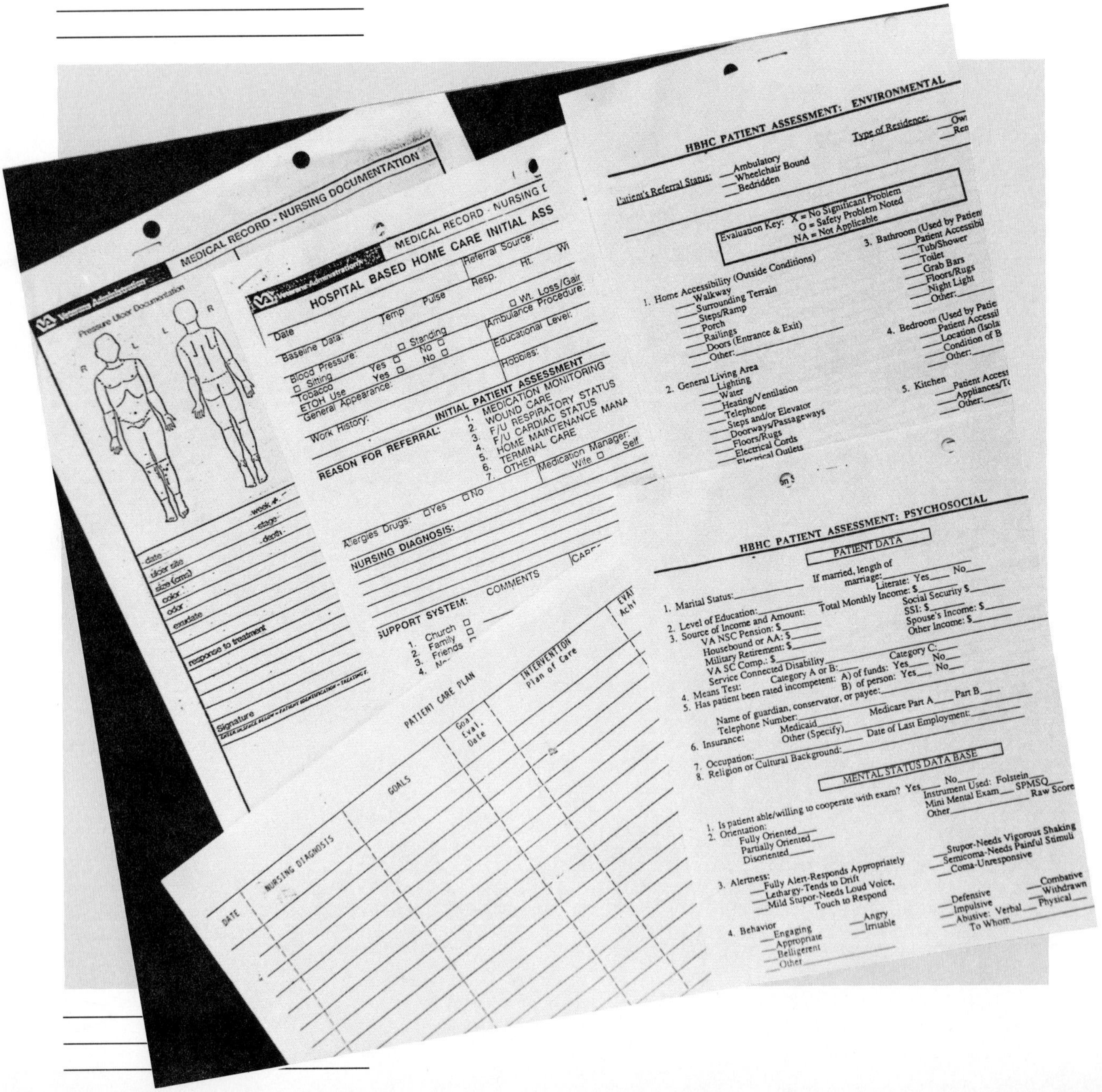

CHAPTER OUTLINE

OBJECTIVES

After completing this chapter, the reader should be able to:

1. Describe how the use of the nursing process in a community setting differs from clinical settings.
2. Identify skills needed to initiate the nursing process in the community setting.
3. Apply the five stage nursing process model—assessment, nursing diagnosis, planning, implementation, and evaluation.
4. Explain how quality assurance and utilization review of nursing care are carried out.

THE NURSING PROCESS is not a new concept. The term began appearing in nursing literature in the late 1950s and early 1960s. The concept was used in nursing education as a framework for teaching students how to think about, plan, and carry out nursing care. By the mid-1960s, a book on the nursing process had been published (Yura and Walsh, 1983).

Since its inception, the use of the nursing process as a conceptual planning and action tool has increased at a phenomenal rate. Not only are there numerous books that address the nursing process per se, but most clinical nursing textbooks also address the subject. The nursing process is used as a framework for research in nursing and the development of nursing theories. It provides the outline for the National Nursing Licensure Examination. Most important, the nursing process has become a practical tool for providing nursing care in clinical settings and is being used more and more as a basis for documenting the care given to a client.

This chapter discusses the nursing process as it applies to community nursing situations. It is important to realize that the nursing process is not unique to any clinical setting. It is a generic tool with numerous commonalities across all clinical boundaries but with specific applications that may differ. Although the nursing process is a tool that may be useful for all clients of home health care and community health nurses (individual, family, and community), this chapter focuses primarily on the nursing process as it applies to the care of the *individual* client. The family and community as clients are discussed elsewhere in this book.

NURSING PROCESS

Yura and Walsh describe the nursing process as

> a designated series of actions intended to fulfill the purposes of nursing—to maintain the client's wellness—and, if this state changes, to provide the amount and quality of nursing care the situation demands to direct the client back to wellness, and if wellness cannot be achieved, then to contribute to the client's quality of life, maximizing his resources as long as life is a reality. (Yura and Walsh, 1983)

The nursing process is a method for diagnosing, planning, delivering, and evaluating the effectiveness of nursing care based on the assessed health status and health concerns of the client. It is as important for the nurse in the community setting to engage in these activities as it is for the nurse in acute care or long-term care settings.

The scope of the nursing care required by the client in the community is much broader. The goal of care for the client is the highest level of wellness or functioning possible. Clients may be at various stages on the health-sickness continuum. It should be obvious that a healthy, or well, client has different needs for nursing care from someone who is newly discharged from an acute care hospital or is a chronically ill, long-term care client living at home. The nurse deals not only with health problems, or health deficits, but also with positive health behavior. Thus the goal of the nurse in the community is not only to help *restore* health functioning, but to *maintain* clients where they are, to *prevent* disease or deterioration, and to *promote* health. The nursing process, as it is applied to the client in the community, must be able to address all these issues (Fig. 3-1).

The nursing process uses a basic problem-solving methodology and applies it to the need for nursing care. The result is a specific care plan designed to meet the needs of a particular client or group.

Using the nursing process provides structure and organization to nursing care. It helps ensure that the client's health concerns or problems do not fall through the cracks. The nursing process must be changed and updated not only when mandated by agency policy or regulations, but whenever indicated by the assessed needs of the client.

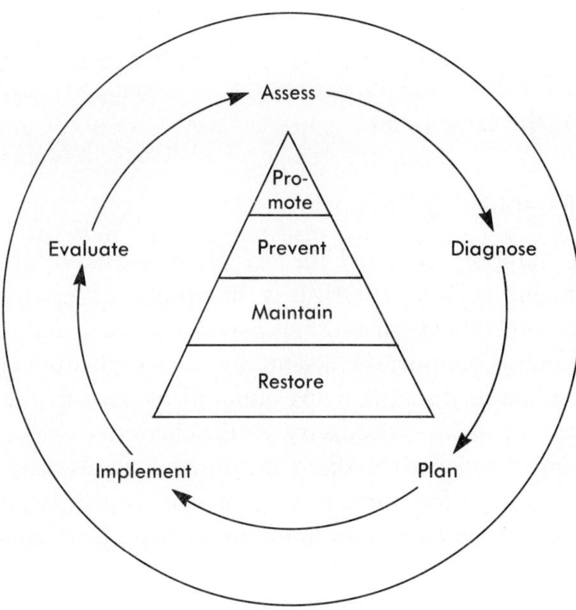

FIG. 3-1. Nursing process in community.

It helps make nursing care deliberate, rational, and based on sound, scientific principles. Doing all of this contributes to the quality of nursing care the client receives. When used properly, the nursing process can help in the measurement of the quality of care. The nursing process is not only an intellectual activity, but a prescription for action as well.

Initiating the Nursing Process

For the nursing process to begin, the nurse and the client must meet. The client is frequently referred to the nurse by someone who thinks the nurse can help the client. Referrals to home health care nurses are made by hospital discharge planning nurses, physicians, case managers employed by other agencies, and families. Referrals to community health nurses are made by these same groups. In addition, health departments are funded to provide programmatic care to certain categories of persons, including people with communicable diseases, prenatal clients, low–birth weight infants, disabled persons, and aged clients. Care for members of these groups may be initiated by a referral, or community health nurses may initiate case finding activities to locate the clients.

Usually the first encounter is in person, although on occasion it may be over the phone or by correspondence. If possible, it is helpful for the nurse to prepare for the first meeting in advance. This can be done by reviewing the written reports, records, or referrals that exist. The nurse can talk to the referral sources to get more information about the client. Viewing this information with an open mind helps keep bias out of the initial encounter. Depending on the amount of preencounter data available, the nurse may want to consult with books or experts who can provide information on the client's health condition(s). Standardized care plans for selected problems may be available also.

Preparatory empathy or so-called tuning-in is a technique that can be used before the first encounter to help get in touch with and develop empathy for the client (Shulman, 1979). It is important for this tuning-in to be affective and not merely intellectual. That is, the nurse tries to actually experience feelings the client may be having by recalling similar personal experiences such as dealing with authority figures, meeting strangers, needing help, and feeling inadequate, fearful, helpless, disapproved of, or frustrated. This is extremely important in situations involving such issues as child abuse and neglect or venereal disease. The results of the tuning-in process are always viewed as tentative.

It is usually possible to schedule the initial encounter. Telephoning the client to make an appointment enables the nurse to begin the nursing process on the phone. The telephone is one of the most important tools the community health nurse possesses, and skill in using it must be developed. The nurse should state clearly who is calling and why and should be friendly and helpful on the phone. The goals of the initial encounter are the following:

1. To meet and define roles
2. To reach consensus on the purpose of the encounter
3. To establish rapport

Meeting and Defining Roles

Professional encounters are not social encounters, although social amenities must be observed. The nurse who visits a client in the home is a guest and should act accordingly. This does not mean, however, that the nurse does not assertively take charge of the interaction.

Nurses introduce themselves by name, role (nurse), and agency represented. This is a good opportunity to present a calling card if one is carried. It is important to clarify whether the nurse is speaking to the client or someone else. Clients and family members are called by their proper names until the nurse has been given permission to do otherwise. A client should never be called by a first name or a nickname such as Gramps or Honey. It is important for nurses to present credentials to the client and to sell themselves. The simple term "nurse" or "registered nurse" may be all the credentials the client needs, but it may also be important for the client to know that the nurse has had experience in caring for new babies or taking care of sick people at home.

Consensus on Purpose

It is often helpful to find out what the client thinks is the purpose of the encounter. For example, a nurse on a home visit might ask, "Mrs. Jones, did the doctor (clinic, agency) explain that I would visit you?" or "Mrs. Jones, the doctor asked me to come to see you. How do you think I can help you?"

The nurse also shares perceptions of the purpose of the encounter. For example, "Mrs. Jones, your doctor asked me to visit to help you learn how to give yourself insulin. Is that what you were told?" or "Is that your understanding?"

This initial consensus and orientation to the purpose is extremely important because it enables both client and nurse to begin the nursing process at the same point.

Establishing Rapport

Rapport is called the act of respectful informality (Elkins, 1984). It is the process of getting comfortable with another. Establishing and maintaining rapport is essentially a first-encounter problem. Rapport helps build client trust in the nurse, which is necessary for the client to disclose data needed to make a meaningful assessment. Therefore the nurse focuses on the rapport issue before launching into more formal aspects of data collection.

Important attitudes and qualities in establishing rapport include the following:

1. Respectfulness
2. Courtesy
3. Objectivity
4. Caring
5. Warmth
6. Concern for client's welfare
7. Interest
8. Attention

Certain communication skills are also helpful in establishing rapport. These include the following:

1. Staging the environment for comfort and freedom from distraction
2. Beginning the interaction slowly
3. Giving the client broad opening statements or questions
4. Letting the client set the pace of conversation
5. Exploring nonintrusive, nonthreatening areas first
6. Using silence appropriately
7. Using nonverbal listening skills—eye contact, open posture, same level and face-to-face interaction
8. Relaxing

The first encounter between nurse and client is a time for mutual sizing-up. It is important for the nurse to perform well, since first impressions are often lasting. A poor impression may delay or indefinitely postpone an effective nursing process.

Assessment

Assessment is the cornerstone of the nursing process. It is the process of compiling a data base about the client's health status. Taking nursing action without first doing an assessment is costly, inefficient, and nonprofessional. For example, teaching insulin-dependent diabetics how to administer to themselves makes no sense without first finding out the following:

1. Whether the client is physically able
2. Whether the client is willing to administer insulin
3. How much the client already knows

Assessment makes the difference between deliberative and automatic nursing action (Orlando, 1961). It is essential if nursing is to be a rational, professional activity.

Compiling a Data Base

In nursing the client has traditionally been viewed as an integrated whole made up of many components or parameters that relate and interact with each other in such a way that the whole person becomes greater than the sum of his or her parts. This integrated human being also relates and interacts continuously with the environment. This is called a *holistic* approach to clients. Nursing's particular area of concern is what impact these internal and external relationships and interactions have on the client's health.

Nowhere does the holistic nature of the client affect nursing care more than in the community. It is critical that the community health nurse be committed to and skilled in assessing all dimensions that have an effect on a client's health. Focusing on one dimension, for example, the physical, may not be appropriate for a particular client.

The problem for the nurse is to determine which dimensions should be stressed and how much data to gather at the initial encounter. If the nurse tries to gather extensive and in-depth data, it can be an operational hazard that requires too much time, too much form filling, or too much probing of the client for information. It may be necessary for the nurse to delay some of the data gathering until a future encounter, flagging those areas where more in-depth information is needed.

To make data gathering manageable and operationally efficient, the nurse can use the following guidelines to focus the initial encounter.

1. What is the problem or situation from the client's point of view? What is the chief complaint? What help is the client seeking from the nurse or from someone else?
2. For what reason was the client referred? What does the other health professional or agency want the nurse to do? Why is the client being referred to the nurse?
3. Are there agency policies or forms that require certain data?
4. Has in-depth assessment in certain areas been done recently by someone else (for example, physical examination)? Is that data available to the nurse?

Data-Gathering Tools

Certain tools or instruments can assist the community health nurse in assessing the client's needs for nursing care. These include the health history, data-gathering protocols and guidelines, self-tests, and diagnostic and screening tests.

HEALTH HISTORY. Using the client as the principal resource, the health history is a systematic and detailed chronicle of the health status. It is an organized method for investigating and recording events in the client's life that are significantly related to health.

Standard health history formats frequently accompany physical assessment protocols. The focus is often on the physical problems of the client. However, nurses may want a broader focus, so questions about social relationships, cultural background, and the environmental aspects of the client's life can be added. On the other hand, a health history protocol that is too lengthy or takes too much time to complete becomes an operational hazard to fill out. In obtaining a health history there may be no need to ask the client for up-to-date data that are already available from another reliable source. Frequently data are available from old records or the referral and can be transferred to the new record. However, it may be necessary to verify some of the data from these sources with the client.

Sometimes clients, because of cultural or personal reasons, are reluctant to provide certain information until the relationship with the nurse has developed into a more trusting one. Examples of these sensitive areas include information about sex, finances, and religion. Postponing the more sensitive questions to the end of the interview or to another time may be the best approach.

PROTOCOLS, GUIDES, AND FORMS. Nurses in the community are often burdened with agency and government forms that must be filled out. Some agencies have specific and detailed formats that must be used in gathering assessment data about a client. Other agencies require specific demographic information about the client but may allow the nurse to follow a more loosely structured format in gathering data about the client.

For the new community health nurse who is unfamiliar with the scope of data that must be gathered, a specific format can be quite helpful. The form can serve as a guide to jog the nurse's memory and can provide an organized method for recording the data. However, the format should not be used so rigidly during the course of an interview that spontaneity cannot develop between the client and the nurse or that the nurse cannot pursue another direction not specified in the form.

SELF-TESTS. As the consumer movement has moved into health care and the wellness movement has gained momentum, increasing numbers of self-tests have been developed to assess the client's state of health. Self-tests are short tests that a client can self-administer and evaluate. Frequently the tests center on one or several life-style behaviors. The client receives a score based on the answers to a series of questions. This score is interpreted as healthy or unhealthy behavior. Theoretically this serves as a motivating force to change health behavior.

Self-tests have been developed for a combination of life-style behaviors, as well as specific behaviors such as stress and coping, alcohol consumption, smoking, nutrition, and exercise. Self-tests can provide the nurse with important data for assessing the client's needs for health promotion or disease prevention activities.

SCREENING TESTS. Screening tests are procedures that give a reasonable assurance of the presence or absence of a health problem. They differ from diagnostic tests in that they are not as definitive or accurate. A positive screening test indicates the need for further diagnostic workup to rule out or confirm the suspected problem. Screening is a valuable tool for secondary prevention.

School nurses frequently carry out multiphasic screening on their school-aged clients. Common school screening tests include height, weight, vision, hearing, scoliosis, blood pressure, and tine testing. Screening tests that are commonly performed on adults include weight, blood pressure, diabetes, anemia, tine or purified protein derivative (PPD), vision, hearing, Papanicolaou smear, and breast and testicle examination.

Screening tests are often performed inexpensively or free as a community service. Community nurses working with clients who have had screening tests need to explain the tests and the meaning of the results. Follow-up is an essential component of any screening procedure. Clients with positive results should be referred for further diagnostic workup.

Sources of Data

The client is the principal source of data in the community health setting. Other important sources include family, informal supports, formal supports, health care team members, records, laboratory reports, and referral information. Normal and abnormal laboratory data can provide important baseline information to use for later comparison. The nurse may need to send formal requests to agencies or professionals for specific laboratory information about the client. Often this can be obtained over the telephone. The client also may know the values of specific laboratory tests or can be asked to obtain these at health care visits. Sharing this information between client and nurse offers an excellent opportunity for health teaching about the purpose of tests and the meaning and implications of results.

Data-Gathering Skills

Gathering data in the community setting involves many nursing skills. The three most important are observation, physical examination, and communication.

OBSERVATION. Observation is a basic skill that nurses learn early in their careers. Observation employs the senses to obtain data about the client.

Observations may focus on the client's physical condition and function. For example, activities of daily living (ADLs) have become an important indication of the physically impaired client's ability to remain out of an institution. Community nurses are increasingly asked to observe and evaluate the client's ADLs to make level-of-care determinations. Skill in making observations becomes a critical part of these determinations.

Observations may also focus on psychologic status factors such as facial expression, ability to express oneself, and appropriateness of affect.

Observations about the client's social and cultural life include the nature and quality of familial interactions and the existence of cultural artifacts in the home.

Parts of the physical environment that should be observed include the presence of safety hazards, the type of neighborhood and housing, environmental comfort factors, and material possessions.

PHYSICAL EXAMINATION. Physical examination is a hands-on skill that focuses on body systems. It involves inspection, palpation, percussion, and auscultation. It is a skill that takes time and practice to acquire. Nurses who work in the community find this a particularly useful tool for both initial and ongoing assessments. The ability to perform an accurate physical assessment on these clients is an important asset.

COMMUNICATION. Communication skills are essential at every stage of the nursing process. Communication can be oral, nonverbal, or written. Writing skills are especially important at the planning stage of the nursing process for the nurse to write clear, concise care plans. At the implementation stage, verbal skills may be used to direct others in giving care, coordinating team efforts, or health teaching. Both verbal and nonverbal skills are employed as the nurse therapeutically counsels clients and offers emotional support. At the evaluation stage, written documentation and feedback are essential in providing the data needed to determine the effectiveness of a care plan.

At the assessment stage of the nursing process, communication skills that facilitate rapport are important. These skills are discussed previously in this chapter. Communication is required to gather the data needed to make an assessment. The principal communication method used is the interview. An interview is a goal-directed conversation between a professional person and a client. The goal of an interview may be to collect data, teach or counsel a client, or provide the client with emotional support and facilitate problem solving. These different purposes call for different interviewing techniques. If the primary goal is to collect data, the nurse must structure the interview to achieve that goal. Allowing a client to ramble or providing too much health teaching may be inappropriate at an initial interview where data must be obtained. The client's needs to ventilate or to learn about health matters may be facets of a problem the nurse identifies through assessment. It may be more appropriate for the nurse to incorporate counseling or health teaching into a plan of care than to deal with them in depth during the data-gathering interview.

The problem for the nurse in conducting a data-gathering interview is to balance the amount of structure. Too much structure, such as asking only predetermined questions and writing down the answers, may appear too mechanical to the client. This can stifle interaction and jeopardize rapport and the quality of the information obtained from the interview. It is easy to miss important data with an interview that is too structured.

A loosely structured interview can also miss important data, since this kind of interview lets the client lead and only information that the client thinks important is brought forth. A loose structure can also be time consuming and therefore inefficient and costly.

The obvious solution is to vary the styles within a given interview, depending on the quality of information being obtained as the interview progresses. It is important to remember that an interview is a two-way conversation. Clients vary in their responses to different styles. Some clients give excellent information in a loosely structured interview. Others are not able to respond to open-ended questions and require considerable structure. Most interviews progress best when the styles are varied according to the type of information being obtained.

Part of skilled interviewing includes ensuring a comfortable, distraction-free environment for the interview. The client must be in a comfortable chair, there should be no interruptions, and the room temperature should be comfortable. It is better for client and nurse to sit face-to-face at the same level. The nurse must not sit behind a desk or table, since that immediately introduces a power factor into the interview. In the home, it is more difficult to structure the environment, since the nurse is a guest. Nevertheless, the nurse can ask the clients where they would be most comfortable talking. It may also be advisable to ask permission to turn off the television or radio.

Scope of the Data

Client dimensions that may be significant and call for data-gathering efforts on the part of the community health nurse include the physical, sexual, psychologic, developmental, socioeconomic, cultural, spiritual, and environmental dimensions.

PHYSICAL DATA. Physical assessment data include significant information about the client's past and present health situations that may indicate a problem requiring community health nursing intervention. Protocols for obtaining the health history and also for reviewing systems and performing the physical examination follow a medical model and are readily available. Although laboratory data are important, they may be difficult to come by in the community setting.

Life-style and nutritional data yield information about potential health problems and the need for health teaching to prevent disease and improve health. Data about medications are important, especially for chronically ill, frail, elderly clients who metabolize medications poorly and are often taking many drugs at the same time. The potential for adverse drug reactions and noncompliance problems is extensive in this group. The community health nurse may have to intervene to prevent exacerbation of symptoms, complications, or death caused by inappropriate medication administration.

Dependence on others when performing ADLs is rapidly becoming a reliable indicator of the need for placement, level of care needs, intensity of service required, and reimbursement costs. Community health nurses may be asked to focus assessment on this area alone. The availability of

ADL resources such as equipment or people must be considered in determining an index of client independence.

Physical assessment is often a good place to begin the data-gathering process. Many clients expect the nurse to be an expert in this area and think the questions or procedures about this are legitimate. Other dimensions related to the client's health status can often be assessed at the same time the physical assessment is performed.

SEXUAL DATA. Sexual data include more than what is determined on physical examination, although the physical sphere is often a nonthreatening place to begin when gathering in-depth sexual information. It is important to approach sexual assessment matter-of-factly and without embarrassment or judgment of the client. Nurses should be aware of their own personal feelings and values regarding sex.

Sexual jargon may present special problems when communicating with clients about sexual matters. Therefore the nurse may need to become familiar with the use of slang and so-called street expressions when discussing sexual data.

When gathering sexual data, the community health nurse is also aware of data that may indicate other kinds of problems or needs that have a profound effect on the client's well-being and that call for nursing intervention. These might include physical, psychologic, social, cultural, or spiritual problems or health concerns.

PSYCHOLOGIC DATA. Psychologic assessment includes gathering data about the client's emotional state, interaction patterns, mental status, attitudes, coping patterns, and past or present history of psychopathologic problems. To use this information, it is important to find out whether the client's behavior is adaptive or maladaptive and whether the current pattern is lifelong or in response to a crisis situation.

These data can help the community health nurse determine the existence of actual or potential psychologic problems, as well as provide information about the availability of resources and social supports. Psychologic data also help identify client strengths and weaknesses and provide clues to intervention strategies. Knowing that a client is suspicious and hostile, for example, can be important information in determining how to approach and interact with that client.

DEVELOPMENTAL DATA. Gathering data about the growth and development of infants and children through adolescence has traditionally been an important community health nursing function. Growth is usually viewed in the physical sense of increase in size. Development is the integration of emerging and expanding capacities into biopsychosocial functioning that varies in complexity and focus. Development is basically a lifelong process in which there are changes in ability and behavior associated with age.

In recent years, interest has grown in extending the notion of growth and development to the adult person. With the adult, growth is conceived of as change rather than cellular expansion. Clearly, physical changes, such as aging, can have a profound effect on biopsychosocial functioning.

Several sophisticated and detailed instruments exist for doing in-depth developmental assessment of children (Stanhope, 1988). Developmental assessment of adults relies more on conceptual models such as developmental tasks (Duvall, 1977), stages in the life cycle (Erikson, 1963), or passages through predictable crises (Sheehy, 1976).

SOCIOECONOMIC DATA. The socioeconomic data base consists of information about the client's social relationships and economic status. Some of this information may be easily obtainable through questioning or observation at the time of the initial contact. Other information may become available only with further contact or more in-depth probing for the information.

Some of this information is quite sensitive, and clients may be unwilling to discuss it. Often however, financial disclosure must be dealt with up front by the nurse to determine the fee for service or eligibility for third party reimbursement.

Nurses must deal with both the client's and their own feelings about financial disclosure. It is best to tell the client why the information is needed and to stress the confidentiality of the information.

CULTURAL DATA. Many clients are a part of the mainstream of American culture. For these individuals a cultural assessment may not be necessary. Other clients, however, may be culturally distinct to the degree that cultural practices or conflicts with the dominant health care delivery system may generate health problems. For these individuals a cultural assessment should be performed. Important clues to the potential need for a cultural assessment include ethnic background, family names suggesting an ethnic identity, race, language, place of residence, country of birth, social class, life-style, and economic status.

Cultural data may be useful in a variety of ways throughout the nursing process. They may indicate an actual or potential health concern or situation that requires nursing action. They may be used to develop a care plan with which the client complies; they may be used to carry out the care plan in a more culturally sensitive and effective way, which minimizes the social distance between the nurse and the client.

SPIRITUAL DATA. Health and illness are fundamental, profound events that human beings have tried to explain through the ages. Religious systems and spiritual explanations and rituals have commonly been employed to do this. Because of this connection between spiritual expression and health, a holistic approach to the client necessitates a spiritual assessment.

Information that deals with the spiritual dimension includes more than data about organized religious affiliation and practices. It may also include the client's philosophic orientation toward life (life view) and whether there is some dimension beyond the human that gives meaning to the client's life and functions to organize behavior.

The religious belief system of the client can affect the health of the client in numerous ways including the following:

1. Religious explanations of what is health (being in harmony with God, being without sin) and what is illness (God's will, punishment for sin) can affect whether a client seeks treatment and from whom, how the client responds to the treatment regimen, and what disease prevention or health promotion activities the client is engaged in.
2. Religious prescriptions for moral behavior can conflict with modern medical science. Issues regarding birth control and abortion are examples of this.
3. Spiritually oriented systems often provide support during illness or adversity. Lack of this support may cause the client to feel alone, guilty, depressed, or angry and can increase stress and illness. The spiritual dimension is complex and not easily accessed.

Clients are often reluctant to discuss religious or life view orientations with strangers. The nurse should be open to religious information but avoid probing questions that may jeopardize the nurse-client relationship or the reliability of the data that is obtained.

PHYSICAL ENVIRONMENT DATA. The impact of the physical environment on the client is considerable. An adequate living environment is important in endeavors to promote a healthy life-style. The existence of air or water pollution at home, for example, makes the attainment of high-level wellness difficult. Living in a high crime area compromises not only clients' physical safety but their mental health as well. With more ill and disabled clients being cared for at home, the assessment and adaptation of the physical environment become critical. Sometimes the decision whether a client can remain at home or be discharged from the hospital hinges on whether the physical environment is adequate and safe. The community health nurse may be asked to make a special predischarge home visit to ascertain this.

Nursing Diagnosis

The second stage of the nursing process is a focusing stage. It involves analyzing and interpreting the collected data by comparing them with norms and previous patterns, evaluating whether comparisons are normal or abnormal, determining the reasons or causes of the deviation if pertinent, and formulating a diagnostic or summative statement. This summation, called the nursing diagnosis, is stated concisely and clearly in language that is understandable to all nurses and other health professionals who may use or contribute to the care plan.

Edel defines nursing diagnosis as "a statement of a potential or actual altered health status of a client(s), which is derived from nursing assessment and which requires intervention from the domain of nursing." She explains that the term "health status" avoids the negative connotation of the term "problem" and allows for positive evaluation of individuals, families, and communities (Edel, 1982).

The diagnostic statement consists of two parts. The first part describes the client's health state, condition, or situation. This may be the actual response (where the concern or problem is present at the time of assessment) or a potential response (where there is risk of a problem developing). The first part may also be a statement of a positive health status that the nurse wants the client to maintain or improve.

The second part of the statement is etiologic, not in a causal but in a relational sense. It is a verbalization of the contributing or influencing factors that are related to the description of client responses. Often the first and second parts of the nursing diagnosis are linked with the phrase "related to."

The nursing diagnostic statement is shared and verified with the client. This encourages the client's participation in the care and fosters independence.

It is important to remember that in community health the nurse not only deals with maladaptive or dysfunctional responses and situations, but with adaptation, wellness, and functional responses as well. The community health nurse in particular has a goal to maintain or promote health and to prevent disease, as well as to restore health. Consequently the nurse needs to use nursing process concepts and terminology with these goals. Diagnostic statements that focus only on problematic issues and ignore the preventative and promotional aspects of the client's health may not reflect the broad scope of nursing in the community adequately.

Originally, nursing diagnosis was seen as the end point of the assessment stage or the beginning point of the planning stage in a four-stage model of the nursing process. However, nursing diagnosis, as a separate stage, is now widely accepted in nursing.

The concept of nursing diagnosis has come into its own in the 1980s. The 1970s saw a proliferation of literature on the nursing process, and more and more books and articles in recent years have focused on the nursing diagnosis part of that process. This nursing diagnosis literature has refined the conception, brought enlightenment to the subject, generated interest, and stimulated controversy (Alex, 1986; Campbell, 1984; Carnevali, 1983 and 1984; Carlson and others, 1982; Edel, 1982; Gordon, 1987; Iyer and others, 1986; Kelly, 1985; Kim and others, 1984; Simmons, 1986; Ziegler, 1986). Some of that controversy revolves around the usefulness of standardized diagnostic labels (taxonomies) of nursing diagnoses.

The best-known taxonomy is published by the North American Nursing Diagnosis Association (NANDA). This group began in the mid-1970s and since then has met approximately every two years to refine and update the taxonomy.

This taxonomy is useful to community nurses. However, its scope is not broad enough to encompass all areas of practice and types of clients encountered in community settings. For example, most of the diagnoses relate to individual responses. Few of the diagnoses relate to family responses, and none relates to other kinds of groups or the larger community. The issues surrounding the development of nursing diagnoses for the community are addressed by Hamilton (1983) and Muecke (1984).

In addition, the NANDA taxonomy is skewed toward health problems, deficits, and negative states. Although the home health care nurse cares for clients who are responding to these types of situations, the community health nurse focuses more on monitoring, reinforcing, and encouraging positive health behavior and on preventing negative situations from occurring.

Nurses with a community focus can help make the NANDA taxonomy more responsive to their particular area of practice by critically examining the NANDA system and using those labels that are appropriate or developing original labels in situations that are not covered by NANDA. Probably the best way to improve the NANDA list is for nurses who work in the community to contribute to its development (Alex, 1986). As an alternative, the Omaha Visiting Nurses' Association has developed a problem/diagnosis classification system that may be more responsive to the community situation (Simmons, 1986). Other community-based nursing agencies around the country are also using this system.

One last point should be noted about the diagnostic stage. It is important to remember that not every client's concerns, problems, or situation needs nursing intervention. The nurse needs to recognize what nursing can do and what other people or agencies in the community can do better.

Planning

Planning is the core of the nursing process. It is the reason why assessment is done, and it provides the rational basis for nursing actions. Planning is a goal-oriented activity in which the nurse and client prioritize health concerns, establish goals and objectives for dealing with the concerns, develop techniques and strategies for meeting the objectives, apportion tasks, and formalize the plan in writing. It is a way of translating the nursing process into a written document.

Types of Care Plans

Planning in the community can be a complex process. Not only are plans made for a wide range of clients, but the nurse contributes to several different kinds of care plans as well. These different plans are similar, but because they are designed for different uses, they vary in some respects. The three types of care plans are nursing care plans, multidisciplinary care plans, and care plans for nonprofessionals.

Nursing Care Plans

Nursing care plans are written prescriptions to enable other *nurses* to care for a client. They may be prepared in clinical language that professional nurses understand, but that may not be easily understood by other health professionals or the general public. The nursing process focuses on this type of care plan.

Multidisciplinary Care Plans

It is not unusual to find care plans developed by all members of the health team who are involved with the client. This is especially true in large home health agencies that employ a variety of health care personnel, including special therapists, as well as nurses. In situations like this, a format that facilitates joint planning is helpful. The problem-oriented record, discussed later in this chapter, is an example of such a format.

Joint planning may also be required as a condition for making level-of-care determinations or for allocating funds for service needs. In these situations nurses and social workers may be involved in making joint assessments and negotiating services to be rendered within budgetary constraints.

Care Plans for Nonprofessionals

Care plans for nonprofessionals become necessary when some aspects of the client's care are done by the client, the client's family or friends, volunteers, or nurses' aides. In this instance the plan is written differently. Only those aspects of care for which the nonprofessional is responsible are written. However, what is written needs to be done in greater detail to comply with job descriptions and training background of employed nonprofessionals such as aides. For example, because of limitations placed on the kinds of tasks an aide may perform, it is not sufficient to write on the care plan "Assist with self-administration of medication at 10 AM qd." Rather, the care plan should state "Bring container labeled Digoxin 25 mg to client at 10 AM daily, read label to client, and open container cap." Furthermore, the care plan instructions should be written in layperson's language, not in professional jargon or with medical abbreviations.

Steps in Planning

Planning involves the following steps:

1. Prioritizing nursing diagnoses
2. Establishing goals and objectives
3. Searching for solutions, activities, and strategies
4. Apportioning tasks
5. Writing the plan

Prioritizing Nursing Diagnoses

To begin planning, all the nursing diagnoses are listed and prioritized to determine which will be dealt with first. The following criteria may be helpful in establishing these priorities:

1. What are the client's main concerns? Starting with the client leads to a much greater chance that the plan will work.
2. Are there any diagnoses in which the client's safety or survival is at risk?
3. Do any diagnoses involve meeting basic human needs as opposed to higher level needs?
4. What is the potential for successful intervention? Begin with the diagnosis that has a high potential for success.
5. Are there any diagnoses that place the public health or welfare at risk? For instance, does the client's noncompliance with communicable disease management regimen place the public at risk?
6. Are there any diagnoses that agency policy dictates must be dealt with first?

In deciding the nursing diagnoses for which to develop plans, the nurse tries to get the client's input and verification that this is indeed a concern that needs to be addressed. Although prioritization means that some preference is given, it does not mean that other diagnoses are excluded from consideration or that more than one plan cannot be developed at the same time.

Establishing Goals and Objectives

Planning involves establishing goals and objectives for each diagnosis the nurse and client decide to address. A goal is a broad statement of purpose, expected outcome, or desired end point. It relates to the diagnosis, focuses the health care team's thinking, and gives direction to the planning process.

Objectives are statements of expected or desired client behaviors; that is, these behaviors are "clinical manifestations that will indicate that the problem is being resolved, is resolved, or has been prevented," and that the goal has been reached (Mayers, 1983). An objective statement is specific, precise, clear, and understandable. It includes a statement of when the objective should be reached. This specification of time is a checkpoint or deadline. An objective should be realistic and attainable, and it should be within client abilities, limitations, strengths, and resources.

The objective statement describes exactly what the nurse can observe to measure or determine whether the objective is met. Thus the objective contains the criteria for evaluating the plan of care. Writing the objective in this manner greatly simplifies the evaluation stage of the nursing process. Using action verbs in the objective statements ensures an objective that is measurable.

Searching for Solutions, Activities, and Strategies

The nurse uses a knowledge base and experience to arrive at a list of actions with potential for solving the problem. The client's ideas for solution are also incorporated. Other sources of input include the following:

1. Professional literature
2. Standardized care plans
3. Advice from colleagues or supervisors
4. Solutions that have worked in similar circumstances

At this point it is helpful to accumulate as many ideas for resolution of the nursing diagnosis as possible. Brainstorming is a technique borrowed from the creative problem-solving field. The aim of brainstorming is to develop quantity, not quality of ideas; thus judgment is withheld while the list of ideas is being generated. Brainstorming can be done with one person, but the more people involved, the greater the potential for innovative and creative solutions. The client and family can easily be included in a brainstorming session if they are comfortable with it and understand the requirement to withhold judgment. The need for client and family input into solution finding cannot be stressed too much, especially if the solution involves their cooperation and activity.

After a list of solution options is generated, judgment is brought into play and one or two viable solutions are chosen. In making this judgment the nurse considers the client's and family's acceptance of the solution, their motivation and commitment, the scientific basis for the solution, the degree of risk involved, the level of risk acceptable, agency policy or law that may mandate solutions, feasibility and practicality, and availability of resources.

Apportioning Tasks

Following the decision regarding solution(s) to the problem or situation, the nurse and the other people involved in the solution decide who will do what. This may involve delegation, negotiation, contracting, and collaboration.

DELEGATION. If the solution is a *nursing* care plan, many aspects of the solution to the problem involve nursing action. The planning nurse may implement the plan or may delegate selected activities to other professional or nonprofessional nursing personnel. Delegation means that certain functions, duties, or tasks are assigned to someone else. However, responsibility and accountability inherent in the assigned work is not delegated completely, and the planning nurse retains some responsibility and accountability for the tasks.

Sometimes housekeeping, personal care, and other so-called assisting tasks can be assigned to nurse's aides who have the necessary training and skills to do these tasks. The availability of this type of assistance to help with housekeeping, cooking, shopping, bathing, grooming, dressing, and eating can make the difference between a client being able to remain at home or having to go into a health care institution. In delegating care to an aide, the planning nurse must have a good understanding of what the aide is *allowed* to do (as stipulated by government or agency policy) and what the aide is *trained* to do.

Adequate supervision of the aide is an important nursing responsibility. In situations where the nurse and the aide are from the same agency, this is more easily accomplished. However, as systems for meeting the home care needs of clients are made more complicated by a variety of contractual arrangements, the assessing/planning nurse may not be the same nurse who implements the plan, supervises the nonprofessional in the home, or both. The implementation and supervision functions may be delegated to another nurse from the same or another agency. Nursing administrators responsible for nursing service arrangements of this type must ensure that the following are done:

1. Responsibility and accountability for nursing care are clearly specified.
2. Fragmentation and duplication of service are minimized.
3. Coordination is facilitated.

NEGOTIATION. Negotiation is a process whereby two or more individuals who are not in agreement reach consensus or agreement about something. A mutual process or discussion that leads to consensus must be undertaken. Community health nurses may find themselves negotiating with family members about the performance of caretaking tasks or with social workers about the necessity of increasing aide services.

Negotiation is an art, but it is also a skill that can be learned. The Harvard Negotiation Project has developed a method of negotiation called "principled negotiation." The goal of the method is to help people decide issues on their merits rather than on the power of the participants or their arguments. Both sides are encouraged to look for mutual gains whenever possible. When interests conflict, the decision should be based on fair standards that are independent of the will of either side. Principled negotiation helps people achieve a measure of success and yet be fair (Fisher and Ury, 1981).

Four principles of negotiation are described by the project. *Separate the people* (negotiators) from the problem. Take care of the people factors as an issue separate from solving the problem. The negotiator must recognize and understand both the perceptions and feelings of other parties in the negotiation. Communication must be open with a lot of active listening. Efforts must be made to state differences explicitly. *Focus on interests,* not positions. A position is basically a solution to a problem. The interests or concerns are the reason for the position. Taking a position on an issue forces negotiators into a corner and makes a change of mind difficult. Negotiators who seem to disagree may find mutual underlying interests if they take the trouble to explore their interests (for example, better care for a client). *Invent options* for mutual gain. This is the familiar idea of generating a list of possible solutions to a problem without judging them or deciding which is best. *Insist on objective criteria.* The negotiators search for acceptable standards, or criteria, by which to judge the solution. This prevents the use of personal power or other situational or people factors from becoming the basis of the decision.

The community nurse finds negotiation skills useful in contracting with clients and in collaborating with other health professionals.

CONTRACTING. Contracting within the framework of the nursing process is the process of specifying the respective responsibilities and activities of the nurse, the client, and the significant others relative to a particular problem or nursing diagnosis. Contracts may be written or oral, but they must be clear and explicit so that all parties understand the contract terms. Contracts of this nature are not legally binding and are always negotiable.

Contracting has several advantages. First, it ensures that the client is involved in planning and implementing the care. This encourages independence and self-care and moves the client to a higher level of health. Contracting also forces commitment, and commitment can be an important motivator of behavior change.

Contracting is an effective tool to help plan the care provided to the client. As cost containment policies place constraints on availability and eligibility for service, it becomes necessary to involve clients and their informal supports in providing care if the client is to remain in the community. For example, it may be possible to maintain a disabled person at home for less than it would cost in an institution if informal supports are willing to provide certain kinds of care, such as cooking or shopping, or being present in the home during certain hours. The contracting mechanism ensures an explicit understanding of who does what and makes commitment to those tasks much more likely.

COLLABORATION. Whenever community nurses interact with other health care personnel as a team of equals to reach a goal, they are collaborating. Collaboration may involve a team planning care for a client, a committee developing a program, or a task force investigating a problem and making recommendations. Collaboration is an important activity in nursing, but especially in community settings.

Collaboration is not something that just happens when members of the health team get together. It is something that must be worked at—a skill to be developed much like other nursing skills. Members of a team must educate themselves in the various team roles and responsibilities and in group dynamics. This mutual education is one of the first activities that occur when team members interact for the first time.

In approaching a team interaction, it is helpful to keep an open mind. One of the most difficult issues a team must deal with is that of professional territoriality. Because there are such large gray areas of functional overlap among the health professions, teams can often become embroiled in professional encroachment problems. It is important not to get into a "we-they" mode of thinking and interacting.

Territorial turf issues are to be expected. It is important not to feel threatened by them. Rather, the team should bring them into the open for discussion. In deciding who is to do what for a client, it is helpful to use some rational criteria including the following:

1. What is best for the client?
2. What is cheaper?
3. What is more efficient?
4. Who knows the client best?
5. Who sees the client most often?
6. Who has the best rapport?

Territorial turf issues can be major stumbling blocks to team effectiveness, and they can make attempts at collaboration unpleasant if they are not handled directly. The best thing to do is be open minded and positive, reward and support others, and above all refocus group interaction on the goal of the team—better service for the client.

Another important aspect of teamwork and collaboration is to recognize the place of expertise. This involves not only recognizing the expertise of other professionals, but also your expertise. People representing different professions bring a wealth of education and experience to the collaborative effort. Each member of the team accepts and appreciates the expertise of the others and above all encourages its expression. The nurse must recognize and feel comfortable with personal expertise and assert that expertise in an articulate, self-confident manner.

In addition to the roles involving expertise that the team members bring to the collaborative effort, the roles of leader and follower must be worked out. Traditional power sources should not be the criteria for choosing a leader. The physician member of the team may not be the best leader. Leadership may better be served by someone who has easy access to other team members and the client, who understands and fosters the expertise of others, and who can organize and coordinate the work. Thus leadership becomes a situational issue that is decided on a case-by-case basis.

The driving force behind any collaborative interaction is the goal or purpose. In teamwork involving planning client care, the purpose and focus are always the well-being of the client. This is something all health professionals can relate to and value, regardless of professional background.

Writing the Plan

The nursing care plan is a way of translating the nursing process into a written document in which goals and activities are articulated clearly and specifications as to who will do what, when, and with what expected result are made. How this is formatted depends on agency procedure. The problem-oriented record format, which is discussed later in this chapter, is an excellent method because it follows the nursing process closely and enables the plan for each diagnosis to be developed and grouped in its entirety.

Ideally there is a plan of care for each nursing diagnosis. All plans should be neat, clear, concise, organized, and written in language appropriate for the people using them. For nonprofessionals it may be necessary to write instructions, or nursing orders, with considerable precision and detail.

Implementation

Implementation is that stage of the nursing process in which the activities and strategies that were planned are actually carried out. Broadly speaking, the community nurse's endeavors center on activities that promote, maintain, or restore health or prevent disease and disability. Implementation includes direct nursing intervention, indirect nursing intervention, and referral.

Direct Nursing Intervention

In many situations the nurse does something directly for or with the client. Increasingly, nurses who work in the community are being called on to provide hands-on nursing care. Changes in the health care delivery system to promote early hospital discharge, ambulatory surgery, and increased home care have expanded the need for technologically skilled nurses in the community. The needs of long-term care and terminally ill clients are also frequently met through hands-on care and assistance. Hands-on care can involve treatments, administration of medications, rehabilitation procedures, and personal hygiene activities.

Improvising Equipment

Medical equipment and supply companies are becoming increasingly sensitive to the need for health care technology in the home. Products that were formerly used solely in institutions are now available for home use. However, these may be too expensive for some clients, and the nurse may need to help clients adapt or improvise equipment out of material available. Equipment and supplies that can be improvised easily and inexpensively in the home include backrests, footboards, bed trays, bed cradles, side rails, pull ropes, elevated beds, bed pads and protectors, bedpans, urinals, commodes, hot water bottles, icebags, call bells, and sterile dressings (American Red Cross, 1979). Even ready-made equipment may require creative and innovative approaches to incorporating it into the home environment. Medical equipment companies supplying the products often have trained consultants who act as resources to the nurse and the client.

Health Supervision

Health supervision is an all-encompassing term used to describe the teaching, counseling, and monitoring function of the nurse.

Health teaching/health education is an important direct nursing intervention. In every interaction with a client, the nurse is alert for the so-called teachable moment and is ready to teach. Health education involves more than imparting information, however. An understanding of learning theory and the principles of adult learning is important, as well as knowledge of available teaching resources and how to use them.

In all health education endeavors, the aim is to promote or maintain health or to prevent disease.

TABLE 3-1 Social Readjustment Rating Scale

Rank	Life event	Mean value	Rank	Life event	Mean value
1	Death of spouse	100	23	Son or daughter leaving home	29
2	Divorce	73	24	Trouble with in-laws	29
3	Marital separation	65	25	Outstanding personal achievement	28
4	Jail term	63	26	Spouse begins or stops work	26
5	Death of close family member	63	27	Begin or end school	26
6	Personal injury or illness	53	28	Change in living conditions	25
7	Marriage	50	29	Revision of personal habits	24
8	Fired at work	47	30	Trouble with boss	23
9	Marital reconciliation	45	31	Change in work hours or conditions	20
10	Retirement	45	32	Change in residence	20
11	Change in health of family member	44	33	Change in schools	20
12	Pregnancy	40	34	Change in recreation	19
13	Sex difficulties	39	35	Change in church activities	19
14	Gain of new family member	39	36	Change in social activities	18
15	Business readjustment	39	37	Mortgage or loan less than $10,000	17
16	Change in financial state	38	38	Change in sleeping habits	16
17	Death of close friend	37	39	Change in number of family get-togethers	15
18	Change to different line of work	36	40	Change in eating habits	15
19	Change in number of arguments with spouse	35	41	Vacation	13
20	Mortgage over $10,000	31	42	Christmas	12
21	Foreclosure of mortgage or loan	30	43	Minor violations of the law	11
22	Change in responsibilities at work	29			

Modified from Holmes TH and Rahe RH: The Social Readjustment Rating Scale, J Psychosom Res 11:213, 1967.

Anticipatory guidance is a type of educational activity that sensitizes clients to the advent of events that have the potential for precipitating problems or crises. The nurse provides information and assists clients in developing coping strategies. For example, nurses often prepare mothers of infants for anticipated developmental levels and the potential for accidents that may occur when an infant can roll over, crawl, or walk.

In addition to anticipating developmental changes and potential problems, the nurse can inform the client about significant life events, situations, or circumstances that can generate stress. The Social Readjustment Rating Scale in Table 3-1 is a tool that measures the amount of stress associated with significant life events and predicts the onset of physical or psychologic disease or disability caused by the accumulation of stress (Holmes and Rahe, 1967). Using this rating scale, the community health nurse can help clients anticipate stress and prepare coping strategies in advance.

Teaching also involves specific technical skills related to self-care. Examples would be self-injection of medication, changing dressings, monitoring urine or blood values, or bathing and personal care. The nurse may teach these skills to clients or to an informal support person who assists the client.

The goal of all health teaching is to increase or stabilize the client's capabilities. This is an important cost containment strategy because it can decrease the amount of formal nursing care required by the client.

Direct nursing intervention can also involve *counseling* or problem-solving activities with the client. The nurse guides the client through the problem-solving process by suggesting and clarifying. The client, however, arrives at appropriate solutions and makes decisions. The nurse does not impose solutions on the client and must accept the client's decisions, even if they seem inappropriate.

There are many levels of counseling, and there are many health care professionals, such as psychologists and other mental health professionals, social workers, clergy, and nurses, who can provide this service. Sometimes counseling involves probing into the unconscious or the background of the client to help the client develop insight or even a significant reorganization of the personality. This complex, in-depth counseling requires a level of expertise that is gained through specialized advanced education. The client who needs this type of counseling is referred to a qualified health professional.

Closely related to counseling is the provision of emotional support. The nurse who has developed an effective and therapeutic interaction style provides this easily. Emotional support is basic to the therapeutic nurse-client relationship.

The supportive nurse is nonjudgmental and empathetic toward the client. This involves the use of appropriate nonverbal communication skills, such as active listening, use of eye contact and body language, and verbal responses to facilitate expression of the client's thoughts or feelings. The nurse must be a professional ally whom clients can trust and with whom they are comfortable.

The client or family is supported in self-care endeavors. Encouraging knowledgeable self-care and independence can contribute to an eventual decrease in nursing time and a consequent reduction in the cost of care. Encouraging the client to make choices is an effective way of fostering independence.

Community health nursing involves *monitoring* the condition of clients frequently and regularly. A hypertensive client may be seen weekly for blood pressure and symptom checks, an anorexic client may be seen weekly for weight checks, or a postsurgical client may be checked every other day for wound healing.

Monitoring involves focusing observations to determine whether the status or progress of the client is within normal limits. Since not all clients are motivated or capable of self-monitoring, monitoring by the nurse can prevent unnecessary hospitalization, deterioration, and other problems. Observations may be made about the client's disease state, symptoms, or response to treatment. The nurse makes a professional judgment regarding the normalcy or appropriateness of what is observed. Corrective action may need to be taken if observations are abnormal or unexpected. This may include reporting the observations to an appropriate person or agency, referring the client for needed services, or developing a new or revised plan of care to handle the new problem.

Environmental Modification

The nurse may also assist clients and their families directly in modifying the home environment. Clients who are temporarily or permanently disabled or who are terminally ill may need suggestions about how to reorganize or restructure the physical environment. This may include moving the client to a room on the first floor or near a bathroom to make caregiving easier, removing safety hazards or obstacles, rearranging furniture and traffic patterns, restructuring common living space, and accommodating large pieces of equipment such as hospital beds, wheelchairs, lifts, oxygen equipment, and commodes. The client, family, and nurse may need to discuss the availability of durable medical equipment to make the caregiving or self-care activities easier. Some community agencies have equipment available for loan or minimal rental fees. Also, the client may be eligible for third-party reimbursement for durable medical equipment. The nurse who is aware of the client's potential eligibility refers the client to appropriate agencies or health care personnel for help in securing it.

Casefinding

Casefinding is another important direct nursing activity. Screening and recognition of early symptoms are important aspects of casefinding. In providing care to a client, the nurse is also sensitive to the health complaints and behavior of significant others around the client. Thus the wife or husband of a bed-bound client who complains of occasional dizziness and blackout spells should immediately alert the nurse to a potential health problem that needs further assessment. A quick blood pressure check (screening tool) can confirm suspicions and stimulate further action if necessary. In this way a possible stroke can be prevented and hypertension can be controlled.

Indirect Nursing Intervention

The implementation stage of the nursing process may also involve indirect nursing activities; that is, it may involve activities done on behalf of the client, but not directly with the client.

Teaching and Supervision of Caregivers

One of the most important indirect nursing activities that the community health nurse may undertake is the teaching and supervision of the client's caregivers. In this situation it is not the nurse who gives care to the client, but someone else who must be taught these skills. Usually these caregivers are members of the client's family (informal supports) or nonprofessional nursing personnel (home care nursing aides). Each of these groups presents different challenges for the nurse.

The family or informal support caregiver is a volunteer who is frequently tied to the client by affection or a sense of duty. The caregiver is provided with information on how to provide physical care for the client. Information on energy-saving strategies, community resources, and coping with behavior problems may also be necessary.

Caretaking responsibilities can become overwhelming for family caregivers. It is important for the nurse to monitor caregivers for signs of stress and burnout. Mental health visits to the caregiver may be necessary to allow for ventilation of feelings and to provide emotional support. It is important to monitor the quality of relationships in the family, being especially alert for deterioration that may occur as the result of burnout. It may be necessary to arrange for respite care to give the family caregiver some relief and prevent the permanent institutionalization of the client.

The aide caregiver is paid and may be employed by an agency providing such services. The aide should come to the home care situation with some basic training. It is important for the community health nurse to understand what the aide has been *trained* to do and is *allowed* to do by government or agency regulation. Basic information received in training must be supplemented with on-the-job training specific to the care requirements and personality of the particular client. For example, the aide may have some basic knowledge about colostomy care, but the specific task requirements vary from client to client, and the community health nurse must orient the aide to each specific client. As a nonprofessional, the aide may also require emotional support and counseling when handling difficult care situations.

Supervision is the process of overseeing the work of someone else to determine if it meets some standard. Supervision involves observing or monitoring the care given, comparing it with the standard (evaluation), and taking corrective action if necessary. The nurse can actually watch the care being demonstrated, look at the results of the care, ask about client satisfaction with the care, or ask about the caregiver's feelings in giving the care. If corrective action must be taken, this can be in the form of reeducation, counseling, and occasionally substituting another caregiver.

Although the nurse delegates aspects of nursing care to the caregiver in the home, total accountability to the client is not delegated. The nurse who writes the plan of care, delegates nursing activities, provides direct care to the client, and supervises the care of others should be the same person. Delivery systems that parcel these activities among different nurses dilute and fragment the care given, jeopardize its quality, and weaken the responsibility and accountability for the client's care.

Coordination

Coordination is a management function that entails the appropriate use of all care providers to achieve continuity of care for a client. Coordination involves making the activities of two or more people interact to achieve an effective result. In health care this means that the work efforts of all team members function smoothly and harmoniously to benefit the client. Coordinated effort can decrease fragmentation of care, ensure continuity of care, prevent duplication and overlap, and prevent overuse or underuse of services. This in turn prevents inefficiency, decreases cost, and improves quality of care.

Coordination is an important indirect nursing activity, and the nurse is an ideal person to function in the coordinator role. The nurse's qualifications for this role include a generalist background, in-depth and frequent contact with the client, ability to interpret and interact with the client at the appropriate level, knowledge of the community, a holistic focus, and familiarity with the nursing process.

"Case management" is a term used to describe an increasingly distinct role in the field of long-term community care. The professional qualifications for this role are still fluid, and it is possible to find nurses, social workers, and other human services workers functioning in this capacity. The case manager functions as the gatekeeper to the long-term community care system. The purpose of the management role is to lower the risk of institutionalization and thus contain the costs of long-term care. Following is a summary of case management duties:

1. The case manager should assess the client's needs for health service and authorization of access to those services. This includes determining eligibility, setting financial limits, and authorizing payment.
2. The case manager should develop a plan of care that is comprehensive, tailored to the client's needs, and designed to maintain or restore independent function. Arrangements are made for providing services through an assessment of available resources (formal and informal) and appropriate referral.
3. Case managers should provide, monitor, and coordinate service delivery. This may also involve advocacy for the client.
4. Case managers should evaluate the effectiveness of the care plan, including the client's progress and response.
5. Case managers should reassess and replan as necessary.

The case management model is similar to the nursing process except that it is broader in scope and more complex. Table 3-2 compares the two models.

As home care expands and becomes more complex because of changes in the health care delivery system, it is likely that the case management model will become functional for other levels of care that require multiple services. Community health nurses and home health care nurses, by

TABLE 3-2 Comparison of Nursing Process and Case Management Models

Nursing process	Case management
Assessment	Assessing need for service; determining eligibility
Diagnosis	Problem listing
Planning	Plan of care; arranging for services
Implementation	Service delivery
Evaluation	Evaluation
Reassessment	Reassessment

virtue of their background and experience, are ideally suited to fill case manager roles.

Referral

Referral becomes necessary when the nurse cannot, either by direct or by indirect nursing interventions, completely meet the client's needs. This may be due to time factors, agency or programmatic policies and regulations, or lack of expertise. Referral is a process that facilitates the client's and family's use of available resources to meet their needs.

Referral is a complex process involving much more than filling out a form and sending it to the appropriate agency. After establishing the need for referral, the nurse determines whether there are any existing client resources that can be used. The client may have an informal support system that can be used or may be affiliated with community institutions, such as a church or school, that can provide needed service. Often clients have used or are already using agencies in the community. For example, a client who is using a family service agency to manage problematic behavior in a child may be able to obtain marital counseling from that agency as well.

The nurse also determines the accessibility of formal community resources. This involves knowing about services provided, eligibility requirements, admitting procedures, fees, geographic proximity to the client, and availability of transportation. Many communities have compiled directories of health and welfare agencies that include some of this information. Even the yellow pages can serve as a partial resource. In addition, the nurse can compile an annotated file of different agencies in the community. More detailed information can be kept there, including names of specific contact people. It is always preferable to make contact with other agencies through a specific person. It humanizes the referral processes and increases the likelihood of a favorable outcome.

The nurse may need to help the client recognize the need for referral (consciousness raising) through problem solving, counseling, and articulation of the problem. Information about available resources and what they can realistically do can be given. The client's basic right of self-determination also ensures the right to refuse referral. As frustrating as this may be for the nurse, referring a client who does not follow through is even more frustrating.

Most referrals are formalized with special referral forms. In some communities, health and welfare agencies have adopted the use of a standardized, interagency referral format. Information required on the form includes the name and address of the agency to whom the referral is being made, the client's name and identifying information, the reason for the referral, and the name and identifying information about the person and agency making the referral. If extensive background information on the client is included in the referral, the nurse should obtain the client's written consent to share this information. Many referral forms also include a blank space for responding to the referral. In addition to sending a written referral, the nurse may want to alert the agency or person by telephone that a referral is coming. Some clients wish to make referral arrangements themselves after they have been given

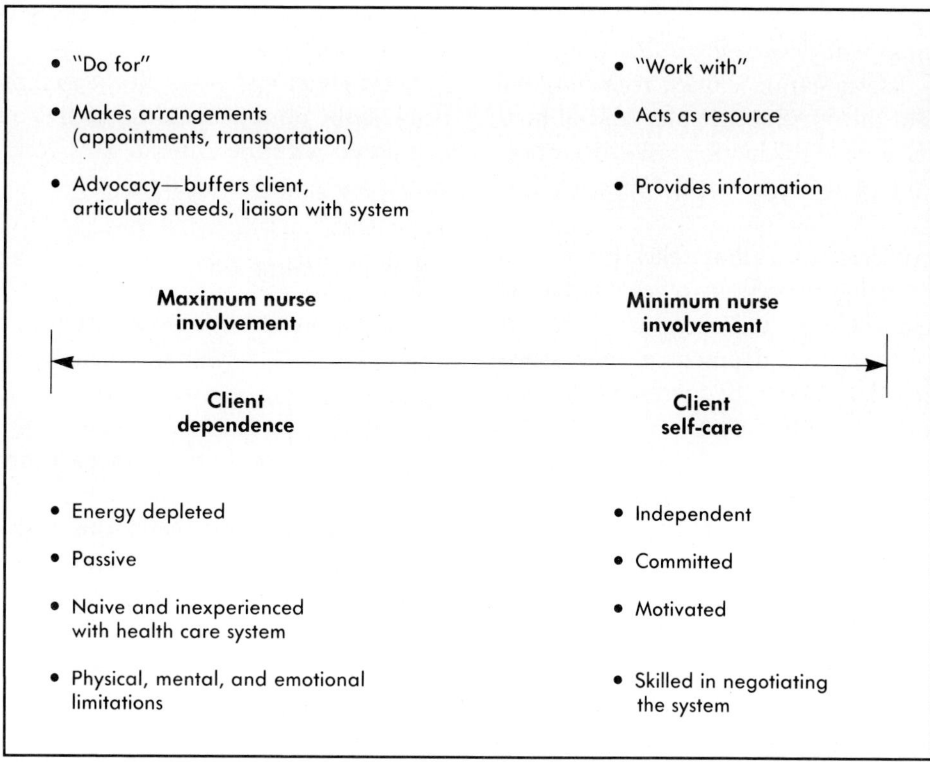

FIG. 3-2. Amount and type of nurse involvement relates to client independence.

the information. This is encouraged because it fosters independence, self-care, commitment, and follow-through. Even in this situation the nurse may want to share information with the referral resource. Client permission is required for this.

Other clients need considerable assistance and support in negotiating the referral process. The amount and type of nursing involvement and the degree of client independence can be viewed on a continuum in Fig. 3-2. In general, the greater the dependence of the client, the more active and involved the nurse must become in the mechanics of making the referral.

The process of referral also requires that the nurse prepare the client to use the services of the referral resource. This includes the resource's name and address, directions to the resource, instructions on what to take along, such as special documents and receipts, how long the wait might be, and what the first visit will be like, that is, whether the client will be questioned or examined. It is much better for clients to prepare to spend a morning than for them to expect to finish in an hour and become angry or anxious because of the wait.

The last part of the referral process is follow-up. This involves finding out whether the client contacted the referral resource and what the outcome was. The nurse needs to determine whether the client's needs were met, and if not, why not. Resources to whom referrals are made respond in writing to the person or agency making the referral stating when the client was seen, what the result was, and what future treatment plans are. If the referral outcome was unsuccessful, the nurse may need to refer again.

Evaluation

Evaluation, as it applies to the nursing process, means that a determination is made regarding the effectiveness of the nursing care plan and of how it was implemented. Evaluation asks the questions, "Did the plan work?" and "Was it effective?"

The type of evaluation that takes place as a stage in the nursing process involves comparing the actual with the expected outcomes or results of the plan of care. A judgment is then made regarding the value, worth, or success of the care plan based on this comparison.

There are several purposes of evaluation at this stage. The first is to make a determination about the effectiveness of the plan. Is it working, and should it continue as is? Is the problem solved, and should the plan be terminated? Another purpose is to determine whether the plan, in whole or in part, needs revision. For example, it may be that the nursing diagnosis is still accurate, but the objectives are unrealistic or the interventions are inappropriate.

Effective evaluation is not a haphazard activity. The key to evaluation is to establish criteria. Nursing process criteria are observable units of client behavior that can be measured in some way. This means that the nurse can determine the presence or absence of the behaviors by what is seen, heard, touched, tasted, or smelled.

The behaviors that a nurse can measure include the following types of client responses with examples:

1. Physiologic—change in client's blood pressure, weight, or laboratory results
2. Functional—client dresses or feeds self
3. Educational—client explains diabetic diet or plans menus using exchange list
4. Psychomotor—client draws up insulin or injects insulin
5. Psychologic—client talks of feeling less depressed, cries less, or goes out more
6. Social—client states siblings help more with aged parent or siblings are observed talking to each other

These client responses, behaviors, or indicators become the objective and subjective data that are compared with the criteria. This comparison becomes the measurement.

Steps in Evaluation

Evaluation involves several steps.

Specifying Criteria

The evaluation criteria for each nursing diagnosis are stated. If the criteria are stated explicitly in the objective statement, this task is easy. If appropriate, evaluation criteria provide a time frame within which the client response (behavior) must be manifest.

Gathering Relevant Data

Data that are relevant to the criteria are gathered. For example, if the criterion is "weight loss of five pounds within four weeks," the appropriate relevant data needed for comparison are the weight of the client, not the daily calorie intake or the exercise regimen.

The type of data needed and the methods for gathering the data are planned from the beginning. If evaluation data are left to chance or to the last minute, the measurement is inaccurate and the evaluation is meaningless. Evaluation data and methods for gathering it must be practical. Evaluating weight loss by comparing a client's actual weekly weight with some standard may not be possible in the home care setting if a client does not have a scale.

Measurement

The relevant data that have been gathered are interpreted and compared with the criteria. The

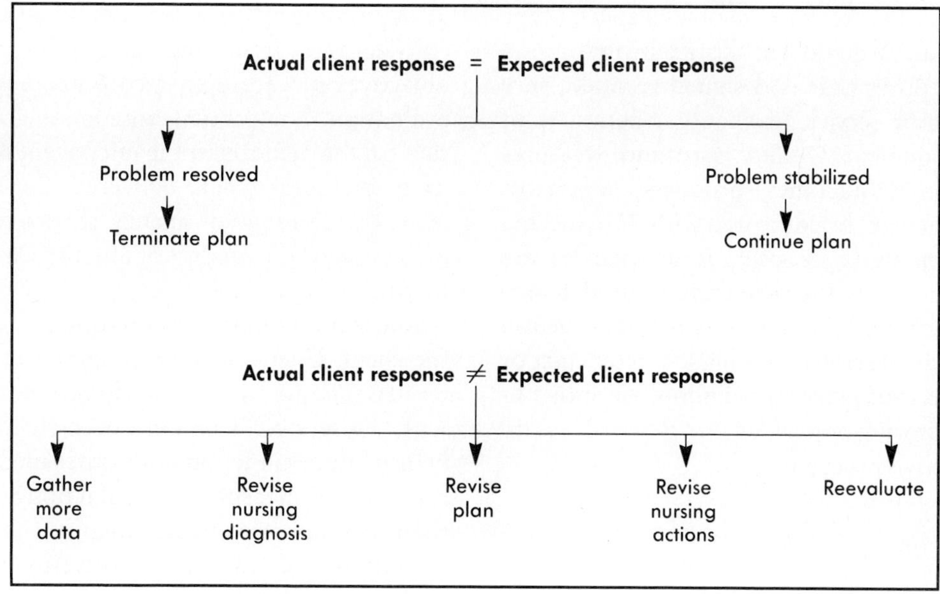

FIG. 3-3. Client response to nursing intervention is evaluated to decide whether further intervention is needed.

actual client behavior or response is compared with what was expected or desired in the planning stage.

Judgment and Decision Making

The nurse makes a judgment (evaluation) as to whether the actual response measures up to or equals the expected response to parts of a treatment regimen. If the two are equal, the nurse may decide to terminate that part of the plan because the problem is solved or the nurse may decide to continue the plan as is. If the client's response does not measure up to what is expected, the nurse reassesses the situation and begins the nursing process all over. In this case the evaluation data become the assessment data for the revised plan (Fig. 3-3).

Evaluation of the nursing care plan is an ongoing activity. Each time nursing care is delivered, the client is evaluated for progress toward goals and objectives. However, evaluation checkpoints at intervals are also built in as part of the care plan. Sometimes these checkpoints are mandated by agency policy or government regulation. For example, Medicare clients must be evaluated every 60 days. Other agencies may also require evaluations after a certain number of visits or months of service, as well as at transfer or termination of service.

Documentation of nursing actions and client responses to those actions becomes critical for evaluation. A record-keeping system that relates progress notes to the care plan simplifies the evaluation process. As discussed in the next section, this kind of documentation is essential for quality assurance programs and is becoming increasingly relevant to cost reimbursement and cost containment issues.

Quality Assurance

No discussion of evaluation would be complete without reference to quality assurance or quality control. Quality assurance involves a special type of evaluation. A quality assurance program is a set of procedures that is designed to make sure the product or service of an organization is of acceptable quality. Quality assurance requires that the actual outcomes (products or services such as client care) be compared with the expected outcomes (goals of service). If deficiencies are identified, methods for correcting these deficiencies are instituted. Examples of remedial action might include in-service training, conferencing, or even dismissal of personnel. Follow-up and continued monitoring of problem areas are necessary for an effective program.

Quality Assurance Tools

Quality assurance is no easy task. It would be prohibitive to try to evaluate nursing care in all its dimensions. Consequently, most tools concentrate on a specific aspect of nursing care. Selected aspects of the nursing process are frequently used as the framework or standard to which actual nursing care is compared.

A popular quality assurance tool that is used frequently in community health is Phaneuf's *Nursing Audit.* The nursing audit is "a method for evaluating quality of care through appraisal of the nursing process as it is reflected in the patient care records for discharged patients" (Phaneuf, 1976). A determination of quality is made by examining the scores after the audit is completed. Record audits may be conducted internally or externally. Most professional nurses feel strongly that audits of nursing records should be conducted by other nurses. This is a peer review and is consistent with the ideal of professional self-regulation that was discussed earlier. For the same reason, it is preferable to conduct internal audits rather than rely on external agencies to perform them. However, government regulation and policies regarding certain programs, such as Medicare, do not always permit this.

Another way of determining quality is to look at the results of care for individual clients and consider these in the aggregate. By comparing the objectives of care (expected outcomes) with the evaluation data (actual outcomes) a determination can be made as to the effectiveness and quality of the nursing care delivered. Evaluating this over a wide range of agency clients can provide indicators of the quality of nursing care delivered by the agency.

Another method for evaluating service is to ask the client. Clients can be questioned through interviews or questionnaires about their satisfaction with the service. This kind of evaluation should be used in conjunction with other methods, since it is more a measure of satisfaction with service than a measure of actual quality. As was mentioned previously, judging professional quality is something only a peer can do because of the expert knowledge involved.

Record Keeping

In assessing the quality of care and the use of services that are delivered to clients, community health agencies rely on the client's record. In some agencies only nurses may be contributors to the record; in broader service agencies, all professional staff may contribute. In looking for evidence of quality care in the record, nurses assume that if something is not written in the record, it was not done. Therefore documentation is important.

A record-keeping format that facilitates finding information required by the nursing audit procedure saves time, energy, and money for the agency. One method that is frequently used in community health agencies is the problem oriented record (POR). This format closely corresponds to the nursing process.

The POR system was originally designed as a method for organizing medical data and preventing the loss of patient information in the hospital. As this was being developed and used in medical circles, the writing of care plans based on the nursing process was coming into its own in nursing. The combination of the two systems has resulted in an effective and efficient recording tool that can be used by any health professional giving service to a client. The POR not only enables data to be recovered easily for auditing purposes, but equally important, it contributes to quality of care by improving interdisciplinary communication about the client and thus improving problem identification and solution. The POR also facilitates nursing accountability and the ability to pinpoint the effect of nursing.

Information is recorded in the record according to problems. (In the nursing process model this would be the nursing diagnosis.) All information that pertains to a given problem is kept together in the record, and the problems are numbered. The problem-oriented recording process includes establishing a data base, developing a numbered problem list, planning diagnostic, treatment, or educational activities in response to the problems, and recording progress notes that reflect actions taken and client responses. SOAPIER is an acronym used to designate the recording process, with a notation made for each of the letters.

S = subjective data
O = objective data
A = assessment
P = plan
I = implementation (action taken)
E = evaluation data
R = reassessment and problem restatement if necessary

Table 3-3 shows the relationship between the nursing process, POR, and SOAPIER.

TABLE 3-3 Relationship Between the Nursing Process, POR, and SOAPIER

Nursing process	POR	SOAPIER
Assessment	Data base	*S*ubjective data *O*bjective data
Nursing diagnosis	Problem list	*A*ssessment
Plan	Plan	*P*lan
Implementation	Action as documented in progress notes	*I*mplementation
Evaluation	Response as documented in progress notes	*E*valuation *R*eassessment

Utilization Review

Utilization review and utilization management constitute an evaluation process that is aimed primarily at cost containment. It is an attempt to judge the appropriateness of the type and length of service provided by an agency and the cost of that service. Funding sources, especially the government but increasingly insurance sources as well, mandate this type of agency-wide evaluation as a condition of payment for services. Improved quality of care can be a by-product of this type of evaluation.

The federal government has taken a central role in the quality, cost containment, and utilization review issues pertaining to health care. A large number of U.S. citizens are beneficiaries of health care through Medicare and Medicaid programs. Increases in the aged population are causing these programs to expand at an unprecedented rate. This makes the federal government responsible not only for the cost of services, but for the quality of services provided as well.

The Health Care Financing Administration (HCFA) is the federal agency responsible for administering the Medicare/Medicaid programs. HCFA has established Professional Review Organizations (PROs) as the watchdogs for quality within cost containment parameters. Each state has a PRO, and any physician or agency that is reimbursed with these moneys is subject to a formalized review procedure to ensure compliance with federal standards.

Quality of care and cost containment are the two important issues the health care delivery system must deal with. Although these are not necessarily opposing and conflicting concepts, recent changes in health care delivery appear to put quality and cost of care on a collision course.

Community health nurses may find themselves caught between these issues. It is essential for the nurse to understand the health care delivery system and to be aware of the philosophies and politics that drive that system. It is also important for the community health nurse to recognize personal values and opinions regarding the quality and cost of health care.

Although the nurse, along with other health professionals, is held accountable for cost containment in health care, the special contribution of nursing to health care delivery is to ensure that the quality of care provided to the client is not compromised. This can occur through a personal relationship with a client, through assumption of the advocate's role for those clients to whom the system is not responsive, or through a broader political activist response. The nursing process, as a proven and effective problem-solving instrument for planning and implementing nursing care, becomes an important tool for ensuring quality care in all of these spheres.

SUMMARY

The nursing process is a problem-solving method for assessing, diagnosing, planning, implementing, and evaluating nursing care in all clinical settings. To provide nursing care that meets each client's needs and that is well organized and scientifically based, the nurse adapts the process model to the community setting.

Initiating the nursing process with the community-based client takes skill and preplanning. First encounters between nurse and client involve defining roles, reaching consensus on the purpose of the encounter, and establishing rapport.

The assessment stage of the nursing process involves compiling a data base about the client's health status. Data-gathering tools and skills useful in other settings are adapted and refined for use in the community setting. Ideally, data are holistic in scope and involve biopsychosocial dimensions of the client's health, as well as environmental aspects of the client's situation.

The second stage, nursing diagnosis, enables the nurse to focus on the actual or potential health problems or concerns of the client in addition to positive health status. Diagnostic statements derived from existing taxonomies such as the one developed by NANDA are useful in the community health setting. However, the community-based nurse may also develop original diagnostic statements because standard taxonomies have not addressed the breadth of health concerns and client situations encountered in the community.

The planning stage involves prioritizing the nursing diagnoses, establishing goals and objectives, searching for solutions, apportioning tasks, and writing the plan. The client is involved in planning as much as possible. Client participation encourages independence and facilitates commitment to the plan. Other professional and nonprofessional health services personnel may also be involved at this stage. Skills involving delegation, negotiation, contracting, and collaboration are used in developing the client's written care plan.

Implementation of the care plan means that the activities and strategies designed to address the nursing diagnoses are actually carried out. Implementation includes direct nursing activities such as hands-on care, equipment improvisation, health supervision, environmental modification, and casefinding. Implementation also includes indirect nursing activities (teaching and supervising others and coordination) and referral.

The evaluation stage compares expected outcomes (objectives) with the actual outcomes as reflected in the evaluation data. Evaluation, like data gathering, is an ongoing activity. Quality assurance and utilization review are evaluation procedures that look at the entire caseload of a community health agency, not just individual client care. Agencies often adapt the nursing process model to their planning and recording procedures because it facilitates the measurement of quality and cost containment.

QUESTIONS FOR DISCUSSION

1. How would you go about compiling a data base for a 15-year-old client who was referred to you after discharge from the hospital as an insulin-dependent diabetic?
2. Using imaginary data compiled for the client in question, suggest one or more nursing diagnoses.
3. Planning for care in the community is sometimes more complex than planning for care in the hospital. Why might this be so?
4. Provide examples of direct and indirect nursing interventions.
5. What processes could you use to evaluate the nursing care in a large community clinic?

REFERENCES

Alex WM: Nursing diagnosis with the family and community. In Logan B and Dawkins C, editors: Family centered nursing in the community, Menlo Park, Calif, 1986, Addison-Wesley Publishing Co Inc.

American Red Cross: Family health and home nursing, ed 8, Garden City, NY, 1979, Doubleday & Co.

Campbell C: Nursing diagnosis and intervention in nursing practice, ed 2, New York, 1984, John Wiley & Sons Inc.

Carlson J, Craft C, and McGuire A, editors: Nursing diagnosis, Philadelphia, 1982, WB Saunders Co.

Carnevali D: Nursing care planning: diagnosis and management, ed 3, Philadelphia, 1983, JB Lippincott Co.

Carnevali D and others: Diagnostic reasoning in nursing, Philadelphia, 1984, JB Lippincott Co.

Duvall E: Family development, ed 4, Philadelphia, 1977, JB Lippincott Co.

Edel M: The nature of nursing diagnosis. In Carlson J, Craft C, and McGuire A, editors: Nursing diagnosis, Philadelphia, 1982, WB Saunders Co.

Elkins CP: Community health nursing: skills and strategies, Bowie, Md, 1984, Brady.

Erikson E: Childhood and society, ed 2, New York, 1963, WW Norton & Co Inc.

Fisher R and Ury W: Getting to yes, Boston, 1981, Houghton Mifflin Co.

Gordon M: Nursing diagnosis, process and application, ed 2, New York, 1987, McGraw-Hill Inc.

Grau L: Case management and the nurse, Geriatr Nurs 5:372, 1984.

Griffith JW and Christensen PJ, editors: Nursing process: application of theories, frameworks and models, ed 2, St Louis, 1986, CV Mosby Co.

Hall J and Weaver B, editors: Distributive nursing practice, ed 2, Philadelphia, 1985, JB Lippincott Co.

Hamilton P: Community nursing diagnosis, ANS 5:21, 1983.

Holmes T and Rahe R: The social readjustment rating scale, J Psychosom Res 11:213, 1967.

Iyer PW, Taptich BJ, and Bernocchi-Losey D: Nursing process and nursing diagnosis, Philadelphia, 1986, WB Saunders Co.

Jarvis L: Community health nursing, Philadelphia, 1981, FA Davis Co.

Kelly MA: Nursing diagnosis source book, Norwalk, Conn, 1985, Appleton & Lange.

Kim MJ and others: Classification of nursing diagnosis: proceedings of the fifth national conference, St Louis, 1984, CV Mosby Co.

Kozier B and Erb G: Fundamentals of nursing, ed 3, Menlo Park, Calif, 1987, Addison-Wesley Publishing Co Inc.

Kritek PB: Nursing diagnosis: theoretical foundations, Occup Health Nurs 33:393, 1985.

Kritek PB: The struggle to classify our diagnoses, AJN 86:722, 1986.

Leahy K, Cobb M, and Jones M: Community health nursing, ed 4, New York, 1982, McGraw-Hill Inc.

Leonard B and Redland A: Process in clinical nursing, Englewood Cliffs, NJ, 1981, Prentice Hall.

Logan BB and Dawkins CE: Family centered nursing in the community, Menlo Park, Calif, 1986, Addison-Wesley Publishing Co Inc.

Lunney M: Nursing diagnosis: refining the system, AJN 82:456, 1982.

Mayers M: A systematic approach to the nursing care plan, ed 3, Norwalk, Conn, 1983, Appleton & Lange.

Miaskowski CA: Nursing diagnosis within the context of the nursing process, Occup Health Nurs 33:401, 1985.

Muecke MA: Community health diagnosis in nursing, Public Health Nurs 1:23, 1984.

Murray RB and Zentner JP: Nursing assessment and health promotion through the life span, ed 3, Englewood Cliffs, NJ, 1985, Prentice Hall, Prentice Hall Press.

North American Nursing Diagnosis Association: 21 New diagnoses and a taxonomy, AJN 86:1414, 1986.

Orlando I: The dynamic nurse-patient relationship, New York, 1961, The Putnam Publishing Group Inc.

Phaneuf MC: The nursing audit, ed 2, New York, 1976, Appleton & Lange.

Sheehy G: Passages, New York, 1976, EP Dutton.

Shulman L: The skills of helping, Itasca, Ill, 1979, FE Peacock Publishers Inc.

Simmons DA: A classification scheme for client problems in community health nursing, DHHS Publication No HRA 80-16, 1986, National Technical Information Services (NTIS No. 14).

Stanhope M and Lancaster J, editors: Community health nursing, ed 2, St Louis, 1988, CV Mosby Co.

Yura H and Walsh MB: The nursing process, ed 4, New York, 1983, Appleton & Lange.

Ziegler SM, Vaughan-Wrobel BC, and Erlen JA: Nursing process, nursing diagnosis, nursing knowledge, Norwalk, Conn, 1986, Appleton & Lange.

BIBLIOGRAPHY

American Nurses' Association: Standards of community health nursing practice, Kansas City, Mo, 1973, The Association.

Archer SE and Fleshman RP, editors: Community health nursing, ed 3, Monterey, Calif, 1985, Wadsworth Inc.

Carpenito LJ: Nursing diagnosis: selected dilemmas in practice, Occup Health Nurs 33:397, 1985.

Carpenito LJ: Nursing diagnosis, Philadelphia, 1987, JB Lippincott Co.

Challela M: The interdisciplinary team: a role definition for nursing, Image 11:9, 1979.

Chance K: The quest for quality: an exploration of attempts to define and measure quality nursing care, Image 12:41, 1980.

Clark MJ: Community nursing, Reston, Va, 1984, Reston Publishing Co.

Clemen SA, Eigsti DG, and McGuire SL: Comprehensive family and community health nursing, New York, 1981, McGraw-Hill Inc.

Creason NS: How do we define our diagnoses? Am J Nurs 87:230, 1987.

Dougherty CM, editor: Symposium on nursing diagnosis, Nurs Clin North Am 20:609, 1985.

Freeman R and Heinrich J: Community health nursing practice, ed 2, Philadelphia, 1981, WB Saunders Co.

Fromer M: Community health care and the nursing process, ed 2, St Louis, 1983, CV Mosby Co.

Pendelton SH: Clarification or obfuscation, AJN 86:944, 1986.

Potter P and Perry AG: Fundamentals of nursing: concepts, process and practice, ed 2, St Louis, 1989, CV Mosby Co.

Pridham KF and Schutz ME: Rationale for a language for naming problems from a nursing perspective, Image 17:122, 1985.

Schmadl J: Quality assurance: examination of the concept, Nurs Outlook 27:462, 1979.

Schoolcraft V, editor: Nursing in the community, New York, 1984, John Wiley & Sons Inc.

Shamansky S and Yanni C: In opposition to nursing diagnosis: a minority opinion, Image 15:47, 1983.

Shoemaker JK: Characteristics of a nursing diagnosis, Occup Health Nurs 33:387, 1985.

Simonson W: Medications and the elderly, Rockville, Md, 1984, Aspen Publishers Inc.

Sorensen KC and Luckmann J: Basic nursing: a psychophysiologic approach, ed 2, Philadelphia, 1986, WB Saunders Co.

Spradley BW: Readings in community health nursing, ed 2, Boston, 1982, Little, Brown & Co Inc.

Spradley BW: Community health nursing, ed 2, Boston, 1985, Little Brown & Co Inc.

Tripp-Reimer T, Brink P, and Saunders J: Cultural assessment: content and process, Nurs Outlook 32:78, 1984.

CHAPTER 4

Epidemiology

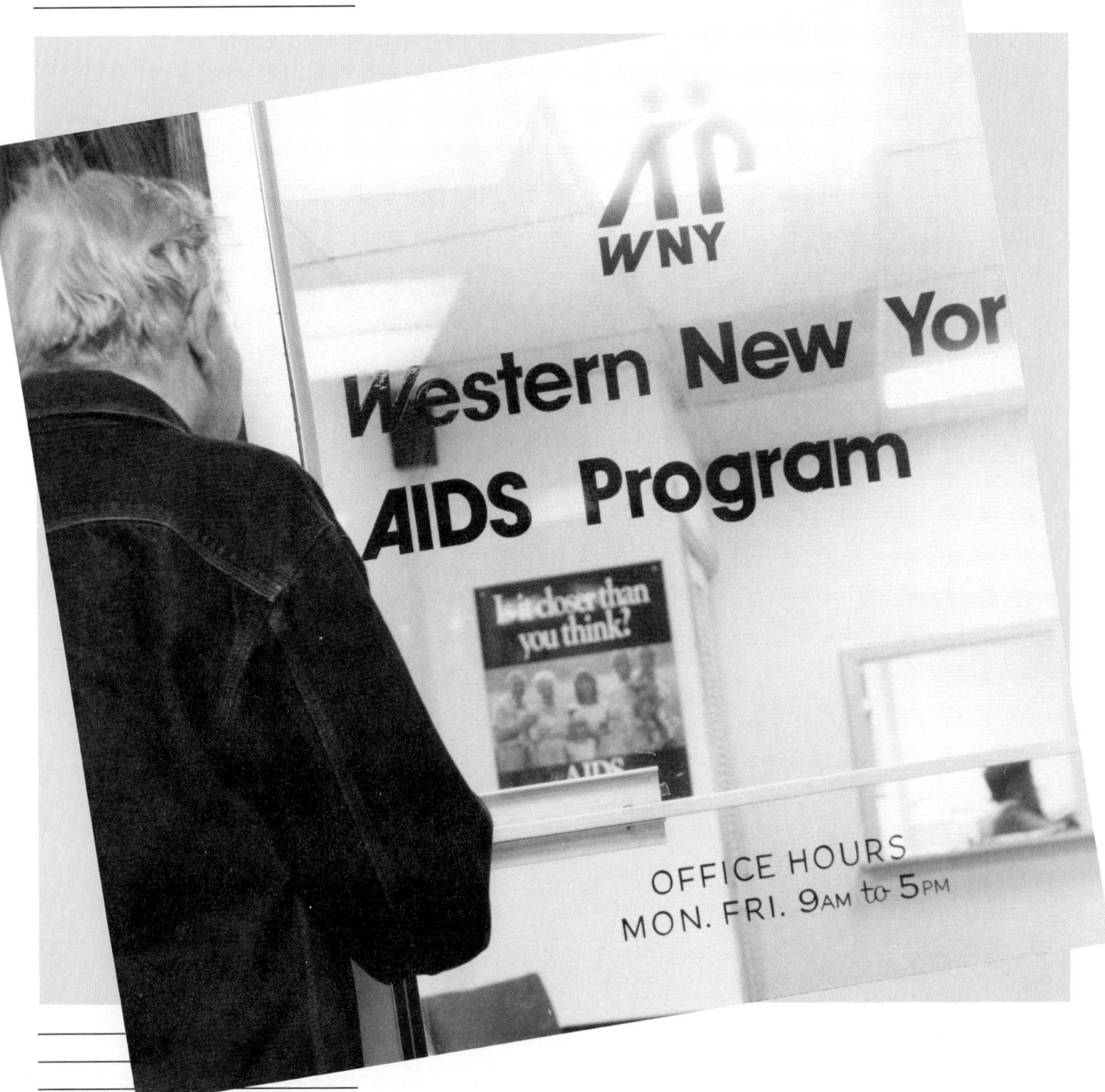

CHAPTER OUTLINE

OBJECTIVES

After completing this chapter, the reader should be able to:

1. Discuss the history of the science of epidemiology.
2. Understand the importance of Edwin Chadwick and other pioneers of epidemiology.
3. Recognize the importance of keeping records and establishing standard diagnoses.
4. Define epidemiology and explain why it is an interdisciplinary science.
5. Define key terms such as incidence, ratio, probability, death rate, mortality difference, mortality ratio, relative risk ratio, and secondary attack rate.

HISTORY OF EPIDEMIOLOGY

Epidemiology is both an old approach to disease and a new science. Many terms in health sciences are derived from Greek. The word epidemiology is derived from the Greek *epi,* meaning on, *demos,* meaning the people, and *Logos,* meaning science or knowledge. Thus epidemiology literally means the study of things that occur on a people. In this broad definition of the term, the study of epidemics dates from the beginning of the study of human health. Much of the writing attributed to the Greek physician Hippocrates, a semilegendary person of the fifth century BC, was concerned with the genesis of epidemics and various acute febrile diseases. Hippocrates believed, from his study of epidemics, that they were caused by a constellation of weather conditions, since only this could explain epidemics' seasonal and annual incidence.

This astrologic-weather approach continued to be the dominant theory through the medieval period into early modern times, and it was carried to its furthest by the great English clinician Thomas Sydenham (1624-1689). Sydenham held that febrile diseases fell into two major groups: the epidemic distempers produced by atmospheric changes and the intercurrent diseases dependent on the susceptibility of the body. Plague, smallpox, and dysentery were attributed to atmospheric changes, whereas scarlet fever, quinsy (a severe pharyngitis), pleurisy, and rheumatism were among those dependent on the body's susceptibility. Sydenham never understood exactly what the association of disease and atmosphere change was, but he believed it was due to a miasma, a sort of vaporous exhalation emanating from the earth, which was associated often with some astrologic changes.

Even though the atmospheric-miasmatic view is clearly erroneous, it was important in the long run, since it had a great deal of influence on what could be regarded as public health measures. Such things as human excrement, garbage, polluted water, and similar materials were believed to give off an unhealthy miasma, and thus the Sydenham view gave a kind of reasoned impetus to the movements to build sewers, drain swamps, and improve sanitation long before the germ theory of disease was accepted.

Coexisting with the atmospheric-miasmatic view, at least from the late medieval period, was the belief by a large number of people that some kind of contagion was a factor in the spread of epidemic disease. The contagion ideas differed from those we hold today, since a more complete understanding was dependent on the discovery of bacteria and viruses in the late nineteenth and early twentieth centuries. Nonetheless, a theory of contagion based on observation developed. Among the most influential in promoting this concept was the Italian Girolamo Fracastoro (1478-1553). His treatise, *On Contagion, Contagious Disease, and Their Treatment,* stated that epidemic diseases were caused by minute infective agents ("seeds" [*seminaria*] was the term he used) and that these were transmissible and self-propagating. Fracastoro believed the seeds were specific to each disease and disease resulted when these seeds acted on the humors and vital spirits of the body. However, to Fracastoro, seeds were not what we now understand by germs but instead were probably conceived of as chemical substances or ferment. These seeds were transmitted by direct contact from person to person, through intermediate agents, and through the air. This last hypothesis allowed Fracastoro to include the atmospheric miasmatic view as part of his seed theory. He believed widespread epidemics, or pandemics, were caused when the general atmosphere became infected, perhaps caused by unusual atmospheric or astrologic conditions.

It was not until the microscope was invented that the minute forms of life assumed to exist by Fracastoro were detected. The first person to observe bacteria and other microscopic organisms was the Dutch lens grinder, Anton van Leeuwenhoek (1632-1723). He communicated his discovery to the Royal Society of London in October 1676. Leeuwenhoek modified Fracastoro's seed theory when he first observed so-called little animals (animacula) under the microscope. He described cocci, bacilli, and spirilla observed in rain water, soil, human excrement, and other materials he put under his microscope. His discovery, however, did not eliminate other theories of disease, since there was a tendency to look on these little animals as the products rather than the causes of the disease.

In fact, history demonstrates that one of the problems in dealing with disease was the lock on imagination that earlier assumptions about disease had. The organisms Leeuwenhoek described were often found in easily decomposable substances such as sour milk and rotting meat, so the controversy could continue, since these substances could be regarded as diseased and the organisms as products of the disease.

Two assumptions came to be accepted by most medical investigators as empirically proved. Some diseases, such as smallpox and plague, had the power to spread from one person to another; others, such as malaria, appeared to be endemic in certain parts of the world but were not clearly transmittable by personal contact. The first of these modes of transmission was called contagion, and the second was called infection or miasma. Contagion, however, was not thought of as an organism but as an emanation from the body of a person who had the disease or from that of a person who had died of it, or from the bodies of healthy people who were crowded together without enough ventilation. Only with the discoveries of Koch, Pasteur, and others was the germ theory accepted. The germ theory gained its final victory when it was realized that yellow fever parasites were carried by mosquitoes. The discovery of animal and other vectors allowed the miasma and contagion theories to be brought together. Even after such discoveries, however, some, including Florence Nightingale, were slow to support the germ theory. She did, however, accept the miasma theory and thus believed in cleanliness.

Modern epidemiology depended not only on a better understanding of the disease process, but also on the development of so-called political arithmetic, the forerunner of what later came to be known as vital statistics. The study of death rates, sex ratios, birth rates, and similar phenomena began in England in the seventeenth century, and it was the ability of those engaged in political arithmetic to demonstrate the effectiveness of their measures that consolidated some of the successes of the early public health movement in improving such things as water supplies and city sanitation.

More sophisticated methods developed in the nineteenth century, and in the English-speaking world these methods are associated with Edwin Chadwick, a disciple of Jeremy Bentham, one of the founders of a movement known as utilitarianism. Bentham and his disciples attempted to deal with public problems on a rational scientific basis, and he spent the last part of his life working out a scheme for a utopian government, which took many measures to improve the general health of its people. One of his supporters was Chadwick, who managed in 1832 to be appointed as assistant to a royal commission to inquire into the operation and administration of the English Poor Laws. Chadwick soon moved from being an assistant to serving on the commission itself, and he took as his special province the health of the poor, which he believed was affected by the physical and social environment in which they lived.

Chadwick applied his theories to his job of commissioner, and the result was the *Report . . . on an Inquiry into the Sanitary Condition of the Labouring Population of Great Britain*. The report, in a district-by-district survey, attempted to correlate living conditions with variations in mortality and economic status. The result was a plausible epidemiologic theory that fitted many of the known facts and served as a basis for community health actions for several generations. Although Chadwick did not subscribe to the germ theory, which had not yet been proved, he recognized that communicable disease was related to filthy environmental conditions, lack of drainage, inadequate water supply, and the piling

CHADWICK AND VITAL STATISTICS

Chadwick's great contribution to epidemiology was in establishing the importance of collecting vital statistics. He listed the following reasons to justify the collection of such data:

1. The registration of the causes of disease can give data to devise remedies or means of prevention.
2. Comparing data would permit the determination of the salubrity, or healthiness, of places so that individual settlements and public establishments could be built in the most healthy areas.
3. Comparative degrees of salubrity could take place, not only within an occupation, but among the same occupation in different locations and circumstances. Thus it might be better to establish certain occupational groupings in certain areas or to try to imitate the conditions where there was the least mortality.
4. Mortality rates could also allow persons to invest money to their best advantage or to the advantage of persons near and dear to them.
5. Population rates could be obtained at different periods and under differing circumstances to draw up effective public policy.
6. Vital statistics would also make it more likely to uncover calamities, casualties, concealed murders, and deaths from heedlessness or negligence.

up of refuse and garbage on the streets and near residences. The great preventives he advocated were "drainage, street and house cleansing," improved sewerage, and introduction of cheaper and more efficient means of removing all noxious refuse from towns and cities.

Chadwick's method proved so effective that it was applied to other areas. With the bacterial knowledge gained in the last part of the nineteenth century, preventive measures for epidemics included not only environmental control, but immunization as well. Most of the preventive efforts concentrated on infectious diseases until well into the twentieth century, but epidemiologists soon observed similarities with other patterns of illness and began to extend their field. Epidemiologists assumed it was far more effective to prevent pathologic changes from occurring than attempting to reverse the damage these changes had caused after their appearance, and thus a whole new series of problems came in for study. The result was what has been called the second epidemiologic revolution. During the past few decades, enormous advances have been made through epidemiologic studies of cancer, heart disease, stroke, and other major noninfectious diseases.

MODERN EPIDEMIOLOGY

Epidemiology is an interdisciplinary science, drawing its basic data from the health sciences, sociology, demography, statistics, geography, engineering, meteorology, and history (for comparative purposes). It relates facts to one another, to previous knowledge of a subject, and to biologic phenomena in general in a consistent way. From this, epidemiology can draw inferences and test those inferences using statistics. The inferences are limited to the study population, so they may focus on a localized epidemic or on some peculiar phase or incidence, or at the grand level epidemiologists may attempt to develop a theory applicable to the occurrence of epidemics in general. In the widest sense, epidemiology deals with the study and interpretation of mass phenomena of health and disease, and its unit is the population group rather than the individual.

Like many other disciplines, epidemiology was closely related to developments outside the field. The successful development of epidemiology required machinery for notification of morbidity and mortality; that is, development required well-organized health departments. In 1876 only eight of the 38 states and nine territories, the unorganized territory of Oklahoma, and Washington, D.C., had health departments. By 1920 all of the then 48 states had health departments as did the Hawaiian and Alaskan territories. There were no county health departments until 1880, but by 1920 there were 131. Several of the large cities

DEFINITION OF EPIDEMIOLOGY

For the purpose of this book, *epidemiology* is defined as the study of the distribution and dynamics of health and disease in populations.

Distribution implies the selection of people for attack by a disease in relation to age, sex, race, occupational and social characteristics, place of residence, susceptibility, exposure to specific agents, contact with other persons, and other characteristics.

Dynamics refers to the distribution in time and is concerned with trends, cycles, or other patterns and intervals between exposure to inciting factors and the onset of disease.

Health and disease covers not only overt morbidity, but also disease-related attributes such as immunologic status, nonapparent diseases defined only by laboratory tests, physiologic abnormalities, such as elevated blood pressure, and other health-related characteristics. Epidemiologic methods can be applied to study any health-related characteristic of a population from genetic traits to accidents, from injuries to emotional states, from health to sickness.

entered the twentieth century with health departments, and by 1920 nearly all had them. The first public health laboratory was established in New York in 1892, but the first official epidemiologist was not appointed until 1909 when the Minnesota Board of Health appointed H.W. Hill to this position. In 1910 the Minnesota Division of Epidemiology was established.

On the federal level, the Public Health Service was authorized in 1893 to cooperate with state and local health departments to prevent the spread of human diseases between the states. Federal laboratories—the precursor to the National Institute of Health—were established in 1902 and allowed the service to research diseases. Registration of births goes back to the middle of the nineteenth century in a few areas but was not made compulsory until the twentieth century. Other data were only sparsely collected in the nineteenth and first part of the twentieth centuries, and although historians can estimate incidences of various diseases from the past, the statistical source materials are not really adequate until well into the twentieth century. In fact the medical examinations of men drafted by the United States during World War I (1917-1918) provided statistics of prevalence of defects and diseases on a nationwide basis for the first time, even though it was essentially restricted to males 18 to 30 years of age.

One of the first positive consequences of the development of epidemiology was an agreement on diagnoses. Many of the early pioneers in epidemiology found it difficult to collect data because the same disease was known in different areas by different names; often there was not always agreement on which symptoms accompanied which disease. Standardized diagnostic criteria were developed to overcome this. It was also necessary to train professionals to deal with epidemiologic issues. The first special laboratory in America devoted to teaching and research in hygiene was established at the University of Michigan in 1889, and this was followed by laboratories at the University of Pennsylvania and Massachusetts Institute of Technology. The first School of Hygiene and Public Health was not established until 1916 at Johns Hopkins University, and it was in this school that the first department of epidemiology appeared.

All of this background is important in arriving at a definition of epidemiology, since it is a term that some people define differently, even though there is increasing agreement on what is meant.

Causes of Disease

The understanding of the causes of disease, which is the major object of epidemiology, involves several steps, the number of which might vary according to which author one reads. In this text three steps are used in epidemiology, but the important thing is not the number 3 but the process involved.

The first step is the description of the frequency and distribution of disease, with comparisons of its frequency in different populations and in different segments of the same population. This is sometimes called *descriptive epidemiology*. From these observations, causal hypotheses can be constructed and information given to understand the nature and extent of a particular problem.

The second step is the formulation of hypotheses, using descriptive epidemiologic data and clinical and laboratory observations to link the disease with the more or less specific population characteristics or modes of exposures.

The third step is the testing of the hypotheses through experimental or observational studies of specific groups of individuals. This is sometimes called *analytic* or *experimental epidemiology*.

Some texts also refer to *substantive epidemiology*, that is, the known epidemiologic characteristics of a particular disease or illness. Epidemiology is a method of describing a disease, but there are also other methods. For example, one can give a clinical description of a disease (the onset and progression of symptoms in individuals similarly affected). Epidemiology looks at the data collectively using variables such as age, sex, and other physiologic characteristics, probabilities, averages, geographic location, and other demographic information.

This epidemiologic method can be illustrated with a classic case of food poisoning that broke out in Chicago in the early 1980s. The clinical approach began when a patient with gastroenteritis appeared either in the physician's office or in the emergency room of the hospital and was seen by a nurse practitioner, physician, or others who took a careful history, observed the signs and symptoms, performed a physical examination, ordered laboratory tests, made a diagnosis, prescribed treatment, observed the patient's progress, and sent a report of the illness to the county health officer.

Epidemiologists monitoring the area noticed a disproportionate number of clients with gastroenteritis being hospitalized. Epidemiologists wanted to know what was causing this statistical change. Since the cases were spread throughout Chicago but not throughout Illinois, it was clear it was due to a localized incident. They then extended the search, examining the time and onset of the disease and the dietary patterns, as well as specific foods ingested, the places the patients had bought their groceries or the restaurants in which they had eaten, the kinds of activities they engaged in, and any number of other factors. By tracing the various leads, they discovered that the one factor the patients had in common was that they had purchased dairy products from one particular store chain. Since the dairy products throughout the chain appeared to have been contaminated (or at least some of them were), they determined that the dairy products must come from a common source. They went to the dairy to take samples, but initial testing did not detect the source. Still, since the epidemiologic investigation pointed to the one source, the dairy products were removed from the shelf and testing continued. Finally it was found that there was a seldom-used bypass in the sterilizing process in the dairy, and when the process was not used, the dairy products were not contaminated. In this case the disease was apparently spread by failure to clean and sterilize part of the equipment; in other cases it might be transmitted by a person, or the disease might result from a combination of factors. Thus epidemiologists prefer to use the term "determinants of disease" rather than focusing on any single cause. Although any infectious disease may be said to have a single necessary cause—the infectious agent—there are numerous contributing factors or secondary agents.

Determinants of Disease

Lead poisoning (plumbism) is a good example of multicausal factors of a disease. Although lead can enter the body through the mouth or skin and may be inhaled with fumes from burning storage batteries, exhaust from automobiles that use leaded gasoline, or any number of other environmental factors (see Chapter 6), it is most common among toddlers, 18 months to three years, who ingest it. It is more common in older sections of cities or countryside where lead-based paint was used to paint houses or where old cribs still have lead-based paint. Toddlers who are teething are likely to bite crib rails or pick up flakes of lead paint in the house or yard. Lead poisoning is more likely to occur in the summer than winter because a hot sun dries up old paint and increases the likelihood of sweet flakes falling off. Thus lead poisoning is more likely to occur among the poor than the rich because the poor cannot afford to paint as often and because many poor persons live in old tenements, which have high–lead content paint on the interiors. Indoor paint in the past generally had a higher lead content than outdoor paints.

The clinical manifestation is insidious except in cases of acute poisoning. Progressive poisoning usually occurs as the result of slow lead absorption or accumulation of lead in blood and soft tissues, where it is slowly transferred to the bones for storage. Acute lead poisoning is most likely to take place in summer from ingestion of large amounts of lead salts or inhalation of lead fumes. In children encephalitis is often a result because of vulnerability of a child's nervous system. The outbreaks are closely associated with low economic status, poor living conditions, proximity to freeways, and any number of other factors that might be regarded as secondary causes.

Often the distinction between primary and secondary determinants can come only after an investigation. Skin cancer, for example, can develop from long exposure to actinic rays, such as those from the sun, intense and prolonged exposure to ionizing radiation, or exposure to carcinogenic chemicals. One determinant therefore is climate and geography, but the other two factors might be occupational. In fact occupational level is a major factor in death rate, with higher death rates in almost all categories of diseases among laborers. The meaning of this statistic, however, is not as clear as it seems, since it might be that sicker workers tend to drift into laboring occupations. On the other hand, a healthy, vigorous, ambitious worker may move upward in occupational structure, whereas a sickly one tends to stay in lower occupations or may be downwardly mobile. Laborers in the past have experienced significant excesses in mortality as compared with other workers in such categories as tuberculosis, diseases of the respiratory system, cirrhosis of the liver, and accidents. Some occupations are much more dangerous than others for certain kinds of diseases. Asbestos workers, for example, have a high incidence of cancer of the lungs. Workers in machine shops had a higher incidence of deafness before ear plugs became widespread. Lead miners often absorbed lead dust through the skin or through their noses (National Vital Statistics Division, 1963).

STATISTICS

The analysis of the variables uses statistical methods. It was through statistical analysis that the dangers of smoking first came to be recognized. Clinical observations of the possibilities of a relationship between smoking and lung cancer date back almost to the beginning of the twentieth century. Lung cancer, however, was an infrequent cause of death during the early years of this century, and the alarm bells did not begin to go off until midcentury when it was realized that deaths from lung cancer were rising, whereas death rates from other forms of cancer and respiratory diseases were declining. Since the incidence of smoking had been rising, there was an apparent correlation, which led to further studies first in England and then in the United States (Smoking and Health, 1962; Smoking and Health, 1964).

Both the English and American researchers used animal studies, clinical and autopsy studies, and population or epidemiologic studies to establish a correlation. In animal studies, several chemical compounds and tars in tobacco smoke were established as cancer producing. Autopsies also demonstrated that smoking produced noncancerous damage that lowers the threshold to known carcinogens. Neither of these kinds of studies, however, was as important as the retrospective and prospective epidemiologic studies. In the retrospective studies, persons with lung cancer were matched with control groups not having lung cancer, and the smoking habits of the two groups were compared. In prospective studies, large groups were followed over time to discover which persons developed lung cancer. At the time of the original 1964 American report, data were available from 29 retrospective studies carried out in a variety of countries and with different research methods and design. All found a link between smoking and lung cancer, a correlation that has continued to be demonstrated. Since the original studies, there have also been a number of prospective studies. One of the things that epidemiologists have now predicted is that the rate of lung cancer in women will increase more rapidly than for men because women as a group increased their smoking habits later than men (Burnham, 1989).

Framingham Study

The best-known prospective study in the United States has been the Framingham study, which is concerned with the epidemiology of atherosclerotic disease. This study emphasizes the value of epidemiologic clinical studies. Atherosclerosis is concerned with changes in the arterial wall. Deposition of lipid material in the intima of the medium-sized and larger arteries eventually leads to atheromatous deposits and ulceration of the intimal surface in contact with the circulating blood. The early process is almost entirely asymptomatic and may take many years. It is not until near the end of the process that the deposits of the atheromatous material encroach on the lumen enough to interfere with blood supply to the heart muscle, brain, lower extremities, kidneys, or other organs. When the atheromatous lesion on the arterial wall ulcerates, the integrity of intimal surface is destroyed, and there is a possibility of clot formation. Although it is possible by arteriography to determine the degree of the narrowing of the arterial lumen before the development of symptoms of ischemia, the invasive nature of such a test makes it impractical and unethical except in the presence of symptoms suggestive of significant ischemia, and then only if there are procedures at hand to relieve the ischemia. Thus it seemed the most effective way of doing an epidemiologic study was to observe characteristics of a population before the disease became overt and try to determine the characteristics and factors involved in a disease. The town of Framingham, Mass., had been chosen for various reasons. A sample of 6507 individuals was chosen for the study—roughly two out of every three residents in the town, which then had a population of about 10,000. Only 68.5% of the selected subjects chose to participate, but there were additional volunteers. Some of those in the sample, however, already had coronary heart disease and therefore were eliminated from the study. The final sample was 5127 individuals—2282 men and 2845 women. The original study ended in 1970 after 20 years, but private funding continued it for another five years, after which the government picked up the cost again.

Periodically reports of the Framingham data were issued, and from these reports the following six major factors in coronary heart disease were identified (Dawber, 1980):

1. Hypertension
2. High blood lipid levels
3. Cigarette smoking
4. A low level of physical activity
5. Obesity
6. Diabetes mellitus

The Framingham study turned out to be another major factor in linking cigarette smoking with a series of diseases and in general in emphasizing life-style as an important factor in preserving wellness. Smoking, for example, has been determined to be a primary cause not only of lung cancer, but of cancer of the larynx, pharynx, oral cavity, esophagus, pancreas, and bladder. It doubles the risk of heart attack in males, and it interacts with certain substances such as asbestos to further increase the death rate. Smokers report more acute and chronic conditions such as chronic bronchitis, emphysema, peptic ulcers, and arteriosclerotic heart disease. Often the data are startling. The American Cancer Society, for example, studied 73,763 men from 1967 to 1976 and used death certificates to find out the cause of death (Slikoff, 1980). Smoking turned out to be a significant factor in the cause of death. From a study of 12,051 asbestos workers, it was determined that cancer rates were even higher in smokers who were exposed to asbestos.

Several conclusions appear obvious from Table 4-1. Smoking poses dangers to one's health as does exposure to asbestos. A person who must work with asbestos can still cut down the probability of an early death by not smoking, since smoking is more dangerous than working with asbestos. If the two are combined, however, the rates escalate far beyond what might have been assumed if the two variables, smoking and asbestos exposure, had been examined separately. The two variables interact with each other instead of simply being additive.

TABLE 4-1 Death Rates, Mortality, and Mortality Ratios for Smokers and Nonsmokers, with and without Asbestos Exposure

Group	Death rate per 100,000	Mortality difference	Mortality ratio
NO ASBESTOS EXPOSURE			
Nonsmokers	11.3	0	1.00
Smokers	122.6	111.3	10.85
ASBESTOS EXPOSURE			
Nonsmokers	58.4	47.1	5.17
Smokers	601.6	590.3	53.24

Some Statistical Terms

Perhaps several factors that appear in Table 4-1, such as death rate, mortality difference, and mortality ratio, need to be explained. The first item is rate, a value that in this case is figured by the following mathematic formula: the number of deaths in a specific period, divided by the population at risk for death. Death rates are always between zero and one but can be multiplied by a factor of 10 to make their meanings clearer. This can be illustrated with a hypothetic example.

There are an average of four on-the-job deaths per year at plant X, which employs 2000 people, and only one on-the-job death per year at plant Y, which employs 5000 people.

Without doing any calculation, the reader can determine that plant X has a higher rate than plant Y. The rate can be determined by using the formula. Four, the number of events (deaths), is divided by 2000, the population at risk of death. This gives a total of .002 in plant X, whereas 1 (death) divided by 5000 (the population at risk in plant Y) gives a total of .0002. If it is listed as rate per thousand, one of the standard comparisons, the rate would be multiplied by 1000. This would give two deaths per 1000 workers in plant X, but if the death rate of workers in plant Y was multiplied by 1000, the result would be .2. This makes the rates difficult to compare, so in this case the rates must be multiplied by a factor of 10 that will give a whole number as the numerator of the rate for plant Y. The calculation then would result in a rate of 20 per 10,000 in plant X and 2 per 10,000 in plant Y.

The next step is to figure the mortality difference—in this case 20 minus 2, or 18. The mortality ratio uses the lowest figure as its base number; thus, figuring ratios, 2 is to 1 as 20 is to x. In this case x would turn out to be 10. Thus working at the first factory is 10 times more likely to lead to death than working at the second one.

All other things being equal, if one had a choice, it would be statistically important to survival to work at plant Y rather than at plant X.

Probability

Probability is a statistical statement. Probability theory was, to a large extent, developed in response to demands by gamblers who sought to lessen the element that chance might play. For example, if a coin is tossed in the air, it should come to rest in one of two ways (unless it falls into a crack and stands upright)—with heads facing up or with tails up. There seems no reason why either heads or tails should come up more often than the other, and if a coin was tossed 1000 times, it could be anticipated that heads would show up about 500 times and tails would show up the rest. This is a statement of probability. Probability, simply defined, is a prediction that may be anything from certainty that a given event will occur to certainty that it will not. If it is relatively certain that a specific event will occur, such as a person ingesting some sort of liquid in the next three days to survive, the probability of its occurrence approaches one. If there is virtually no chance that it will occur, the probability approaches zero. Probabilities run between zero and one and are expressed as fractions, decimals, or percentages.

A good example is the probability of a person inheriting a genetic disease. Cystic fibrosis, as an example, is a severe genetic disorder in which the body's mucus-secreting glands function abnormally, producing large quantities of thick mucus that often localize in the lungs, pancreas, and digestive tract. Currently there is no cure, and afflicted children require a high level of concentrated care during life spans that often do not exceed 18 years.

Cystic fibrosis is inherited as a recessive gene. That means that the normal noncarrier is homozygous for the dominant gene (CC), the normal carrier has a heterozygous genotype (Cc), and the affected child is homozygous for the recessive gene (cc). Since those holding the double dose of the recessive gene rarely reproduce, the typical cross that produces a child with cystic fibrosis is Cc × Cc, which, following the Mendelian assortment and recombination of genes, yields the following offspring possibilities:

CC Cc Cc cc

The probability of having a child with cystic fibrosis is one chance in four, .25, or 25%. The probability that the child will be normal is three chances in four, .75, or 75%. The chance of the child being normal yet a carrier is one in two, .50, or 50%. Probability has no memory, and these same laws apply to each and every birth. Just because a couple had one child with cystic fibrosis does not mean that their next child will not have the disease.

Other terms are also important in the epidemiologic discussions, particularly the study of incidence and study of prevalence. Incidence is the number of new cases (or incidents) of disease that occur within a specified time period among a specified population. Poliomyelitis can serve as an example. In city A, with a population of 100,000 in 1960, there were 20 cases of poliomyelitis reported as compared with 8 cases reported in city B, which had the same population. Some conclusions can be drawn about the nature of immunization taking place in city A versus city B because, with the development of the polio vaccines, the predicted incidence was expected to be about 8 per 100,000. The public health officials immediately knew their vaccination program in city A was not as effective as expected.

Prevalence is different from incidence because it refers to all known cases of a disease in a specified population during a particular period, irrespective of when they first began. The prevalence of polio in city A, again hypothetic, was 700, including all those people who still had the disease and who contracted it before vaccination, and in city B it was 60.

Each of these measures provides important but different information. Prevalence measures the amount of disease present in a particular population, whereas incidence provides a picture of how new cases are distributed in the population. Measures of prevalence of disease are most useful in estimating the magnitude of various health problems. Knowing how much disease there is in the population and how disease spreads itself regionally and among different social segments and age groups allows more effective planning to deal with the issue. Measures of incidence, in contrast, provide a basis for studying the cause of disease, since these measures show how a disease first occurs in a population and whom it strikes. Prevalence data are not so good for this because they group together the results of factors producing the disease and factors affecting the course of the disease, including its severity, access to treatment, adequacy of treatment, and health habits.

One of the single most important and most productive guides to prevention and control is the relative risk ratio (RR). Risk ratios estimate the risk of acquiring a disease when exposed to a causal agent or risk factor. Risk ratio is derived by dividing the disease rate of a group that has been exposed to a factor by the disease rate of another group, the control group, that has not been exposed to the factor. For example, by dividing the rates of lung cancer in smokers by the rates in nonsmokers, the relative risk can be calculated as 9:1. However, when risks are based on prevalence model research, they are called prevalence ratios (PR) instead of risk ratios. When they are derived from case control studies, the relative risk ratio is expressed as an odds ratio (OR).

Case fatality rate is the death rate of persons with particular diseases. It is a significant statistic when the clients are actually followed from disease outbreak until death or recovery. It is less valuable if it is based on a defined period, since the full mortality rate of the disease might not be completely clear during any single phase of the disease process.

Secondary attack rate is calculated by observing families from the time of the introduction of the first case of the disease for the period during which related (secondary) cases might occur. The number of such secondary cases divided by the number of persons at risk in all of the families being studied gives the secondary attack rate. For the rate to be valid, however, it is necessary to know which family members might be at risk in a particular family, since some members might have contracted the disease earlier and become immune or might have been given immunity by administration of immune globulin or other means.

Mortality Statistics

A key to epidemiology is effective mortality statistics. The main reason that a law was passed to require the signature of a medical professional on a death certificate before cremation, burial, or other actions could be performed was to lay a basis for mortality statistics. In addition to the cause of death, the laws now require that sex, race, marital status, birthdate, usual occupation, birthplace, service in the armed forces, and Social Security number be included in mortality statistics.

Responsibility for the reliability of any statistic is on those doing the reporting (still usually the physician). This method of reporting leaves many things we would like to know to subjective judgment, as well as to the whim of fashion in diagnosis. This is particularly true with deaths related to illnesses or events that large sections of society look on with disfavor or that might bring onus on the family. A good example of this is the failure to list as cause of death any sexually transmitted diseases (STDs), particularly AIDS and syphilis, or of diseases brought about by these STDs. Another example is suicide. Health departments do not have the personnel or resources to cross-check all cause-of-death reports, so results are sometimes inaccurate. Even with such factors as illegitimacy, women whose socioeconomic status is low are more likely to be reported as single mothers than are other single mothers.

The data can be erroneous in other ways. A study was performed that traced addresses from 1177 birth certificates drawn randomly and found that on 68 of the birth certificates the addresses were nonexistent or the family name on the birth certificate was unknown to the people who lived at the address or even in that neighborhood (Bullough, 1972). Since much data are based on geographic location, whether census tract or school district, this adds another source of error to the vital statistics. It does not negate their value but suggests some caution in their use.

Death rates are computed and published for all causes and ages and in many combinations of place, race, age, and sex (Health, 1982). The crude death rate is calculated for a designated period, usually one year. The numerator of the rate is all deaths in the period. The denominator is the number of persons who were in the population in which the death occurred, but who were estimated to be living at the midperiod. Death rates are calculated by political subdivisions, since this is the way census data on which population figures are based are calculated. As indicated previously, there is obviously room for error, but it is hoped the percentage of error remains somewhat constant. There are special kinds of statistics such as cause specific; that is, the number of deaths for which the underlying cause given on the death certificate is a particular condition, such as cancer of the esophagus. Age-specific rates are derived from the number of deaths in a specified age range, whereas place-specific rates apply to those in a particular geographic area. All of these can give insights to epidemiologists, since if there is a larger ratio of deaths from one cause in a particular area than in most other areas, this suggests an abnormality. This is true for any of the other specified ranges.

In general, broad categories of death are more accurately certified than death from specific diseases. Although death certificates try to distinguish between immediate and underlying cause and there is usually a space for reporting other conditions, the philosophic approach of the person signing the death certificate—usually a physician—is all-important. Not all physicians are aware of the advancing medical knowledge, nor are all findings, even when an autopsy is performed, readily available when the death certificate is completed. Although it is possible to correct the certificate later, this is seldom done. Usually only the condition listed as the underlying cause of death is coded routinely in the published reports, and only recently has attention been given to other conditions as well.

This subjective approach to filling out a death certificate emphasizes the dangers of international comparisons because there are also cultural differences in diagnostic terminology. Chronic bronchitis is more often listed as a cause of death in the British Isles than in the United States because British practitioners use it as a more all-inclusive diagnosis than do U.S. physicians. Still, mortality statistics are a primary tool in epidemiology and reveal much about the general health of population. It is clear, for example, that infant mortality has a clear relationship to social and economic factors and that it often indicates the existence of severe economic problems or a maldistribution of resources.

Mortality for a specific disease over time can be presented graphically (Fig. 4-1), indicating that lung cancer, for example, increased first in men and then in women, after the introduction of cigarette smoking among members of that sex. The mortality increases with age, although it tends to level off at 70 years of age.

Mortality can also be measured by "cohort," a term developed by W.H. Frost in the 1930s. Cohort is defined as a segment of the population born during a particular period and traced through successive age periods of life (Fig. 4-2).

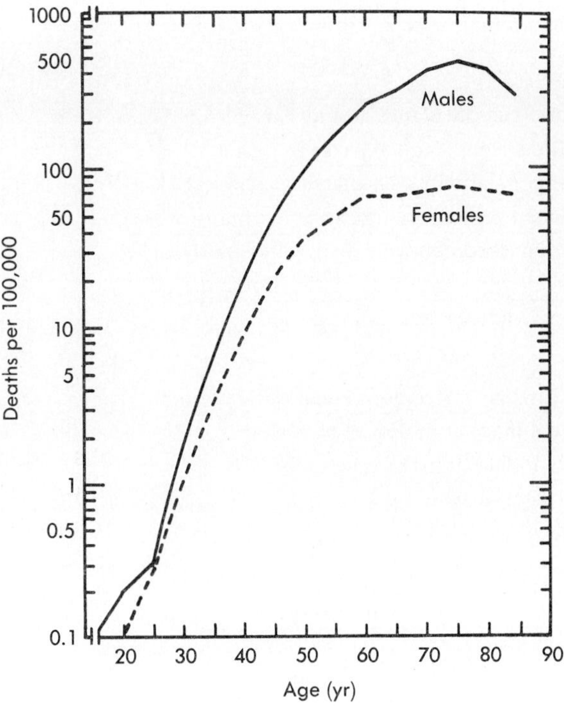

FIG. 4-1. Mortality rate per 100,000 from cancer of lung by age and sex, logarithmic rate scale.

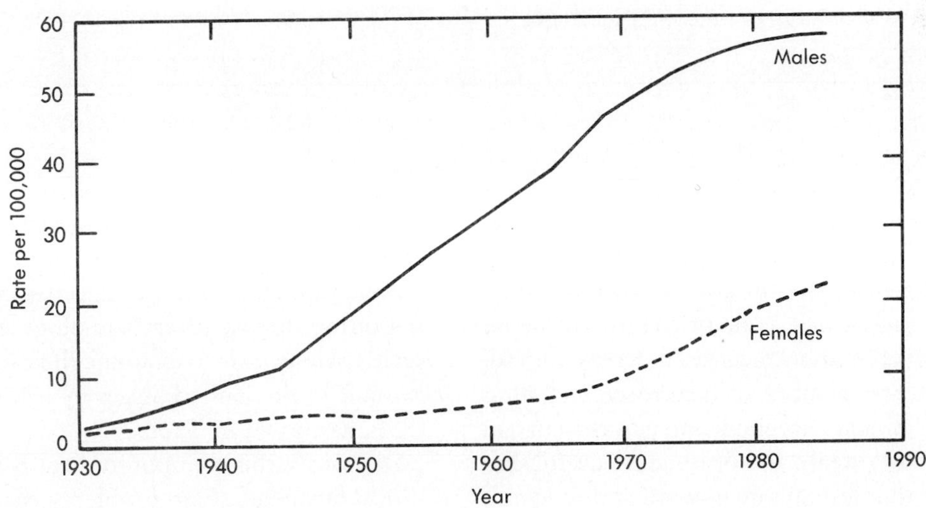

FIG. 4-2. Age-standardized mortality for lung cancer in U.S. whites and U.S. women from 1930 to 1983.

TABLE 4-2 Rates of Some Commonly Used Indices of Community Health

Table type	Population factor
GENERAL MORTALITY	
Crude rate $= \frac{\text{Deaths during a year}}{\text{Average population as calculated at midyear}}$	Per 100,000 population
Cause-specific rate $= \frac{\text{Deaths from a stated cause in year}}{\text{Average population as calculated at midyear}}$	Per 100,000 population
Age-specific rate $= \frac{\text{Deaths among persons in a given age group in year}}{\text{Average population in same age groups (midyear)}}$	Per 100,000 population
Proportional rate $= \frac{\text{Deaths from a specific cause in given time period}}{\text{Total deaths in same period}}$	Per 100,000 population
MORBIDITY	
Incidence $= \frac{\text{New cases of disease in a place during a specific period}}{\text{Persons in a place at midpoint of period}}$	Per 100,000 population
Prevalence $= \frac{\text{Existing cases in a place at given time}}{\text{Persons in a place at same time}}$	Per 100,000 population
MATERNAL AND INFANT MORTALITY	
Maternal (puerperal) rate $= \frac{\text{Deaths from puerperal causes in year}}{\text{Live births in same year}}$	Per 1000 live births
Infant rate $= \frac{\text{Deaths of children younger than one year of age during year}}{\text{Live births in same year}}$	Per 1000 live births
Neonatal rate $= \frac{\text{Deaths of children younger than one year of age in a year}}{\text{Live births in same year}}$	Per 1000 live births
Fetal rate $= \frac{\text{Fetal deaths during year}}{\text{Live births and fetal deaths in same year}}$	Per 1000 live births and fetal deaths
Perinatal rate $= \frac{\text{Fetal deaths at 28 weeks or more and infant deaths younger than seven days of age during a year}}{\text{Live births and fetal deaths at 28 weeks or more in same year}}$	Per 1000 live births and fetal deaths

Although the cohort may be altered by such things as movement across the borders of the area or country concerned, it still gives insight. An individual's changing risk as he or she ages is better indicated by the cohort curve, whereas the administrator and planner of health services finds the cross-sectional curve indicative of the current distribution of disease and death more useful. For a condition that displays no upward or downward time trends, both views usually show the same age pattern. There are various other measures that can be used. Some of those most commonly used by the community health nurse are shown in Table 4-2.

Perhaps one of the more effective ways of demonstrating the use of epidemiology as a guide to health problems is to examine the causes of death by rank in the United States in 1900, 1960, and 1980, as shown in Table 4-3.

Obviously the community health nurse of the 1960s faced different problems than the nurse who was entering public health at the beginning of the twentieth century. As the incidence of contagious diseases decreased, other causes of death

TABLE 4-3 Leading Causes of Deaths by Rank, United States, 1900, 1960, 1980

Rank	Cause of death	Deaths per 100,000 population	Percent of all deaths
1900*			
	All causes	1719.1	100.0
1	Influenza and pneumonia	202.2	11.8
2	Tuberculosis (all forms)	194.4	11.3
3	Gastritis	142.7	8.3
4	Disease of the heart	137.4	8.0
5	Vascular lesions affecting central nervous system	106.9	6.2
6	Chronic nephritis	81.0	4.7
7	All accidents	72.3	4.2
8	Malignant neoplasms (cancer)	64.0	3.7
9	Certain diseases of early infancy	62.6	3.6
10	Diphtheria	40.3	2.3
1960			
	All causes	945.7	100.0
1	Diseases of the heart	366.4	38.7
2	Malignant neoplasms (cancer)	147.4	15.6
3	Vascular lesions affecting central nervous system	107.3	11.3
4	All accidents	51.9	5.5
5	Certain diseases of early infancy	37.0	3.9
6	Influenza and pneumonia	36.6	3.5
7	General arteriosclerosis	20.3	2.1
8	Diabetes mellitus	17.1	1.8
9	Congenital malformations	12.0	1.3
10	Cirrhosis of the liver	11.2	1.2
1980†			
	All causes	878.3	100.0
1	Diseases of the heart	336.0	38.2
2	Malignancies	183.9	20.9
3	Cerebrovascular diseases	75.1	8.6
4	All accidents and their adverse effects	46.7	5.3
5	Chronic obstructive pulmonary disease‡	24.7	2.8
6	Pneumonia and influenza	24.1	2.7
7	Diabetes mellitus	15.4	1.8
8	Cirrhosis and chronic liver disease	13.5	1.5
9	Atherosclerosis	13.0	1.5
10	Suicide	11.9	1.4

Modified from Lerner M and Anderson OW: Health progress in the United States: 1900-1960, Chicago, 1963, University of Chicago Press, and from Vital Statistics, 1980: Hyattsville, Md, 1987, National Center for Health Statistics.

*Rates for 1900 apply to the death-registration states only.

†One reason for the decline in death rate in 1980 was the comparative youth of the population and greater longevity of U.S. residents. These rates began to rise again in 1986. Congenital malformations and diseases of early infancy declined in part because of the lower birth rate during that same period.

‡Before 1980 listed separately as bronchitis, emphysema, asthma.

increased because, even though people lived longer, they still ultimately died. Tuberculosis, for example, had disappeared from the top 10 causes of death, as had chronic nephritis and diphtheria. Diabetes, which certainly was fatal until insulin was discovered in the 1920s, has moved up as a cause of death, perhaps because more people are being diagnosed as diabetic. Cirrhosis of the liver, associated primarily with alcoholism, also gained importance, although some of the cases of nephritis might have been due to the same cause. Congenital malformations were also one of the top 10 causes of death in 1960, indicating better maternal care, which undoubtedly led to many more women carrying infants to term who otherwise might have spontaneously aborted. The rise of cancer is perhaps due to the fact that more people are living longer, but it also, as indicated in the earlier discussion, is associated with such things as smoking and pollution.

ROLE OF THE COMMUNITY HEALTH NURSE

The nurses who work in the community have come to recognize that neighborhoods with a high proportion of infant births present different problems from those with a predominant population of elderly people. Using the available data, a nurse can predict what service might be needed, as well as determine how effective such services might be. In short, epidemiology gives nurses the means for assessment of needs, planning, implementation, and evaluation. It can also give some kinds of data for dealing with individual patients such as heavy smokers, asbestos workers, alcoholics, and diabetics and allow the nurse to take preventive steps. Throughout this book, epidemiologic data are used in specific situations to illustrate the use of such data by the nurse more effectively.

SUMMARY

Epidemiology is an interdisciplinary science aimed at identifying the causes of illness. Although this quest for an understanding of illness dates from ancient times, the modern science of epidemiology was dependent on the nineteenth century development of statistical methodology. Following this development, studies could be done tracing the incidence, mortality, location, and cause of a contagious disease. Twentieth century epidemiologists have broadened their concern to include other types of illnesses, including cancer and heart disease. In the process they have linked lung cancer to smoking and identified the risk factors related to atherosclerotic heart disease.

QUESTIONS FOR DISCUSSION

1. Define the term "epidemiology."
2. What steps might you take to carry out an epidemiologic study of a specific disease in a given population?
3. If the problem you were studying was lead poisoning, what might be the findings of your epidemiologic study?
4. Why are good local and national systems for recording vital statistics extremely important to epidemiologists?

REFERENCES

Bullough B: The non respondents: problems using birth certificates, Med Rec News 46:18, 1975.

Burnham JC: American physicians and tobacco use, Bul Hist Med 63:1, 1989.

Dawber TR: The Framingham study: the epidemiology of atherosclerotic disease, Cambridge, Mass, 1980, Harvard University Press and the Commonwealth Fund.

Health: United States, 1982, DHS Publication No (PHS) 83-1232, Washington, DC, 1982, US Government Printing Office.

Lerner M and Anderson OW: Health progress in the United States: 1900-1960, Chicago, 1963, University of Chicago Press.

Slikoff IJ: Scientific basis for control of environmental health hazards. In Last JM, editor: Maxcy-Rosenau public health and preventive medicine, ed 11, New York, 1980, Appleton & Lange.

Smoking and health, A report by the Royal College of Physicians, London, 1962, Pitman Medical Publishing Co.

Smoking and health, DHS Publication No (PHS) 1103, Washington, DC, 1964, US Government Printing Office.

National Center for Health Statistics National vital statistics division, Mortality by occupational level and cause of death among men 20 to 64 years of age, US Special Reports 53:105, 1963.

Vital statistics, 1980: Hyattsville, Md, 1987, National Center for Health Statistics.

BIBLIOGRAPHY

Abramson JH: Re: definitions of epidemiology, Am J Epidemiol 109:99, 1979.

Frost WH: The age selection of mortality from tuberculosis in successive decades, Am J Hygiene 30:91, 1939.

Lilienfeld D: Definitions of epidemiology, Am J Epidemiol 107:87, 1978.

Miettinen OS: Theoretical epidemiology, principles of occurrence, New York, 1985, John Wiley & Sons.

Valanis B: Epidemiology in nursing and health care, East Norwalk, Conn, 1986, Appleton & Lange.

Winslow CEA: The history of American epidemiology, St Louis, 1952, CV Mosby Co.

CHAPTER

5

Health Education

Marietta Stanton

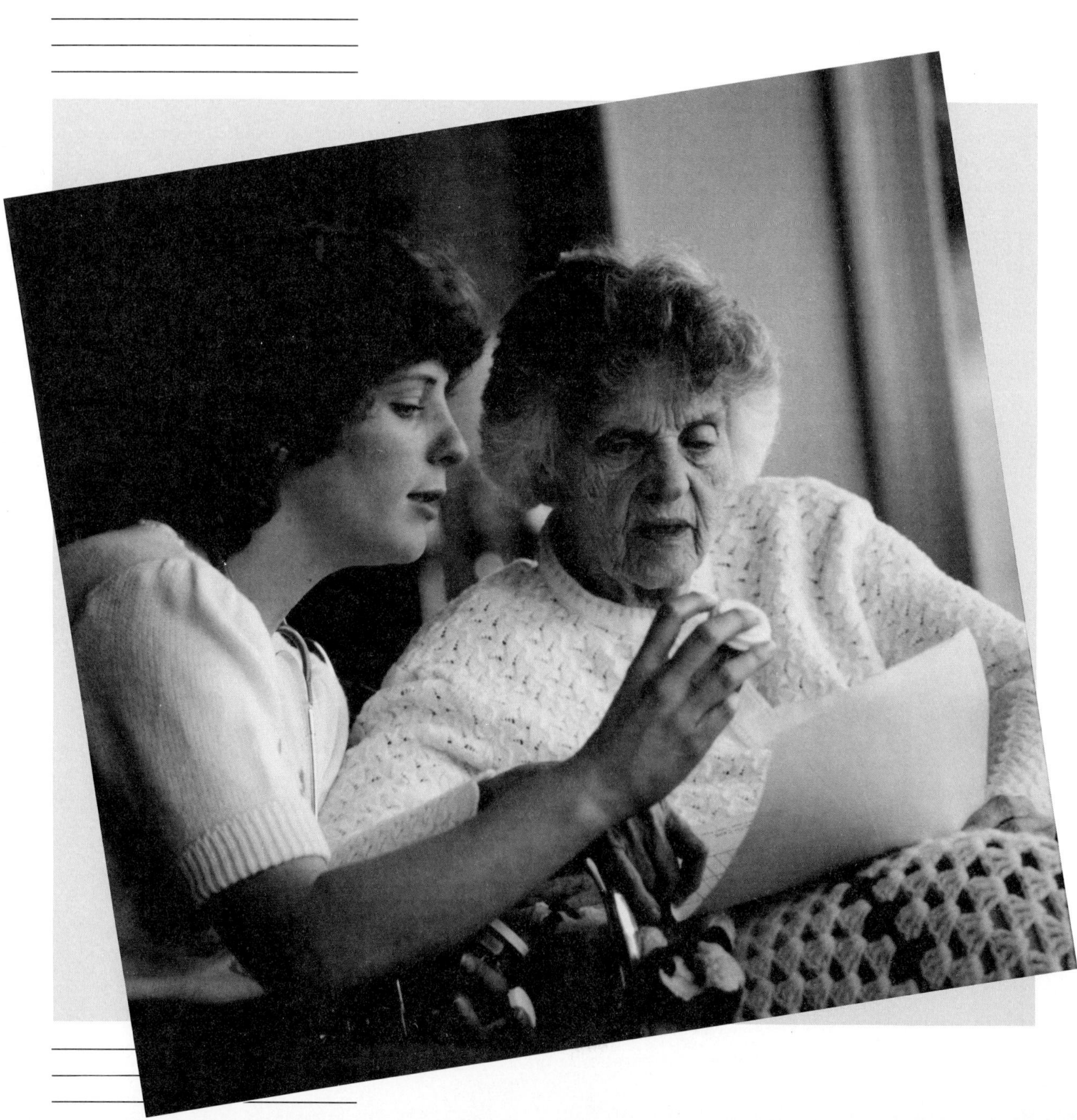

CHAPTER OUTLINE

Learning theories
Health belief model and individual health behavior
- Compliance
- Motivation
- Readiness to learn

Theories of communication
Nursing process and client education
Nurse and a plan for educating clients
- Design phase
- Implementation and evaluation

Nurse's educative role in health promotion and disease prevention
Nurse's educative role in overt illness
Nursing the community
Nurse and other members of the health care team
Summary

OBJECTIVES

After completing this chapter, the reader should be able to:

1. Formulate a theoretic approach to the development of client education programs.
2. Develop a teaching program for a specific client.
3. Integrate the nursing process into the client education continuum.
4. Discuss an approach to health education at the community level.
5. Determine the nurse's role in coordinating client education.

HEALTH EDUCATION in a community environment requires a four-pronged thrust to maximize health potential. Health promotion, preventive health teaching, client education about disease processes, and client involvement during the rehabilitation phase must occur. Since intervention might be required at any point in the health education cycle (Fig. 5-1), a community health nurse must have not only a full repertoire of knowledge and skills but a realization that educational processes are an integral component of nursing.

Health education can be either formal or informal. Informal teaching focuses on the unique needs of clients as different needs arise, usually on a one-to-one basis. On the other hand, formal health teaching is defined as organized classes for one or more individuals where both the content and strategies are preplanned. Usually teaching plans are drawn up to meet specific educational needs, but when the nurse encounters a previously unassessed educational need, on-the-spot teaching should also be used and refined later as time permits. Since the community health nurse encounters a wide variety of individuals with unique values and needs, teaching must be accommodated to deal with a range of potential health behaviors, as well as levels of compliance.

Inevitably the community health nurse has a real opportunity to affect health behaviors and practices, but to meet these responsibilities, the nurse must obtain a sound training in health teaching and be able to apply it to the community environment. Some knowledge of the learning theories is basic to gaining understanding of teaching.

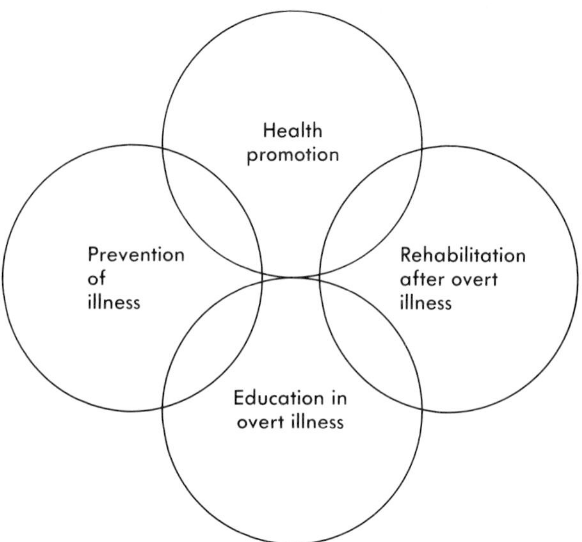

FIG. 5-1. Health teaching cycle.

LEARNING THEORIES

Learning is the process whereby changes in knowledge or attitudes occur. Theories of learning postulate how those changes occur. These theories also provide some insight into the mechanisms by which thinking, behavior, or attitudes are changed. Many theories of learning have evolved in this century, and traditionally these have been applied to the more formalized school settings. They can, however, also provide a foundation for health education, since every learner and learning situation is different and an understanding of diverse theoretic approaches increases ability to teach.

Twentieth century learning theories generally encompass two major schools of thought. The first comprises the conditioning theories of the behavioristic family, and the second comprises the cognitive theories of the Gestalt-field family.

For behaviorists or conditioning theorists, learning is a change in behavior. It occurs when stimuli and responses become related according to mechanistic principles (Bigge, 1976). A change in behavior produces patterns of activity that emerge from a series of responses and stimuli. Stimuli from the environment produce a specific response or increase the probability of a specific response. Behaviorist theorists interpret learning in terms of changes in behavioral tendencies. Early behaviorists such as Thorndike had a concept of learning involving a process termed "stamping in," an accidental form of response modification (Bigge, 1976). In other words, the focused repetition of an activity becomes part of an individual's normal behavior pattern if the behavior is consistently rewarded and reinforced. These pioneer behaviorists were interested in the neural physiology of behavior change. In addition, they focused on the specific circumscribed elements of the stimulus-response situation. More contemporary behavioristic theorists, or neobehaviorists, place less emphasis on the actual physiologic operation of the neurologic system but instead focus on response and modification. Neobehaviorists attempt to explain purposeful behavior—something the earlier behaviorists did not do. They also focus on a more complex stimulus-response configuration. Some neobehaviorists, such as Gagne and Skinner, emphasize successive, systematic changes in the learner's environment, producing change through reinforcement and response. Behaviorists see the person as an organism; they focus on the physical environment and interpret change as action or reaction to specific stimuli.

For Gestalt-field theorists, learning is a process of changing insights, outlooks, expectations, or thought patterns (Bigge, 1976). These theorists are more concerned with the individual's psychologic environment than the physical one. Learning is visualized as an interactive rather than a perceptive process. In fact, learning is described in terms of a reorganization of perceptual sets. Students change behavior through an understanding of significant problems in a given situation, and this enables them to manipulate and change their environment to their own advantage. A well-known theorist who supports this approach is Lewin. The organism is still conceived of as a person, but the focus is on the individual's psychologic environment. Change is interpreted as a mutual, simultaneous interaction by the organism with the environment.

Although the descriptions of these two schools of thought represent some of the differences between the two, they do not fully reflect the vast amount of literature available for both sets of theory. Moreover, despite the apparent differences between the two approaches, the following are learning principles acceptable to both:

1. Motivation plays a central role in learning. Whether motivation springs from physiologic or psychologic needs, it plays a crucial role in the success of the learning process.
2. Intrinsic motivation is superior to extrinsic motivation. In other words, motivation that arises from an individual's inner needs (intrinsic motivation) better facilitates learning than motivation stimulated by an external source (extrinsic motivation).
3. Praise or blame is usually more effective in promoting learning than ignoring the achievement or lack thereof.
4. Mutual goal setting between teacher and student in terms of learning needs and goals facilitates learning.
5. Readiness to learn is necessary for the achievement of learning goals.
6. Practice is important to learning.
7. Learning that is made meaningful to the individual and has applicability to the individual's situation increases the retention of learned material.
8. Overlearning contributes to retention. This implies that continued practice after initial mastery of knowledge or skill is important.
9. Spaced review is superior to so-called cramming.

In addition to the accepted principles listed previously, Knowles (1980) has proposed other conditions of learning that should be incorporated into any planning for client education. Many of these are simple commonsense axioms. The learning environment should be characterized by physical comfort, mutual trust and respect, freedom of expression, and acceptance of differences. Learners should perceive the goals of the learning experience and have a sense of progress toward these goals. When goal setting is shared between teacher and learner, both have accountability for the outcome. Although these general principles are directed toward the adult learner, they can also be applied to children or adolescents.

In addition to the preceding discussion of learning theory, the nurse should be aware that many theorists differentiate between the teaching of children and the teaching of adults. Adult learners are problem oriented and use their own experiences as a basis for learning. The younger learner is more dependent and malleable. The teaching role in the adult situation is more facilitative, whereas with the child the teacher is more controlling and provides direction. Evaluation of the adult is geared primarily toward self-diagnosis, whereas with the child there is more of an emphasis on adherence to standards within a judgmental environment (Knowles, 1980).

What does all this mean to the nurse who must provide learning situations that promote health, prevent disease, or promote optimum health potential? Quite simply, it means that the theories of learning provide a foundation for health education. They provide principles on which one can build a teaching-learning situation. A variety of theories are needed because nurses may encounter various types of learners with varying levels of skills and because nurses must instruct learners on a variety of subjects that vary in complexity and intensity. In some situations the nurse may not be able to use the cognitive, or field, approach to the learning situation. Perhaps the patient needs knowledge or skills to survive, and these must immediately become a conditioned response. The nurse in this situation does not have the benefit of time to enable the patient to explore the rationale for survival skills. Initial teaching may emerge from a behavioristic philosophy for the client to do one thing and the nurse to do another. Later, as the nurse encounters sociocultural blocks or attitudes that interfere with further convalescence, it might be important to provide insightful, problem-solving learning situations proposed by the Gestalt-field theory. A behavioristic approach might work better when the patient needs to master psychomotor skills. A cognitive-field approach may facilitate the acquisition of new knowledge or attitudes. None of the previous material is prescriptive; it merely states that the nurse may need to use both types of learning theories when planning approaches to unique individuals. For example, in the discussion differentiating the child from the adult learner, one perceives that different approaches to the learners based on age were emphasized. However, in some situations when an adult is ill and more dependent, principles from the pedagogic model designed for children may be most useful in determining teaching strategies. Some adults, whether they are ill or not, want control of their environment. One would not succeed in using a pedagogic model in that specific teaching-learning situation. Children because of their immaturity need more structure and limits than most adults require or desire.

Additionally, both approaches may be applicable to the same client. For instance, in teaching a client a self-care procedure, the nurse may demonstrate and redemonstrate a certain activity such as self-irrigation of a wound. The nurse demonstrates the procedure and has the client redemonstrate the procedure while reinforcing appropriate actions. As clients become more adept at this, the nurse may begin explaining more complex information to assist them in making decisions about modifications to the procedure. The nurse, in dealing with the client, continually assesses the client's abilities and uses the approach inherent in either type of learning theory to facilitate the client's mastery of this aspect of self-care. This can also be applied to the family members or significant others assisting with care.

HEALTH BELIEF MODEL AND INDIVIDUAL HEALTH BEHAVIOR

Understanding health care behavior is also important to the nurse involved in community health care. The health belief model (Rosenstock, 1966)

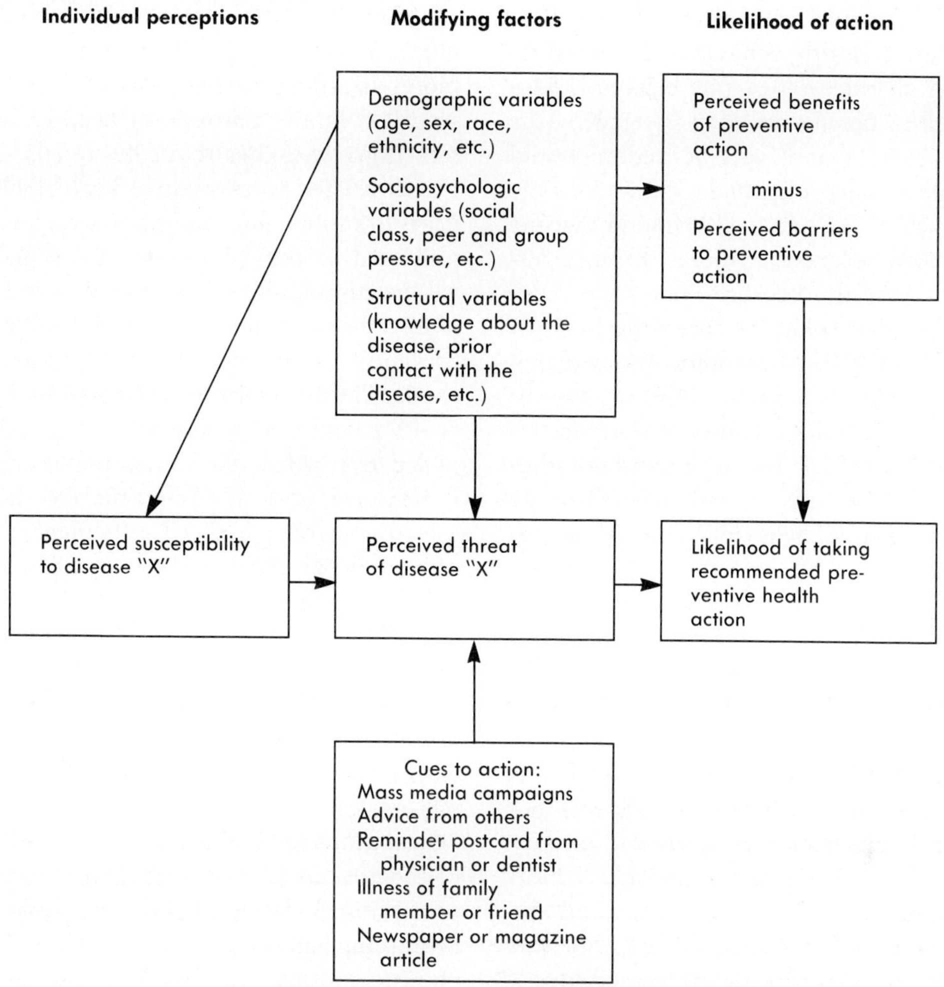

FIG. 5-2. Health belief model.

helps the health care provider predict health care behaviors and helps identify approaches that influence health care outcomes.

As originally developed, this model describes actions taken by a healthy individual to prevent illness. It depicts theories of decision making and relates these to various health behaviors. The behavior motivation part of this theory is attributed to Lewin, a social psychologist (Davidhezar, 1983). According to Lewin (1935), behavior is dependent on the value placed by an individual on an outcome and on the individual's perception that a certain behavior will produce that outcome.

In Fig. 5-2 the Rosenstock (1966 and 1974) model of this theory is represented. Following this model, a decision to take a health action is based on perceptions of susceptibility to a condition and the severity of the consequences resulting from that condition. The decision to pursue a particular health action is influenced by the potential benefits of preventing or reducing susceptibility to or severity of a sickness and the psychologic, as well as the financial and other, costs for pursuing a particular health action. The model also includes cues to action that are internal or external stimuli to a particular health behavior.

Although this model was initially designed to study preventive health behaviors, it has since been used to investigate sick-role behaviors. Activities aimed at getting well are affected by the individual's belief that a specific action would ameliorate illness, an individual's estimate of the severity of that illness, and the likelihood that the individual could reduce that threat through personal action (Janz and Becker, 1984).

The health belief model has been the focus of a considerable number of theoretic and research investigations. Janz and Becker (1984) have reviewed 46 of these and found different significant dimensions of the model. Twenty-four of the studies investigated preventive health behaviors, 19 investigated sick-role behaviors, and three researched clinic use.

According to their summary the most powerful dimension of the health belief model was the so-called perceived barriers. Although both were important overall, perceived susceptibility was a stronger contributor to understanding preventive health behavior, whereas perceived benefits was the most significant dimension in sick-role behavior. Of the four dimensions, perceived severity produced the lowest overall significance for all the studies examined; this dimension had the strongest relationship to sick-role behavior but had a weak association with preventive health behavior (Janz and Becker, 1984).

Pender (1987) has modified this classic model in studies of preventive health behavior. Besides perceived threat, perceived susceptibility, and perceived seriousness of the original model guiding individual perceptions, two other factors are added to the health belief model. According to Pender, research appears to support the addition of perceived importance of health and perceived control. The emergence of importance of health as an additional factor may be related to the American public's increasing orientation to prevention rather than disease. Internal versus external locus of control has also been found to be predictive of preventive health behaviors in selected studies. Other variations in the health belief model are suggested by Pender with regard to the modifying factors. These modifying factors are so-called family patterns of health care and interactions with health professionals. Again research related to preventive health behavior appears to support these additional factors. Pender's proposed modifications have many implications for the community health nurse because the community health nurse has a front-line position in preventive health care. Pender has also proposed changes in the health belief model with regard to health promotion. Cognitive-perceptual variables added that affect the decision-making phase of health promotion are importance of health, perceived control, perceived self-efficacy, definition of health, perceived health status, perceived benefits of health-promoting behaviors, and perceived barriers to health-promoting behaviors. Pender additionally discusses interpersonal, demographic, biologic, and situational factors that are modifying factors of the health belief model with regard to health-promoting behaviors. Interpersonal factors within this model include the expectations of significant others, family patterns of health care, and interactions with health professionals. Situational determinants of health-promoting behavior appear to include health-promoting options available and ease of access to health-promoting alternatives. Demographic characteristics, such as age, sex, and race, are seen as affecting health-promoting behavior indirectly through their affect on cognitive and perceptual mechanisms.

Biologic characteristics are modifying factors in health promotion behaviors. For instance, body weight seems to be a significant predictor of intention to engage in exercise (Pender, 1987).

A community health nurse is continually involved in all aspects of health education, health promotion, and disease prevention for the client with overt illness. In dealing with overt illness, the nurse must focus on severity of illness and the consequences to the individual client. By focusing on the severity of symptoms and demonstrating the implications for the client's particular life-style, the nurse can have improved results in changing unhealthful behaviors. At the same time, it is important to find out if there are barriers to the client adapting these more healthy behaviors. If these barriers are apparent, the nurse can plan strategies to circumvent these obstacles.

In working with clients on promotion of health and disease prevention, the community health nurse must focus on susceptibility and examine its consequences in terms of the patient's culture, life-style, and value system. Again, barriers such as cost and accessibility must be evaluated. Even if clients believe susceptibility is a problem, they may perceive the cost as both personally and financially too great to justify changing the behavior.

The health belief model and Pender's modified prevention and promotion models are useful tools for community health nurses, since they encourage nurses to examine an individual's unique set of circumstances and design health care and client education accordingly.

Compliance

Client compliance with treatment plans is a widespread problem in the treatment of medical disorders (Ross and Guggenheim, 1983). Kiesler and Kiesler (1970) make a distinction between compliance and private acceptance. Compliance involves a change in behavior but may not be based on attitudinal change. Personal acceptance involves a change in health behavior, as well as a change in attitude.

Kelman (1969) has expanded the concept of compliance further. He maintains compliance is related to two more types of personal and social influence—identification and internalization.

Identification appears to involve a certain adaptation of another's behavior because the relationship with that person is positive. This low-level type of compliance persists as long as the relationship between the influencer and individual is positive. Therefore behavior change is reversible and subject to social interference.

A higher-order aspect of compliance is internalization. With internalization the health behavior fits into the individual's existing value system. At this point behavior is resistant to change. It would appear paramount to move compliance from an identification to an internalization process. There are other more universal factors that affect compliance. Individuals for the most part have a need to fit in with their particular peer group. In addition, they need to be popular and conform to cultural norms, or behave like other people (Kiesler and Kiesler, 1970).

Festinger (1953) discusses a theory of dissonance. According to this theory, the decision to comply is made once. Choosing compliance or noncompliance produces dissonance in both instances. Compliance on one hand involves perhaps approval by an influential group of health care providers. Noncompliance involves perhaps a conflict with personal values and experiences.

Becker and others (1972) explain compliance with sociopsychologic theory of value expectancy. This purports that compliant behavior is governed by the value of its results to the individual.

Motivation plays a part in compliant behavior (Lewin, 1935). This theory has been used with various health behaviors.

Caplan and others (1976) maintain that knowledge of one's disease and motivation to achieve control are predictors of compliance. Support and attention from the caregiver are reported to promote adherence (Haynes, Taylor, and Sackett, 1979). Home visits (Earp, Ory, and Strogatz, 1982) and contracts have also improved compliance (Steckel and Swain, 1977). Kerr (1985) found that self-monitoring increased adherence. The usefulness of self-monitoring techniques is reiterated by Epstein and Masek (1978) and Gabriel and others (1977).

So-called tailoring and use of prompts and reminders have been cited as a manner in which compliance may be increased (Schmidt, 1979). Tailoring refers to coordinating, for example, medication administration times with the client's daily schedule. Direct prompts used include leaving the pill bottle on the television set so that it is in view when the news, for instance, comes on. Indirect prompts include leaving messages on frequently used items such as a watch or salt shaker.

Contingency management is another method for improving adherence behaviors (Dapcich-Miura and Hovell, 1979). This intervention employs a system of rewards that are gained with compliant behavior. Conversely a response-cost system can be used where demerits are given for noncompliant behavior.

Nagy and Wolfe (1984) found that when patients were satisfied with the care they received and rated their physician high in terms of competence and responsiveness, they were compliant.

Schultz (1980) found that poor family functioning, little social support, and low self-esteem of the client or a significant other were indicators of high risk for noncompliance.

Cerkoney and Hart (1980) found that clients who have symptoms and who perceive their illness as severe tend to be more compliant. Buchanan and others (1979) found that, as symptoms disappeared, noncompliance became more frequent.

Although sociodemographic factors are predictive of entry into the health care system, they are not predictive of compliance levels once treatment is initiated (Haynes, 1976).

Many factors seem to affect compliance, as well as noncompliance. It is evident in the literature that the health belief model can be used to predict compliance to a certain degree. It is equally apparent that this is a complex issue requiring a great deal more research and analysis.

In summary, compliance can be approached from two levels—the theoretic and the practical levels. On the theoretic level the community health nurse becomes aware that true compliance involves an internalization of the value of the health care behavior. An integration of the activity or concept into the client's repertoire of behaviors is requisite for true compliance. On the practical level, even if the client makes a conscious decision to comply, helpful reminders and prompts might be of great assistance. Support, understanding, and creative approaches on the part of the community health nurse may help the client achieve compliant behaviors.

Motivation

Any discussion of compliance without reference to motivation and readiness to learn on the part of the client can be fruitless.

Motivation to perform a certain activity is produced by a system of extrinsic (external) or intrinsic (internal) rewards. Extrinsic motivation occurs when a reward that is valuable to the client is provided to stimulate a particular behavior. Some examples might be a child prompted to stop crying by the offer of a lollipop, a student studying all night to obtain a passing grade, and a man slowing his car to below the speed limit when seeing a police car to avoid receiving a ticket. All of these activities are prompted by an external source. Internal motivation is of a higher order in that behavior is prompted by a system of internal rewards rather than the external rewards previously described. The client performs or exhibits a particular behavior because personal satisfaction is gained from its completion. For instance an individual pursues a research project because of personal interest in finding facts related to the project. A person works diligently on a painting project and finds personal satisfaction in the result.

The major difference between the two types of motivation is that with external motivation the desired behavior occurs only as long as the external reward system is available. With internal motivation the behavior recurs indefinitely as long as personal satisfaction occurs. Obviously, internal motivation is the more desirable alternative.

However, how a person fosters this type of motivational pattern is highly individualized and dependent on that person's individual system of values and needs.

As was discussed with compliance and the health belief model with adaptation, many factors affect decisions to perform specific health behaviors. Behavior that is consistent with a specific value system is more likely to be exhibited. Therefore motivation is contingent on persuading or demonstrating to the individual client that a particular behavior is beneficial and consistently reinforcing until the activity becomes internally satisfying to the individual. How does one accomplish this? It is a highly individualized process, and the nurse must really assess the clients' needs but also be in tune with their sociocultural values and mores. A useful approach applied to other fields that may be valuable here is a marketing approach to client care (Stanton, 1979).

In marketing, four principles are applied regarding product, price, promotion, and place (Kotler, 1976). All four factors affect the success of any particular product. The product must be attractive to the consumer; it must be psychologically and financially priced right; it must be accessible; and the person must know about it and understand that it is beneficial. Only when the price, product, promotion, and place are consistent with needs will someone be motivated to buy the product. Nurses can be health education marketers. Any company that has a successful marketing campaign carefully assesses the values and needs of the consumer and creatively seeks approaches to motivate consumers to buy that company's product. Nurses can do this. It is useful to know the difference between marketing and selling. Selling is short term. It does not consider needs and values, but the promotion is so pervasive that people buy the product. Selling does not concern itself with customer satisfaction because it is interested in a one-time investment on the part of the consumer. On the other hand, marketing carefully analyzes satisfaction with the product because marketers value return business. Motivating an individual to "buy" a health care action or behavior takes creative marketing of that behavior and careful analysis of how it fits into the individual's value system. There are many approaches to motivation, which is generally considered a prerequisite to learning. However, these four marketing principles can assist the nurse in determining individual needs, meeting those needs, and initiating change in health care behavior.

Readiness to Learn

Besides motivating people to learn throughout the health education continuum, nurses must consider readiness to learn. If an individual is not motivated and open to or ready for the learning situation, the teaching-learning process may be less effective. This is important in health promotion and prevention but critically important to the individual with an overt illness.

Crate (1965) discussed psychosocial adaptation to illness and client teaching. The stages in this adaptation are denial, developing awareness, reorganization, resolution, identity change, and ultimately successful adaptation. During these various stages the approach to client teaching differs (Bille, 1981). The teaching-learning situation in the denial stage has a characteristic present tense focus. In this stage, it is helpful for the nurse to cultivate trust with the family and carefully explain procedures and routines. As clients enter the developing awareness stage, they may vent hostilities. At this point present tense teaching continues to be most suitable. Support, listening, and one-to-one interaction while avoiding conflict with the client is appropriate. As clients begin to wonder in the reorganization stage about life changes resulting from the illness, they may wish more information from the nurse. The client and family need to be encouraged to communicate. The nurse may begin to teach future-oriented material. As the client becomes more comfortable in the resolution stage, perhaps group instructional settings become more appropriate. During the identity change phase, the client may actively seek more information about the illness. The nurse may need to explain and clarify material while encouraging maximum independence. When the client has successfully adapted to the disease process, perhaps referral to community resource groups where additional learning can take place is appropriate.

This model is used to show how attention to stages in the disease process must be considered in the determination of readiness to learn. Careful attention must be paid to these stages during an overt illness, as well as to barriers to learning such as fatigue, sensory deficits, anxiety, pain, and environmental distractions that may distract the learner. These must be considered in determining readiness to learn. Determining readiness to learn does not simply mean delaying teaching; it means using strategies that accommodate the stage of illness and potential barriers to learning.

THEORIES OF COMMUNICATION

An important consideration in health education is communication. The nurse in the teaching role must be cognizant of the dynamics involved in human interaction. Communication involves both verbal and nonverbal use of language. Language is one code that individuals use to express themselves, but facial expressions and movements of the hands and arms are also used (Birdwhistell, 1954). Hall (1959), in his book *The Silent Language,* discusses other signals by which individuals express attitudes through their personal use of space.

What is the purpose of communication? Probably the basic purpose of communication is to influence someone or something (Berlo, 1960). Communication is a two-way street that involves the production of a message, as well as the receipt of that message. The production of this message takes many forms and is molded and engineered by a sender, as well as filtered and interpreted according to the perceptual set of the receiver. The source of the message has a purpose for communicating, and the receiver has a purpose for listening. When these purposes become inconsistent, communication breaks down.

Since communication is affected by social system values and mores, there are many different ways of saying the same thing. The existence of a social system, in fact, evolves from the communication of these values and mores among members of a given social system. This macrosystem has ramifications for communication exchanges between the nurse and client. Communication is a highly complex process. A nurse must consider the impact of communication on the teaching role. Kasch (1984) suggests that to effectively communicate with unique individuals from differing social systems, it is necessary to adopt a process called perspective taking. Perspective taking involves more than role-taking in that it implies sensitivity to the individuality of the client's point of view (Kasch, 1984). It also considers the unique characteristics of the wellness or illness role. Kasch goes on to explain that nurses must be able to use perspective taking in their communication with clients to be adaptable and flexible.

Communication within the nursing role involves two major components as indicated earlier—information giving and teaching. Wilson-Barnett (1985) insists that success in the teaching role requires not only that the nurse recognize the client's major personal concerns but that the nurse educator accept teaching as a two-way process that generates unplanned questions and topics that must be addressed.

Why is communication important? It is important because in health care it has the potential to affect outcomes. Yoos (1981) states that many factors influence compliance. Some of these cannot be changed by the nurse. However, the quality of interaction between the caregiver and client may be an important way the nurse can influence client adherence. Improving the quality of nurse-client interaction depends in part on maximizing the quality of the nurse-client interaction (Kasch and Knutson, 1985). Kasch goes on to discuss the following two styles of interaction that exert interpersonal influences: position-centered and person-centered speech.

Position-centered speech is based on the assumption that effective communication depends on everyone following a script and playing a role. This style assumes that the nurse and client have similar expectations of the other's respective role. Nurses using position-centered speech tend to use rule-based and role-based strategies that suggest how a client should behave (Kasch and Knutson, 1985). This type of communication does not encourage mutual goal setting but focuses on the nurse's expectations of the client's role and behavior. This would seem closely aligned with the nurse in an authoritarian role.

In a person-centered orientation, the nurse considers roles from both an individual and institutional perspective. In this type of communication, the nurse becomes cognizant of the individual's beliefs and values. This type of communication implies an adaptability to the client's unique demands and needs (Kasch and Knutson, 1985). Communication of this nature relies more on persuasive elements. It appears more democratic in that it assumes that clients need to understand their treatment and that this treatment regimen must take unique attributes of the client into consideration. The style of interaction may be less threatening to many clients.

Wolfe (1982) in a study about attitudes toward the nurse-patient relationship found that nurses with a basic expressive orientation did not agree that there should be an emphasis on task, symptoms of disease, and firm control of patient learning. According to this investigator, an expressive orientation implies a concern for client goals and expectations. A nonexpressive orientation implies a concern for tasks and structure.

Therefore communicating is a highly complex process. Language and movement are basic codes for communicating. These codes are affected by personality development, as well as the social system from which one emerges. Any communication has a purpose, as well as a sender and receiver of a message. The interpretation of these messages is influenced by the unique characteristics of those involved in the communication. There are verbal and nonverbal behaviors that affect communication. Persons may interpret this behavior and react to inferred feelings and cues (Riley and Riley, 1972). Communication and subsequent interaction are highly complex. The nurse in the educative role must be aware of the impact of communication on the success of a teaching intervention.

Nurses can facilitate communication by perspective taking and can facilitate compliance with teaching goals by a person-centered orientation of communication. A crucial step in this process is for nurses to understand their own attitudes toward the teaching role. It has been suggested that many nurses are highly uncomfortable with this role. Some possible reasons for this may stem from a perceived lack of support for nurses in a teaching function (Stanton, 1986). Awareness of a problem is necessary for its amelioration, and nurses must strive to enhance their communication strategies in the teaching role.

NURSING PROCESS AND CLIENT EDUCATION

The nursing process is an important conceptual model that is relevant to client education in the community health setting. This process allows the nurse educator to use a decision-making model for the design, implementation, and evaluation of the individual's health education needs.

The initial step in the nursing process is assessment. This is gathering pertinent information about the client with a variety of techniques and traditionally involves nursing judgment regarding identification of clients' developmental level, health status, culture, physical environment, and interpersonal relationships (Jasmin and Trygstad, 1979).

Once these data are gathered, the nurse can make an educational diagnosis. This diagnosis as it relates to health teaching includes a statement of the educational need and factors that might create this need and the impact this educational need may have on daily living.

Once the nursing educational diagnosis is made, the nurse designs goals for the educational process. Once these goals are set and shared with the client, the nurse begins to plan strategies for accomplishing these educational goals. At this point it is obvious that the community health nurse must be cognizant of the many theories discussed in this chapter and comfortable with conducting a teaching-learning situation. The development of an actual teaching plan is discussed further later in this chapter. Once the plan is derived, it is implemented and evaluated.

Evaluating one's teaching and another's learning is a significant component of this process. Evaluation may take many forms; however, it is essential that techniques that assess attainment of previously specified goals be used. Modifications to the teaching plan can then follow.

Therefore the nursing process can serve as an important blueprint for the design, implementation, and evaluation of community health education. This blueprint for client education can be supported if the nurse is cognizant of techniques involved in the structuring of an educational experience; the next section assists in the actual development of a lesson plan.

NURSE AND A PLAN FOR EDUCATING CLIENTS

Educating the client is an integral part of professional nursing. Whether community health nurses are effective as educators depends on how comfortable they feel with this particular component of their role. Just as nurses must learn certain technical procedures, they must learn to be educators. It is not just teaching talent that makes someone an effective teacher. It is knowledge and implementation of that knowledge in a meaningful manner that usually produces the best results.

Gaining some familiarity with different learning theories and selecting a theory or theories that are consistent with the educational goals of the client teaching are prerequisites to planning any educational experience. Additionally the nursing process serves as the guiding structure for client education. Within the context of this process, the planning of educational experiences is facilitated by using what is termed a "technology of instruction" (Gagne and Briggs, 1979). This involves certain critical steps in the preparation of a lesson plan. These steps can be divided into three basic tasks—design of the program (analogous to the assessment, diagnosis, and planning steps of the nursing process), implementation (implementation), and evaluation (evaluation) (Stanton, 1983).This technology of instruction provides a conceptual framework for nurses who are teaching clients within a variety of community health care settings. The concurrent phases of the nursing process are noted.

Design Phase

The design phase of program development involves all the initial steps the nurse educator uses in planning a learning experience. Characteristically, planning or designing a program involves determining learning needs and learner characteristics (Redman, 1976). The educator can determine learning needs by assessing the client's present status and concluding what knowledge, skills, and attitudes still require some type of formal learning experience. This learning-needs assessment can be either oral or written depending on what the nurse educator feels is more appropriate. For instance, written or oral tests to evaluate clients' knowledge of their disease processes might be beneficial, or asking the client to demonstrate a particular technique might be the most appropriate approach. Interviewing the family might also yield information about the client's present level of knowledge and compliance with treatment plans. The nurse, however, has a great deal of latitude in determining the strategy for assessing learning. No matter what strategy is selected, it must provide the necessary data base about what the client still must learn. The nurse educator also must assess learner characteristics (Huckaby, 1980; Yoder-Wise, 1980). Assessing learner characteristics implies that the nurse evaluates the client's physiologic, psychologic, and sociologic attributes. For instance, the client's age greatly influences a nurse's approach to the learning experience. For example, as previously discussed the adult learner usually prefers self-directed activities, whereas children need more structured learning experiences. Before actually planning any educational experience, the nurse must take into consideration what clients need to know and their individual values and characteristics, as well as their motivational level and readiness to learn. The use of any available data source for this assessment is important. Once this is completed, a formal plan of instruction is developed.

The next step in this design process is to determine goals and objectives. Much confusion exists about the difference between goals and objectives. Put simply, a goal is a statement of the preferred outcome of instruction. It is a statement that does not have to be written in terms of the learner but in terms of what the nurse desires to accomplish. The objectives, on the other hand, are specified for the learner and should include action verbs that can be properly evaluated. One good source to assist the novice in the art of specifying behavioral objectives is Mager (1975). Most learning tasks or objectives can be divided into three domains. These three domains, or classifications, are called a taxonomy. This taxonomy helps the program developer determine which domain a particular learning task is most related to. Most learning tasks deal with knowledge, skills, attitudes, or a combination of these. In choosing the proper taxonomic classification, one must reflect on what learning tasks are to be accomplished. Knowledge objectives would deal with the mastery of facts and theories or the cognitive domain. Any type of skill performance would be contained within the psychomotor domain, and any attitude change would be included in the affective domain. The importance of separating behavior on the basis of a taxonomic classification is that often the methodology and strategies of instruction, as well as the evaluation, would differ accordingly (American Hospital Association, 1979). An excellent method for developing objectives in the health education area is to use the ABCD list (Adelson, Watkins, and Caplan, 1985). The "A" is for audience. In most cases it is the client and family. The "B" is for the specific behavior the client should exhibit as a result of the teaching. This should be an action verb that is observable by the nurse-teacher. "C" is for the conditions under which the behavior is performed. For example, will the client need a specific piece of equipment to accomplish the objective? Conditions should be incorporated into the objective statement. The "D" stands for degree as in the degree of accuracy or performance according to preselected criteria that are acceptable and observable measures of performance. This ABCD system helps the nurse set objectives.

Another important consideration in the design of an instructional program for the community health nurse is the development of a content outline that is related to the behavioral objectives. Each objective implies a certain body of content, and this content should be written out in clear, concise terms not only to assist the nurse designer but to promote consistency and follow-up by professional colleagues. Once the objectives and content are delineated and a determination of the taxonomic classification of the objectives is completed, a specific teaching strategy can be determined. A taxonomic classification divides all possible learning behaviors into three categories—thinking, or the cognitive domain, feeling, or the

Program goal (1)					
Objectives (2)	Related content (3)	Teaching strategy (4)	Instructional and/or audiovisual materials (5)	Evaluation methodologies (6)	Bibliography and resources (7)
1	1	1	1	1	1
2	2	2	2	2	2
3	3	3	3	3	3
4	4	4	4	4	4

FIG. 5-3. Format for client lesson plan.

affective domain, and doing, or the psychomotor domain. Instructional adjuncts, such as brochures, pamphlets, and films, should also be selected. The use and evaluation of these instructional materials should be made by the nurse educator only after careful review of the behavioral objectives. An excellent guide for choosing and using various strategies, as well as developing instructional materials, is available through the American Hospital Association and titled *A Media Handbook* (1979). Strategies and materials are useful only if they aid the accomplishment of the behavioral objectives and are consistent with the objectives' taxonomic classification. These strategies and instructional materials should be included in a formal lesson plan so that again there is consistency and follow-up among colleagues. The final step in the design phase of program development is the compilation of a resource bibliography. The importance of this is that other individuals when implementing a program or using a lesson plan would benefit greatly from these resources for review. This again promotes consistency and accurate implementation of the lesson plan. In Fig. 5-3 the suggestions regarding the initial program design are formulated into a lesson plan format that can be included in a notebook or chart or on a large index card, whichever suits the nurse's particular needs. This lesson plan format includes all the steps that are discussed in association with the design phase of program instrumentation. This plan is completed after the professional nurse has determined the learner needs and individual learner characteristics. A sample lesson plan is shown in Fig. 5-4.

Implementation and Evaluation

Once a formal plan of instruction is developed, based on individual or collective learning needs and characteristics, and initialed, the instruction can begin. Several considerations are important. If the instruction is geared to an individual, the scheduling of the event should be mutually planned by the nurse and the client. However, if the nurse is planning the educational experience for a larger group, a schedule of classes should be established. In addition, if the program that is designed will be implemented by several different individuals, some preplanning among the staff should take place. During the implementation phase, all aspects of the program should be continually evaluated to determine information retention and see what adjustments must be made. This is especially helpful if a variety of individuals from the same organization are implementing the same program (Gagne and Briggs, 1979). All audiovisual materials should be evaluated to determine whether they are pertinent to the purpose

Program goal (1)					
Objectives (2)	Related content (3)	Teaching strategy (4)	Instructional and/or audiovisual materials (5)	Evaluation methodologies (6)	Bibliographic resources (7)
1. At the completion of this teaching episode, clients will be able to accurately take their own radial pulse.	1. Definition of pulse. 2. What produces pulse. 3. Why pulse is important. 4. Factors that affect pulse. 5. Fingers used. 6. Placement of fingers on wrist. 7. Palpating pulse procedure. 8. Counting pulse. 9. Use of second hand of watch in determining pulse. 10. Calculating pulse. 11. Differentiating resting pulse vs. pulse after activity.	1. Use diagram of heart and circulatory system for content 1 to 3. 2. Have clients listen to their own hearts while resting and after activity for content 4 and 9. 3. Demonstrate use of fingers and placement; have clients find pulses in both their own wrists and yours for content 5, 6, and 7. 4. Have client calculate pulse for 15-, 30-, 45-, and 60-second intervals, content 5 to 11.	1. Diagram of heart and circulatory system. 2. Stethoscope. 3. Watch with second hand. 4. Handouts on procedure.	1. Have client take pulse. Keep daily log. 2. Have clients take pulse at same time as nurse and verify their count.	1. Pamphlet: *Monitoring Pulse.* 2. Prepared handouts—available central office.

FIG. 5-4. Sample client lesson plan.

of the program. This type of evaluation could be included in the written evaluation of the program completed by the client and staff. Another important aspect of the evaluative process for the nurse educator is the development of instruments to determine the level of learner accomplishment (Redman, 1988). These instruments or measures should match the behavioral objectives in content, type of taxonomic classification, and level of sophistication (Green, 1975). The evaluative process must not only provide feedback on the program and the degree of learner accomplishment but also determine the success of the program in accomplishing its overall goals. If a program is developed to increase compliance with some type of preventive health measure, it must be determined how successful the program was in accomplishing that goal. This implies that some research related to the program's effectiveness should always be considered a matter of vital concern to professional nurses and to the clients with whom they interact. If indeed nurses wish to develop successful teaching plans and strategies, they must be able to document the plans in a legitimate manner. Research and validation also enable nurses to share success with others involved in similar professional endeavors. Evaluation should include research on the effectiveness of teaching efforts on a short- or long-term basis.

This discussion does not imply that if this process is formalized it cannot accommodate more on-the-spot teaching plans. As with the nursing process, one can assess a teaching need, design a plan of teaching, and implement the plan, as well

Criteria	Yes	No
1. Program goals are specified in writing.		
2. Behavioral objectives for the program are specified in writing.		
3. A taxonomy is used in the development of objectives.		
4. An outline of content is developed in relation to defined objectives.		
5. Strategies and learning activities are defined in accordance with the written plan of objectives and content.		
6. Audiovisuals are previewed and included in the written program plan.		
7. A bibliography of materials used in the development of the program is included with the program package.		
8. There is a plan for staff development when a specific program is implemented.		
9. A written schedule for classes in the program is available to the groups' staff members, clients, and clients' families.		
10. Learning activities related instructional materials are available as outlined in the formal written program.		
11. The specific program has enough flexibility to allow for individual modifications.		
12. Formative evaluation, or ongoing evaluation, is conducted by the staff involved in the implementation of a specific program.		
13. Formal research is conducted to evaluate the client's mastery of program content.		
14. Written objectives and performance tests are used to evaluate the client's mastery of program content.		
15. There are written evaluation forms for evaluation of the program by clients and their families.		
16. There are summary or final evaluation sessions for staff to accomplish review and revision.		
17. There are written forms for staff involved in teaching the program to evaluate the program.		
18. There are evaluation forms for client and family evaluation of learning material and audiovisuals.		

FIG. 5-5. Criteria for evaluating formal client education programs.

as evaluate it quickly. For instance, if the nurse assesses on a home visit that a diabetic client needs further teaching regarding urine testing and is misreading the contrast chart, some action is needed. The nurse can formulate a teaching objective, design a miniteaching session, and evaluate its effect.

This presentation deals with the three major components of program development—design, implementation, and evaluation. It discusses steps that are thought to be necessary at each phase of the program development process. A format for a lesson plan is presented, although this could vary according to the particular agency's situation or needs. Also provided is a criterion for evaluating existing programs to determine whether or not they have considered the steps that have been discussed within this presentation. This criterion provides a baseline for assessing whether or not the program has a technologically sound basis for its subsequent use. It is hoped this will provide the nurse with the tools required to effectively implement successful client education programs, as well as evaluate those currently in existence. A sample plan is portrayed in Fig. 5-5.

Ultimately all designs, plans, and evaluation need some type of documentation process. This documentation of client teaching can be integrated into major systems of documentation by an agency. Many examples of client education documentation exist. However, they are only as useful as the nurse makes them. Simplicity and accessibility are key elements to the documentation of client care.

NURSE'S EDUCATIVE ROLE IN HEALTH PROMOTION AND DISEASE PREVENTION

Nurses as educators of the health consumer have an obligation to be familiar with health promotion and disease prevention strategies in the United States. They also should be ready to collaborate with other health care providers to improve the health of the population.

The first step is to be familiar with the surgeon general's goals set in 1980 (U.S. Department of Health and Human Services, 1979). The goals are shown in the following box, and the target date for accomplishment is 1990.

The surgeon general's report also identified improvements needed in 15 priority areas for the accomplishment of these goals. These priority areas fall into three major categories—personal preventive services, health protection, and health promotion.

Preventive services are provided by physicians,

THE SURGEON GENERAL'S GOALS ON HEALTH PROMOTION AND DISEASE PREVENTION, 1990

For infants, the goal is 35 percent lower death rate than the 14.1 deaths per 1,000 live births that occurred in 1977. That would mean less than 9 deaths per 1,000 births by 1990. By 1982, we were already halfway there. Deaths were down to 11.2 per 1,000 live births.

There are also two subgoals for infants:
- to reduce incidence of low birth weight infants;
- to reduce birth defects.

For children, ages 1-14, the goal is a 20 percent lower death rate. That would be less than 34 deaths per 100,000 population by 1990, compared with 43 in 1977. By 1982, we were closing fast on this goal with deaths down to 36 per 100,000.

Subgoals for children are:
- to enhance childhood growth and development;
- to reduce childhood accidents and injury.

For adolescents and young adults, ages 15-24, we seek a 20 percent lower death rate, from 117 per 100,000 population in 1977 to less than 93 in 1990. The figure in 1982 was down to 105.

Subgoals in this age group are:
- to reduce death and disability from motor vehicle accidents;
- to reduce the misuse of alcohol and drugs.

For adults, ages 25-64, our goal is a 25 percent lower death rate, from 540 in 1977 to less than 400 per 100,000 population in 1990. In 1982, the figure had already declined by more than a hundred to 436 deaths per 100,000 population.

Subgoals for adults are:
- to reduce heart attacks and strokes;
- to reduce the incidence of cancer.

For older adults, ages 65 and over, the goal is a 20 percent reduction in days of restricted activity, to less than 30 days per year.

Subgoals for older adults are:
- to increase the proportion of older people who can function independently;
- to reduce premature death and disability from influenza and pneumonia.

Modified from US Department of Health and Human Services: Healthy people: the surgeon general's report on health promotion and disease prevention, Washington, DC, 1979, US Government Printing Office.

hospitals, and other health care providers. The target areas are hypertension, family planning, pregnancy, infant health, immunizations, and control of sexually transmitted diseases.

Health protection involves efforts by government, industry, and other agencies to control toxic agents in the environment, enhance accident prevention and safety, improve dental health, and decrease infectious diseases.

Health promotion includes programs that educate the public about the risks involved in health abuses and that increase public commitment to sensible life-styles that can add years to life (U.S. Department of Health and Human Services, 1984).

After these goals were published, a series of objectives was developed by various public and private groups. Specific agencies are overseeing these efforts and collaborating on their accomplishment.

In February 1984, a conference titled "Prospects for a healthier America: achieving the nation's health promotion objectives" convened in Washington, D.C. Work groups representing five pivotal components for national health were represented. These work groups discussed the objectives and made specific recommendations (U.S. Department of Health and Human Services, 1984). The recommendations from the Health Professions' Group are presented here. One set of recommendations is directed at the Public Health Service (PHS), and the second set is directed at health professions' organizations. Recommendations for the PHS include the following:

1. The PHS should review and revise the 1990 objectives when necessary with participation by health professions' organizations.
2. The PHS should consider specific changes in the existing 1990 objectives or the development of new objectives, including setting specific goals for increasing seatbelt use, reducing mortality in the population older than 65 years (with a subdivision for older than 75 years), narrowing the gap between segments of the population by setting goals for such high-risk groups as blacks and the poor, and developing objectives for early detection of diseases in which early intervention can reduce mortality.
3. The PHS should support research to expand the science base in health promotion and disease prevention, with particular attention to applied research of effective interventions and patient-provider interaction.
4. The PHS should help combat provider skepticism by supporting efforts to provide better access to, and sufficient quantities of, health promotion materials of proven quality and effectiveness.
5. The PHS should take the lead in developing a health professions' organizations task force on health promotion and disease prevention along the lines of the National High Blood Pressure coalition, which is cited as an example of cooperation and coordination by different organizations and groups.
6. The PHS should consider the need to oppose unproven or harmful methods of health promotion, if not by direct means then certainly by stronger advocacy of proven effective methods.

Recommendations for health professions' organizations include these:

1. Endorse the 1990 objectives. Some modification of certain objectives is desirable, but as a whole they are basically sound and should be endorsed.
2. Participate in an ongoing health professions' organizations task force to develop a cooperative and coordinated approach to health promotion.
3. Divide objectives among different groups to make efficient use of available resources and then pool the results. (The proposed task force would facilitate this approach.)
4. Participate in the further development of national objectives. Organizations are more likely to support objectives if they participate in their development.

5. Participate in the development of effective health promotion tools and methods through research and demonstration projects (subject to available funding).
6. Pursue efforts to encourage third-party payers to reimburse for health promotion and preventive health care services.
7. Foster more effective education and training for health professionals in health promotion and disease prevention, with particular focus on how health promotion can be integrated into conventional health care (for example, finding the teachable moment); how different providers can work together to achieve health promotion goals; and how providers can participate effectively in community-based, health promotion coalitions.

Health promotion and disease prevention are important components of consumer education. Nurses, because of their unique continual proximity to clients, have a major role in this effort. Nurses must be as committed to health promotion and disease prevention as they are to the more rehabilitative aspects of educating clients who have overt disease processes. Some specific strategies that may increase the community health nurse's impact on health promotion and disease prevention include the following:

1. Nurses become committed to meeting the nation's health care goals in their own community by active involvement in their professional associations.
2. Nurses become familiar with health care programs and agencies and other providers that address target areas of concern and will then use them and refer clients to them.
3. Nurses seek self-development in the design, implementation, and evaluation of health promotion and prevention programs.
4. Nurses incorporate this type of health education counseling in their daily dealings with clients and do not restrict teaching efforts to illness or overt disease processes.
5. Nurses collaborate with other health care providers to deliver consistent and comprehensive health education that addresses health promotion, disease prevention, and education of clients with overt illness.

NURSE'S EDUCATIVE ROLE IN AN OVERT ILLNESS

The nurse's educative role in an overt disease process is a responsive one. The nurse assesses the educational needs and designs, implements, and evaluates a program to meet those needs. This educative process is based on the type of knowledge, skills, and attitudes the client requires to survive. It is possible to meet those needs through a more formal client education program or through more individualized efforts.

During a disease process, nurses must begin the educative process by providing information. This entails the exploration of care and treatment to provide an immediate response to client concerns. This more informal interaction, although more flexible and individualized, still has specific goals and content.

As clients become convalescent and move out of the hospital, their educational goals may be more complex. It is at this point that the community health nurse must assess the level of knowledge regarding the disease process and treatment the client has received in the hospital. It may be practical to integrate clients into groups for instruction. This instruction should be adjusted to an individual or group setting, although objective content, strategies, and resources should be consistent so that continuity continues as the patient progresses toward integration of the new learning into ADLs. As the overt disease process is controlled and clients begin to integrate these ramifications into their life-styles, the community health nurse can begin to address health promotional and preventive educational needs.

During this entire process the full repertoire of theories discussed in this chapter can be used.

NURSING IN THE COMMUNITY

Nurses not only teach individual clients or groups but may collaborate in or lead the development of community education. This entails sectors of general populations. The decision-making model inherent in the nursing process is equally applicable to the development of new programs or activities to address community health problems. However, these activities are approached on a larger scale. Assessment of needs at this level would probably include the following:

1. Reviewing secondary sources of data (for example, census reports or National Vital Registration System)
2. Reviewing service use records
3. Conducting a community survey
4. Using key members of the population
5. Conducting a community forum

A useful approach to formulating plans for community programing is again borrowed from marketing (Berkowitz and Flexnor, 1979). These steps include the following:

1. *Research the market for potential clients.* Conduct studies that define the characteristics, needs, and wants of the target population.
2. *Develop segment-specific strategies.* Develop your product, price, promotion, and place marketing strategies based on information described in step 1.
3. *Determine goals and objectives.* Goals and objectives for project implementation should reflect information from steps 1 and 2.
4. *Implement the program.* In this stage the project is implemented according to plan proposed in step 3.
5. *Evaluate the program regularly and in a formal manner.* Use input from this evaluation to revise, continue, or delete programs.

This process parallels the nursing process and is indeed the bare bones of a marketing audit or survey. It may provide a useful guide to the nurse contemplating programing for specific community groups.

NURSE AND OTHER MEMBERS OF THE HEALTH CARE TEAM

The nurse is a vital member of the health care team. The role of educator is an equally important component of the nurse's total care provision. The interaction evident between the nurse and other allied health care professionals in other aspects of care is similar to that evident in the teaching role. The nurse, as the professional having the greatest amount of contact with the client, assumes a major role in this process. However, consulting and using the knowledge of other health team members in the teaching process is advantageous and even efficacious to learning.

The nurse, because of continual direct contact, can reassess patient learning needs, redesign teaching plans, implement teaching episodes, and evaluate results. At any point within this teaching process, other professionals can be consulted for input or used to implement segments of the program.

SUMMARY

An understanding of one or more learning theories can facilitate the teaching process. Twentieth century learning theories are usually either behavioristic in orientation or focused on cognitive processes.

Behaviorists focus on conditioning as a mechanism for changing behavior. Cognitive theories see learning as a method to change expectations or thought patterns.

Using learning theory as a basis, the nurse can develop a variety of approaches to client education in the community. One approach is to use a three-step lesson plan—designing a program, implementing the program, and evaluating the program.

A knowledge of the teaching and learning process is important not only in the care of acutely and chronically ill clients, but also in health promotion and disease prevention in the community.

QUESTIONS FOR DISCUSSION

1. How would you apply a behavioral theory of learning to teaching a client how to change a specific behavior? For example, how could you help a client quit smoking using a behavioral theory?
2. Nine generally accepted learning principles are suggested in Chapter 5. List at least five of these principles.
3. What does the health belief model predict?
4. Provide examples of the teaching nurses might carry out in the community.

REFERENCES

Adelson R, Watkins F, and Caplan R: Continuing education for the health professional, Rockville, Md, 1985, Aspen Systems Corp.

American Hospital Association: A media handbook, Chicago, 1978, The Association.

American Hospital Association: Implementation of patient education, Chicago, 1979, The Association.

Becker MH, Drachman RH, and Kirsch JP: Predicting mother's compliance with pediatric medical regimes, J Pediatr 81:843, 1972.

Berkowitz E and Flexnor W: The marketing audit: a tool for health service organization. In Cooper P, editor: Health care marketing, Rockville, Md, 1979, Aspen Systems Corp.

Berlo D: The process of communication, New York, 1960, Holt, Rinehart & Winston, Inc.

Bigge ML: Learning theories for teachers, ed 3, New York, 1976, Harper & Row, Publishers Inc.

Bille DA: Practical approaches to patient teaching, Boston, 1981, Little, Brown & Co. Inc.

Birdwhistell R: Kinesics and communication—explorations, vol 3, Toronto, 1954, University of Toronto Press.

Buchanan N and others: Factors influencing drug compliance in ambulatory black urban patients, S Afr Med J 10:368, 1979.

Caplan RD and others: Adhering to medical regimens, Ann Arbor, 1976, University of Michigan Press.

Cerkoney K and Hart L: The relationship between the health belief model and compliance of persons with diabetes mellitus, Diabetes Care 3(5):594, 1980.

Crate MA: Nursing functions in adaptation to chronic illness, Am J Nurs 65:72, 1965.

Dapcich-Miura E and Hovell MF: Contingency management to a complex medical regimen in an elderly heart patient, Behav Therapy 10:193, 1979.

Davidhezar R: Critique of the health belief model, J Adv Nurs 8:467, 1983.

Earp JR, Ory M, and Strogatz D: The effects of family involvement and practitioner home visits on the control of hypertension, Am J Public Health 72:1146, 1982.

Epstein LH and Masek BJ: Behavioral control of medicine compliance, J Appl Behav Med 11:1, 1978.

Festinger L: An analysis of compliant behavior. In Sherif M and Wilson MO, editors: Group relations at the crossroads, New York, 1953, Harper Brothers Publishing.

Gabriel N, Gagnon JI, and Bryon CK: Improving patient compliance through the use of daily reminder charts, Am J Public Health 67:968, 1977.

Gagne R and Briggs L: Principles of instructional design, ed 2, New York, 1979, Holt, Rinehart & Winston Inc.

Hall E: The silent language, New York, 1959, Doubleday & Co.

Haynes RB: A critical review of determinants of patient compliance with therapeutic regimens. In Sackett DL and Haynes RB, editors: Compliance with therapeutic regimens, Baltimore, 1976, The Johns Hopkins University Press.

Haynes RB, Taylor D, and Sackett D, editors: Compliance in health care, Baltimore, 1979, The Johns Hopkins University Press.

Huckaby I: A strategy for patient teaching, Nurs Admin Q 4(2):47, 1980.

Janz N and Becker M: The health belief model: a decade later, Health Educ Q 11(1):1, 1984.

Jasmin S and Trygstad L: Behavioral concepts and the nursing process, St Louis, 1979, CV Mosby Co.

Kasch C: Interpersonal competence and communication in the delivery of nursing care, Adv Nurs Sci 6(2):71, 1984.

Kasch C and Knutson K: Patient compliance and interpersonal style: implications for practice and research, Nurse Pract 10(3):52, 1985.

Kelman HC: Compliance, identification and internalization, J Conflict Resol 2:51, 1969.

Kerr J: Adherence and self-care, Heart Lung 14:24, 1985.

Kiesler CA and Kiesler SB: Conformity, Reading, Mass, 1970, Addison-Wesley Publishing Company Inc.

Knowles M: The modern practice of adult education from pedagogy to andragogy, Chicago, 1980, Association Press, Follett.

Kotler P: Marketing management, ed 3, Englewood Cliffs, NJ, 1976, Prentice Hall.

Lewin K: A dynamic theory of personality, New York, 1935, McGraw-Hill Inc. A collection of articles that Lewin wrote before 1935 and a new survey chapter.

Mager RF: Preparing objectives for instruction, Belmont, Calif, 1975, Fearon.

Nagy UT and Wolfe G: Cognitive predictors of compliance in chronic disease patients, Med Care 22(10):912, 1984.

Pender NJ: Health promotion in nursing practice, Norwalk, Conn, 1987, Appleton & Lange.

Redman B: The process of patient teaching in nursing, ed 6, St Louis, 1988, CV Mosby Co.

Riley J and Riley M: Sociology: an approach to human communication. In Budd R and Ruben B, editors: Approaches to human communication, Rochelle Park, NJ, 1972, Hayden Book Co.

Rosenstock I: Why people use health services, Milbank Q 44:94, 1966.

Rosenstock I: Historical origins of the health belief model. In Becker M, editor: The health belief model and personal health behavior, Thorofare, NJ, 1974, Charles Stock.

Ross D and Guggenheim F: Compliance and the health belief model: a challenge for the liaison psychiatrist, Gen Hosp Psychiatry 5:31, 1983.

Schmidt JP: A behavioral approach to patient compliance, Postgrad Med 65:39, 1979.

Schultz S: Compliance with therapeutic regimens in pediatrics: a review of implications for social work practice, Soc Work Health Care 5(3):267, 1980.

Stanton M: Patient and health education: lessons from the marketplace, Nurs Management 16(4):28, 1979.

Stanton M: An instructional technology for patient education, Patient Counselling Health Education 14(4):208, 1983.

Stanton M: Nurse attitudes towards patient education, Nurs Success Today 3(3):16, 1986.

Steckel SB and Swain MA: Contracting with patients to improve compliance, Hospitals 51:81, 1977.

US Department of Health and Human Services: Healthy people: the surgeon general's report on health promotion and disease prevention, Washington, DC, 1979, US Government Printing Office.

US Department of Health and Human Services: Proceedings of prospects for a healthier America: achieving the nation's health promotion objectives, Washington, DC, 1984, Public Health Service, Office of Disease Prevention and Health Promotion.

Wilson-Barnett J: Principles of patient teaching, Nurs Times, p. 28, Feb 20, 1985.

Wolfe M: Dimensions of nursing students' attitudes toward the nurse-patient relationship in a patient education setting, Psychol Rep 51:1165, 1982.

Yoder-Wise PS: Adult teaching strategies, J Cont Ed Nurs 11(6):15, 1980.

Yoos L: Compliance: philosophical and ethical considerations, Nurse Pract 6(5):27, 1981.

BIBLIOGRAPHY

Green JA: Teacher mode tests, ed 2, New York, 1975, Harper & Row Publishers Inc.

Lewin K and others: Level of aspiration. In Hunt J, editor: Personality and the behavior disorders: a handbook based on experimental and clinical research, New York, 1944, Ronald Press.

CHAPTER 6

Environmental Issues

Matthew Leopard and Vern Bullough

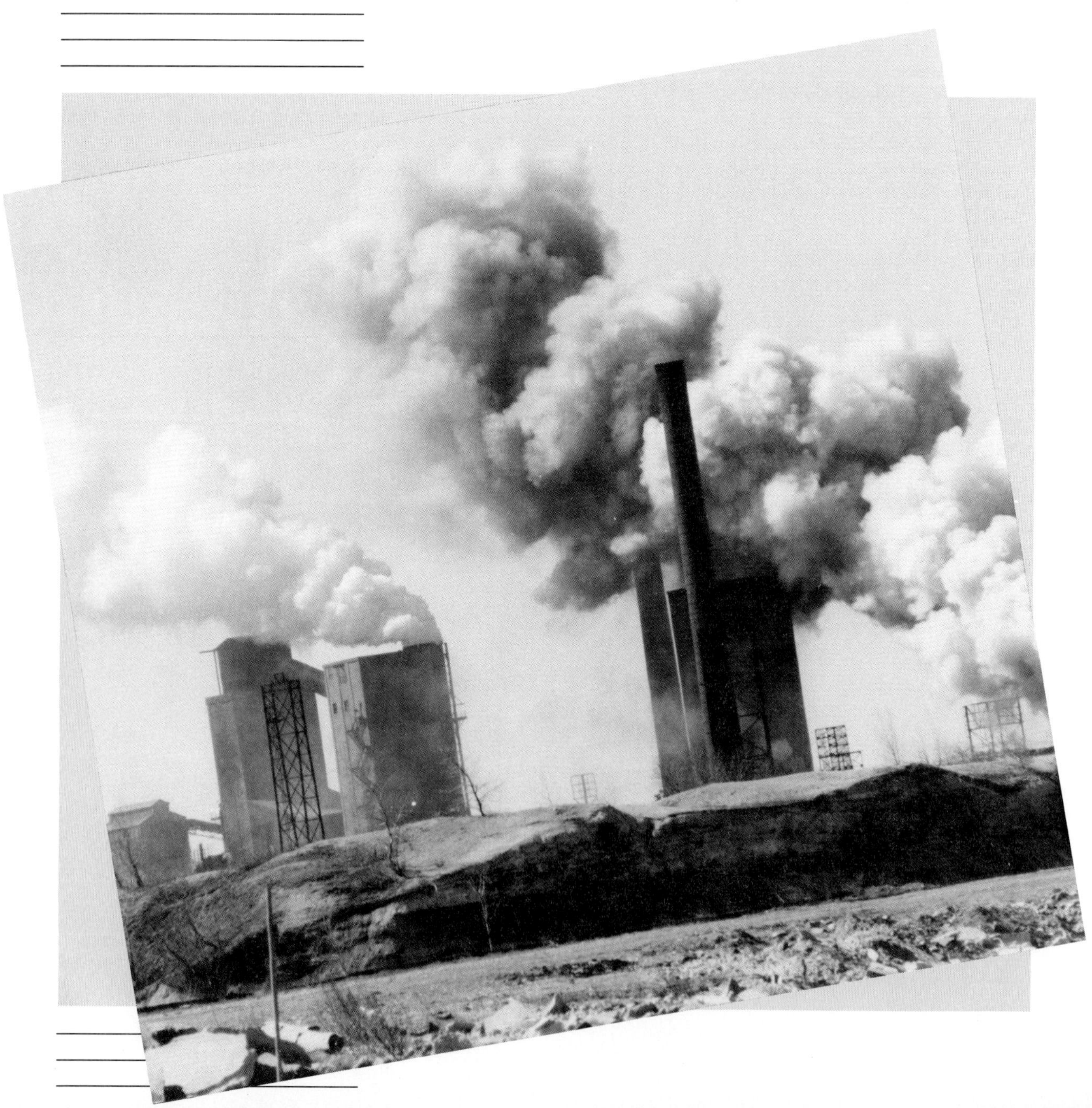

CHAPTER OUTLINE

OBJECTIVES

After completing this chapter, the reader should be able to:

1. List the courses of the major environmental health hazards and describe the threat they pose to clients.
2. List some of the behavioral properties of pesticides and the reasons they bring added danger.
3. Discuss the health problems associated with toxic waste dumps.
4. Know who Rachel Carson was and what she accomplished.
5. Know some of the technical terms associated with radiation and understand the standards for measurement.
6. Know what toxic metals are.

ENVIRONMENTAL ISSUES, like so many other things in this book, are both old and new. Some environmental issues (and illnesses), such as coal miner's black lung (an affliction brought on by inhaling coal dust), concerned nurses decades ago but are no longer major health problems. Unfortunately, other previously unknown or unrealized contaminants have risen to confront us. Waterborne typhoid fever, which killed many in the past, has been more or less eradicated in the United States, but other diseases produced by water contaminated by pesticides or heavy metals plague us.

Much of the public concern about the vast array of environmental pollutants grew out of the ecology movement of the 1960s and 1970s. Ecology, however, represents a much older concern. The term was coined more than 100 years ago by combining the Greek words *okos* (house) and *logos* (the science or study of). The first popularizer of ecology was the German philosopher Ernest Haeckel, who defined it as "a body of knowledge concerning the economy of nature and the investigation of the total relation of the animal to its organic or inorganic environment" (Kormondy, 1965). A simpler definition was given by Rachel Carson, the mother of the modern environmental movement, who called ecology "the study of the web of life" (Carson, 1962).

Pollutants have a universal scope. Children's lives are endangered when they eat paint chips that contain lead or inhale exhaust fumes from cars that use leaded fuel. Adults often work, eat, and breathe in areas that are contaminated with industrial vapors or where the noise level is so high that it interferes with concentration. Pollutants are found in the food we eat, the water we drink, and the hospitals in which our children are born. A chapter such as this can only scratch the surface of the problem, but by concentrating on some of the issues, readers will have enough background to explore the subject more deeply. They will also know enough to consider the dangers of pollutants when nursing their clients.

PESTICIDES

A major class of pollutants is grouped together under the term "pesticides," a variety of chemical poisons designed to eliminate various pests. It is estimated that without pesticides about one third of the world's annual crop production would be lost to pests. This emphasizes the importance of pesticides and why farmers have long sought ways of eliminating pests. The ancient Greeks, for example, used arsenic as an insecticide, and it is used even to this day (Edwards, 1972). Pyrethrum (copper acetoarsenite), also known as Paris green, received its first widespread use in the United States in the 1860s when it was used to kill the Colorado potato beetle. In 1887, with the establishment of agricultural experiment stations in the United States in conjunction with state land-grant colleges, the search for pesticides became a national commitment. A major breakthrough took place in 1918, when it was found that a fine dusting of calcium arsenate on crops poisoned the notorious adult boll weevil, a rapidly spreading insect that threatened the U.S. cotton industry (Dunlap, 1981).

The effects of pesticides seemed so miraculous that initially there was little opposition to their use. One of the first warnings against their indiscriminate use came from Anton J. Carlson, a famous physiologist at the University of Chicago, who in 1917 wrote that the insecticides could have deleterious effects on human protoplasm. Efforts to establish control over pesticides, however, proved difficult. When the U.S. Department of Agriculture tried to set a maximum limit on the use of arsenicals in fruit sprays, the outcry was so great that it was forced to retreat from the initial standards. These initial defeats on efforts to control pesticides had long-range effects because they helped mold a compliant attitude among both government enforcers and the public toward the use of pesticides and other pollutants. After being forced to modify, amend, or even withdraw many early efforts at regulation, regulatory bodies moved more and more cautiously to intervene even though researchers increasingly became aware that the residue effects of pesticides remained long after their initial application. A whole vocabulary developed to explain these potential dangers (see box).

It has been possible only in the last two decades to study effectively the various behavioral properties of many of the chemicals used in pesticides. Unfortunately, most of the knowledge about such dangers has come after the fact; that is, after effects are observed only after pesticides have been applied. A good example of this is the case of dichlorodiphenyltrichloroethane (DDT), the miracle pesticide of World War II. Although DDT was discovered in 1874, its pesticide qualities were not realized until 65 years later (Brown, 1978). Researchers then found that if they sprayed the pesticide against a wall not only did it kill the insects on the wall, but insects could not land on the wall safely for six months after the initial spraying. The first widespread use of this miraculous new pesticide was in World War II. It seemed the ideal insecticide, since it was lightweight, inexpensive, and gas soluble and had low toxicity to mammals but extreme toxicity to insects (Dunlap, 1981). In 1943 when Naples faced a typhus epidemic, the U.S. occupation forces sprayed more than 3 million individuals with DDT and halted the epidemic in its tracks. This was the first time in history that such a large-scale outbreak was stopped by using a pesticide. This and similar successes gave DDT widespread publicity as a wonder chemical, and when it was released for public use in August 1945, many predicted that the housefly and hornfly would soon disappear (Dunlap, 1981). There were a few dissenting voices to this new panacea, and as time went on, the dissenters gathered strength. One of the first problems surfaced in specially prepared infant foods. In 1947 the Beechnut Babyfood Company reported difficulty in finding food sources free of DDT, something it was required to do by law. Soon after, a researcher in Princeton,

TERMS USED TO DESCRIBE BEHAVIORAL PROPERTIES OF PESTICIDES

Environmental persistence denotes the ability of a chemical to remain unchanged in the environment. The longer the chemical remains intact, the greater is its persistence. A highly persistent pesticide can contaminate an area for years.

Bioaccumulation is the ability of a pesticide to build up, or concentrate, within certain tissues of a living organism. This can take place in two different ways. The pesticide may be incorporated through the food chain. In this case, even though the pesticide may have been applied in low concentrations, the concentration increases as the smaller organisms containing the pesticide are consumed by larger organisms. The larger predators at the top of the food chain ultimately can accumulate lethal doses of pesticide even though it was originally sprayed in "harmless" amounts. Bioaccumulation may also occur through direct absorption of the pesticide from the environment. Fish, for example, may absorb poisons in the water through their gills and store them in their body fat, so the person eating such fish receives high poison concentrations (Foehrenbach, 1972).

Specificity decribes the number of types of organisms a particular pesticide may harm or kill. A nonspecific pesticide is capable of destroying a whole range of organisms that are both beneficial and harmful, since it kills not only the insect pest but other insects, as well as the predator that feeds on the insect. Unfortunately, insects usually recover more quickly than the predators. The pests develop tolerances and require more pesticide, which ultimately kills many other creatures (Brown, 1978).

Migration describes the ability of a chemical to move through one or more media. The degree a chemical moves depends on its own chemical properties. Water-soluble chemicals may end up in drinking wells or may be carried with water vapor for thousands of miles (Risebrough, 1968).

Environmental interaction is one of the most frustrating problems to deal with, since certain chemicals may break down and combine with other chemicals in the environment to form pollutants that are much more dangerous than the original pollutant. The effects of sunlight, rain, and temperature are just a few factors that may transform relatively harmless chemicals into poisons. A good illustration of this danger is the ability of a pesticide known as aldicarb to join with naturally occurring nitrites and form carcinogens that can create mutagenic effects in infants (McWilliams, 1984).

N.J., reported that the widespread use of DDT against the Dutch elm disease had led to a radical decline in the survival of bird nestlings. Perhaps because DDT was considered such a wonder chemical, these early warnings were largely unheeded. Evidence of its dangers, however, continued to mount and were brought to public attention by Rachel Carson in her influential book, *Silent Spring* (1962).

The widespread publicity given Carson and her book made her an emotional and factual rallying ground for the anti-DDT advocates. The forces she set in motion soon moved from discussions of environmental issues to the political front. Within a year DDT was the primary topic of scientific and congressional hearings. Despite such widespread discussion, no immediate action resulted at the national level. This led opponents of DDT to move to state legislatures and courts. One of the leaders in the struggle was a new organization, the Environmental Defense Fund (EDF), which successfully campaigned for the abolition of DDT in Wisconsin and later in Michigan. Adding fuel to the fight was an announcement by the National Cancer Institute in 1969 that DDT might be cancer causing. In the 1970s the National Scientific Advisory Committee began a series of deliberations about the use of DDT. Although there was a growing number of problems linked to the use of DDT, such as abnormally thin eggshells among the bird population and abnormal enzymatic activity in humans, as well as its cancer-causing potential, the committee was reluctant to come up with a final recommendation until more scientific studies had been performed. The Wishy-Washy Report caused such a public uproar that the head of the newly formed Environmental Protection Agency (EPA), William Ruckelshaus, decided to ban its use in the United States effective December 31, 1973. He justified his decision on the grounds that a court decision had upheld the right of the state of Wisconsin to ban it (Dunlap, 1981). Banning something, however, did not fully eliminate the problem. In the 1980s, for example, it was found that an Italian pesticide with the trade name Dicofol included as much as 12% to 14% DDT (Graham, 1984). Although the manufacturer of Dicofol quickly offered to make cuts in the DDT content (Hager, 1985), other pesticide problems remain. In 1985, for example, the pesticide aldicarb (Temik) caused what the press called the "Great Watermelon Disaster." Temik was not authorized for use on watermelons, but some farmers sprayed them anyway, perhaps accidentally. Some of these sprayed melons were served on the Fourth of July, and about 300 people required medical treatment after displaying symptoms similar to those of influenza (dizziness, nausea, perspiration, shaking, and blurred vision). As a result of the contamination more than 1 million watermelons had to be destroyed (Melon contamination, 1985). This misuse of the pesticide did not lead to its elimination by Union Carbide, which manufactured Temik. Instead the company urged stiffer penalties for misuse and published more effective directions for its use.

Sevin is chemically related to Temik and is also manufactured by Union Carbide. Sevin killed or injured thousands in a chemical leakage in Bhopal, India, in 1985 (Marshall, 1985c). The Indian courts have awarded more than $200 million to the various Indian claimants against Union Carbide.

Sometimes it seems as if no pesticides are safe in the long run. Larvadex, a chemical fed to chickens as a means of preventing the growth of insect larvae in the fowl's fecal matter, may induce bladder stones in humans. Melamine, a by-product of Larvadex's active ingredient, is known for this and is found in the eggs and meat of chickens that are fed the chemical (Weis, 1984). Paraquat, another insecticide, is cited as inducing the symptoms of Parkinson's disease (Lewis, 1985), and when taken internally it is lethal to humans (West Germany bans, 1984). Baking mixes contaminated by ethylene dibromide (EDB) in 1984 led a number of states to pull such mixes from the grocery stores (Science, 1984). Although it was believed earlier that the chemical dissipated into harmless amounts during processing, further research disclosed that it persisted for 300 to 500 days in sufficient amounts to cause cancer in mice. It has also been implicated in the death of two workers who directly absorbed a 0.1% to 0.3% solution through their skin, and it contaminated some 500 wells in Florida (Raloff, 1984b). In 1988 many lawn-spraying companies were forced to change pesticides because they caused allergies.

The controversy about pesticides will continue for some time. There is no easy solution to the dangers they pose, and no good alternative to eliminating pests exists. This means that the nurse in the community must be aware of the inherent dangers of even the most commonly used pesticide and alert to possible allergies they cause.

TOXIC WASTE DUMPS

The pesticide problem has another dimension that also has implications for the community health nurse, namely their disposal. There has been a long tradition in the United States of using vast, empty areas as a receptacle for unwanted, often hazardous wastes without thinking about or anticipating the consequences. The dangers of such practices came to public attention in the 1970s, largely through the problems of the Love Canal area in Niagara Falls, New York. The canal itself was an abandoned ditch started at the turn of the century by William T. Love to divert water from the Niagara River to produce cheap electricity.

Later the ditch was used as a toxic waste dump by the Hooker Chemical Company. In the 1950s the property was sold to the Niagara City Board of Education for $1. Hooker officials claimed to have warned the city about the intrinsic dangers of the dump, but city officials later denied such a warning had been given (Brown, 1980). It is clear, however, that the chemical company required the city to sign disclaimers absolving Hooker of any responsibility for accidents sustained on the property. The city divided the land into two parts, one for a school and playground and another that was sold to a private developer for family housing. Construction was completed in the 1950s. The only problem noticed at that time was chemical sludge that appeared when the foundations were being excavated. In 1976 the owner of a home adjacent to the canal presented the EPA with ooze from her basement that was found to contain 82 industrial chemicals, at least 11 of which were believed to be cancer causing. Matters worsened during the next several months, in large part because of the extremely heavy precipitation recorded in the area, culminating in the blizzard of January 1977, which closed the city. The high water levels forced a wide variety of toxic wastes to the surface, but neither city nor county officials proved helpful in dealing with the problem. One local health official tried to calm anxious families by stating that the effects of the chemicals were only the equivalent of smoking one cigarette per day (Gibbs, 1981). As residential protest mounted, the New York State Health Commissioner in 1978 authorized a series of epidemiologic and physiologic studies. These studies found a higher rate of miscarriages, stillbirths, and low–birth weight infants in the area compared with state averages. After these studies the commissioner ordered all pregnant women to be relocated, and the problems of Love Canal hit the national headlines. After the results of a chromosome test indicated that 11 of 36 residents sampled had sustained chromosomal damage, President Jimmy Carter declared the situation an emergency, and the remainder of the residents were relocated (Chromosome change, 1980).

Matters are not always so simple as they seem, and Love Canal remains controversial. The validity of the Love Canal studies continues to be questioned by some members of the scientific community. Although there has been an increasing willingness to accept the results of epidemiologic studies, the sample was regarded by many as too small and not long term enough to make the kind of conclusions that were made. Economics was also involved, since the city of Niagara Falls was reluctant to lose the tax base in the area and many residents did not feel they received a fair price for their homes. The media pressured the Niagara Falls government to come up with precise answers, but research scientists could present only probabilities, further increasing the anxiety of many inhabitants of the Love Canal area. The event, moreover, was a new phenomenon, requiring guidelines for legal action, health studies, and potential damage assessment. There was no uniform agreement on how to conduct the studies or what they might mean.

The more than 700 families caught between the politicians, scientists, and media in the Love Canal incident represent only the beginning of the hidden problem that has been created by centuries of careless dumping. It also serves to remind us nurses of the pitfalls that await us as we try to deal with problems of environmental hazards to health.

One of the more beneficial results of the uproar about Love Canal was the passage of the Comprehensive Environmental Response and Liability Act in 1980, often called the superfund. The legislation allocated $1.6 billion over five years to identify and clean up wastes (U.S. Congress, Congressional Budget Office, 1985). Initially a list of 600 U.S. priority sites requiring superfund expenditure was compiled, and efforts were made to begin the cleanup. By 1985 only 12 sites had been cleaned up (Shortfall, 1985), and to speed progress the superfund was increased to $7.5 billion in 1986. This probably is still not enough, since as of this writing it is estimated that there are more than 20,000 hazardous waste dumps with cost of cleanup estimates ranging from $23 billion to more than $100 billion (House passes, 1985).

One of the things community health nurses should research is the existence of toxic waste sites in their community. Since many of the effects of exposure to toxic substances, such as cancers, liver and kidney disorders, and skin problems, may not appear until decades later, a familiarization with the epidemiologic histories in the area would be helpful. Such data would also indicate if there was an unusual number of miscarriages, stillbirths, or low–birth weight infants that could not be explained by other factors. Since one of the reactions of people who find they live near a toxic dump site is hysteria, the nurse must be prepared with accurate information to deal with community members. This is more difficult than it seems, since hard data on adverse health effects are not always as precise as nurses would like them to be.

RADIATION

The dangers of exposure to radiation were demonstrated to the world with the meltdown of the Soviet atomic energy plant at Chernobyl in 1986. Before this there had been accidents in a number of countries, including the United States and the Soviet Union, but the consequences had been minimized by those in authority. There was no great fear of such accidents; the fear was of nuclear bombs. The initial lack of information about the Soviet accident fueled unrest that resulted in panic and in some cases violent protest. Estimates of the number of people suffering radiation damage from the Chernobyl incident vary, but the numbers might run into the millions. Again one of the major difficulties in assessing risk is that some of the chronic health disorders that occur might not become apparent until 20 years after the exposure (Gofman, 1981).

Radiation is a more complicated issue than exposure to fallout from a defective atomic plant, since radiation energy or radiant energy includes such diverse forms as light, heat, radiowaves, and microwaves. The motion of these energies is both wavelike and particlelike with each wave or par-

FORMS OF IONIZING RADIATION

Gamma rays—Photons from the nuclei of an atom.
X-rays—Photons emitted from the nuclei but produced from two protons and two neutrons.
Beta radiation—High-speed, negatively charged (electrons) or positively charged (positrons) particles.
Neutron radiation—Neutrons emitted as a result of radioactive decay.

ticle consisting of energy. Since the amount of energy might vary with different particles or waves, the effects do also. Ionizing radiation occurs when energy particles, such as photons, possess enough energy to produce an ionizing effect. Ideally, an atom is composed of equal numbers of negatively charged electrons and positively charged protons. A highly charged particle such as a photon has enough energy to knock an electron out of an atom, making the atom imbalanced. Ionizing radiation is made up of high-energy particles that displace electrons in an atom, thereby creating the imbalanced ion. There are a variety of forms of ionizing radiation (see box above).

The types of radiation described come from a variety of sources. In the immediate post–World War II era most attention was focused on strontium 90, a principal component of radioactive fallout from nuclear weapons testing. Strontium 90 was produced at the first atomic explosion in New Mexico and is still found in countries that do their nuclear weapons testing aboveground. Before nuclear weapons testing in the United States, Great Britain, and the Soviet Union went underground, there was fear that strontium 90 would be absorbed as a calcium substitute and become incorporated into the bone tissues of young children. Court trials based on the effects of fallout from nuclear testing in Nevada indicate that this was a theoretical possibility not only for children, but for adults as well. A Salt Lake City judge in the early 1980s awarded \$2.66 million to the survivors of nine cancer victims (eight who died of leukemia, and one who died from breast cancer) and \$100,000 to a victim of thyroid cancer. The verdict was based on the failure of government officials monitoring the blasts to warn inhabitants of nearby areas of the potential dangers (Raloff, 1984a).

MEASURES OF IONIZING RADIATION

Roentgen is the amount of radiation producing a given number of ions in a given quantity of air. It is used to measure x-rays and gamma rays.
Rad is the standardized quantity of radiation absorbed by a particular material or tissue.
Rem (roentgen equivalent man) is the dose of various kinds of radiation; the rem is equivalent to the rad but is used to measure x-rays. It is usually used for doses of less than 10 rad.
RBE (relative biological effectiveness) is a conversion from rad into rem: rem = RBE × rad.
Half-life is the amount of time required for a substance to decay to half its original amount.

The Nuclear Defense Agency contested the decision of another government agency, the General Accounting Office (GAO), to award money to 42,000 military and civilian personnel who had been exposed to radiation during a nuclear testing operation that took place on or near the Bikini atoll. The defense agency claimed that personnel were not overexposed, whereas the GAO argued that the monitoring of radiation was insufficient (Radiation exposure, 1985).

The box above defines various terms used in the measurement of radiation.

Underground testing contributes about 4 to 5 mrem (millirem or one thousandth of a rem) to the yearly total radiation exposure of the average person. Nuclear power plants, another synthetic source of radiation, contribute about 1 mrem to the annual total but pose additional problems with accidental spills and waste storage (Rosenthal, 1984). Surprisingly, the largest single source of synthetic radiation comes from medical applications with x-rays constituting roughly 90% of these nonnatural sources. A chest x-ray study adds about 30 mrad (one thousandth of a rad), whereas gastrointestinal fluoroscopy can add up to 100 times that amount (Rosenthal, 1984). The significance of these numbers comes from the fact that about 240 million x-ray studies are taken each year in the United States, or about one per person. The Committee on the Biological Effects of Ionizing Radiation (BEIR) of the National Academy of Sciences classifies low-level radiation as 10 rad or less, but this standard has been challenged in recent years. Originally it was believed that a dose less than 10 rad would have no chronic health effects, and doses were plotted on a curve from the most significant effect to no effect. Many radiation experts now believe the relationship between dose and effect is better shown by a linear plot, and only when there is no exposure at all can it be said there is no possibility of radiation-induced effects (Land, 1984). The current controversy is extremely important to nurses, not only in their relationship with their clients but in their own professional capacity. They must monitor their own exposure to x-rays, as well as the exposure of their patients. Machines producing radiation should be carefully examined each year, and every means possible should be taken to minimize dosage. Fortunately, as researchers became aware of the potential danger of even minimal dosages, the amount of radiation used by x-ray machines declined to only 20% of what it was in 1940 (Gofman, 1981). New techniques such as ultrasonography do not use x-rays at all and probably will increase in popularity because of this.

The most feared aspect of peacetime radiation use stems from the accidental release of radioactivity into the atmosphere as either a result of improper waste disposal or a safety breakdown in a power plant. The spread of a radioactive cloud through Europe from the Chernobyl incident created a tremendous uproar; fresh agricultural products were temporarily banned in several countries, children and pregnant women were evacuated in areas of Poland and the Ukraine in the Soviet Union, and the death toll resulting from this has continued to mount (Raloff and Thomsen, 1986). In the United States a partial meltdown occurred at Three Mile Island. This released an unknown amount of radiation into the atmosphere, although it is estimated that the largest amount received by any one person was about 0.10 rad, the equivalent of four x-ray studies. Workers in radiation plants are exposed to not more than five rad per year (Marshall, 1984a). One result of both the Chernobyl and Three Mile Island accidents has been to cast doubt on the safety of generating electric power through nuclear plants, a matter that is now much in the political arena.

A major problem adding to the dangers of the use of radiation, including its use in the health care industry, is disposal of wastes. A tragic example of careless disposal of nuclear wastes occurred in Juarez, Mexico, in 1984. An irradiation machine used in cancer therapy at a Texas hospital was sold to a Juarez clinic that stored it in a warehouse from which it was stolen. Inside the machine were more than 6000 pellets of cobalt 60, each containing about 70 microcuries of radiation. The burglars opened the machine on their truckbed, spilling some of the pellets and receiving exposure of 300 to 450 rem—enough to cause death in half the burglars. The machine was then sold as scrap metal at a local junkyard. Many of the pellets were melted with the scrap, and this metal was made into a variety of products, which found their way into houses and even furniture on both sides of the border. To add to the complications, the truck used in the theft scattered radioactive pellets on the highways where they became imbedded in the tire treads of other cars that further scattered the pellets. Overall an estimated 200 individuals received exposure from 1 to 50 rad, increasing their risk of cancer several times (Marshall, 1984b).

RADON

Not all radioactive wastes are caused by humans. It can also occur naturally from the decay of earthbound materials, and some geographic areas have higher exposure than others. Radon gas, a natural decay product of radium, is found not only in mine tailings (that is, residuals) in Colorado and Florida but in what has been labeled the "radon prong," a specific area of eastern Pennsylvania, northern New Jersey, southern New York, and western Massachusetts. One house located on the prong was found to have 100 times the radon levels allowed in uranium mines. The accidental discovery of this exposure occurred when the owner set off detectors at the nuclear plant where he worked. Some experts theorize that radon may be the second leading cause of lung cancer in the United States, and the EPA is currently monitoring some 20,000 homes in the radon prong to determine more specific threats to health. Although there is little anyone can do to reduce the natural emission of radon gas, the problem can be greatly lessened by ventilating basements in afflicted areas. Community health nurses living in this area must take the existence of radon gas into account in assessing their clients and, until more is known, make certain that basements are well ventilated (How to check, 1985).

Certain occupations subject workers to more exposure than do others. Radium miners are a good example, and the Navaho miners who worked in uranium mines in the 1960s are 14 times as likely to have cancer (Samet and others, 1984). Commercial pilots and flight crews might also be more susceptible to cancer as a result of exposure to cosmic radiation at the higher altitudes for long periods (Raloff, 1985).

As the dangers of radiation have been recognized, governments and other institutions have taken steps to lessen them. Aboveground testing of nuclear weapons has been discontinued by the United States, the Soviet Union, and the United Kingdom. The United States enacted the Nuclear Waste Policy in 1982 to select and develop a high-level waste facility. At the time of the act there were roughly 12.6 metric tons of spent waste that needed to be stored; by 1998 it is estimated there will be an additional 30,000 metric tons, not counting the wastes developed by the defense department. As of this writing, Nevada has been designated as the site of storage. Even transporting such wastes is hazardous, and to deal with this problem there has been considerable effort to find ways to make wastes less hazardous (Peterson, 1985a; Sales and Boatner, 1984). Obviously much more needs to be done, but based on what researchers now know, radiation exposures will continue to be a problem confronting the community health nurse.

TOXIC METALS

Lead

One of the least publicized and most widespread potential health problems is metal toxicity. Some metals, such as sodium and potassium, are essential to biologic functioning, whereas doses of other metals, such as lead and mercury, can result in severe brain damage and even death. It is not possible to cover all the effects of metals on health in a brief chapter such as this, but a knowledge of some of the problems is critical to community health nurses.

A typical case involved a two-year-old black boy who was admitted to a hospital with vomiting, intermittent abdominal pains, and constipation. Blood tests revealed, among other problems, hypochromic anemia, and x-ray films displayed dense metallic markings in the bone tissue. Despite efforts to detoxify the patient and arrest the convulsions, the child died the day after admission (Oehme, 1978). The boy was a victim of lead poisoning. He could have ingested lead from a variety of sources such as paint chips on an old crib, old food coloring or paint that is now banned, or old dishes made from pewter that contained lead (Needleman, 1980). Lead poisoning can lead to encephalopathy if taken in sufficient quantities, but even in small quantities it can lead to hyperactivity and short attention span.

One of the early studies of lead poisoning described a so-called lead belt that consisted primarily of poor urban areas in the East and Midwest where lead-based paints had been used on houses and furniture earlier in this century. The 1966 study reported that 20% to 40% of the children in these areas had elevated lead levels in the blood. As a result of such findings, Congress in 1971 enacted the Lead Prevention Act, which allocated funds for the establishment of screening facilities under the direction of the surgeon general and the removal of lead paints from dwellings in poor areas and prohibited any addition of lead to paint (Needleman, 1980). However, caution in working with the old lead paint and other sources of lead contamination is important because workers who rehabilitate houses can also absorb too much lead.

Still another source of lead is the emissions from automobiles using leaded gasoline. To counter this danger the EPA called for a phasedown in the lead content of gasoline, the phasing out of cars that required leaded gasoline, and the manufacture of new cars that could use unleaded fuel. Seemingly as one source of lead contamination was found and steps were taken to eliminate it, other sources appeared. Lead is found in solder, which often connects pipes that carry our drinking water, many of the toy soldiers, miniature cars, and molded utensils of the past, in pottery glazes, and in gunpowder. The average adult consumes about 150 to 300 μg (a millionth of a gram) from food each day and inhales about 20 μg from the air. For children the average ingestion rate per day is about 100 μg, but the absorption into the tissues is much higher (Needleman, 1980).

Chronic lead exposure occurs most frequently among children younger than five years of age. Children who exhibit symptoms such as tiredness, pallor, appetite loss, irritability, sleep disturbances, and even behavior changes may have been ingesting lead for three months. The first areas to sustain damage are the pathways of heme (the iron protoporphyrin constituent of hemoglobin), and then the kidney and liver. Prolonged high-level exposure results in nerve damage caused by the degeneration of the axons and the demyelination of the peripheral nerves (Oehme, 1978).

Treatment of lead poisoning is a three-step process involving the reduction of lead in the body, location and minimization of the sources of lead intake, and lessening of the vulnerability to lead intake through better nutrition. To lower concentration, chemicals such as calcium disodium edectate (EDTA), British antilewisite (BAL), and D-penicillamine are given. These chemicals either chelate or bind to lead and allow it to pass through the body.

Finding the source takes some detective work by the nurse and requires an inspection of the house and yard, although the most common source is paint chips from windowsills or cribs. Diet is important because diets poor in calcium, phosphorus, and iron result in greater absorption of lead by the body (Oehme, 1978). The Centers for Disease Control in 1984 recommended further reduction of lead levels in the blood from 30 to 10 μg per 100 ml of blood, a goal that will be difficult to achieve without further reductions in automobile emissions (Marshall, 1984b).

Mercury

Another metal that poses difficulties is mercury, which in the past was often used for medicinal purposes. In fact it was the standard treatment for syphilis until well into the twentieth century. Mercury's dangers have been known for some time as indicated by the expression "mad as a hatter," which referred to the sequelae of inhaling mercurial vapors by hatmakers who used mercury in their manufacturing process. As late as World War I, studies suggested that some 60% of the members of the French guild of hatmakers were experiencing some form of mental derangement from inhaling mercury fumes (D'Itri, 1977).

Although hatmakers are no longer victims of mercury poisoning, others are. One of the new sources of mercury poisoning came to the attention of Japanese observers along Minimata Bay in Japan who documented what they termed "dancing cat disease," the zigzag, whirling motions of cats in their death throes. A similar disease was soon noted in humans, particularly children, and the source was eventually traced to a local industrial firm dumping mercury into the ocean. The mercury was absorbed by the fish and other sea life as methyl mercury, and this seafood was harvested and consumed by locals. Action to remedy this problem was slow, and by 1974, 103 deaths had been attributed to mercury poisoning in the area, 18% of the children were mentally retarded, and more than 3000 cases of poisoning had been recorded (Oehme, 1978).

Unfortunately, mercury poisoning has not been restricted to one rural area in Japan. In the United States alkyl mercury was often used as a fungicide in some areas and in others as a treatment to protect seeds from spoilage during storage. In New Mexico, a farmer was given some waste seeds from a local grain repository. He fed these seeds to his 14 pigs, one of which he then slaughtered. Two of his children who ate the pork became comatose, another became semicomatose, 12 of his pigs died, and the surviving pig was blinded. Analysis of the pig that had been slaughtered and partially eaten by the family revealed 29.4 parts per million (ppm) of mercury. The U.S. Department of Agriculture acted more quickly than the Japanese government, and the result was a ban on the use of alkyl mercury products in the United States (D'Itri, 1977).

Interestingly, mercury in its most elemental form is not particularly toxic. The mad hatters inhaled mercurial nitrate, and the other cases of mercury poisoning involved the ingestion of organic (carbon-based) mercury solutions. Methyl mercury is particularly dangerous and is converted from less toxic forms of certain bacteria. Many forms of sea life then absorb it, leading to concentrations in the food chain that approach toxic levels in humans. Once methyl mercury is ingested or absorbed, it binds to red blood cells from which it spreads to the bone marrow and nerve cells, and causes damage either to these areas or to the spinal cord. Symptoms of low-level chronic exposure include anorexia, salivation, and foul breath. Acute poisoning can cause gastrointestinal hemorrhaging, bloody diarrhea, and, in the most severe cases, death. Treatment involves emptying of the stomach, use of antibiotics, and the use of chemical binders or chelators to mercury.

Arsenic

Arsenic is another naturally occurring mineral that has toxic qualities and can accumulate in an organism. Seawater normally includes some arsenic, about 2 to 5 μg per liter, so some creatures can accumulate it in their systems. In the ocean off the coast of southern California, some crabs have been found to have concentrations between 14 and 43 ppm arsenic (Oehme, 1978), but the FDA limits arsenic to 2 ppm in animal by-products and 0.5 ppm in muscle tissue.

Arsenic is normally a by-product of smelting factories, coal plants, and geothermal emissions. It can be either inhaled or ingested into the body, and once in the system it is concentrated in the kidney, liver, spleen, skin, hair, and nails. Children living near smelters have been found with three and a half times the normal concentration in their nails and hair. Since arsenic resembles phosphorus, it may be mistakenly used by the body for such things as chromosomal repair (Goyer and Mehlman, 1977). Chronic symptoms include weight loss, skin sores, and hair loss. Acute symptoms include damage to the production of red blood cells, severe gastroenteritis, hemorrhaging, and death. Some arsenic forms may be carcinogenic, since higher cancer rates have been noted among users of arsenic-contaminated wells in Taiwan. Treatment of arsenic victims is similar to that of mercury or lead victims (Oehme, 1978).

Selenium

Selenium is a newcomer to the list of well-known dangerous metals. It is an essential nutrient in humans and in minute concentrations is believed to reduce the risk of some cancers, lessen the chance for periodontal disease, and lower the rate of sudden infant death syndrome. The average intake in the diet is about 1.8 mg per day, whereas adult blood levels of selenium are 10 to 34 μg. The body's need for selenium has resulted in some health food companies marketing selenium tablets, which are also extolled for their presumed anticancer properties. Unfortunately, the toxic dose of selenium is not much more than the normative amount. The FDA has forced some of the selenium tablets off the market on the grounds that their concentrations were too high (Lead in imported, 1985). Naturally occurring selenium may also reach toxic levels through the combustion of fossil fuels or the smelting of a variety of scrap alloys. Hydrogen selenide is one of the toxic forms created by interaction with industrial acids on organic matter. Seleniferous soil runoff is devastating to wildlife in areas where such soil is abundant. Such devastation took place in the Kesterson Wildlife Refuge when it was contaminated by wastewater runoff from the San Joaquin Valley in California. The result was growth in the number of deformed waterfowl and loss of a previously thriving gamefish population. Analysis found 53 ppm selenium in mosquito fish and 4700 ppm (four times the level that is set for mandatory placement in a toxic dump) selenium in the surrounding water district (Marshall, 1985a and b).

Nickel

Nickel, which is absorbed through the skin, results in what has been termed the "nickel itch." It also causes a rash on the hands when it is absorbed over time. Nickel carbonyl is a colorless industrial liquid that is toxic; symptoms include headaches, fatigue, and insomnia. Often there is a temporary remission of these symptoms, followed by a relapse marked by a cough, chills, muscular pain, and general weakness. Prolonged exposure to nickel may also be linked to some forms of cancer. Treatment for acute exposure is a combination of sodium bicarbonate and dithiocarb (Oehme, 1978).

Copper

Copper in excess quantities is also toxic. Wilson's disease is a metabolic disorder in which the liver is unable to remove copper from the body. The Kayser-Fleischer ring is a condition in which a green or brown ring appears around the cornea and is symptomatic of nerve damage and of toxic accumulations of copper in the liver and kidney. Copper sulfate can be fatal if ingested.

Cadmium

The list could go on to include cadmium, which causes what is termed "itai-itai disease" in Japan and which appears naturally in some drinking water (Oehme, 1978).

WATER POLLUTION

Most contaminants have been uncovered only in the last few decades. Since many of them are associated with specific geographic areas, nurses must pay special attention to problem metals in the areas in which they practice. Fortunately, as we have uncovered new areas of public health concern, some of the older ones have lessened. Typhoid fever killed 31.3 per 100,000 population at the turn of the century, whereas today the death rate is almost zero. This change was brought about by improvements in water treatment and more effective disposal of human wastes. Similarly, chlorination of water has led to declines in a host of waterborne diseases. Still, infectious pathogens that exist in water continue to pose a threat to human health, whereas the pollution of the water supply by organic and inorganic chemicals has just begun to be addressed. The passage of the Clean Water Act in 1972 and the subsequent amendments to the act have worked to eliminate direct discharges of pollutants into navigable waters. There are still problems with groundwater supplies, however, and such sources supply the drinking water for 50% of the population. A major source of difficulty is that water sources serving fewer than 25 individuals and 15 service connections are generally not monitored by water quality agencies (USGS, 1984), and this means that people living in rural areas are often at risk. Nurses in rural areas must be aware of the potential problems associated with groundwater contamination but, for that matter, so must nurses in such areas as Long Island where much of the population depends on groundwater.

AIR POLLUTION

Another source of pollutants is the air we breathe. Air pollution is an extremely generalized term depicting a hodgepodge of gaseous, vaporous, and particulate substances that can damage our health under the right conditions (see box). In 1970 Congress enacted the Clean Air Act, which, among other things, placed tighter emission control standards on industrial air emissions and required the development and implementation of catalytic converters on automobiles.

Although the EPA has effectively concentrated much of its efforts to minimize the dangers of these airborne pollutants, under special conditions they still pose problems for which the community health nurse should be on the alert.

Air pollutants are found not only outdoors but indoors, often in higher concentrations than outside. Recent research indicates that the modern climate-controlled buildings with windows that

FIVE KINDS OF AIR POLLUTANTS OF CONCERN TO COMMUNITY HEALTH NURSES

1. Total suspended particles (TSPs) are discharged from industrial and other sources at the rate of 100 million tons annually. The bulk of particulates comes from fuel combustion, gravel crushing, grain processing, and steel manufacturing. The composition of particulates ranges from tiny asbestos fibers to coal dust; the smaller the particles, the greater the likelihood of their penetration to the lung. Tiny particles penetrate the alveoli and enter the lymphatic system as potential carcinogens, often carrying toxic metals or radioactive substances with them (Stone and Smallwood, 1974).
2. Sulfur dioxide results mainly from the combustion of high sulfur coal fuels for electric power. It is irritating to the eyes, nose, and throat and may precipitate asthmatic attacks or severe respiratory disorders. In certain atmospheric conditions, it may be transformed into sulfuric acid, one of the components of acid rain, which is destroying the lakes and forests of the United States, Canada, and Europe.
3. Nitrogen dioxide is derived from automobiles and fossil fuel–burning electric plants. It can be damaging to the respiratory tract but is much more visible when it interacts with atmospheric carbon compounds to form ozone and other photochemical oxidants that make up smog (Abelson, 1985).
4. Carbon monoxide is the colorless and odorless gas that binds with the heme of the red blood cells almost immediately after inhalation. The result is a deprivation of oxygen, which induces headaches, dizziness, a slowing of reflexes, and in a relatively short period, death. Automobile exhaust is the largest source of carbon monoxide, and in cities such as Los Angeles temperature inversions have resulted with carbon monoxide levels of 100 ppm, a level that leads many to feel dizzy and to suffer a headache (Stone and Smallwood, 1974). Carbon monoxide is an ever-present danger when an automobile is left running. In fact, the widespread knowledge of this makes carbon monoxide poisoning a common form of suicide.
5. Ozone is the primary component of smog, and it is produced in a reaction involving nitrogen dioxide, hydrocarbons, oxygen, and sunlight. It is a contributing factor to the destruction of vegetation, particularly conifers. It also, as indicated, produces a general irritation to the eyes, nose, and throat (Karen, 1985).

do not open are particularly prone to difficulty because pollutants can be circulated through the heating and cooling systems. Smoking raises particular problems, and it is for this reason that airplanes are increasingly forbidding smoking on short flights and that smoking is allowed only in designated areas of restaurants, theaters, factories, and office buildings in many government jurisdictions. Even in the home, air pollution is a problem, and children reared in homes where both parents smoke have a 30% greater chance of respiratory illnesses. Other indoor pollutants include asbestos (from insulation), benzene (from solvent cleaners), styrene (from plastics and carpets), and fungal bacteria (from air conditioners and humidifiers). Since asbestos has been demonstrated to be a factor in lung cancer, there is a national movement to remove asbestos from schools, churches, and other such buildings. Formaldehyde is found in more than 3000 different building products, and new limits have been placed on its use, since it causes headaches and irritates the respiratory tract. Benzene and styrene are believed to be factors in leukemia, as well as kidney and liver damage. The so-called Legionnaires' disease was the most notorious result of a rare type of bacteria that grew in the air-conditioning units of the Philadelphia hotel hosting an American Legion convention in 1976 (Carey, 1985).

NOISE POLLUTION

Often overlooked as a hazard to health is noise pollution, defined as any unwanted sound found within the environment. This rather broad definition can include anything from the unwanted crickets at a summer concert to a portable radio blasting at the beach. For noise to be classified as a health hazard, however, level, frequency, and length of exposure should be taken into account. At the lowest level a noise can be annoying, whereas at other levels it can result in the disruption of activities (such as reading this book), loss of hearing, and ultimately mental and physical deterioration. Noise level is measured by decibels (dB) and dB scale is based on the power of 10, so 60 dB is 10 times the intensity of 50 dB. The danger level for hearing loss is 80 dB, although the EPA has set the current standards for the workplace at 90 dB. It plans to lower the level to 75 dB (UAW Sound Security Department, 1979). Even the 90 dB level, however, is far less than the levels that some rock bands reach, although it is odd to think of music as a noise pollutant. Sound frequencies are measured in hertz (Hz), units representing cycles per sound. The audible range for humans is between 20 and 20,000 Hz. Continual exposure to high noise levels such as the sound of machinery can severely impair hearing over several years.

Although noise can be annoying, the real danger is a loss of hearing, which may be temporary or permanent. Research has shown that an aggravating noise can disturb sleep patterns, lower the body's resistance to disease, and cause nausea, headaches, and other physical symptoms of illness (Cohen, 1981). Nurses who are conscious of the dangers noise poses to their clients can urge the use of ear plugs, the establishment of sound barriers (such as many highway departments have built alongside the throughways), the wrapping or muffling of the cause of the noise, the planting of trees and shrubs (both act as noise mufflers), or other similar activities. Often clients are not fully conscious of the problem of noise pollution because they become accustomed to it. In these cases the nurse may have to encourage remedial action for problems the client might have ignored (Bruce, 1985).

SUMMARY

The purpose of this chapter is to make the nurse aware of the effect of environmental issues on public health. The environmental movement of the past two decades, despite criticisms for exaggeration and overreaction, has been a potent force in changing the nation's attitude toward the environment and has made the public aware of the dangers to their health that pollution can cause. Just as a natural community is regarded as a finely woven web of life, so is the human community. The actions and attitudes of the nurse in recognizing the potential dangers of various forms of environmental pollutants can help bring about a much healthier community.

QUESTIONS FOR DISCUSSION

1. Why are pesticides hazardous to human health?
2. List three sources of radiation exposure for humans.
3. Who was Rachel Carson, and what did she accomplish?
4. Which metals are hazardous to human health? List one possible source of exposure to three of these metals.

REFERENCES

Abelson PH: Air pollution and acid rain, Science 230:617, 1985.

Brown M: Laying waste: the poisoning of America by toxic chemicals, New York, 1980, Pantheon Books.

Brown WA: Ecology of pesticides, New York, 1978, John Wiley & Sons Inc.

Bruce RD: Noise pollution. In Jarvis LL, editor: Community health nursing, ed 2, Philadelphia, 1985, FA Davis Co.

Carey J: Beware of sick building syndrome, Newsweek, p 5860, Jan 7, 1985.

Carson R: Silent spring, Boston, 1962, Houghton-Mifflin.

Chromosome change in Love Canal victims, Science News 117:325, 1980.

Cohen S: Sound effects on behavior, Psychol Today 15:38, 1981.

D'Itri PA and D'Itri FM: Mercury contamination: a human tragedy, New York, 1977, John Wiley & Sons Inc.

Dunlap TR: DDT: pesticide policy and US history, Princeton, NJ, 1981, Princeton University Press.

Edwards CA: Persistent pesticides in the environment, Cleveland, 1972, CRC Press.

Foehrenbach F: Chlorinated pesticides in estuarine organisms, J Water Pollution Control Federation 44(4):619, 1972.

Gibbs LM: The Love Canal: my story, as told to Murray Levine, Albany, NY, 1981, State University of New York Press.

Gofman JW: Radiation and human health, San Francisco, 1981, Sierra Club Books.

Goyer RA and Mehlman MA: Toxicology of trace elements, New York, 1977, Halsted Press.

Graham F: DDT is alive and well, Audobon 86:367, 1984.

Hager M: DDT: the pesticide that didn't go away, Newsweek p 10, March 4, 1985.

House passes tough superfund bill, Science News 128:390, 1985.

How to check for radon, Consumer Reports 50:601, 1985.

Indoor pollutants, Washington, DC, 1981, National Academy Press.

Karen N: Pollution: now the bad news, Newsweek p 26, April 8, 1985.

Kormondy EJ: Readings in ecology, Englewood Cliffs, NY, 1965, Prentice Hall, Prentice Hall Press.

Land CE and others: Childhood leukemia and fallout from the Nevada nuclear tests, Science 223:5947, 1984.

Lead in imported pottery, FDA Consumer 19:4, 1985.

Lewis R: Parkinson's disease: an environmental cause? Science 229:257, 1985.

Marshall E: Juarez: an unprecedented radiation accident, Science 223:1152, 1984a.

Marshall E: Legal threats halt CDC meeting on lead, Science 223:672, 1984b.

Marshall E: San Joaquin flooded with water researchers, Science 230:920, 1985a.

Marshall E: Selenium poisons refuge, California politics, Science 229:144, 1985b.

Marshall E: The rise and decline of Temik, Science 229:1369, 1985c.

McWilliams L: A bumper crop yields growing problems, Environment, vol 26, 1984.

Melon contamination, toxic effects raise pesticide use issue, Chemical Engineering News 63:3, 1985.

Needleman HC: Low level lead exposures, New York, 1980, Raven Press.

Oehme FW: Toxicity of heavy metals in the environment, New York, 1978, M Dekker

Peterson I: Finding a resting place for radwaste, Science News 127:6, 1985a.

Radiation Exposure at Crossroads, Science News 128:397, 1985.

Raloff J: Court rules US responsible for some fallout cancers, Science News, 125:308, 1984a.

Raloff J: EPA to limit, then ban EDB in citrus, Science News 125:151, 1984b.

Raloff J: Air crew radiation doses climbing, Science News 127:357, 1985.

Raloff J and Thomsen DE: Chernobyl may be worst nuclear accident, Science News 129:276, 1986.

Risebrough RW and others: Pesticides: transatlantic movements in the northeast trades, Science 159:1233, 1968.

Rosenthal E: The hazards of everyday radiation, Science Digest 92:38, 1984.

Sales BC and Boatner LA: Lead iron phosphate glass, Science 226:45, 1984.

Samet J and others: Navahoes signal uranium mining hazards, Science News 126:9, 1984.

Shortfall at Superfund, Science News 128:215, 1985.

Stone R and Smallwood H: Intermediate aspects of air and water pollution, Washington, DC, 1974, US Government Printing Office.

US Congress: Congressional budget office report—US government policy, Washington, DC, 1985.

United Auto Workers Sound Security Department: What every representative should know about health and safety, Pub No 449:6, Detroit, UAW.

US Geological Survey: National Water Summary, 1983, Washington, DC, 1984, US Department of the Interior.

Weis JS: Pesticide policies change slowly, Bioscience 34:549, 1984.

West Germany bans paraquat, New Scientist 103:7, 1984.

BIBLIOGRAPHY

Abelson PH: Ground water contamination, Science 224:673, 1984.

Alternatives urged for several pesticides, Chemical Engineering News 63:5, 1985.

Black JA: Water pollution technology, Reston, Va, 1977, Reston Publishers.

Borchardt JA: Viruses and trace contaminants in water and waste water, Ann Arbor, Mich, 1977, The University of Michigan Press.

Brodine V: Air pollution, New York, 1973, Harcourt Brace Jovanovich Inc.

Clark DR Jr and Kryhitsky AJ: DDT: recent contamination, Science 225:2731, 1983.

Compensation for low level radiation, Science News 125:297, 1984.

Conservation Foundation: State of the environment: an assessment at mid-decade, Washington, DC, 1984, The Foundation.

Crawford M: Outside review urged for waste debate, Science 230:9245, 1985.

Eisenbaud M: Sources of ionizing radiation exposure, Environment 26:611, 1984.

Health hazards and chemical dumps, Science News 126:313, 1984.

Janerich DT: Cancer incidence in Love Canal area, Science 212:1404, 1981.

Keough C: Water fit to drink, Emmaus, Pa, 1980, Rodale Press.

Medvedev ZA: Nuclear disaster in the Urals, New York, 1978, WW Norton & Co.

Muffin mix scare, Time, p 20, Feb 13, 1984.

Nader R and Brownstein R: Beyond Love Canal, Progressive, p 28, May 1980.

Peterson I: Radwaste program: a delay in plans, Science News 125:5, 1984.

Peterson I: Standby storage for nuclear waste, Science News 127:27, 1985b.

Pye VI and others: Groundwater contamination in the US, Philadelphia, 1983, University of Pennsylvania Press.

Ricklefs E: Ecology, New York, 1973, Chiron Press.

Selenium tablets recalled, FDA Consumer 18:2, 1985.

Spengler JD and Sexton K: Indoor air pollution: a public health perspective, Science 223:6, 1984.

Sun M.: EDB contamination kills federal action, Science 223:464, 1984.

Tomato scare Italian style, Time 126:34, 1985.

US Office of Technology Assessment: Superfund strategy, Washington, DC, 1985, US Government Printing Office.

White-Stevens R: Pesticides in the environment, New York, 1971, Marcel Dekker Inc.

CHAPTER

7

Nutrition: An Integral Part of Community Health Care

Alma Blake

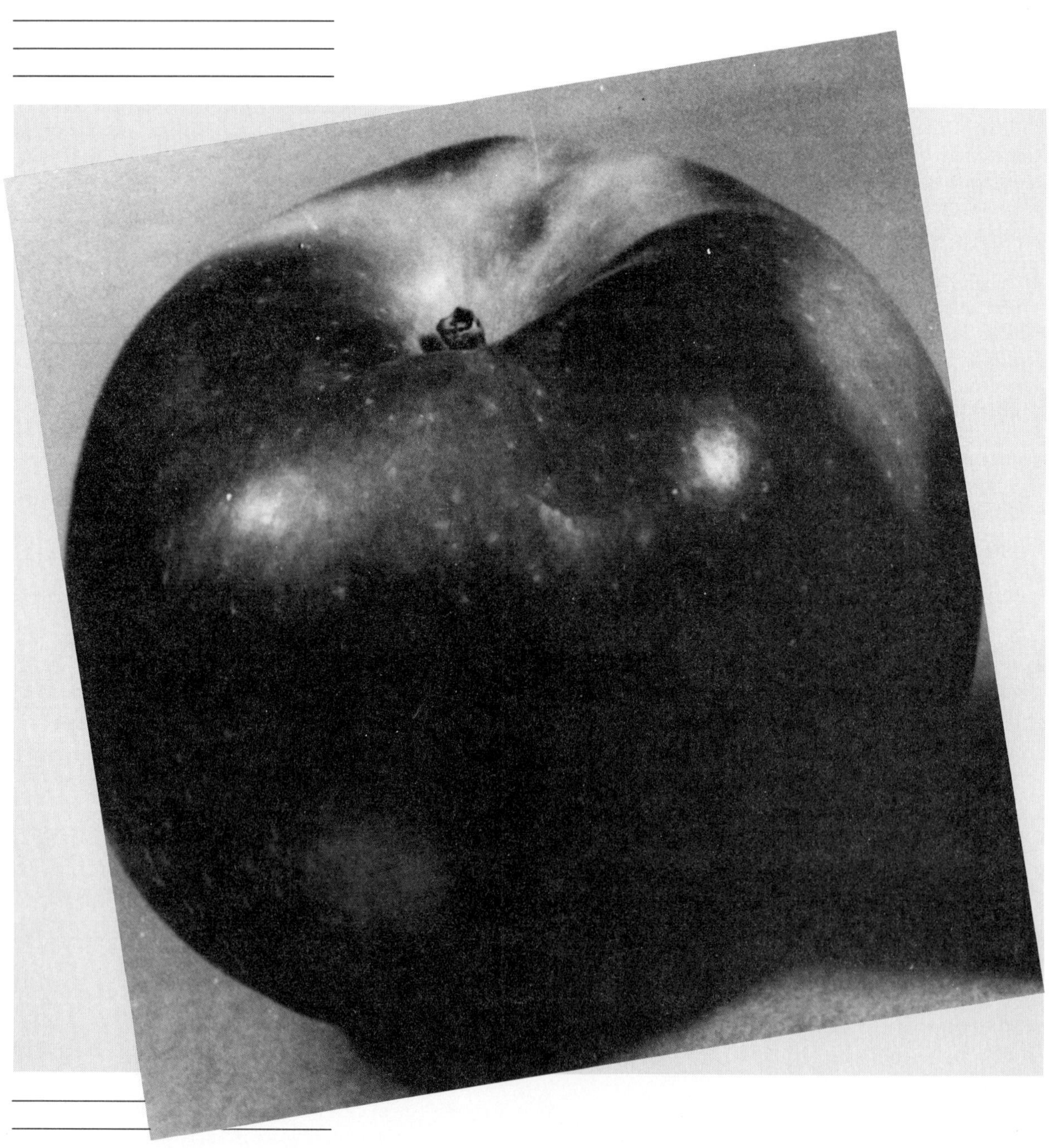

CHAPTER OUTLINE

OBJECTIVES

After completing this chapter, the reader should be able to:

1. Define the major nutrition-related health problems in the United States.
2. Identify populations at nutritional risk.
3. Identify and appreciate the role of food and nutrition in preventing or treating major health problems.
4. Identify common nutrition attitudes, beliefs, and practices of the general public.
5. Refute common nutrition fallacies with facts.
6. Use food and nutrition information to assess nutrition needs and provide appropriate counseling and referrals.

AT ONE TIME, GETTING ENOUGH FOOD TO EAT was the concern of a major portion of the U.S. population. There was little scientific information indicating that food had a significant role in chronic disease development except as it related to starvation or overeating. Currently food or food components are implicated in every major chronic disease considered a leading cause of death in the United States.

The awareness, interest, and concern of the public about the role nutrition plays in health maintenance has increased tremendously during the past decade. The public now demands nutrition information that will help them maintain health and prevent disease.

Qualified nutritionists or dietitians (registered dietitians, or RDs) are attempting to meet nutrition education needs of the public. However, RDs are few compared with the population served. Other health professionals are increasingly assuming responsibility for educating the public about nutrition, and government agencies are attempting to dispense nutrition information in a timely, well-publicized manner.

Food manufacturers, drug companies, and the media, as well as so-called health advocates, capitalize on the desire for knowledge by bombarding the public with information. The health advocates often present their theories, as well as a product to sell, in the following context: "The scientific establishment rejects my theories because I am not part of organized health." The proof of their theories usually consists of anecdotal, individual testimonies. They fail to mention that their theories have not been scientifically tested or have been tested and disproved.

Although the media increasingly seek advice from qualified nutritionists and other health professionals, they give a tremendous amount of publicity to individuals advocating unproven, unscientific nutrition practices. Another problem is the often precipitous publication of new information in the popular press without full peer review. This contributes to public confusion. Food companies have long made nutritional claims about food products such as "low in cholesterol" and "rich in vitamins and minerals." However, the new trend that concerns the nutrition community includes statements such as those strongly implying that a product prevents cancer.

This atmosphere presents a major challenge to anyone attempting to provide credible nutrition information to the community.

Health professionals must screen nutrition information appropriately, based on scientific evidence. Nurses need to understand basic nutrient roles and needs, as well as facts about food content. In other words, the current situation places demands on health professionals to keep up with basic knowledge and remain aware of available resources. Nurses need to help the public sort out issues facing them and provide the public with or direct them toward reliable information.

The purpose of this chapter is to provide an overview of the public's nutrition attitudes and practices, the nutritional and health status of the population, the role of nutrition in preventing or treating major health problems, and an update of nutrition knowledge. The ultimate goal of the chapter is to provide the nurse with basic information to make general decisions about the nutrition needs of clients in the community, provide general nutrition advice, and seek consultation from and refer patients to qualified nutrition professionals for in-depth nutrition advice and counseling.

ASSESSMENT OF NUTRITIONAL STATUS AND DIETARY INTAKE

Overall Assessment

The unique contribution of dietitians and nutritionists to health care is their knowledge of food, food components, nutrients, food's use, and its relationship to health and disease. The ultimate concern of nutritionists and dietitians is the nutritional and health status of the individual. Nutritional status is defined as an individual's health as influenced by the intake and use of food. As-

TABLE 7-1 Selected RDAs*

Category	Age (years)	Energy (kilocalories, or kcal)†	Protein (gm)	Iron (mg)	Vitamin C (mg)
Children	1 to 3	1300 (900 to 1800)	23	19	45
Females	11 to 14	2200 (1500 to 3300)	46	18	50
Males	23 to 50	2700 (2300 to 3000)	56	10	60

Modified from Food and Nutrition Board: National Research Council, Recommended dietary allowances, ed 9, Washington, DC, 1980, National Academy of Sciences.
*Values expressed as daily amounts.
†The energy value of food is expressed in terms of a unit of heat, or kilocalorie (abbreviated kcal). Kilocalorie and calorie are often used interchangeably. Kilocalorie is defined as the amount of heat required to raise the temperature of 1 kg of water 1°C, for example, from 15°C to 16°C.

sessment of nutritional status must include evaluation of clinical, biochemical, anthropometric, and dietary intake data. Nurses must consider appearance of the individual, for example, skin integrity and wound healing (clinical), whether an adult has lost or gained a significant amount of weight in a short period (anthropometric), if a hemoglobin level is low (biochemical), and whether nutrient intake is adequate (dietary). Biochemical, clinical, and anthropometric indices of nutritional status are discussed in basic nutrition nursing texts. Therefore the emphasis here is dietary evaluation.

Diet Assessment

A discussion of guides for diet evaluation provides an overview of tools used to assess dietary practices of individuals and the public, a prediction of the impact on physical function (through biochemical, clinical, and anthropometric indices), a framework for nutrition discussions throughout this chapter, and a description of tools that can be used by the nurse to provide sound nutrition information.

When evaluating nutritional status or dietary intake, providing general nutrition information, or counseling, nurses must make every effort to use the best scientific information available, as well as the prevailing interpretation. A major portion of the information used in formulating evaluations and giving dietary advice is found in the recommended dietary allowances (RDAs) of the Food and Nutrition Board of the National Research Council. The RDAs are published in manual form and revised approximately every four years (Food and Nutrition Board, 1980).

Recommended Dietary Allowances

RDAs are the daily levels of intake of essential nutrients considered adequate to meet the known nutritional needs of most healthy persons. These levels are based on available scientific knowledge. Examples of selected RDA values appear in Table 7-1. Except for energy, the RDAs contain a safety factor, an amount above requirements. The safety factors have been added to allow for variations in individual needs, absorption, and use and therefore cover most of the population (Food and Nutrition Board, 1980). Generally, diets containing less than two thirds of RDAs are considered inadequate to sustain good health.

Since the RDAs are for healthy persons, special needs for nutrients arising from such problems as premature birth, inherited metabolic disorders, infections, chronic diseases, and the use of medications require special dietary and therapeutic measures.

Food Guides for Diet Assessment

Obviously evaluation of nutrient intake using the RDAs is relatively complex and time consuming. As a result, nutrition experts recognize the need for less complex, less time-consuming methods of evaluating diets. Methods are needed to make general judgments about overall diet adequacy and whether diets provide a foundation for adequate nutrition or potentiate health problems or disease. In this context, two basic questions must be answered—how can evaluation be accomplished in a reasonably accurate and practical manner, and once a health professional makes an evaluation, or assessment, and determines the needs, how can this information be translated into language the average person will understand?

Basic Four Food Guide

Publications such as *The Basic Four Food Guide* and *Dietary Guidelines for Americans* set nutritional goals well.

Basic Four Food Guide. The *Basic Four Food Guide* contains recommended amounts of four basic food groups for children, adults, and pregnant and lactating women. The goal of this guide is to provide the foundation for an adequate diet; the goal seems to have been met except for calories for adult men and iron for women. Health professionals must provide additional guidance for intake of nutrients as well as for appropriate fat and fiber intake. *The Basic Four Food Guide* is a useful tool particularly for working with individuals who have no disease and are not at a high risk for disease but have poorly balanced diets because of lack of knowledge and experience with food selection and meal planning.

Nevertheless, critics say *The Basic Four Food Guide* is too simplistic, does not meet all micronutrient needs, and is too high in fat and too low in fiber. However, no one has developed an acceptable substitute plan that is suitable as a basic foundation for an adequate diet and easily understood by the average person. Therefore continued use of *The Basic Four Food Guide* as a foundation for planning adequate diets seems appropriate for now.

TABLE 7-2 Basic Four Food Guide

Food	Number of servings for adults	Suggested serving sizes
Milk and cheese	2 to 4	1 cup milk, 1½ oz cheese, 1¼ cup ice cream (for equivalent calcium)
Meat, poultry, fish, beans, and eggs	2	2 oz meat, 2 eggs, 2 oz cheese, 1 cup dried beans or peas
Fruit and vegetables	4	½ cup juice, ½ cup cooked vegetables, 1 cup raw vegetables
Whole grain breads and cereals	4	1 slice bread, 1 cup ready-to-eat cereal, ½ cup rice
Miscellaneous: fats, sweets, and alcohol	(eat sparingly)	1 tsp margarine, 1 tsp sugar, 1 tbsp salad dressing, mayonnaise, or jelly

Modified from National Dairy Council: How to eat for good health, Rosemont, Ill, 1985, National Dairy Council.

The Basic Four Food Guide appears in various formats and with varying amounts of information. One version of selected examples of the guide appears in Table 7-2.

Dietary Guidelines for Americans

The Dietary Guidelines for Americans, published by the United States Department of Agriculture (USDA) and Department of Health and Human Services (DHHS), is a lesser-known guide that is gaining recognition. The focus of the guidelines is prevention of major chronic diseases. Health professionals can use the guidelines as a general tool to evaluate dietary practices and translate them easily for the general public.

The guidelines are not without criticisms and controversy. One criticism is that they are too vague and general. However, a more substantive controversy surrounds their efficacy. A number of the nutrition experts conclude that available

DIETARY GUIDELINES FOR AMERICANS

1. Eat a variety of foods daily.
2. Maintain a desirable weight.
3. Avoid too much fat, saturated fat, and cholesterol.
4. Eat foods with adequate starch and fiber.
5. Avoid too much sugar.
6. Avoid too much sodium.
7. If you drink alcohol, do so in moderation.

Modified from USDA, DHHS: Nutrition and your health, dietary guidelines for Americans, ed 2, Washington, DC, 1985, U.S. Government Printing Office.

data are inadequate to support the recommendations for the general population. For example, the experts question the efficacy of suggesting that individuals not at high risk for heart disease benefit from a low–saturated fat, low-cholesterol diet. Individuals not at high risk for heart disease include those with normal blood lipids, no family history of heart disease, no cardiovascular disease, and normal weight. Nevertheless, the prevailing belief held by nutrition experts is that changes recommened in the guidelines are based on sound scientific data and that the changes are prudent and may be protective for most of the population. The boxed material shows the seven guidelines. The detailed published guidelines are available from the U.S. Government Printing Office (USDA, DHHS, 1985).

The discussion in the following paragraphs on nutritional status and nutrition and health attitudes, beliefs, life-styles, and specific practices provides a framework for the eventual consideration of actual nutrition and health problems prevalent in the community and how they might be prevented or treated.

Nutritional Status and Dietary Intake of U.S. Population

The Department of Health and Human Services (DHHS) and the National Center for Health Statistics collect nutritional status data in the National Health and Nutrition Examination Survey (NHANES) every four years from a probability sample of the U.S. population. A recent evaluation of that and other existing health and food consumption data is summarized below.

Some Americans in extreme poverty (migrant workers, Indians on reservations, and the homeless) may not have sufficient amounts of food, and 3% of Americans who responded to a survey about perceived food adequacy said that sometimes or often there was not enough to eat. However, clinically significant nutritional deficiencies for which the diet is responsible are relatively rare. The principal nutrition-related health problems of Americans come from overconsumption of fat, saturated fatty acids, cholesterol, and sodium. A concomitant nutrition problem is obesity. On the other hand, underconsumption is apparent in subgroups of the population. Women have low calcium intakes; dietary and biochemical data indicate that vitamin C intake is low in some groups; and impaired iron status seems a particular problem for young children and females of childbearing age (USDA, DHHS, 1986).

A recent evaluation of U.S. diets from NHANES data shows trends in intake that contribute to some of the existing health problems; for example, some leading sources of calories listed on the survey included white bread, cake, and pastries, which are low in fiber and high in fat and calories. Pastries, alcohol, and soft drinks constituted 15% of the total calories reported in the survey. According to the survey, whole milk is consumed twice as often as 2% milk or skim milk (Block and others, 1985).

Nutritional Risk Factors

Many factors or situations predispose individuals or groups to poor nutritional status and disease. The prevalence of health conditions directly or indirectly related to nutritional status is generally highest among low-income groups. Specific additional predisposing factors include any disease that severely interferes with absorption and metabolism of nutrients, severely restricted therapeutic diets, especially in children and the elderly, severe limitation of eating habits for religious, cultural, or philosophic reasons such as vegetarianism, and alcoholism, which interferes with food use but also results in poor diets.

POVERTY, RACE, AND NUTRITIONAL HABITS

One must always be cognizant of the fact that poverty plays a major role in diet adequacy. However, it is a mistake for the nurse to approach the traditionally poor clients with the preconceived notion that poverty is the sole reason for food habits and attitudes that contribute to poor health. Actually, evaluation of our best up-to-date data on food intake in the United States indicates that income level is no longer consistently a *primary* determinant of nutrient intake (Senauer, 1986). It is necessary to add that those who live in extreme poverty have poor diets and are at risk for malnutrition. It is also known that the elderly who have low incomes often have inadequate diets.

Nevertheless, it is important to recognize the major influence of food choices on diet adequacy. Some low-income individuals have inadequate diets because of the way they choose to spend resources. Some maintain that in the United States, the land of plenty, no one should be deprived of the material things possessed by the majority. As a result, a major portion of income is spent on nonfood items. Other low-income individuals feel they have the right to choose foods they like, and even though they are on general public assistance or food assistance programs they feel that health professionals do not have the right to dictate their food choices.

A major question posed by health professionals that is being researched aggressively is why health messages do not reach the low-income population. Researchers have as yet found no definitive answer; however, there are many contributing factors. One is the limited educational level of many persons below the poverty line. Another factor is that the messages are often in language, style, and forms the poor do not relate to or use.

A broader issue however, is that the poor often lead crisis-oriented lives. They worry about how they will manage the near future but have little time to consider how habits and choices will affect them in one year let alone several years, and many do not feel they have a viable future relative to economics or longevity. It is also well documented that health beliefs play a major role in society's decision to effect healthful practices. Researchers have found that many poorly educated persons do not believe they will be affected by problems cited by health professionals. Others often present the following fatalistic attitude: "If something is going to happen, it will; therefore why should I deprive myself of foods I like?" In addition, many ethnic groups do not regard health problems, especially obesity, as a major social or health issue.

Finally, since blacks and Hispanics make up a large percentage of the poor, nutrition habits cannot be attributed only to poverty—ethnicity affects nutrition. Traditional foods are extremely important to many ethnic groups, and even though the foods may have low nutrient density or high fat or sugar levels, they refuse to relinquish them. This refusal is noted even in individuals who have moved up the educational and economic ladder. Some groups resent the fact that their food habits are often categorically labeled as unhealthy and see this evaluation as prejudiced.

Available research is rampant with data indicating that poor members of all races and the poorly educated in general do not take health preventive measures as do high-income, well-educated persons. However, any dogmatic reasons given are speculative. Nutrition and health researchers, educators, and nutritional health agencies realize that causes and viable solutions to nutrition problems must be determined.

ATTITUDES, BELIEFS, AND LIFE-STYLES

Life-styles, population composition, attitudes and beliefs about food, and health determine food intake and eating behaviors. In turn, these factors influence nutrition and health education and intervention needs of the public, as well as the knowledge required to meet the needs.

Attitudes and Beliefs

Results of a nationwide survey by the USDA demonstrated nutrition concerns. Almost two thirds of those surveyed had adjusted food selection in the three years before the survey. The adjustments included reductions in dietary levels of sugar, fat, cholesterol, sodium, and calories.

The survey also found that individuals are concerned about food safety. The population in general believes our food is safe. However, some population segments believe it is unsafe and practice risk avoidance to extremes. For example, many attempt to avoid all preservatives and additives used for such things as thickening and color, including those that have been used safely for decades (DHHS, USDA, 1986). A discussion of selected concerns follows.

Additives and Cancer

According to one researcher, about 10% of the population believes that food additives are the leading cause of cancer. Many people read in popular magazines that 35% of all cancers are related to diet and think this means additives. However, the figures in the magazines refer to lack or excess of food components, many of which are naturally occurring; that is, they refer to diets high in fat and low in fiber, for example (Whelan, 1985). Occasionally, additives or products formed with additives, such as nitrosamines (found in some cured meats), are found to be carcinogenic, but this is not a widespread occurrence.

Food Components and Cancer

Caffeine has been investigated in relation to breast cancer. However, researchers have found no causal relationship.

Additives and Adverse Reactions

The belief that food additives cause widespread adverse reactions has not been substantiated. However, although not widespread, severe or fatal reactions occasionally occur as with sulfites. Sulfites caused some deaths, as well as acute asthma attacks and anaphylactic shock, before the FDA banned sulfites in August 1987 (Taylor, 1986). On the other hand, researchers reviewed approximately 517 reports of alleged aspartame (artificial sweetener) toxicity and found no evidence of a widespread health hazard (Bradstock and others, 1986).

Life-Styles and Eating Behaviors

Life-styles influence U.S. food consumption patterns and therefore the knowledge needed to provide nutrition guidance.

Eating Away from Home

Researchers suggest that the percentage of the food dollar spent eating out currently exceeds 40% (Morgan and Goungetas, 1986). Although researchers report that meals eaten out tend to be lower in nutrient density, they make up a small portion of the daily intake. Therefore eating out does not have a significantly negative effect on nutrient adequacy. Some reports indicate that $2 of every $5 spent eating out is spent in fast-food restaurants—a fact that concerns many in the nutrition community. However, the advent of salad bars in these establishments has made it possible for the consumer to choose a varied and more nutritional meal. Nevertheless, individuals on special diets, especially low-cholesterol, low–saturated fat, or low-sodium diets, as well as those concerned about cardiovascular disease prevention, should limit the meals they eat in fast-food restaurants.

Vegetarianism

Vegetarianism remains a fairly popular practice with nontraditional groups termed the "new vegetarians." These are younger persons who have recently become vegetarians and who have alternative life-styles and philosophies (Helman and Darnton-Hill, 1987). A 1978 Roper poll estimated the number of persons in the United States who practiced some form of vegetarianism to be 7 million (Freeland-Graves and others, 1986). The following list defines the three major types of vegetarianism.

1. *Vegetarian:* One who lives wholly or principally on vegetable foods and avoids any form of animal food
2. *Lacto-ovo vegetarian:* One who avoids meat but consumes eggs, milk, and milk products, as well as grains, fruits, and vegetables
3. *Vegan:* A person who eats only grains, fruits, and vegetables

A well-balanced vegetarian diet (especially that of a lacto-ovo vegetarian) can include all essential nutrients. However, vegans may have problems obtaining adequate amounts of vitamin B_{12}. Anyone who intends to follow a vegetarian diet should be well read on the subject and should have a good concept of protein sources and grain mixtures that complement each other to provide adequate essential amino acids. People who approach vegetarianism casually are at risk of an inadequate diet.

Ethnic Eating Patterns

Every ethnic group has its own particular food heritage. Nurses should know the traditional pattern of groups with which they work, but they must not assume that the groups adhere to the ethnic patterns totally or in part. Examples of such stereotypes are that Chinese Americans always eat traditional Chinese foods or that blacks always eat diets high in pork and cured foods. All food habits have positive and negative implications for health. Another side of the ethnic food issue is that it is currently popular to eat foods of other ethnic groups fairly regularly and even to adopt those foods. In the more cosmopolitan areas, this occurs mainly because of specialty restaurants and grocery stores. In areas of the country where a particular group constitutes a significant percentage of the population, such as Mexican Americans in the Southwest, there is a total integration of various habits and influence on all aspects of eating in the region. In addition, of course, there is a common thread of so-called American food habits. Therefore a counselor providing nutrition education and advice needs to consider the environment in which individuals live as well as their ethnicity.

FACTS, DIET FADS, AND FALLACIES

The attitudes, beliefs, and life-styles of the population discussed in the previous section dictate how the population attempts to deal with real or perceived problems.

In the following paragraphs, some of the more common specific practices carried out because of erroneous, often misguided beliefs are discussed. For example, many believe such things as most essential nutrients and dietary components are missing from our food supply, many foods contain poisonous additives, nutrient deficiences and excesses or specific foods cause behavioral and psychologic problems, supplementation with specific nutrients improves physical and sexual performance or increases one's life span, and only special food combinations effect weight loss.

During the past 15 years, many Americans have made good, basic changes in the way they eat, and many of the diet changes made were based on sound nutrition information. Nevertheless, some changes are based on false premises or a distortion or exaggeration of scientific information. Those groups mentioned earlier that take advantage of the public's quest for knowledge usually take recommendations made by credible health organizations a step further than scientific data support, or they advocate shortcuts.

A major example of this practice by the business world is the proliferation of calcium supplements and calcium-fortified foods after the amazing media blitz caused by the highly publicized reports that calcium plays a major role in protection against osteoporosis. It is a fact that the diets of adult and teenage women are low in calcium and that most women's calcium intake needs to be increased through diet and possibly through calcium supplementation. But it is also a fact that calcium is not the only factor involved in protection against osteoporosis.

Nevertheless, manufacturers have saturated the media with advertisements dramatically implying that unless women in America take calcium supplements, they will be devastatingly crippled by osteoporosis in later years.

Vitamin and Mineral Supplementation

General Information

Surveys show that those who supplement their diets with vitamins and minerals tend to be white, female, and well educated and tend to have diets higher in nutrients than those who do not supplement (Koplan and others, 1986). In addition, the elderly make up a large percentage of those spending large amounts of money on supplements. In a telephone survey of approximately 3000 individuals, vitamin C was reported to be the most frequently consumed nutrient, followed closely by the B vitamins, vitamin E, vitamin A, and vitamin D. Megadoses are defined as doses 10 or more times the RDA. Megadoses reported in the survey ranged from 10 to 50 times the RDAs for individual nutrients (Stewart and others, 1985).

Vitamin C

Since publication of Linus Pauling's book *Vitamin C and the Common Cold,* enormous quantities of vitamin C have been consumed by the public. Doses ranging from 1 to 10 g are taken to prevent a cold and as much as 15 g is taken to treat one. To put this in perspective, 10 mg daily prevents scurvy and the RDA is 60 mg per day. Many controlled studies have indicated that vitamin C does not prevent colds but may have some small effect in reducing the severity of the symptoms. The amounts taken act as a drug similar to an antihistamine (Nutrition Myths and Misinformation, 1985).

Vitamin E

Vitamin E is a known antioxidant, and antioxidants are free radical scavengers. Some experts on aging theorize that free radical reactions and lipid perioxidation produced during normal metabolism lead to cellular damage and aging. Extrapolating from this knowledge, many life extension proponents advocate routine daily supplements of various antioxidants including vitamin E. There is no empiric evidence supporting the effectiveness of supplements for this purpose.

Vitamin Toxicity

Many substances that are harmless in small or moderate doses can cause harm in large amounts or by gradual buildup over many years. Even water-soluble vitamins cannot be taken in megadoses with impunity. Individuals with high serum vitamin C levels caused by excesses ($\geq$ 2g) over time can develop a catabolic enzyme that destroys vitamin C. Thus an abrupt reduction in vitamin C intake in these individuals results in rebound scurvy. One of the more toxic effects of megadoses of vitamin C is that they may contribute to kidney stone formation. Excessive doses of niacin can cause severe flushing, itching, and liver damage. Fat-soluble vitamins are well known for their toxic effects, since they are deposited in major organs. For example, megadoses of vitamin A can cause lack of appetite, retarded growth in children, and enlargement of the liver (Herbert and Barret, 1982).

Supplementation for Specific Health Problems

The premenstrual syndrome (PMS) is manifest as irritability, depression, water retention, and food cravings with attendant hypoglycemic symptoms. Some nutrition experts believe the condition is due to a hormonal imbalance of estrogen and progesterone. A few health professionals support a controversial nutrition theory that the imbalance and the resultant PMS are due to a deficit of pyridoxine (vitamin B_6) or magnesium or to intake of certain foods such as sugar. Those supporting the theory suggest that treatment should include supplementation with deficient nutrients and avoidance of sugar. Controlled studies have had mixed results, and most researchers in the area do not feel there is adequate evidence to recommend a specific dietary regimen (Shangold, 1986).

Hypoglycemia

The small but vocal segment of the population who believe that food causes most of our ills have popularized the theory that hypoglycemia is a disease. These advocates believe that sugar and refined carbohydrates cause hypoglycemia. Furthermore, they blame hypoglycemia for many maladies including PMS, hyperactivity, and criminal behavior.

But hypoglycemia is not a disease, it is a symptom. It is true that spontaneous hypoglycemia is a rare and often serious condition in which abnormal amounts of insulin or other hormones are secreted. As a result, a hypoglycemic person's blood glucose level is constantly or episodically too low. Symptoms are vague and nonspecific and include anxiety, sweating, light-headedness, and fatigue (Whitney, Hamilton, and Sizer, 1985). The diagnosis should be made only if circulating glucose levels are low (usually ≤50 mg/dl) as tested with mixed meals, if hypoglycemia is shown to be the basis of the symptoms, and if the symptoms are relieved by carbohydrate (American Diabetes Association, 1983; Charles and others, 1981).

Hypoglycemia should not occur in the normal person except transiently because of irregular inadequate calorie intake, which leads to frequent low glucose levels. The situation can be easily remedied by regular meals and adequate kilocalorie intake (Cataldo and Whitney, 1986). This is not to say that individuals who have low blood glucose levels cannot be helped by frequent meals or snacks with protein and by moderate carbohydrate intake.

Diet and Behavior

Hyperactivity

Controlled studies show no relationship between sugar and hyperactivity in children. There is a placebo effect of any regimen that focuses on individuals, and it can influence behavior. For example, persons registered for weight loss diet programs lose weight even if they are only on a waiting list.

The Feingold diet is also ineffective in controlling hyperactivity. Feingold's theory, which is based on anecdotal reports that food coloring and dyes, salicylates, and preservatives cause hyperactivity, has been repeatedly refuted in controlled research studies.

Criminal Behavior

The claim that a diet high in sucrose and other refined carbohydrates produces dramatic mood swings, feelings of hostility and aggression, and therefore criminal behavior has no factual support (Diet and Behavior, 1985).

Weight Loss Regimens

Providing resources for people to become thin is big business. The president of a national weight group organization reported that more than 60% of American women diet at some time every year. Market researchers estimate that Americans spend more than $10 billion a year on diet drugs, exercise tapes, diet books, diet meals, weight classes, and other weight-loss devices. Of the money spent, $200 million was spent on nonprescription diet pills. One disreputable diet book advocating limited foods plus special food combinations for weight loss sold 1.8 million copies.

IDENTIFICATION OF A FAD DIET

1. Promise of weight loss practically overnight with little effort
2. Promise of excessive amounts of weight loss in a short period, for example, 10 lb a week for 10 weeks
3. A product is sold directly to the public
4. Kilocalorie levels of 600 or less or diets limited to a few foods to which special biologic powers are attributed
5. Little or no emphasis on behavior change or exercise
6. No major research to support theory or results—only anecdotal reports from a few individuals
7. Claim that established medical and health professionals are attempting to hide this major discovery

Guidelines for Weight Loss

A successful weight reduction program is one that helps the individual lose weight and keep it off. Many Americans are weight conscious but are fairly inactive and reluctant to moderate long-term food intake. Therefore many are tempted to take the purported easy way. Even some medical professionals fall into the trap. However, there is no magic, easy way to lose weight and maintain the loss despite what late-night television advertisements or advocates of miracle diet plans say. In fact, many of these extreme plans, such as liquid protein meals sold in the late 1970s, have caused health problems and have even proved fatal. Weight loss and maintenance of that loss are difficult and require commitment and a long-term effort. An appropriate weight reduction program should foster a long-term decrease in kilocalorie intake, a change in eating behaviors, and an increase in exercise and should be supervised by a qualified health professional. The low-kilocalorie diet should be no less than 900 to 1000 kcal. The diet should include all food groups and should be nutritionally well balanced.

Fad Weight Reduction Methods

Fad weight reduction methods fall into several categories, but this section focuses only on diet pills, limited food diets, and diet books. The most common forms of diet pills that are currently sold include pills from food products, such as grapefruit, that advertisements promise will melt fat away, but of course do not work, and over-the-counter diet pills that contain small amounts of appetite suppressants. The appetite suppressant works for a limited time and then loses its effect. Proponents of limited food diets usually state that foods allowed must be eaten at the right time and in the right combinations. The suggested combinations supposedly have a special metabolic effect causing weight loss, and combinations of foods other than those recommended supposedly prevent weight loss. Companies offering limited food diet plans often claim that the diet is associated with some major health institution or government organization. Most individuals cannot follow these regimens for more than a week because of boredom, hunger, or side effects. Weight is lost because the individuals are on a semistarvation diet and have all the attendant side effects. If they attempt long-term adherence, irritability, dizziness, and fatigue follow. Some of the more unacceptable diet books follow limited food plans and theories similar to those of limited food diets. In addition, they provide rigid daily or weekly schedules of eating and menus that are extremely low in kilocalories, for example, 600 kcal. Some of the books include a limited discussion of behavior modification and exercise. The same problems identified for limited food diets hold true for these diet books. In the final analysis the authors are recommending extremely low-kilocalorie diets with a gimmick. The boxed material gives guidelines for recognizing fad diets.

MAJOR NUTRITION-RELATED HEALTH PROBLEMS

Available data indicate that diet and nutritional status are related to several leading causes of death of Americans such as cardiovascular diseases, some cancers, and diabetes mellitus, as well as obesity, the major health problem. Although the public tends to focus on possible diet inadequacies, many of the real problems, as stated earlier in this chapter, are due to dietary excesses. The next discussion focuses on the clinical description, associated risk factors, and preventive measures for some of the problems previously mentioned.

Obesity and Health

Evidence is overwhelming that obesity adversely affects health and longevity. Obesity is the excess accumulation of body fat. The more commonly used methods of determining weight problems and obesity follow.

Relative Weight

Relative weight = actual weight ÷ ideal weight × 100. Ideal weight is defined by Metropolitan Life Insurance (1983) as the midpoint of a range of ideal weights for medium-framed individuals of a given height. Relative weight is the most common and practical definition of weight for everyday use. Relative weight has been used historically to define obesity as ≥ 20% of ideal weight. Another common method of measuring and defining obesity is the body mass index (BMI) such as the Quetelet Index (weight/height^2). Values for BMIs are compared with data from NHANES for the population aged 20 to 29 years.

According to NHANES II data, 28% of the population aged 25 to 74 years (approximately 32 million persons) are overweight. Overweight is defined as BMI ≥85th percentile for men and women aged 20 to 29. Of these 32 million overweight people, 11.7 million are severely overweight—BMI ≥90th percentile for men and women aged 20 to 29 years. Weight problems are more prevalent among black women and women below the poverty line. Many factors possibly contribute to high rates in this group, including intake of high-calorie, low-nutrient density foods such as sweets and soft drinks, as well as starches, which are often less expensive, lack of associated control measures such as exercise, and lack of stigma attached to obesity. The underlying cause of obesity is an imbalance between energy intake and output. Environmental and genetic factors likely to be involved in the development include excess energy intake, low physical activity, and metabolic and endocrine abnormalities (DHHS, USDA, 1986).

A fair amount of available data shows that many obese people do not eat more than their counterparts of normal weight. However, many questions exist about the accuracy of intake data acquired from large population surveys, as well as the appropriateness of using group averages of kilocalorie intake to determine a relationship between food intake and obesity in individuals. The preceding notwithstanding, any prevention or resolution of the problem must consider decreased kilocalorie intake, changes in eating behavior, and increased physical activity.

Hypertension

Both heredity and environmental factors are implicated in the cause of hypertension. Dietary sodium, calcium, potassium, and several other nutrients may be involved in biochemical mechanisms that regulate blood pressure. Many experts in the field propose that subsets of the population can be identified as sensitive to salt (sodium) and therefore prone to hypertension, since sodium is considered by many experts a major nutrient involved in the cause of hypertension. The net effect of most nutrients on cardiovascular physiology and hypertension is still unknown (USDA, DHHS, 1986).

Dietary preventive measures include weight loss and maintenance and a decrease in sodium. Many experts also suggest adequate calcium has a role in prevention.

Diabetes Mellitus

Diabetes mellitus is a disorder of the blood glucose regulation mechanism.

The categories or types of diabetes include type I, or insulin dependent diabetes mellitus (IDDM), and type II, or non–insulin dependent diabetes mellitus (NIDDM). NIDDM is the most common form of diabetes and is causally related to diet factors such as high calories, low fiber, and high simple sugars. Diabetes is more prevalent among females, blacks, persons with incomes below the poverty line, and the overweight. NIDDM has its onset during the adult years.

NIDDM has a strong genetic component, but numerous other factors including obesity have been linked to its occurrence. Recent research indicates that overeating and weight gain are associated with increased fat cell size and impaired insulin response. Weight loss increases the response to insulin (DHHS, USDA, 1986). It follows that weight loss to an acceptable level and maintenance of that level is important in decreasing the risk of NIDDM.

Coronary Heart Disease

Atherosclerosis is a type of arteriosclerosis (general thickening of the arterial wall) that is characterized by accumulation of lipids (primarily cholesterol) in the walls of the medium-sized and large arteries. An elevated blood lipid value, or hyperlipidemia, leads to this accumulation.

Serum cholesterol values that place clients at a high risk for coronary heart disease are listed by the 1985 NIH Consensus Development Panel on Health Implications of Obesity as follows: serum cholesterol value ≥220 mg/dl for ages 20 to 29, ≥240 mg/dl for ages 30 to 39, ≥260 mg/dl for clients older than 40 (DHHS, USDA, 1986).

Many experts suggest that ideal cholesterol values for adults fall within 130 to 190 mg/dl. They recommend that individuals with levels greater than 190 mg/dl be treated with appropriate intervention according to level of risk.

Fat and Cholesterol

Researchers (DHHS, USDA, 1986) have found strong associations in large population groups between dietary fat, dietary cholesterol, blood lipid values, and mortality from coronary heart disease. However, they have not identified an independent effect of fat or cholesterol.

Other Dietary Factors

Excess kilocalories seem relevant only as they relate to obesity. Researchers have found no consistent independent relationship between sucrose or starch intake and increase in the incidence or prevalence of coronary artery disease. However, there is growing evidence that water-soluble fibers decrease blood lipids. The association of alcohol intake and atherosclerosis is neither strong nor consistent. Some suggest that 2 oz of alcohol per day or its equivalent is protective. Alcoholism, however, is linked directly to heart disease (DHHS, USDA, 1986).

Cancer

Although there is no absolute proof of a direct cause-effect relationship in humans, cancers of the stomach, colon, rectum, pancreas, breast, and uterus have been associated with diet (Cleveland and Pfeffer, 1987).

Fat and Fiber

Although there is some debate, the prevailing theory is that a positive correlation exists between total fat intake and colon and breast cancer. However, some researchers believe the causative factor may be specific kinds of fat (Nauss and others, 1987), and there is a negative relationship between consumption of dietary fiber and the development of cancer. Insoluble, poorly fermentable fiber such as cellulose, legumes, and wheat bran are considered protective. Others theorize that phytate, an acidic nonnutrient component found in plant seeds, is the protective factor (Graf and Eaton, 1985).

Vegetables (Crucifers)

Epidemiologic evidence suggests that consumption of cruciferous vegetables such as cabbage is associated with reduction in the incidence of several types of cancer in humans (Committee on Diet, Nutrition and Cancer, 1982).

Vitamin A

Epidemiologic evidence suggests that consumption of foods rich in carotenes or vitamin A is associated with a reduced risk of some types of cancer such as lung, bladder, and larynx cancers. No evidence supports the idea that vitamin A supplements reduce the risk of cancer.

Vitamin C

Limited evidence suggests that vitamin C can inhibit the formation of some neoplasms. The consumption of foods containing vitamin C is associated with a lower risk of cancers of the stomach and esophagus in some studies. However, the evidence remains equivocal.

Selenium

Data from epidemiologic and laboratory studies suggest that selenium may offer some protection against cancer. However, the range between safe and toxic levels of selenium intake is narrow. Food sources reflect soil content. Good sources in descending order are organ meats, muscle meats, and cereals.

Alcohol

Epidemiologic studies suggest that even moderate alcohol consumption (at least three drinks a week) increases the risk of breast cancer (Willett and others, 1987).

The boxed material on the opposite page includes preliminary dietary recommendations for reducing cancer risk.

SPECIAL NUTRITION AND HEALTH CONCERNS DURING THE LIFE CYCLE

In this section nutrition concerns of subgroups of the population, such as pregnant and lactating women, infants and children, and the elderly, are discussed. The special concerns and problems of these groups often receive limited attention in a discussion of the total population. Students are referred to a nutrition text for an in-depth discussion of nutrition during the life cycle.

Pregnancy and Lactation

Weight gain in pregnancy, nutritional risk of teenage pregnancy, and nutrition and lactation are topics currently receiving special attention in medical and nursing literature.

DIETARY RECOMMENDATIONS TO REDUCE CANCER RISK

1. Reduce consumption of fat from present level to 40% to 30% of calories.
2. Increase consumption of fruits, especially citrus fruits, and vegetables, especially carotene-containing vegetables such as carrots, cruciferous vegetables such as cabbage, broccoli, and cauliflower, and whole grain cereal products.
3. Minimize consumption of food preserved by salt curing, salt pickling, or smoking.
4. Limit the consumption of alcoholic beverages to moderate levels if it is consumed at all.

Recommendations from Expert Committee, National Research Council. Modified from Cleveland LE and Pfeffer A: J Am Diet Assoc 87:162, 1987.

Weight Gain Guidelines in Pregnancy

Researchers are currently stressing the importance of ranges of normal weight gain (24 to 32 lb) rather than a single narrow limit (Jacobson, 1986). Recommendations and a new chart (Rosso, 1985) for monitoring weight are based on the realization that an underweight pregnant woman needs to gain more weight than an obese pregnant woman. However, all pregnant women should gain weight, and severe weight reduction diets are contraindicated.

Teenage Pregnancy

A pregnancy in adolescence when the mother is less than three years post menarche automatically puts her at nutritional risk. If the mother has not reached her growth potential, nutrient needs for her growth plus that of the fetus must be met (Adolescent Pregnancy, 1986).

Lactation and Energy Needs

Lactating women require additional kilocalories, and the 1980 RDA is 500 kcal above that for nonlactating women. However, growing evidence suggests that lactating women may need fewer extra kilocalories because of enhanced metabolic efficiency (Butte and others, 1984; Illingworth and others, 1986). Nevertheless, extremely low kilocalorie diets, such as 1000 kcal per day diets, which some women follow to lose weight at a faster rate, are ill advised and can decrease the quantity of milk produced.

Infant Feeding

Although commercial cow's milk formulas provide acceptable nutrition, breast feeding remains the recommended feeding method if circumstances permit. A major advantage of breast milk is the protection against infection it provides infants because of antibodies in the milk. Parents are still encouraged to delay introduction of solid foods until the infant is six months old, but many pediatricians suggest that four months is an acceptable age. No statistical relationship between breast feeding, bottle feeding, or solids introduction and obesity has been found.

Childhood Obesity

A 1987 study strongly supports the previous findings that children who are obese at age six to nine years have a higher potential of remaining obese as adults. Freedman and others (1987) found that 43% of children who were obese when first examined at ages two to 14 years were obese eight years later. Those who were severely obese tended to remain obese. The results suggest that some moderate dietary intervention along with exercise should be initiated in severely obese children, since they have a good chance of remaining obese.

Nutrition and Child Athletes

Young athletes have increased energy needs, but the proportion of nutrients needed remains the same. However, special concerns include replacing fluids, which is crucial, since the young have difficulty adapting to exercise in warm environment and meeting calorie and nutrient needs to support optimal growth for elementary school–aged athletes regardless of which sport they play. Easy fatigue and poor performance can result from calorie deprivation (Smith, 1981).

A transient so-called sports anemia occurs in young athletes in early training because of hemodilution. However, the hemoglobin level of these athletes eventually stablizes within the normal range. Nevertheless, it is important to make sure iron-deficiency anemia is not a contributing factor.

Adolescent athletes should be encouraged to eat a well-balanced diet that provides adequate energy. This is especially true for girls who tend to restrict calories severely even when they are not overweight and for male wrestlers who follow severe food and fluid restrictions immediately before matches to make weight.

DIAGNOSTIC CRITERIA FOR ANOREXIA NERVOSA

1. Refusal to maintain a minimal normal weight for age and height, that is, weight loss leading to body weight 15% less than that expected or failure to gain weight during a period of growth, leading to body weight 15% less than that expected
2. Intense fear of gaining weight or becoming fat, even though the individual is underweight
3. Disturbance of body image; that is, the person claims to feel fat even when emaciated and believes that one area of the body is too fat even when obviously underweight
4. In females, absence of at least three consecutive menstrual cycles when otherwise expected to occur (primary or secondary amenorrhea) (A woman is considered to have amenorrhea if her periods occur only after hormone, or estrogen, administration.)

Modified from American Psychiatric Association: Diagnostic and statistical manual of mental disorders, ed 3, Washington, DC, 1987, The Association.

Eating Disorders

An eating disorder is the misuse or perceived misuse of eating in an attempt to solve or camouflage psychosocial problems. Many experts suggest that eating disorders do not spontaneously appear in adolescence and that careful histories indicate early, distorted child-parent feeding interactions in people with eating disorders. Societal pressures that encourage women to pursue extreme thinness are a contributing factor to eating disorders (Satter, 1986).

Anorexia Nervosa

Anorexia nervosa is a disease characterized by voluntary refusal to eat, persistent intentional loss of weight, and maintenance of an abnormally low weight. Refusal to eat persists despite hunger, admonitions, reassurances, or threats. Anorexia nervosa is often precipitated by bouts of restrictive dieting to lose small or occasionally significant amounts of weight.

Although it is increasingly being diagnosed at earlier ages, overt manifestations of anorexia nervosa generally begin at puberty or later adolescence. Less commonly it appears after age 20. Females constitute 95% of anorectic persons. Anorexia nervosa is more commonly found in high-achieving, high-income whites. The severity of the disorder varies from mild conditions that require little treatment to severe forms that require hospitalization. Anorexia nervosa is fatal in 5% to 15% of the cases.

Many anorectic persons practice unusual hoarding or handling of food. Weight loss and food refusal are pleasurable (Munoz, 1984). Often anorectic persons exercise excessively to maintain thinness and attempt to hide the activity. Some also practice vomiting and purging, which are characteristics of bulimia.

Initial treatment for severe anorexia nervosa is hospitalization, psychiatric counseling, and enteral feeding if necessary. Although physicians, as well as dietitians, discounted nutrition counseling for anorectic persons in the past, its role is now recognized. Nutrition counseling at the appropriate point is important in restoring normal eating habits (Huse and Lucas, 1983). For borderline anorectics, nutrition counseling on a continuing basis along with psychologic counseling should be an integral part of the care.

Bulimia

The bulimic syndrome typically begins in adolescence or the early twenties. Bulimics are predominantly white females who are of normal weight or slightly overweight or who were previously overweight. Prevalence data are limited. One group reported that 4% of 1300 college women asked about bulimic behaviors were considered probable bulimics and 2% were bulimic (Pyle and others, 1983).

Many bulimics skip meals, diet, or fast before a binge. Most report being on and off diets continually. Therefore they have few normal eating behaviors. Some clients report binging 10 or more times a day.

Bulimia is characterized by repeated episodes of rapid ingestion of large amounts of food, usually in less than two hours. The number of kilocalories ranges from 1000 to 4000 or more. Foods typically eaten include those perceived by bulimics as absolutely forbidden, such as candy, cake, pastries, ice cream, and crackers. The individual is aware that the binges are abnormal. Many bulimics (40% to 60%) use laxatives and diuretics (Johnson and others, 1984).

Many health professionals question the wisdom of classifying bulimia as a syndrome, since the symptoms occur along a continuum of weight disorders from anorexia to obesity. Bulimia has also been publicized by the media, and this may have led to inflated prevalence rates.

Long-term psychologic and nutrition counseling are indicated for bulimia. The goals of nutrition counseling include helping the patient normalize eating, recognize that food provides nutrients besides those for energy, avoid perceiving any food as absolutely forbidden, and understand that a healthy diet is not necessarily a high-calorie diet.

DIAGNOSTIC CRITERIA FOR BULIMIA NERVOSA

1. Recurrent episodes of binge eating (rapid consumption of a large amount of food in a discrete period)
2. A feeling of a lack of control over eating behavior during eating binges
3. Regular episodes of self-induced vomiting, using laxatives or diuretics, strict dieting or fasting, or vigorous exercising to prevent weight gain
4. Minimum average of two binge eating episodes per week for at least three months
5. Persistent overconcern with body shape and weight

Modified from American Psychiatric Association: Diagnostic and statistical manual of mental disorders, ed 3, Washington, DC, 1987, The Association.

Nutrition and the Elderly

Individuals 65 years of age and older account for 11% (23 million) of the U.S. population (Munro, 1985). The fastest growing segment of the older population is the so-called frail elderly—those older than 75 years of age. The nutritional status of the frail elderly is of particular concern because many among them can no longer plan meals, shop for food, or cook (Streib, 1983). In addition, a survey of a group of frail elderly showed that 36% were on special diets with 1 to 3 restrictions (Ludman and Newman, 1986).

After the previous general statements, it must be repeated that the elderly are not a homogeneous group. Many do not fit the stereotype of eating poor diets or living on tea and toast. Many eat well, and those who can maintain their traditional eating pattern have a better nutritional status (Nutrition and the Elderly, 1984).

However, for those with a poor nutritional status, the primary causes are lack of knowledge, poverty, social isolation, physical disability, including no teeth or dentures, or poor dentures, mental disorders, severely restricted therapeutic diets, and factors that decrease taste and smell. Secondary causes include malabsorption from intestinal disorders, alcoholism, and therapeutic drugs.

NUTRITION NEEDS AND HOME CARE

Technologic advances and concern for cost of inpatient care have allowed and encouraged the management of a greater number of acutely ill clients at home. The implications for nutrition care are tremendous, since most of these clients are at high risk of malnutrition and have difficulty maintaining adequate dietary intake. They often have complex feeding needs and therapeutic regimens, such as enteral feeding or modified diets in the case of dialysis clients, as well as poor appetites. Obviously, the nutrition care in these situations is highly specific (Cataldo and Whitney, 1986; Krause and Mahon, 1984).

It seems more appropriate in this text to provide basic guidelines for dealing with special diet and nutrition needs of patients at home. The guidelines presented are relevant for a chronic or acute problem when caring for any client at home with a therapeutic diet.

The nurse should first understand how the disease affects food intake and nutritional status. Nurses then need to understand the principles of traditionally recommended diets, special nutrient needs, and traditional types of feedings for the problem. The preceding information is necessary for a general knowledge base. Most acutely or severely chronically ill clients have been in an acute-care facility and have a prescribed diet. Therefore it is important to determine and understand such things as exactly what prescription, instructions, information, and menus have been provided by the dietitian *for the specific client.* This means reviewing materials that the client has in the home and seeking advice for clarification from the consulting dietitian, if necessary. Then and only then should the nurse assess the understanding of the client and significant others about such things as the therapeutic diet and special food products needed and provide advice. The nurse should also evaluate the client's and significant others' ability to accomplish the diet plan in the home environment. Because of the long-term nature of care, the nurse needs to reassess

GENERAL COMMUNITY NUTRITION RESOURCES

FOOD ASSISTANCE AND FEEDING

Food stamps. Food stamps are available to low-income, working poor, as well as those on public assistance.

Surplus commodity food. Surplus commodity food such as cheese, butter, and dried milk powder are available free in some states.

Food assistance for women, infants, and children (WIC). Low-income pregnant women and children up to five years of age get selected foods or vouchers for those foods.

School breakfast/lunch. A school breakfast or lunch is free for eligible low-income children.

Congregate meals for senior citizens. Congregate meals for senior citizens are served in various community centers. A minimum fee is suggested, but it is not required.

HOME-DELIVERED MEALS

Meals on Wheels. For a minimal fee meals are provided by state and community Meals on Wheels agencies.

Proprietary home-delivered meals. Check yellow pages for proprietary home-delivered meals.

OTHER SERVICES

The state or volunteer agencies on aging often provide transportation for food shopping and homemaker services for food shopping and meal preparation.

NUTRITION COUNSELING

Nutrition counseling is available from RDs in private practice and ambulatory care divisions of acute care hospitals, HMOs, community health centers, and the cooperative extensions.

TABLE 7-3 Guide for Common Therapeutic Diets

Disease/problem	Basic dietary guidelines	Food sources
Diabetes type I	Maintain a consistent, regular food intake.	
	Maintain weight.	
	Increase consumption of complex carbohydrates.	Complex carbohydrates include rice, pasta, and bread.
	Increase consumption of fiber.	Fiber-containing foods include legumes, whole grain breads, and cereals.
	Consume only moderate amounts of simple sugar.	Foods containing simple sugars include sugar, honey, cake, candy, and cookies.
	Avoid simple sugar as between-meal snacks.	
Diabetes type II	Maintain a low-calorie diet for weight loss and maintenance.	
	Increase consumption of complex carbohydrates.	
	Increase consumption of fiber.	
Obesity	Maintain a low-calorie diet.	
	Include all basic food groups in diet; increase fruit and vegetable consumption; decrease quantity of food intake and portion sizes; and decrease fat intake.	High-fat foods include fried foods, butter, margarine, mayonnaise, gravies, fatty meats, and whole milk.
	Decrease intake of simple sugars, and desserts.	Simple sugars include sugar, honey, candy, sweetened beverages, pies, and cakes.
Hypertension	Maintain low-calorie diet (if needed). Maintain weight. Decrease consumption of sodium.	High-sodium foods include prepared convenience foods, such as frozen potpies, canned or powdered soups, cured meats (hot dogs and ham), and pizza, seasoned salt, and any food with salt on the outside.
	Maintain adequate calcium intake.	High-calcium foods include dairy products, such as milk, cheese, and yogurt, and dark green vegetables.
	Maintain adequate potassium intake.	High-potassium foods include fruits and vegetables such as bananas, oranges, orange juice, and potatoes.

Continued

the client's dietary intake and weight status periodically to identify emerging nutrition problems. For example, changes in appetite or disease process can affect clients' appetite and thus their nutritional status.

Finally, in addition to periodic consultation with the consulting dietitian, it is crucial that the nurse have knowledge of and use community resources such as Meals on Wheels, shopping assistance, or homemaker services that help clients meet their nutrition needs (see box).

DIETARY GUIDELINES FOR COMMON THERAPEUTIC DIETS

The nurse has the responsibility for knowing the general principles of therapeutic diets most often prescribed for clients. This includes knowledge of the traditional general allowances and restrictions of foods, food components, or nutrients. Nurses must also know major sources of relevant food components or nutrients.

Table 7-3 summarizes general guidelines for

TABLE 7-3 Guide for Common Therapeutic Diets—cont'd.

Disease/problem	Basic dietary guidelines	Food sources
Coronary artery disease/ hyperlipidemia	Lose weight and maintain the loss.	
	Decrease consumption of saturated fat and cholesterol.	High-cholesterol and high–saturated fat foods include eggs (yolk), red meat, butter, lard, and cold cuts such as bologna and salami.
	Increase consumption of low-fat foods.	Low-fat foods include fish, chicken, skim milk, vegetables, and fruits.
	Increase consumption of polyunsaturated fats.	Polyunsaturated fats include vegetable oils and margarines (corn, safflower, and sunflower).
	Increase consumption of omega 3 fatty acids.	Foods with omega 3 fatty acids include those with fish oils, especially oilier, fatty fish such as salmon, mackerel, trout, cod, and sardines.
Underweight and undernourished	Eat a well-balanced diet. Increase calorie and protein intakes and between meal snacks that are high in calories and protein.	In addition to regular foods, special liquid supplements are available. Check with resource dietitian for teaching hospital diet manual.
Chronic renal failure	Check ability to afford, shop for, and prepare foods. Diet must include adequate amount of calories.	
	Maintain a moderate- to low-protein diet depending on stage of failure. Decrease consumption of phosphorus depending on state of disease.	High-protein foods include meat, eggs, milk, legumes, cheese, and special low-protein foods on market. Check with resource dietitian or teaching hospital diet manual.
Gastrointestinal problems		
Constipation	Maintain adequate well-balanced diet. Maintain adequate fluid intake. Increase consumption of fiber.	
Diverticulosis (chronic)	Increase consumption of fiber.	Foods containing insoluble fibers include whole wheat breads, bran cereal, vegetables, and fruits (seeds may cause irritation).
Ulcers	Eat three well-balanced meals per day. Avoid eating within four hours of going to bed. Avoid caffeine-containing beverages, decaffeinated coffee, alcohol, excessive pepper or chili powder, and any foods that cause discomfort.	
Hiatal hernia	Maintain a low-fat diet and eat low-fat meals. Do not lie down immediately after eating. Avoid alcohol, spearmint, peppermint, chocolate, and caffeine-containing beverages.	
Dumping syndrome	Maintain a high-protein, moderate-fat diet. Eat small meals. Avoid taking liquids with meals. Use medium-chain triglyceride (oil) if steatorrhea is present.	

therapeutic diet modifications for common chronic diseases. The reader is referred to a diet therapy text for a full discussion of diet therapy (Cataldo and Whitney, 1986; Krause and Mahon, 1985).

SUMMARY

The nursing role in relation to nutrition focuses on client teaching and referral. There are two resources that are helpful in this task—the *Basic Four Food Guide* and the *Dietary Guidelines for Americans*. These basic guides, however, need to be adapted to meet the client's individual situation. Diet can be influenced by a variety of factors including income, ethnicity, race, attitudes, life-styles, and even misinformation. Misinformation is particularly important in the widespread popularity of fad diets, including most of the weight reduction diets. Nutritional needs also vary throughout the life span, and a knowledge of these changing needs enhances nurses' dietary teaching role.

QUESTIONS FOR DISCUSSION

1. What are the advantages and disadvantages of using the *Basic Four Food Guide* as a tool for evaluating the diets of individuals and families?
2. List three types of life-styles that may be implicated in poor eating habits.
3. Analyze the latest fad diet you have heard about for its nutritional value and its probable impact on weight loss.
4. Define anorexia nervosa and bulimia. Do you believe the incidence of these conditions is increasing? Why or why not?

REFERENCES

Adolescent pregnancy: counseling considerations, Nutrition and the MD 12:4, 1986.

American Diabetes Association, Endocrine Society, and American Medical Association: Statement on hypoglycemia, JAMA 223:682, 1983.

Block G and others: Nutrient sources data from NHANES II. II. Macronutrients and fat, J Epidemiol 122:27, 1985.

Bradstock M and others: Evaluation of reactions to food additives: the aspartame experience, Am J Clin Nutr 43:464, 1986.

Butte NF and others: Effect of maternal diet and body composition on lactational performance, Am J Clin Nutr 39:296, 1984.

Carino C and Chmelko P: Disorders of eating in adolescence: anorexia and bulimia, Nurs Clin North Am 18:343, 1983.

Cataldo C and Whitney E: Nutrition and diet therapy, St Paul, 1986, West Publishing Co.

Charles MA and others: Comparison of oral glucose tolerance tests and mixed meals in patients with apparent idiopathic postabsorptive hypoglycemia, Diabetes 30:465, 1981.

Cleveland LE and Pfeffer A: Planning diets to meet the National Research Council guidelines for reducing cancer risk, J Am Diet Assoc 87:162, 1987.

Committee on Diet, Nutrition and Cancer, National Research Council: Diet, Nutrition and Cancer, Washington, DC, 1982, National Academy Press.

Diet and behavior, Dairy Council Digest, 56:21 1985.

Food and Nutrition Board, National Research Council: Recommended dietary allowances, ed 9, Washington, DC, 1980, National Academy of Sciences.

Freedman D and others: Persistence of juvenile-onset obesity over eight years: the Bogalusa heart study, Am J Public Health 77:588, 1987.

Freeland-Graves J, Greninger S, and Young R: A demographic and social profile of age- and sex-matched vegetarians and non-vegetarians, J Am Diet Assoc 86:907, 1986.

Frisch R: Nutrition, fatness, puberty, fertility, Nutr and the MD 12:1, 1986.

Graf E and Eaton J: Dietary suppression of caloric cancer: or phytate? Cancer 56:717, 1985.

Helman A and Darnton-Hill I: Vitamin and iron status in new vegetarians, Am J Clin Nutr 45:785, 1987.

Herbert V and Barret S: Vitamins and "health" foods, Philadelphia, 1982, George F Stickley Co.

Huse D and Lucas A: Dietary treatment of anorexia nervosa, J Am Diet Assoc 83:687, 1983.

Illingworth J and others: Diminution in energy expenditure during lactation, Br Med J 292:437, 1986.

Jacobson H: Nutrition and pregnancy: advances in knowledge of fetal and maternal nutrition, Food Nutr News 58:21, 1986.

Johnson C, Lewis C, and Hagman J: The syndrome of bulimia. Symposium on eating disorders, Psychiatr Clin North Am 7:247, 1984.

Koplan J and others: Nutrient intake and supplementation in the United States (NHANES II), Am J Public Health 76:287, 1986.

Krause M and Mahon LK: Food, nutrition and diet therapy, ed 7, Philadelphia, 1984, WB Saunders Co.

Ludman E and Newman J: Frail elderly: assessment of nutrition needs, Gerontologist 26:198, 1986.

Metropolitan Life Insurance Company: Statistical Bulletin 64:1, 1983.

Morgan K and Goungetas B: Snacking and eating away from home. In Food and Nutrition Board, National Research Council: What's America eating? Washington, DC, 1986, National Academy Press.

Munoz RA: The basis for the diagnosis of anorexia nervosa. Symposium on eating disorders, Psychiatr Clin North Am 7:215, 1984.

Munro H: Nutrient needs and nutritional status in relation to aging, Drug Nutr Interact 4:55, 1985.

Nauss KM, Jacobs LR, and Newberne PM: Dietary fat and fiber: relationship to calorie intake, body growth and colon tumorigenesis, Am J Clin Nutr 45(suppl):243, 1987.

Nutrition myths and misinformation: special report, Nutr and the MD 11:1, 1985.

Pyle RL, Mitchell JE, and Eckert EE: The incidence of bulimia in freshman college students, Int J Eating Disorders 2:75, 1983.

Roe DA: Drug-induced nutritional deficiencies, Westport, Conn, 1976, Avery Publishing Group Inc.

Rosso P: A new chart to monitor weight gain during pregnancy, Am J Clin Nutr 41:644, 1985.

Satter EM: Childhood eating disorders, J Am Diet Assoc 86:357, 1986.

Senauer B: Economics and nutrition—what is America eating? Proceedings of a symposium of the Food and Nutrition Board National Research Council, Washington, DC, 1986, National Academy Press.

Shangold G: Nutrition and the premenstrual syndrome, Nutr and the MD 12:1, 1986.

Smith N: Nutrition advice for the young athlete. In Haskell W, Scala J, and Whittanaes J, editors: Nutrition and athletic performance. Proceedings of the conference on nutritional determinant in athletic performances, Palo Alto, Calif, 1981, Bull Publishing Co.

Stewart ML and others: Vitamin/mineral supplement use: a telephone survey of adults in the United States, J Am Diet Assoc 85:1585, 1985.

Streib G: The frail elderly, Gerontologist 23:40, 1983.

Taylor SL: Food allergies and sensitivities, J Am Diet Assoc 86:599, 1986.

US Department of Agriculture, Department of Health and Human Services: Nutrition and your health: dietary guidelines for Americans, ed 2, Washington, DC, 1985, US Government Printing Office.

US Department of Agriculture, Department of Health and Human Services: Nutrition monitoring in the United States: a progress report from the Joint Nutrition Monitoring Evaluation Committee, DHHS Pub (PHS) 86-1255, Washington DC, 1986, US Government Printing Office.

Whelan E: Diseases and misinformation. In Nutrition myths and misinformation: Special Report, Nutr and the MD 11:1, 1985.

Whitney E, Hamilton E, and Sizer F: Nutrition concepts and controversies, ed 3, St Paul, 1985, West Publishing Co.

Willett WC and others: Moderate alcohol consumption and the risk of breast cancer, N Engl J Med 316:1174, 1987.

IT is important to understand the structure and function of the health care delivery system. It not only influences the development of nursing as a profession, but also has an impact on how nursing services are delivered. American nursing differs from British, Canadian, or Mexican nursing in part because of the differences in the health care delivery systems. Health care delivery systems do not, however, remain static but are continually changing because of the development of new technologies, new scientific discoveries, new demands by consumers, and changing perceptions of what the roles of the workers in the system should be. Too often in the past, nurses have not been the agents of change. Rather, they have been passive participants in the change. One of the objectives of the three chapters in this section is to give nurses the kind of background and information that will enable them to be active participants in bringing about changes that will improve client care.

Change does not occur in a vacuum, and, although it often occurs accidentally, those in a position to seize the potential changes can have an important role in directing them. To do this in the health care arena requires an understanding of the economic and social factors involved in the health care delivery system, the services rendered, and the personnel involved. This kind of information is given in Chapter 8. In the past much of the directed change that occurred took place in a particular area, usually a city, county, or state, and was copied by others. Although this still occurs, change now takes place on a national level, although there are pilot projects that help pretest the effects of change. Chapter 9 looks at many of the factors present that are forcing changes both in the nature of health care and the way it is delivered. Economics is obviously a major force in these changes. This puts nursing in a critical position because it represents the largest group of professionals involved in health care. Although the rapid escalation of costs of American health care has not been caused by a radical increase in the salaries of nurses, one of the ways in which administrators try to economize is to cut personnel costs. In fact, one of the major forces behind the move to home health care has been the widespread belief that it is less costly than hospital care. A major reason home health care has so far proved less costly is that there are many factors other than nursing salaries built into the costs of hospital care.

Changing perceptions and bringing about changes in the health care system are rather complex processes. Chapter 10 looks at some of the theories of social change and illustrates how nurses themselves can be agents of social change. Change can begin with the effort of one nurse, but unless other nurses join together, change is not likely to occur. This is because change really involves a group process and ultimately to be successful nurses must go beyond the ranks of nurses. The first steps to nurse involvement in change are for nurses to know and understand the health care system. They then must begin to take steps to bring about the changes that will most benefit the client in the long run and allow nurses to deliver the kind of nursing care that clients want and need.

Health Care Delivery System

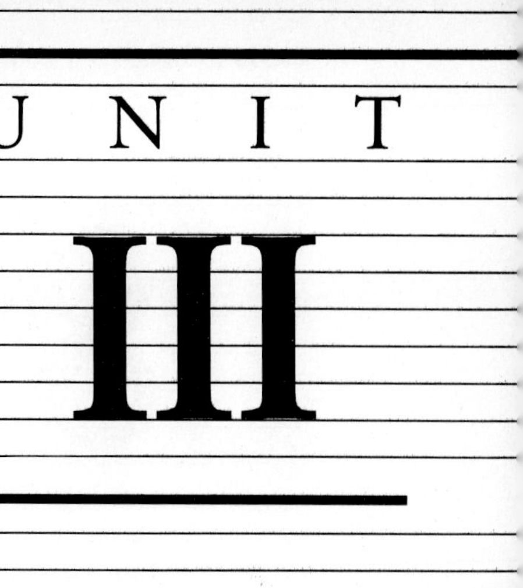

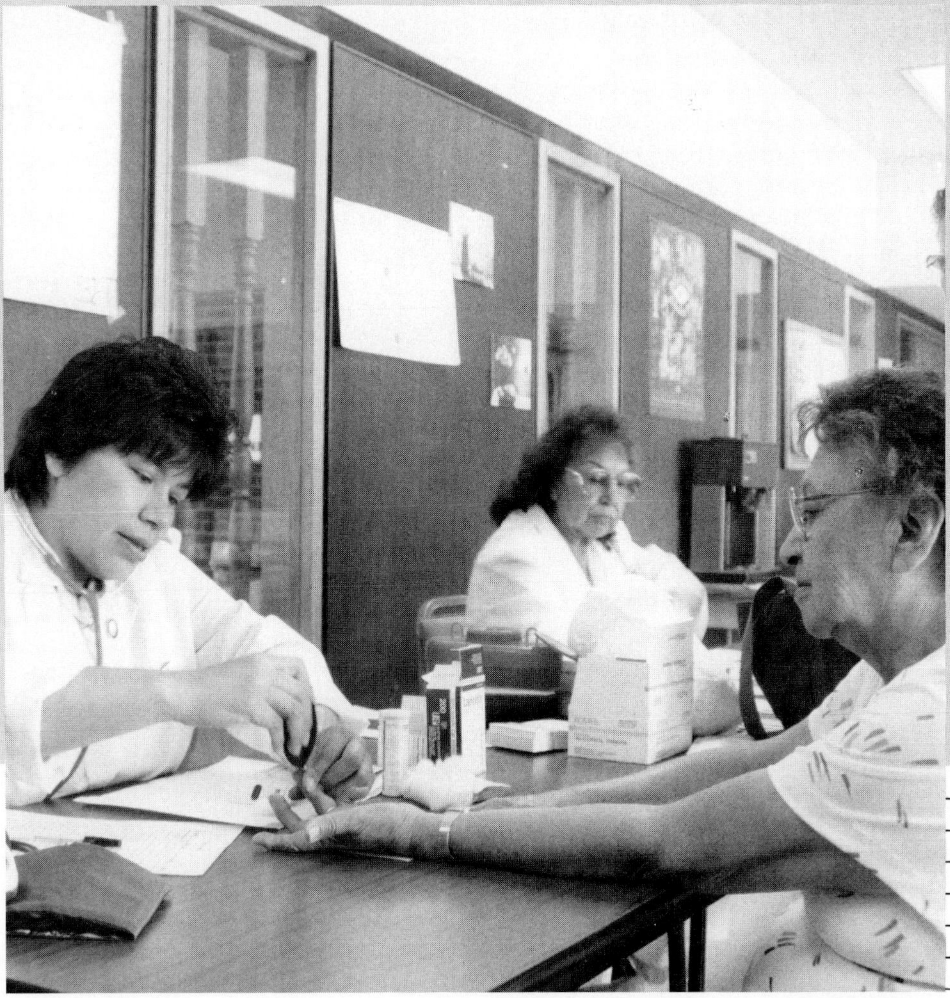

CHAPTER 8

Health Care Delivery System: Its Services, Personnel, and Economic System

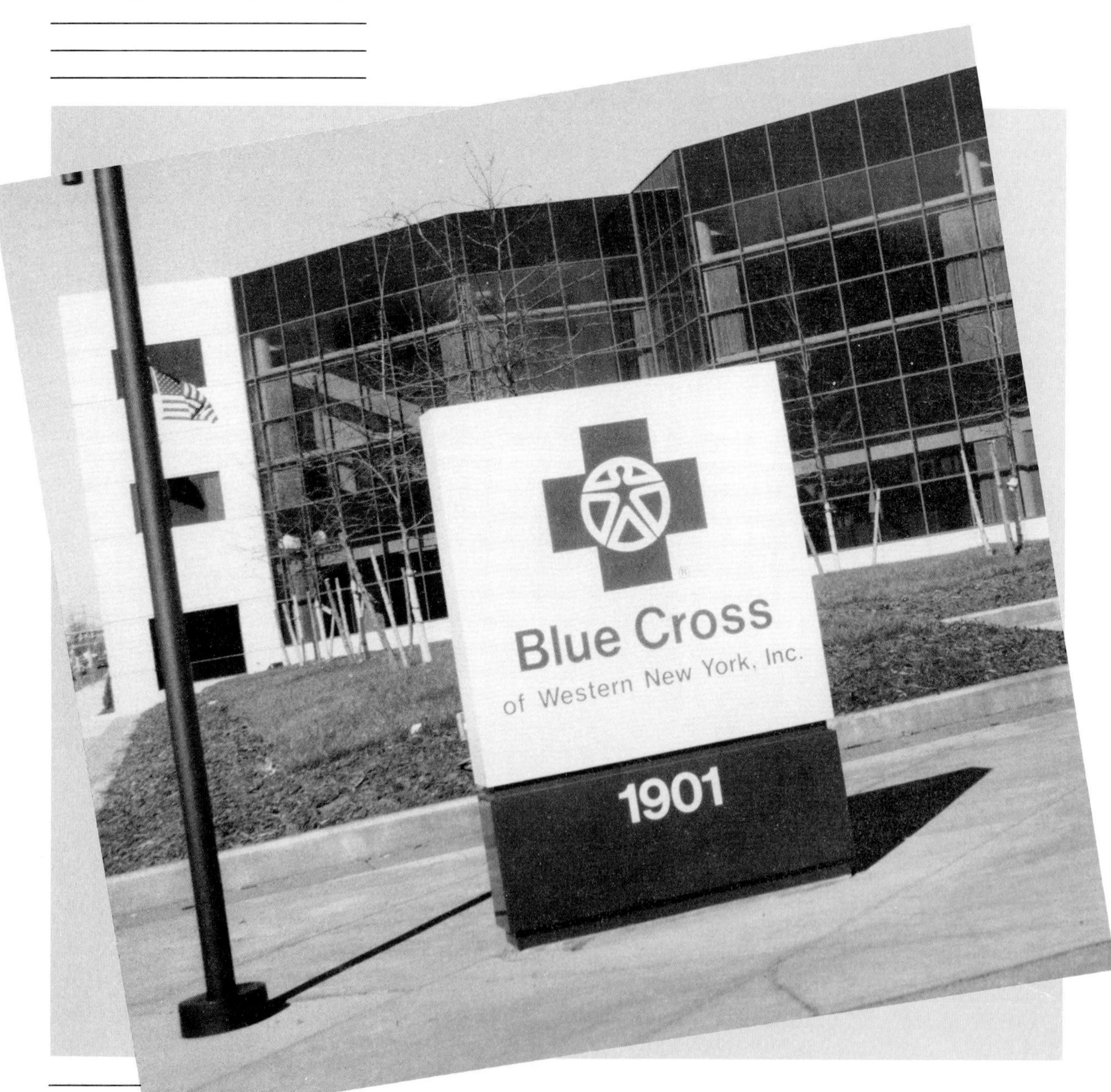

CHAPTER OUTLINE

Primary, secondary, and tertiary care: definitions and discussion

Goals of the system: prevention, cure, and sustaining care

Stratified personnel of the health care delivery system

Economics of the system

- Early campaigns for national health insurance
- Hill-Burton Act
- Private hospital and health insurance
- Health maintenance organizations

Summary

OBJECTIVES

After completing this chapter, the reader should be able to:

1. Define the following concepts:
   a. Primary care
   b. Secondary care
   c. Tertiary care
2. Discuss the goals of the system including:
   a. Prevention
   b. Cure
   c. Sustaining care
3. Trace the historical changes that have made the system more complex.
4. Describe the political issues surrounding government financing of health care.
5. Discuss the economics of the health care delivery system, differentiating between:
   a. Public or private financing
   b. Fee-for-service vs. capitation payment for services
   c. Health insurance that is provided by commercial carriers, health maintenance organizations, or nonprofit carriers

THE TERM "HEALTH CARE DELIVERY SYSTEM" is often used to describe the way in which health care is furnished to people. The term is not without problems. There are so many variations in the American health care delivery system that critics argue it is a nonsystem or at best a collection of poorly articulated competing systems (Torrens, 1984). The most commonly used alternative term, "health care industry," captures the flavor of the size and complexity of the system, but it obscures the fact that services are delivered in contrast to products being manufactured. Because there seems to be no better term, we have chosen to use health care delivery system despite its problems.

In this chapter and the one that follows, the health care delivery system is described and critiqued from a variety of vantage points. That the whole system is analyzed, including its institutional aspects, illustrates another facet of the community health perspective. Community health workers are reformers at heart. They want to improve the health care delivery system and incorporate more preventive care into it. To bring about reform, an understanding of the whole system is needed. Therefore an overview is included here.

This chapter focuses on the services provided by the health care delivery system and its personnel, the changing economics of the system, and a description of the development of health insurance including health maintenance organizations (HMOs). Chapter 9 follows with coverage of Medicare and Medicaid, the current inflationary problems, and a comparison of the American health care delivery system with other health care delivery systems. The two chapters should be read together so that a thorough understanding of the system is gained.

It is possible to classify the services offered by the health care delivery system using a variety of formats. Two major classification systems are presented here. The first approach divides the system by the acuity of the clients' illnesses and the level of specialization of the professionals serving them. Primary, secondary, and tertiary care are the three levels of care described. The second approach classifies care by prevention, cure, rehabilitation, or sustaining care. An understanding of both these dimensions should help clarify the health care delivery system.

PRIMARY, SECONDARY, AND TERTIARY CARE: DEFINITIONS AND DISCUSSION

Primary care is the usual entry point for clients of the health care delivery system. It is oriented toward the promotion and maintenance of health, the prevention of disease, the management of common episodic illnesses, and the monitoring of stable chronic conditions. Primary care ordinarily occurs in ambulatory care settings. Treatment is managed by the client or the family, with health professionals providing diagnostic expertise and guidance.

Secondary care is oriented toward clients with more severe acute illnesses or chronic illnesses that are exacerbated. If hospitalization occurs, it is usually in a community hospital. Most individuals who enter this level of care are referred by a primary care worker, although some people are self-referred. The physicians who provide secondary care are usually specialists.

Tertiary care is the most complex level of care. The illness may be life threatening, and the care ordinarily takes place in a major hospital affiliated with a medical school. Clients are referred by workers from primary or secondary settings. The health professionals, including physicians and nurses, tend to be highly specialized, and they focus on their area of specialization in the delivery of care (DHEW, 1975; Jonas, 1981; Rydman and Rydman, 1983).

Table 8-1 summarizes the three levels of care and provides examples. The following box illustrates how an individual with a chronic illness could move back and forth from one level of care to another. The primary care level is probably the

TABLE 8-1 Levels of Health Care

Levels	Disease stages	Examples of illnesses and treatments	Treatment sites	Professionals
Primary care	Entry into system, well persons, episodic illness, stable chronic conditions	Urinary tract infection, stable diabetes; physical examinations, immunizations	Clinic, physician's office, client's home, nursing home	Family practice physician, nurse practitioner, community health nurse, physical therapist
Secondary care	Acute illness, chronic illness	Appendicitis, out-of-control diabetes; hospital care, surgery	Community hospital, skilled nursing facility	Physician specialists, all types of nurses
Tertiary care	Serious acute illness, life-threatening illness	Myocardial infarction, ruptured peptic ulcer, end-stage renal disease; hospital care	University hospital, highly specialized clinic, specialized hospitals	Physician specialists, all types of nurses

most important for community health nurses because it is usually provided in ambulatory settings. However, nurses also care for persons who are dying at home, and they provide services to persons who are discharged from the hospital while they are still acutely ill. These are instances of secondary or even tertiary care.

GOALS OF THE SYSTEM: PREVENTION, CURE, AND SUSTAINING CARE

The other way to conceptualize the services of the health care delivery system is to divide the services by their goals, including prevention, cure, and sustaining care (Table 8-2). *Prevention* is aimed at stopping the disease process before it starts or preventing further deterioration of a condition that already exists. *Cure* is aimed at restoring a client to health. *Sustaining care* is aimed at lessening the pain and discomfort of illness and helping clients live with disease and disability.

Some sociologists and nurse theorists have conceptualized the nursing role as being focused on sustaining care and preventing disease, whereas

CASE STUDY ILLUSTRATING THE THREE LEVELS OF HEALTH CARE

PRIMARY CARE

As an example of the levels of care consider the case of Mrs. M. At the beginning of the study she had stable type 1 diabetes and was treated through an HMO by a family physician–nurse practitioner team. A community health nurse visited her home to check her technique with insulin administration and diabetic self-care.

SECONDARY CARE

Bronchitis developed in Mrs. M., and she was placed in a community hospital to treat her bronchitis and to recalibrate her insulin dosage because of an elevated blood glucose level. Her physician was an internist who specialized in respiratory problems. He consulted with the family physician and an endocrinologist to manage the insulin. A diabetes nurse discussed Mrs. M's lifestyle and home care with her. She recovered.

PRIMARY CARE

She returned to her home and the HMO for primary care management for three years.

TERTIARY CARE

However, her husband was then killed in an automobile accident. She became depressed and forgot to take her insulin. She was found in a coma by her neighbor and was admitted to the university hospital intensive care unit.

TABLE 8-2 The Goals of the Health Care Delivery System

Goals	Examples
Primary prevention	Immunizations for communicable diseases Teaching a wellness-oriented life-style Eliminating hazards in the work place
Secondary prevention	Hypertension screening and early treatment Teaching breast self-examination Papanicolaou smears to detect cervical cancer Antibiotic treatment of streptococcal pharyngitis aimed at preventing rheumatic fever
Tertiary prevention	Rehabilitation after a spinal cord injury Smoking cessation program for clients with emphysema
Curative services	Antibiotics for a kidney infection Surgery
Sustaining care	Comfort measures Hospice care Medication for pain

medicine is focused on curing illness (Johnson, 1959; Schulman, 1972; Skipper, 1965). Other nurses have argued that there are two groups of nurses. One group is technical and cure oriented, whereas the other group is care oriented. This dichotomy assigns the cure focus to hospital nurses, whereas the care and preventive elements predominate in the more autonomous community roles. The work role of nurse practitioners and home health care nurses would probably span all three of these orientations (ANA, 1965; Bullough and Sparks, 1975; Kramer, 1974). These arguments probably have merit if they are not pushed too far.

Unfortunately for the student who must understand and remember these lists, preventive services are also popularly categorized as primary, secondary, and tertiary preventive health care. *Primary prevention* refers to the prevention of an illness before it has a chance to occur. Immunization against communicable diseases is a major primary preventive measure. *Secondary prevention* includes the early detection of actual or potential health hazards. This allows for prompt intervention and possibly a cure of the disease or condition. *Tertiary prevention* is aimed at avoiding further deterioration of an already existing problem. Rehabilitative efforts are sometimes tertiary preventive measures. Smoking cessation to stop the deterioration of already diseased lungs could be classified as tertiary prevention (DHEW, 1975). Quitting smoking does not cure the disease, but it might lessen future damage (Rydman and Rydman, 1983).

STRATIFIED PERSONNEL OF THE HEALTH CARE DELIVERY SYSTEM

There are approximately 7 million health workers in the United States. This does not include those who manufacture drugs and appliances, those who clean the buildings, or other related workers. These persons would increase the size of the industry to approximately 8 million workers. The system is highly stratified with sharp differentials in income, power, and prestige. Although size and complexity do not always go together, they most often do. The rapid growth of the system has paralleled its growing complexity.

The top-level occupations in the health care delivery system are already highly professionalized, and the professionalization process is continuing. Moreover, as nursing and the other middle-level health care occupations gain power, the continuing professionalization is further widening the gap between the low-level workers and the rest of the health care delivery system.

Although there is a variety of definitions of professionalization, it is basically a process whereby a group of workers gains power, prestige, and income because the workers hold a unique body of knowledge that is not shared by their clients. In part because of this protected knowledge, the public is forced to give professions significant control over their own affairs. (Daniels, 1971; Freidson, 1970; Freidson, 1971). The learned occupations in turn further professionalization by lengthening training programs, organizing collectivities, seeking support from the state through licensure or similar devices, and taking pains to enhance the charismatic mystique that surrounds their expertise (Carr-Saunders and Wilson, 1933; Moore, 1970). Thus professionalization has increasingly separated the high-status health occupations from the untrained or minimally trained health workers and has also increased the social distance between high-status health professionals and their clients. For example, the social distance between modern speciality physicians and their clients is greater than that between the old family doctors and their clients (Bullough, 1988).

A third basis for the broad span of the stratification system is the fact that the health care industry is labor intensive. As the cost of labor has risen, health care costs have escalated. Moreover, the work is often of an emergency nature, so staffing needs are not totally predictable; this in turn leads to overstaffing on quiet days (Georgopoulos, 1972). Technologic advances in health care in the last few decades, including automation and the development of elaborate diagnostic and monitoring devices, have tended to broaden the spectrum of patients who can be effectively treated rather than cutting down the amount of labor needed to care for patients. Some of the machines have in fact increased the requirements for personnel by necessitating a new class of technicians to monitor or use them. Consequently the health care industry has not reaped the cost-saving benefits of recent technologic advances that other industries have.

In an effort to deal with the problem of escalating labor costs, hospital administrators and clinic managers have sought to rationalize the system by breaking down work roles into component parts and assigning the simpler tasks to workers with less formal training. This has led to the development of an army of technicians and assistants. Some of the technical roles, such as those of physiotherapist, x-ray technician, dietitian, health records technician, and inhalation therapist grew out of the nursing role, whereas the laboratory and engineering specialties seem to have had their origins in the older job description of the physician.

The major thrust in the differentiation of the nursing role occurred in the decade following World War II. What previously had been one occupation was divided into at least the nursing aide, licensed practical nurse, and registered nurse levels. In addition, a small contingent of nurses was already earning baccalaureate degrees in this era. The associate degree registered nurse programs started as an experimental project in 1952 (Montag, 1959), and they have grown in popularity. The master's degree specialty level developed as a major element in the system after 1964 when the federal government started supporting graduate nursing education. Thus the current clinical nursing work force includes nursing aides and orderlies, licensed practical nurses and vocational nurses, diploma and associate degree registered nurses, baccalaureate level registered nurses, and master's degree level specialists (Bullough and Bullough, 1983; Kalisch and Kalisch, 1978).

The role of the physician has been more resistant to this type of differentiation than that of the nurse. Although it is true that a myriad of technical specialties has broken from the physician's role, the role has not experienced the same multilevel differentiation as that of the nurse. The total nursing work force is not only the largest component in the system, it is in some ways the most complex (Bullough and Bullough, 1974).

So far in this discussion, the factors creating the hierarchy that characterizes the health care delivery system seem legitimate. New recruits to the health care delivery system need to learn to live with the hierarchy. Less legitimate are some of

TABLE 8-3 Percentages of the Persons Employed in Selected Health Occupations Who Are Black and Female*

Occupation	Number (expressed in 1000s)	Percent Female	Percent Black
Health diagnosing occupations†	735	13.3	2.7
Physicians‡	519	15.8	3.2
Dentists	126	6.7	2.4
Health assessment and treating occupations	1900	85.8	7.1
Registered nurses	1372	95.8	6.7
Pharmacists	158	26.7	3.8
Dietitians	71	90.8	21.0
Therapists	247	76.3	7.6
Physician's assistants	51	36.3	7.7
Managers, medicine and health	91	57.0	5.0
Health technologists and technicians†	1111	84.3	12.7
Clinical laboratory	255	76.2	10.5
Dental hygienists	66	98.6	1.6
Radiology	101	71.7	8.6
Licensed practical nurses	443	97.0	17.7
Health service occupations	1739	89.2	23.5
Dental assistants	154	98.1	6.1
Health aides, except nursing	316	86.8	16.5
Nursing aides, orderlies, and attendants	1269	88.7	27.3
TOTAL	5576	76.5	12.8

Modified from US Bureau of Labor Statistics: Employment and earnings, Washington, DC, 1984. US Government Printing Office.
*Covers civilians 16 years old and older. Annual averages based on data collected by Bureau of the Census as part of Current Population Survey.
†Includes other occupations not shown separately.
‡Medical and osteopathic.

the hidden factors in the stratification pattern. Table 8-3 shows the major health occupations as they are classified in a study done by the U.S. Bureau of Labor Statistics (US Bureau of Census, 1986). The female and black percentages of each occupational group are shown. Notice that the distribution of women is pyramidal, with only a few women in the high-status health professions and heavy representation of women in the low-status occupations.

Although the causal factors in this pattern are many and undoubtedly include all the prejudices against women in the work force, these prejudices have been ingrained through the professional schools. Medical schools and the other high-status professional schools remained resistant to admitting more than a few token women throughout most of the twentieth century. The situation started to change in the 1960s, and by the 1981-1982 academic year 31% of the students accepted to medical school and 20% of the students accepted to dental school were women (Datagram 1982; Solomon, 1982).

Schools of nursing also played a significant role in creating the sex-segregated pattern. According to the 1910 census figures, approximately 7% of student and trained nurses were men. Most of these came from schools affiliated with mental hospitals or from one of the few all-male nursing schools. The early twentieth century efforts of nursing to upgrade educational programs forced the mental hospitals to close, effectively cutting off slots for male recruits.

The general hospital schools excluded men because they required student nurses to live on the hospital grounds in student nurses' dormitories. This was done to maintain surveillance on student nurses' behavior and keep them available for night work. The norms of that period would not allow men to stay in these quarters. By 1950, only 1% of the practicing nurses were men (Bullough and Bullough, 1978). The current changeover to collegiate nursing has again created opportunities for men to enter nursing. Approximately 5% of the registered nurse students are now men (ANA, 1985), and 3% of practicing registered nurses are men (Secretary's Commission, 1988).

The educational system has also been a significant factor in excluding blacks and other minorities from the high-status health professions, although economic deprivation is certainly an added factor. Table 8-3 shows the same type of pyramid for black workers as for women. The education problem for minority students, particularly black students, started at the elementary school level with segregated educational patterns (Bullough, 1972; Coleman and others, 1966; Myrdal, 1944). As long as schools were segregated, minority members were unprepared for admission to professional schools. However, even those who managed to get a good basic education faced overt and covert discriminatory patterns when they tried to enter high-status professional schools. Until the 1960s, when federal legislation outlawed discrimination in publicly supported educational programs, the only significant opportunity to enter medicine or dentistry available for black students was through one of the segregated black schools (Cogan, 1968; Dummett, 1952).

Black nurses could attend Provident Hospital School in Chicago, Freedman's Hospital School in Washington, D.C., or segregated southern schools. A study done in 1925 by Ethel Johns that was sponsored by the Rockefeller Foundation found that the graduates of these schools were employed primarily in segregated black hospitals where they worked as staff nurses with white supervisors. Only rarely was a black nurse employed by a visiting nurse association or in a public health department. When they were hired, they were paid less than their white colleagues and excluded from supervisory positions. The Henry Street Settlement, established by Lillian Wald, was an exception to this generalization. Wald, a strong supporter of equal opportunity, employed 25 black and 150 white nurses, paid them equal salaries, and accorded them equal recognition (Hine, 1988).

The segregation situation started changing during World War II in part because the Bolton Act, which created the Cadet Nurse Corps, included nondiscriminatory provisions. After the war some of the schools retained their nondiscriminatory practices, so the minority exclusion in nursing became less oppressive than it was in the high-status health professions (US Public Health Service, 1950). In 1981, 13.5% of the students admitted to registered nursing programs were members of minority groups. The graduation rate was less impressive—only 8.8% of the graduating nurses represented minority groups (ANA, 1983). Approximately 4.5% of the employed registered nurses were black, 1.6% were hispanic, and 0.3% were Native Americans (Secretary's Commission, 1988).

That salary inequities and discriminatory patterns still remain in such a large and complex system creates pressure for reform, and reform creates upheaval. Some of the changes are coming about through unionization as the unions move from productive industries to service industries, and the professional associations turn to collective bargaining. However, the process of organizing and negotiating is not without trauma for the participants. Nurses with community roles tend to be positioned in the middle of the system. Sometimes they participate in the unionization process as workers, whereas at other times they fill managerial roles. Negotiations can be particularly difficult because the cause of the workers is just, yet increases in labor costs must necessarily be reflected in already inflated client care costs.

ECONOMICS OF THE SYSTEM

The variety of financial mechanisms used to pay for health care in the United States also makes the system complex. In fact, the current economic picture, as well as the transitions taking place, is understandable only when viewed in a historical context. Traditionally hospitals were financed by church bodies or municipal or county governments. Hospitals developed in the Middle Ages as generalized institutions that served the needy, including pilgrims, orphans, the elderly, and the sick. As nursing groups developed in the medieval period, they became the sponsors of many hospitals and the functions narrowed to focus on the sick (Bullough and Bullough, 1978).

In Protestant countries after the Reformation in the sixteenth century some hospitals were taken over by Protestant churches, whereas others were supported by government entities. Nurses in the Protestant countries were minimally trained and paid subsistence wages. Hospitals were the institutions of last resort, housing primarily the destitute sick or persons with communicable diseases.

The late nineteenth century development of nursing schools based on the Nightingale model upgraded hospitals and made them places where people came not only to die, but to recover as well. This upgrading made hospitals attractive to physicians, so the focus of medical care was transferred from private offices to hospitals, and the stage was set for the development of twentieth century health care technology (Rosenberg, 1987). Along with the developments in technology there were also changes in hospital finances with private and governmental insurance systems furnishing the support for the technologic revolution.

The early nursing school movement focused on students as the bulk of the hospital work force. Graduate nurses were employed as private duty nurses in homes and hospitals or as teachers and administrators. Students filled the worker role for more than 50 years, from the foundation of the first Nightingale schools in 1873 to about 1930. The number of nursing schools increased from five in 1873, to 432 in 1900, to 1908 in 1930 (Bullough and Bullough, 1981). It is not surprising that this created an oversupply of nurses (Burgess, 1928). Graduate nurses were forced to compete with unpaid students for work. Some graduate nurses even offered their services to hospitals for room and board. Beginning in the late 1920s the hospital work force began to gradually change to a salaried staff. Correspondingly the number of schools of nursing fell to 1387 in 1940 (Bullough and Bullough, 1981). Unfortunately, this change resulted in nurse salaries so low that a half century later the salaries of nurses still lag behind those of other equally prepared workers (Bullough, 1988).

Hospitals are still the major employers of nurses, using two thirds of the nursing work force (ANA, 1985). Private duty nursing, in which one nurse cares for one client, employed the largest number of graduate nurses in the era of the student labor force. It was not, however, an economical way to deliver nursing care unless the nurse earned a low salary or the client was very ill. Private duty nursing, using a fee-for-service system for remuneration, declined after 1930 as nurses were hired by hospitals. Although still not an effective use of nursing time, private duty nursing is having an interesting revival in the community. Hospital fees have escalated rapidly in the last 20 years, reflecting not only the development of high technology in health care but also the inflationary costs of Medicare and other government programs. Hospital fees are now so high that one-to-one nursing care in patients' homes is often more economical. This movement was escalated by the development of the prospective payment system for Medicare that was instituted in 1983. Few nurses in the home care situation actually nurse. Most are filling the roles of case managers or administrators of nursing teams rather than serving as individualized providers on a fee-for-service basis. Still a small cadre has revived the private duty services in the home.

Even though nurses long ago abandoned the fee-for-service system, physicians tend to regard it as the norm and even the ideal, in part because of a rose-colored vision of the past. Nineteenth century physicians were almost all paid on a fee-for-service basis. Clients purchased advice from doctors when they felt it was needed, which was usually when they were sick. It was an illness-oriented system. Since the United States was smaller, more rural, and less industrialized, the doctor and the patient were often neighbors and friends. Since more physicians were general practitioners, the care was less fragmented. Although physicians' care could cure fewer persons then than is now possible, the work role of the doctor was probably more emotionally satisfying. Consequently many physicians look back to this era as the best of all possible times. By doing so they forget the realities of the economic system of the past in their optimistic view of some of the other attributes of the system. Physician salaries were much lower and less secure, since serious illness tended to make it impossible for people with marginal incomes to pay fee-for-service doctor bills. The whole system worked against practical, preventive medicine.

Fee-for-service survives today as the primary method of financing physician care for a portion of the middle class consumers (Torrens, 1984). This segment is insured for hospital care but not physician care. However, if one follows trend lines, it is clear that more costs are paid by third-party payers each year, so the direct fee-for-service is being modified by insurance. Dentistry probably retained fee-for-service the longest, but union contracts in the last two decades are now bringing dentists into reimbursement systems.

Community health care, including control of communicable disease, sanitation, the collection of vital statistics, broad-scale efforts to improve preventive care, and efforts to control the environment have almost always been financed by either private nonprofit groups or government entities. The history of the public health movement covered in Chapter 1 showed a gradual shifting of this burden to government bodies. This is not an unreasonable situation. Public health measures focus on the welfare of the collective, so public financial responsibility is an expectation.

Early Campaigns for National Health Insurance

Proponents of national health insurance started campaigning as early as 1915 when several of the more advanced industrialized nations had established government plans for health care delivery. This led to the formation of the Committee on the Costs of Medical Care in 1927 under the chairmanship of Ray Lyman Wilbur who was secretary of the interior. For the next five years the committee, with the support of various private foundations, investigated the costs of medical care. The final summary of findings, titled *Medical Care for the American People,* appeared in 1932, when the country was at the depth of the Great Depression (Committee on the Costs of Medical Care, 1970). It included both a majority and a minority report. The majority favored medical and hospital insurance on a voluntary basis, until adequate research could be accumulated to form a comprehensive system based on compulsory tax deductions. The majority also approved group medical practice organized around health centers and grants-in-aid to provide hospitals, physicians, and nurses to poor and thinly populated areas. It also urged government support of the cost of medical care for the indigent, tubercular, and mentally ill (Roemer, 1985).

On the other hand, a minority report written by the physicians and dentists on the committee opposed any kind of prepaid medical care, even on a voluntary basis, and vehemently objected to the proposal for group practice. The minority was willing to accept hospital insurance plans, provided they were sponsored and controlled by organized medicine. In general, the minority view coincided with the emerging view of the American Medical Association (AMA). The hostility with which the majority report was greeted by the medical profession is evident from the pages of the *Journal of the American Medical Association,* which labeled the report as "inciting to revolution." Morris Fishbein, the editor, went so far as to call the recommendation for group practice an attempt to establish medical "soviets" (Cray, 1970).

Franklin Roosevelt was fearful that medical opposition would prevent passage of any social security legislation, so he requested the House Ways and Means Committee to strike most provisions dealing with health care from the 1935 Social Security Bill (Bullough and Bullough, 1982). Title V of the act enhanced the role of the Children's Bureau by providing grants to the states for maternal and infant preventive care. Because these grants were administered by the states, they did much to strengthen state and local health departments and shape community health nursing after 1935 (Jain, 1983).

In 1939, Senator Robert F. Wagner of New York formally introduced a national health insurance proposal to the U.S. Senate. Although it failed to get out of committee, Wagner continued to introduce it in successive sessions. In 1943, he was joined by Senator James Murray and Representative John Dingell, and in this and subsequent years it was known as the Wagner-Murray-Dingell bill. Despite public opinion polls indicating strong national support for governmentally sponsored health insurance, the AMA and its allies were able to prevent the bill from coming to a vote (Corning, 1970).

Hill-Burton Act

The first large-scale entry of the federal government into health care financing came at the end of World War II when Congress passed the 1946 Hill-Burton Act (Title VI of the Public Health Services Act). It provided funds to hospitals to increase their capacity to care for people. It represented a major effort on the part of the government to furnish resources to the underserved (Ginzberg, 1984). Between 1946 and 1979 approximately $4 billion in grants and loans for construction and modernization to care for the poor was allocated to 7000 hospitals, nursing homes, and other health care facilities (Neely and Tigar, 1983).

One of the requirements written into the law by Congress was that hospitals receiving building funds would assume an obligation to provide reasonable services to indigent patients. Since this feature of the law was never operationally defined by legislators, it essentially was not enforced; in effect, any service to the community could be considered reasonable by the government. Starting in 1970, some public interest law groups, including most notably the National Health Law Program, started campaigning for enforcement of this provision. They wrote papers urging enforcement and fought a series of lawsuits. Finally in 1972 (26 years after the writing of the law), the Department of Health, Education and Welfare issued draft regulations suggesting that hospitals use 5% of their total costs or 25% of their net income, whichever was more, to provide services for those who could not pay (Hill-Burton, 1972). This proposal was vigorously opposed by the American Hospital Association (AHA), which had by 1972 emerged by a powerful lobby. The AHA argued that hospitals had a crucial responsibility to stay solvent to serve the community, that such a provision was unnecessary, that the poor could be cared for in some other way, and that even though many hospitals had built new wings under the 1946 Hill Burton Act, which specifically provided for beds for the poor, such beds had never been used. After three years of delays, watered-down regulations were passed (Federal Register, 1975; Hill-Burton, 1975; Rose, 1975). Hospitals now have an obligation to give some services to the poor, but it is still difficult for a poor person who does not have proof of a third-party payer to gain admittance to a hospital.

Private Hospital and Health Insurance

The voluntary health insurance movement is usually traced to a plan that started in 1929 at Baylor University Hospital in Dallas. For $6 per year per person the hospital agreed to provide 21 days of hospitalization to each of 1500 local teachers. The plan proved so successful that it was soon extended to other Dallas residents. Soon similar plans were springing up around the country (Sinai and others, 1946).

By 1935, hospitals had enrolled about 23,000 people in more than 400 different employee insurance groups. By 1937, the AHA had approved various hospital plans that met its criteria by allowing such plans to use its trademark of a blue cross. In the first list of Blue Cross subscribers published in 1938, some 1.5 million persons were enrolled. The Blue Shield plan developed out of plans set up by state medical societies to provide physicians' services. They adopted the blue shield as their trademark in 1945 (Somers and Somers, 1961).

Commercial insurance plans entered the field after Blue Cross and Blue Shield were well established. Collectively commercial carriers sell more than the nonprofit Blue Cross and Blue Shield programs. For a while the commercial carriers could offer insurance at a lower rate by using what are called experience ratings. That is, when they signed a group of healthy young workers, who are not usually ill, they charged less. When a group of older persons were enrolled, the rate was higher. However, that advantage in the marketplace quickly disappeared because the nonprofit carriers also began to use experience ratings. This means that currently people who have a history of illness or are older pay more for health insurance, and people with chronic illnesses are often not covered for that illness. Although 205 million persons in the United States (or 85.5% of the population) are now covered by some kind of public program or private health insurance, the exemptions and other mechanisms that protect the insurance companies make coverage less than perfect for the public (Bodenheimer and others, 1975; Health Insurance Association, 1988).

Health Maintenance Organizations

A Health Maintenance Organization (HMO) is a formally organized delivery system that provides comprehensive services to an enrolled membership for a fixed prepaid fee. It is both an insurance company and a health care provider (Anderson and others, 1985). HMOs are also group medical plans. This makes the Mayo Clinic in Rochester, Minnesota, a precursor to the modern HMOs. The Mayo Clinic has treated seriously ill patients since the nineteenth century. Its example was followed by other specialized clinics, such as Cleveland Clinic, the Ochsner Clinic in New Orleans, and the Lahey Clinic in Boston. These clinics had little opposition from organized medicine, but when the concept of the clinic was combined with the prepaid factor and preventive care and was opened up to a wider public, organized medicine responded negatively. On the urging of their medical associations, many states passed laws prohibiting group practice of any kind.

The matter came to a head in the case of the Group Health Association established in 1937 in Washington, D.C., by employees of the Federal Home Owners Loan Corporation. This nonprofit prepayment hospitalization and medical care program contracted with physicians to serve its members. The physicians employed by the group soon found themselves expelled from the District of Columbia Medical Society and barred from the seven district hospitals because of their lack of AMA certification. The District Medical Society even went so far as to warn physicians of a rule barring medical consultation with nonsociety members. Hospitals were also warned that, if they accepted patients from the Group Health Association, they would lose AMA approval for their intern-training programs. The effect of such action was to deny hospitalization and other benefits to members of such prepaid groups. Because of such actions against the health group, the U.S. government instituted a suit for criminal violation against the AMA and the District of Columbia Medical Society. The resulting conviction was eventually affirmed by the U.S. Supreme Court in 1943. This decision facilitated the development of other group plans (Rosen, 1958).

The Kaiser-Permanente Plan was started by Henry J. Kaiser, a California contractor, as a plan for his employees when he was building Grand Coulee Dam. It was expanded during World War II, as Kaiser turned to building ships. Shortly after the end of the war the system went public and, through contracts with various unions and other organizations, Kaiser-Permanente began offering total prepaid medical care to all subscribers. For those who belong to complete Kaiser plans, everything is paid except drugs used in outpatient care and these are sold at discount prices. From the start, Kaiser-Permanente insisted that all companies and organizations offering their plan also offer competing ones. This tends to keep subscribers from feeling trapped within the Kaiser system, and it also serves as an effective cost-accounting procedure.

The Health Insurance Plan of Greater New York (HIP) was developed at about the same time to insure public employees, and in Seattle, Washington, a group of consumer cooperative HMOs developed. Although the structure of these early prototype HMOs varied somewhat, all combined the insurance and health care provider functions. Since the early HMOs were all prepaid plans, they naturally developed a focus on preventive health care and the avoidance of unnecessary treatment, which also turned out to be a clear cost-saving mechanism (Somers and Somers, 1961).

In a 1966 study of various prepaid group practice plans, it was found that, for each 1000 subscribers, physicians in the group practice performed less than one fourth the number of tonsillectomies, half the number of appendectomies, and only slightly more than half the hysterectomies done by fee-for-service physicians. This same trend appeared with those welfare patients enrolled in group practice plans. In 1962, for example, New York City's HIP began to enroll welfare recipients, and it was found that HIP physicians made one fourth the number of premium-priced home calls and ordered only one half the highly profitable (and highly expensive) laboratory tests that fee-for-service, solo practitioners ordered (Cray, 1970; Tunley, 1966).

The federal government recognized the cost-effectiveness of the approach and in 1973 passed Public Law 93-222, the Health Maintenance Organization Act. The law established minimum requirements for HMOs that allowed them to qualify for grants, contracts, loans, and loan guarantees to offset the costs of planning and establishing new programs. In return for a monthly or annual subscriber fee, the HMO must contract to provide certain types of care. Minimum benefits included physicians' services, inpatient and outpatient hospital services, necessary emergency medical services, short-term ambulatory, evaluative, and crisis-intervention mental health services, medical treatment and referral services for alcohol and drug abuse and addiction, laboratory, diagnostic, and therapeutic radiologic services, home health services, and preventive services, including voluntary family planning services, infertility services, and preventive dental care and eye examinations for children.

Further federal government support was given to HMOs in 1982 when the Health Care Financing Administration (HFCA), the government body administering Medicare and Medicaid, set up a demonstration project featuring the HMO concept. Contracts were negotiated with HMOs and competitive medical plans (CMPs). These contracts brought private physicians into a per capita reimbursement plan. Early analysis of data from 21 of the demonstration projects indicates that in both the HMOs and the CMPs people are hospitalized less often than in the fee-for-service sector. Specifically, the demonstration project clients averaged 1951 hospital days per 1000 persons compared with 3432 days per 1000 persons in the private sector. This constitutes a significant saving and will probably encourage HCFA to continue the program (Rossiter, 1988).

The HMOs are also important because of their emphasis on preventive care. The prepayment mechanism encourages this emphasis. Subscribers contract for services without knowing what illnesses they face. Thus preventing illness or using less costly treatment modalities saves money for the HMO. The HMOs tend to have less costly staffing patterns, including the extensive use of nurse practitioners and physicians' assistants instead of all-physician staffs, optometrists instead of all-ophthalmologist staffs, and clinical psychologists instead of psychiatrists. Moreover, HMO physicians tend to avoid unnecessary surgery.

SUMMARY

The modern American health care delivery system offers a wide variety of services. The personnel are organized into a highly stratified hierarchy that is in the process of changing as the workers at the middle and lower levels professionalize and seek more power in the system. In the nineteenth century the system was made up primarily of nurses and physicians. That dyad has been replaced by a large, complex team of workers. In the nineteenth century a fee-for-service mechanism paid physicians, whereas hospitals used an unpaid student nurse labor force. A fee-for-service approach, however, was also used to pay the graduate nurse who took private cases. Today most workers in the complex health care delivery system are salaried or reimbursed by some type of insurance. The insurance industry is divided into three major groups—the nonprofit organizations, including Blue Cross and Blue Shield, the commercial carriers, and the HMOs, which provide both insurance and health care service.

QUESTIONS FOR DISCUSSION

1. Distinguish between primary, secondary, and tertiary care.
2. Why are health care delivery services extremely stratified?
3. What is meant by the fee-for-service system, and how and why it is being modified?
4. Why was the Hill-Burton Act such an important piece of legislation?
5. What is a health maintenance organization, and how does it work?

REFERENCES

American Nurses' Association, Committee on Education: First position on education for nursing, Am J Nurs 65:106, 1965.

American Nurses' Association: Facts about nursing 82-83, Kansas City, Mo, 1983, The Association.

American Nurses' Association: Facts about nursing 84-85, Kansas City, Mo, 1985, The Association.

Bodenheimer T, Cummings S, and Harding E: Capitalizing on illness: the health insurance industry. In Navarro V, editor: Health and medical care in the US: a critical analysis, Farmingdale, NY, 1975, Baywood Publishing Co Inc.

Bullough B: Alienation and school segregation, Integrated Education 10:29, 1972.

Bullough B: Stratification. In Hardy ME and Conway ME, editors: Role theory: perspectives for health professionals, ed 2, Norwalk, Conn, 1988, Appleton & Lange.

Bullough B and Bullough V: Educational problems in a woman's profession, J Nurs Educ 20:6, 1981.

Bullough B and Bullough V: Introduction: educational issues: background paper. In Bullough B, Bullough V, and Soukup MC, editors: Nursing issues and nursing strategies for the eighties, New York, 1983, Springer Publishing Co Inc.

Bullough V and Bullough B: The causes and consequences of the differentiation of the nursing role. In Stewart PL, editor: Varieties of work experience, New York, 1974, Halsted Press.

Bullough VL and Bullough B: The care of the sick: the emergence of modern nursing, New York, 1978, Prodist.

Bullough VL and Bullough B: Health care for other Americans, New York, 1982, Appleton & Lange.

Bullough B and Sparks C: Baccalaureate vs associate degree nurses: the care-cure dichotomy, Nurs Outlook 23:688, 1975.

Burgess MA: Nurses, patients, and pocketbooks, New York, 1928, Committee on the Grading of Nursing Schools.

Carr-Saunders AM and Wilson PA: The professions, Oxford, England, 1933, Clarendon Press.

Cogan L: Negroes for medicine: report of a Macy Conference, Baltimore, 1968, Johns Hopkins University Press.

Committee on the Costs of Medical Care: Medical care for the American people, Chicago, 1970, University of Chicago Press.

Corning PA: The evolution of Medicare: from idea to law, Washington, DC, 1970, US Department of Health Education and Welfare, Social Security Administration, US Government Printing Office.

Cray E: In failing health: the medical crises and the AMA, Indianapolis, 1970, The Bobbs-Merrill Co.

Daniels AK: How free should professions be? In Freidson E, editor: The professions and their prospects, Beverly Hills, Calif, 1971, Sage Publications, Inc.

Datagram: Applicants to U.S. medical schools 1977-78 to 1981-82, J Med Educ 57:882, 1982.

Department of Health, Education and Welfare: Trends affecting U.S. health care system, DHEW Pub No HRA 76-14503, Washington, DC, 1975, US Government Printing Office.

Dummett CO: The growth and development of the Negro in dentistry, Chicago, 1952, Stanek Press for the National Dental Association.

Federal Register, October 6, 1975.

Freidson E: Professional dominance: the social structure of medical care, New York, 1970, Atherton.

Freidson E, editor: The professions and their prospects, Beverly Hills, Calif, 1971, Sage Publications Inc.

Georgopoulos BS, editor: Organization research on health institutions, Ann Arbor, Mich, 1972, Institute for Social Research.

Ginzberg E: Health reform: the outlook for the 1980s. In Lee PR, Estes CL, and Ramsay NB, editors: The nation's health, San Francisco, 1984, Boyd & Fraser Publishing Co.

Health Insurance Association of America: HIAA health trends chartbook, Washington, DC, 1988, The Association.

Hill-Burton: Health Law Newsletter 13:1, 1972.

Hill-Burton: Health Law Newsletter 55:3, 1975.

Hine DH: They shall mount up with wings of eagles: historical images of black nurses, 1890-1950. In Jones AH, editor: Images of nurses: perspectives from history, art and literature, Philadelphia, 1988, University of Pennsylvania Press.

Jain SC: Policy concerns and the changing role of government in personal health: a perspective. In Jain SC and Paul JE, editors: Policy issues in personal health services: current perspectives, Rockville, Md, 1983, Aspen Publishers Inc.

Johnson DE: A philosophy of nursing, Nurs Outlook 7:198, 1959.

Jonas S: Health care delivery, ed 2, New York, 1981, Springer Publishing Co Inc.

Kalisch PA and Kalisch BJ: The advancement of American nursing, Boston, 1978, Little, Brown & Co Inc.

Kramer M: Reality shock: why nurses leave nursing, St Louis, 1974, CV Mosby Co.

Montag M: Community college education, New York, 1959, Blakiston, McGraw-Hill.

Moore WE: The profession: roles and rules, New York, 1970, Russell Sage Foundation.

Myrdal G: An American dilemma: the Negro problem and American democracy, New York, 1944, Harper & Bros.

Neely GM and Tigar NL: Shifting federal policy and its impact on minorities' access to health services. In Jain SC and Paul JE: Policy issues in personal health services: current perspectives, Rockville, Md, 1983, Aspen Publishers Inc.

Roemer MI and Falk IS: The committee on the costs of medical care, and the drive for national health insurance, public health, then and now, Am J Public Health 75:841, 1985.

Rose M: Federal regulation of service to the poor under the Hill-Burton Act: realities and pitfalls, Northwestern University Law Review 70:168, 1975.

Rosen GA: A history of public health, New York, 1958, MD Publications.

Rosenberg C: The care of strangers: the rise of America's hospital system, New York, 1987, Basic Books Inc.

Rossiter LF, Nelson LM, and Adamache KW: Service use and costs for Medicare beneficiaries in risk-based HMOs and CMPs: some interim results from the National Medicare Competition Evaluation, Am J Public Health 78:937, 1988.

Rydman LD and Rydman RJ: The United States health care delivery system. In Burgess W and Ragland EC, editors: Community health nursing: philosophy, process practice, Norwalk, Conn, 1983, Appleton & Lange.

Schulman S: Mother surrogate after a decade. In Jaco EG, editor: Patients, physicians and illness, ed 2, New York, 1972, Free Press.

Secretary's Commission on Nursing: Interim report, Washington, DC, 1988, The Commission.

Sinai N, Anderson OW, and Dollar M: Health insurance in the United States, New York, 1946, The Commonwealth Fund.

Skipper JK Jr: The role of the hospital nurse: is it instrumental or expressive? In Skipper JK Jr and Leonard RC, editors: Social interaction and patient care, Philadelphia, 1965, JB Lippincott Co.

Solomon E: Trends in female enrollment in health professions schools, J Dent Educ 46:672, 1982.

Somers HM and Somers AR: Doctors, patients, and health insurance, Washington, DC, 1961, The Brookings Institution.

Torrens PR: Overview of health services in the United States. In Lee PR, Estes CL, and Ramsay NB, editors: The nation's health, ed 2, San Francisco, 1984, Boyd & Fraser Publishing Co.

Tunley R: The American health scandal, New York, 1966, Harper & Row Publishers Inc.

US Bureau of the Census: Statistical abstract of the United States 1985, ed 105, Washington, DC, 1986, US Government Printing Office.

BIBLIOGRAPHY

Anderson OW and others: HMO development: patterns and prospects: a comparative analysis of HMOs, Chicago, 1985, Pluribus Press.

Blendon RJ: Health policy choices for the 1990s, Issues in Science and Technology 2:65, 1986.

Coleman JS and others: Equality of educational opportunity, Washington, DC, 1966, Office of Education, Department of Health, Education and Welfare.

Jain SC and Paul JE, editors: Policy issues in personal health services: current perspectives, Rockville, Md, 1983, Aspen Publishers Inc.

Luft HS: 1984. Definition and scope of the HMO concept. In Lee PR, Estes CL, and Ramsay NB, editors: The nation's health, San Francisco, 1984, Boyd & Fraser Publishing Co.

US Public Health Service: The US Cadet Nurse Corps and other federal nursing training programs, 1943-1948, Washington, DC, 1950, US Government Printing Office.

Williamson K: Letter to Elliot Richardson, Secretary of Health, Education and Welfare, April 20, 1972.

CHAPTER

9

Changing Health Care Delivery System

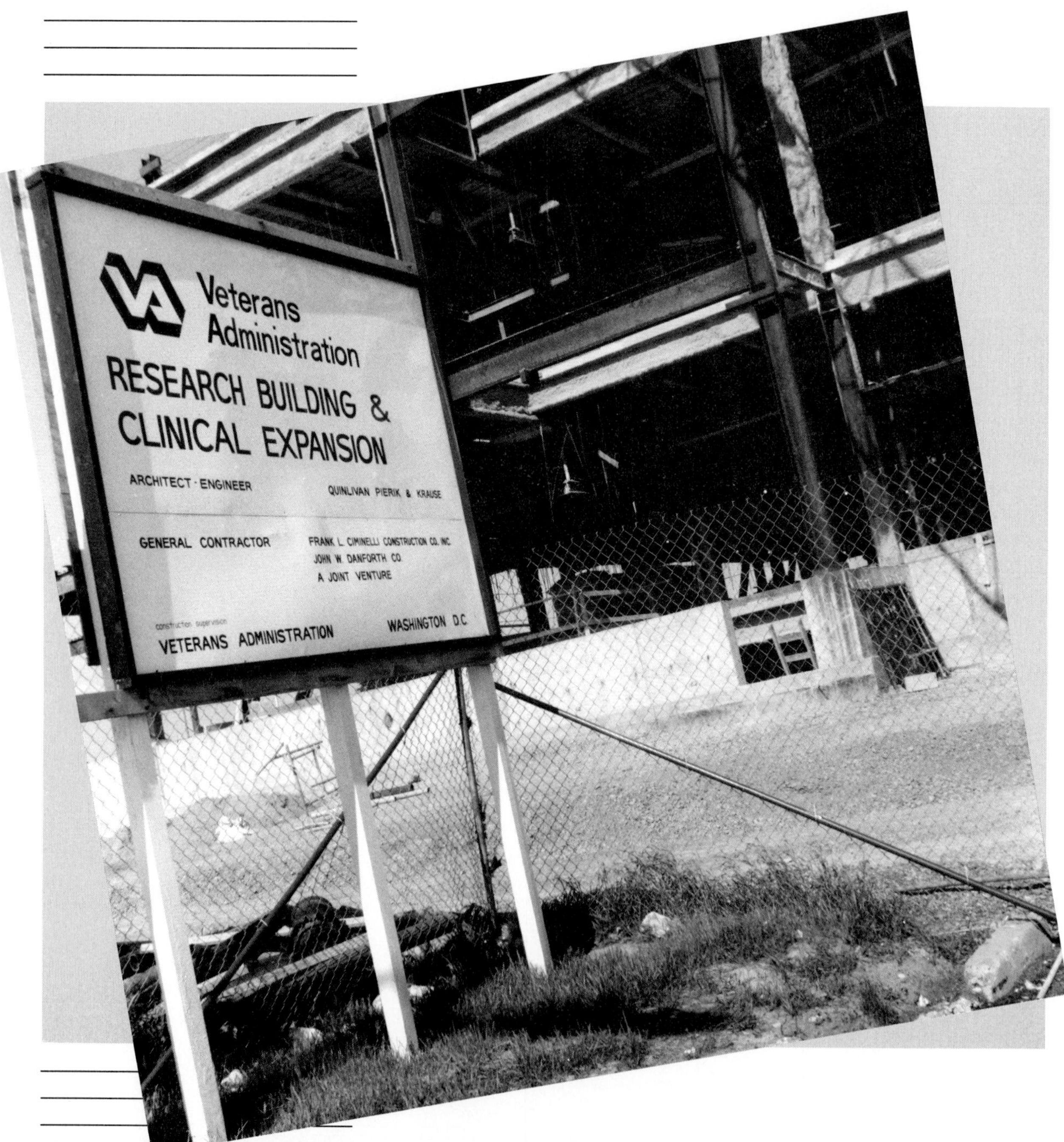

CHAPTER OUTLINE

Factors in the inflation of health care costs
- Federal programs
- Increases in hospital beds
- Increases in health workers
- High technology
- Treatment orientation of the system
- Malpractice lawsuits

Implications of the inflationary cycle

Efforts to control inflation
- Prospective payment system using diagnostic related groups
- Changing structures: home health care

Other contemporary trends
- Nursing shortage
- Hospital reorganization
- Preferred provider organizations
- Community nursing centers

Health care delivery systems in other countries
- United Kingdom
- Germany
- Union of Soviet Socialist Republics
- Canada
- Sweden

Summary

OBJECTIVES

After completing this chapter, the reader should be able to:

1. Describe the political dynamics surrounding the passage of the Medicare/Medicaid legislation in 1965.
2. Discuss the reasons for the subsequent inflation in the cost of health care.
3. Understand the rationale for the institution of a prospective payment system (PPS) of federal reimbursement for health care services.
4. Discuss the implications of the PPS including the increased reliance on home health care.
5. Describe other trends in the health care delivery system including:
   a. The nursing shortage
   b. Hospital reorganization
   c. Preferred provider organizations
   d. Community nursing centers
6. Compare the health care delivery system of the United States with those of selected other countries.

IN THE LAST TWO DECADES THE GOVERNMENT has increasingly entered into the health care delivery system. Although agitation for greater government intervention grew during the twentieth century, in retrospect it seems that the factor most responsible for creating a change in public opinion about national health insurance was the growing number of elderly persons. As a general rule it is the elderly who have medical costs so large that they can wipe out a lifetime of savings. By 1965, 9.5% of the population was older than 65 years (Davis, 1983), and the number has continued to grow.

When Representative Aime J. Forand introduced a bill to furnish hospital, surgical, and nursing benefits to all recipients of Social Security in 1957, opposition came from the American Medical Association (AMA), the National Association of Manufacturers, the Health Insurance Association of America, the U.S. Pharmaceutical Association, and the American Farm Bureau Federation. Supporting the Forand legislation were the National Association of Social Workers, the National Farmers Union, and the American Nurses' Association (ANA). The support of the ANA was crucial because it was the first major group of health professionals to break ranks with the AMA. Its stance encouraged the American Hospital Association (AHA) to reevaluate its position on health insurance. Although the AHA did not immediately support government insurance, they did not oppose the Forand bill. Instead they issued a statement pointing out that something had to be done to help elderly clients pay their bills. Large hospital bills were not only a problem of the elderly. Hospitals were being left with many uncollectable debts (Bullough and Bullough, 1982).

In 1960, Senator Robert Kerr and Representative Wilbur Mills introduced a substitute bill providing for federal subsidies to states to help pay for health care of welfare recipients, including aged indigents. Although this was a weak compromise for the Forand bill, it had the merit of being enacted. The new legislation soon proved ineffective because many states never bothered to institute the programs necessary to use the grants. In 1962 the Medicare bill, a revision of the original Forand bill, was again introduced, but with the full support of President John F. Kennedy. Although it failed to get out of committee in that session of Congress, it gathered support and was enacted into law in 1965 under President Lyndon B. Johnson.

The original Medicare Act was financed through the Social Security system and provided two separate but coordinated coverages. Hospital insurance for most persons aged 65 or older was given, as well as supplemental medical insurance for persons in the same age group who voluntarily enrolled and paid the required monthly premiums. A companion bill, upgrading the provisions of the Kerr-Mills bill, was also passed that year and was generally known as Medicaid, although various states gave it a different name. This bill gave funds to states to set up health care programs for welfare recipients covered under the federal programs for families with needy children, the totally or partially blind, and the totally disabled (Corning, 1969).

FACTORS IN THE INFLATION OF HEALTH CARE COSTS

Federal Programs

The supporters of increased federal support for health care rejoiced with the passage of the Medicare/Medicaid legislation, although the programs were not without problems. They were, in fact, a major variable in the inflation in the cost of health care that followed. Fig. 9-1 shows the increase in health care costs since 1960. Dollar costs of and percentage of gross national product spent on health care are shown. Dollar costs for health care have risen sharply from the 1960 level of $26.9 billion to the 1987 level of $497 billion. The line showing the percentage of gross national

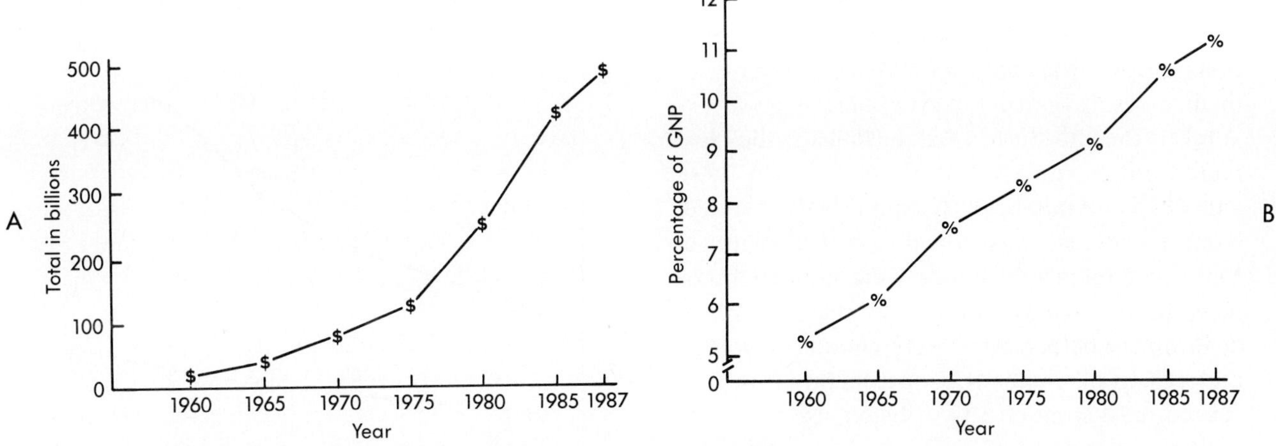

FIG. 9-1. **A,** National health expenditures in dollars. **B,** National health expenditures in percentage of gross national product. (Modified from US Bureau of the Census: Statistical abstract of the United States, 1988, ed 108, Washington, DC, 1987, US Government Printing Office.)

product spent on health care takes into account the generalized inflation of the economy, so it is probably a more accurate measure of true increases in costs. Note that this line also moves up steadily although less dramatically than the dollar figure. The percentage of the gross national product spent on health care has more than doubled from 5.3% in 1960 to the current level of 11.1%. This amounts to nearly $2000 for every man, woman, and child in the United States (Russel, 1981; U.S. Bureau of Census, 1987).

The inflationary aspect of the Medicare/Medicaid legislation was not necessarily inevitable but stemmed in large part from the political compromises that were necessary to achieve passage of the legislation. To gain support of hospitals and physicians, these two groups of providers were allowed to charge their customary fees, a procedure roughly equivalent to allowing cost-plus contracts for defense contractors. Inflation was an inevitable consequence, since there was no means to prevent increases.

The second compromise, calculated to gain the support of the growing insurance industry, mandated the use of an insurance company, usually Blue Cross, as an intermediate carrier for Medicare payments (Bodenheimer, Cummings, and Harding, 1977). This added another layer of administration to the program and made government reform of the system more difficult.

It should be added that even without these compromises, the cost of Medicare would have increased each year because of demographic factors. Both the birth rate and the death rate are decreasing, leading to a disproportionate increase in the elderly population. In 1965, 9.5% of the U.S. population were classified as elderly; in 1980 this figure reached 11%; and an elderly population of 12% is anticipated by 1990 (Davis, 1983). When Medicare was implemented in 1966, it covered 19.1 million persons. In 1983 there were 29.4 million persons eligible for such care (US DHHS, 1983). Since health care costs are calculated to be three times higher for persons older than 65 years than for younger persons, the number of elderly persons who are covered is an important factor in the increased health care costs (Blendon, 1986; Davis, 1983).

Increases in Hospital Beds

There are other factors involved in the increased costs besides Medicare and Medicaid, many of them a result of federal programs. A good example is the Hill-Burton Act, technically the Hospital Construction Act of 1946. Between 1946 and 1975 the number of hospital beds doubled, but this increase was not always well planned. Many community hospitals were granted funds to build new wings without any real attempt to determine whether there were enough people in the area to fill the beds. Consequently hospitals started marketing efforts to better use the overbuilt facilities.

The increase in hospital beds led to an increase in demand for health care workers to staff the hospitals. Most of the health care literature between 1946 and 1975 emphasized the shortage of nurses and other health care personnel. The government responded with the Health Professions Education Assistance Act of 1963, which furnished funds for construction of facilities to train physicians, nurses, dentists, and other health professionals. This was followed in 1964 by the Nurse Training Act, which has furnished funds for more than two decades to assist schools of nursing and nursing students (Kalisch and Kalisch, 1982; Rubenfeld and others, 1981). Although some of these funds were used to upgrade the educational level of nursing, the government programs also significantly increased the number of students schools could admit.

Increases in Health Workers

The number of active registered nurses increased from 370,000 in 1950 to 621,000 in 1965 when the Medicare/Medicaid legislation was passed. That figure has more than doubled with 1.6 million registered nurses now employed (ANA, 1985; Secretary's Commission, 1988; US Bureau of the Census, 1984). The number of practical nurses has also increased dramatically—from 49,000 in 1950 to 539,000 in 1986. Nursing aides and orderlies increased from 221,000 in 1950 to 13 million in 1986 (US Bureau of the Census, 1987; US Department of Health and Human Services, 1986).

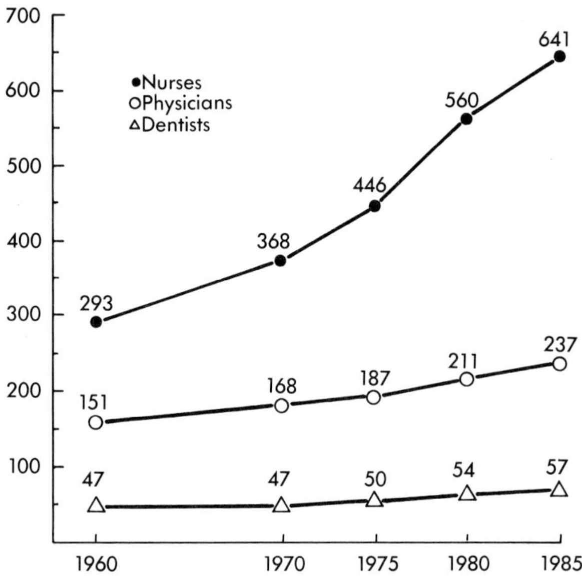

FIG. 9-2. Numbers of registered nurses, physicians, and dentists per 100,000 U.S. population.

Fig. 9-2 shows the increase in the number of registered nurses per 1000 population from 1960 to 1985. This increase is compared with the more controlled growth patterns of medicine and dentistry. The rapid increases in nursing personnel before 1983 reflect primarily an expansion of the institutional work force, including hospitals, skilled nursing facilities, and nursing homes.

Funds for hospital construction were provided by the Hill-Burton program, whereas Medicare and Medicaid paid for the use of the new hospital capacity. Also contributing to the growth in the number of hospital beds was the development of the insurance industry, which paid for diagnostic and treatment procedures only if they were carried out in a hospital. Only the health maintenance organizations (HMOs) avoided this inflationary factor by covering procedures such as gastrointestinal x-rays on an outpatient basis instead of requiring admission to a hospital.

Although the use of nurses increased, the inflationary impact of the growth in the nursing work force was limited by the suppression of salaries. Salaries for registered nurses, practical nurses, and nursing aides did not increase in proportion to those of other health workers or in proportion to the total escalation in the cost of health care. Even today, job worth studies of nursing salaries indicate that the pay is well below that of other workers with comparable levels of skill, effort, responsibility, and working conditions (Barnes, 1980; Remick, 1984).

For a time in the 1960s observers argued that a shortage of physicians was causing the incomes of physicians to escalate. This is because the demand for physician care had grown as medicine was able to do more for clients. A strange paradoxical series of events followed. Massive funding was pumped into medical schools by the federal government. This was partly research money that supported medical faculty members, but it also included a significant portion of the Medicare/Medicaid dollars allocated to hospitals to pay for the training of residents. The supply of physicians increased from 151 doctors per 100,000 persons in 1960 to 237 per 100,000 in 1985 (US Bureau of the Census, 1988). However, the income of physicians increased from a median net income for office-based practitioners of $47,500 in 1975 to $102,000 in 1987 (US Bureau of the Census, 1988). In 1980 the Graduate Medical Education National Advisory Committee issued a report anticipating an oversupply of physicians by the middle of the decade (GMENAC, 1980; McNutt, 1981; Whitney, 1983). As the actual oversupply develops, physicians' incomes may be brought under control, but to date there is no downward trend.

Unfortunately, the increased income of physicians is not the major inflationary factor in raising health care costs. Rather it is the services offered by physicians that have become more expensive. Having a larger supply of physicians increases the cost of care in a community. This is because physicians' services are elastic and determined by the physician instead of the client. Having more physicians in a given area leads to more medical procedures and to more surgery being performed rather than to cost savings (Roemer and Axelrod, 1977). According to a 1975 study, each physician produced approximately $250,000 to $300,000 in additional health care costs in the form of laboratory and hospital costs (Reinhardt, 1975).

High Technology

A fourth factor creating the inflation in health care costs is the development of high technology in health care. Although certain technologic advances are cost saving, others increase costs. For example, antibiotics have lessened the length of many illnesses and shortened hospital stays for surgery by preventing or limiting infections. The recent development of the lithotrite to destroy kidney stones with shock waves is cost saving because it is less expensive than surgery. However, these types of developments are overshadowed by the costly technology of the computed tomography and nuclear magnetic resonance imaging scanners. The scanners not only are expensive to buy and maintain, they are also replaced often because the technology is still being developed and new models come out frequently. Centers that pride themselves on keeping up with the state-of-the-art equipment replace these costly machines every few years.

Dialysis technology has increased health care costs by keeping people in the final stages of renal disease alive and needing dialysis. The Social Security amendments of 1972 furnished the funds for clients needing dialysis, and the cost of the procedure and the number of clients served have increased each year since then. Cyclosporine, which safely suppresses the immune response, has greatly expanded the possibilities for organ transplants since its development in this decade.

Unfortunately, expanded use of transplants is costly, particularly in terms of health care personnel. Thus the high technology of the past few decades has significantly increased the cost of health care.

Treatment Orientation of the System

A more subtle inflationary factor is the fact that the American health care delivery system tends to be treatment oriented instead of preventive care oriented. Although it is well known that preventive health care, including immunizations and health teaching focused on increased exercise, better nutrition, and smoking cessation, can save health care dollars and increase public well-being, the major public funding in recent years has emphasized acute-care services and illness-oriented research. This was particularly true of the Medicare legislation, which furnished hospitalization and physician services for the elderly but did not provide funding for preventive services. Medicaid was somewhat more preventive care oriented, but it reached a smaller population (Davis, 1987).

Malpractice Lawsuits

Malpractice lawsuits are now emerging as a sixth inflationary force. The problem started more than two decades ago and is probably based on public awareness that the American health care system is marked by broad neglect of clients with many iatrogenic, or provider-caused, problems (Meyers, 1987). Physicians, as the most powerful professionals and also the most visibly wealthy, became the first target for lawsuits. To protect their life savings, they countered by buying more malpractice insurance, which made them more attractive as defendants for liability suits. Currently physicians pay annual premiums of $10,000 to $80,000 for malpractice insurance depending on their specialty. Surgeons, obstetricians, and anesthesiologists pay the highest premiums. More recently hospitals and clinics have faced significant increases in their insurance rates, and the nurse specialists are being targeted for increases in premiums, which adds to the problem (Bullough, 1987).

Certainly these rapidly escalating costs have caused health workers to examine their practices to avoid negligence. Hospitals have hired risk managers who search out and correct hazardous practices that could lead to lawsuits. However, the situation has also caused some overreaction. Defensive practices including unnecessary x-rays and laboratory tests have become the norm. This escalates the cost of health care (League of Women Voters, 1985). Legislative relief for this problem is complex and may not be worked out for several years.

IMPLICATIONS OF THE INFLATIONARY CYCLE

These six inflationary factors are in many ways interactive. The government programs have increased hospital beds and personnel and supported the growth of high technology. Defensive medical practices and high technology increase the cost of having a physician in the area, so the total inflationary package is complex. However, it is clear that much of the escalation in costs centers on hospitals. For example, between 1965 and 1975 physicians' fees increased 5.7% per year, whereas hospital costs increased 12.1% per year. During this same period the consumer price index went up 4.5% per year. Average hospital costs went from $50 per person in 1960 to $400 per person in 1980 (Shortell, 1984).

This level of inflation raises some policy questions. How much is too much? Are the improvements in health care that have occurred in the last two decades worth the escalation in cost of health care that has occurred? Since more than 11% of the gross national product is now being spent on health care, compared with 5.3% in 1960, it is important to realize that those funds must nec-

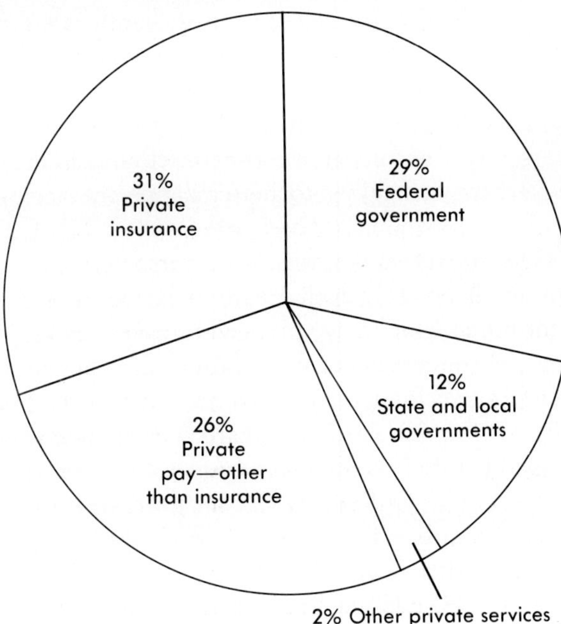

FIG. 9-3. Source of funds for health care.

essarily be drawn from spending for other purposes (Marmor, 1983; Russel, 1981).

While this philosophic discussion takes place, the federal and state governments have appropriately become concerned. This is undoubtedly because government's share of the costs has increased to 41% of the total with 29% of that share borne by the federal government (Fig. 9-3).

EFFORTS TO CONTROL INFLATION

The first major effort to control costs took place in the National Health Planning and Resources Development Act of 1974 (Public Law 93-641). This act replaced the Hill-Burton Hospital Construction Act, the Comprehensive Health Planning Program, and the Regional Medical Program—three federal programs. The goal of the legislation was to monitor federal spending and at the same time see that better and more effective health care was given to more people. To do this, the act set up a series of state, regional, and local boards called health systems agencies (HSAs) that have the power to determine whether new facilities are needed or old ones should keep getting federal funds. To ensure consumer participation in decision making, the law stipulated that 51% of the members of the board be consumers. However, consumers are essentially disorganized, so this has meant that organized groups that are not engaged in health care delivery control a simple majority of the votes. These groups, including labor unions and special community interest groups, have their own special interests. The agencies are more effective in making negative decisions than in doing anything positive to improve health care, and instead of limiting the power of traditional health care groups, the HSAs have given these groups more power. Despite these and other criticisms, HSAs represent a historic step forward because they are the first effort at rational planning for health care. As they gain experience, HSAs are denying certificates of need to some wasteful proposals.

The Reagan administration brought with it drastic antiinflationary measures. Because Medicaid serves primarily disabled persons, children, and poor persons, who do not constitute a voting bloc, it has always been less popular in Congress than Medicare, which serves an elderly voting population. Medicaid became an immediate target for cuts in federal spending starting in 1981. By 1983 $3 billion dollars in federal expenditures had been eliminated. This shifted some of the expenses to state governments, although in many cases needy persons simply went without the care that Medicaid had provided (Wing, 1984). Cuts in programs for women and children were particularly devastating.

Prospective Payment System Using Diagnostic Related Groups

Significant efforts to control Medicare spending started in 1982 when the Tax Equity and Fiscal Responsibility Act was passed. It called for limits on the amount of money that could be paid for Medicare clients, but it used the old retrospective payment system. The situation escalated in 1983 when the trustees of the Medicare fund reported to Congress that, if no changes were made in the level of income or reimbursement, the fund would be depleted by 1987. This stark revelation forced the first major revision of Medicare since its inception. The Social Security Amendments of 1983 replaced the retrospective fee-for-service payment for hospital services with a prospective payment system (PPS). Under the PPS patients are diagnosed on admittance to the hospital, and their diagnosis is assigned to one or more of the 467 diagnostic related groups (DRGs) that have been developed. Payment is calculated using the client's DRG, age, treament procedure, discharge status, and sex. The DRG concept was developed by Yale University under a ten-year contract with the U.S. Health Care Financing Administration (HCFA), which is the section within the Department of Health and Human Services responsible for administering federal funding for health care. The purpose of the original research was to define case types, each of which could be expected to receive similar amounts of services from the hospital. The concept was implemented in New Jersey, where the 467 DRGs were tested. Federal implementation of the PPS using the DRGs started with the first accounting period after October 1, 1983, with full implementation by 1987 (Davis, 1984; Mitchell and Dibble, 1988; US DHHS, HCFA, 1983).

Changing Structures: Home Health Care

The PPS for the first time put hospitals at risk for costly procedures, as well as for the length of clients' hospital stays. To date, the costly high technology trend seems to have continued to advance, but the length of hospital stays has decreased. The average length of stay in 1982 was 7.6 days. By 1984 it had dropped to 6.7 days (Mitchell and Dibble, 1988). This has significantly raised the average acuity of clients who are still in the hospital, since they are being discharged when they still need nursing care, something that was less likely to occur 10 years ago. Hospital nurses have become more cost conscious, and they have been struggling to better define the actual costs of nursing care (Joel, 1984).

The impact on the role of the nurse in the community is possibly even greater. Clients are being sent home while they still need intravenous feedings, chemotherapy, and a variety of other procedures. Technical skills are needed to care for clients who still need acute care. The change was so sudden that the financial basis for the services has not been worked out, but the need for greater federal support has been acknowledged by the U.S. Health Care Financing Administration (Davis, 1987). Home health care is clearly emerging as a major nursing field with opportunities for nurses to develop innovative practices as case managers, direct care givers, and administrators.

The growing importance of home health care as a nursing specialty is well documented in the literature. This important trend calls for a reorientation of nursing education to emphasize the community as a work place with particular emphasis on home nursing (Coleman and Smith, 1984; Davis, 1987; Edwardson and O'Grady, 1988; Griffith, 1987; Harris, 1988; Kleffel, 1988; Lewis, 1987; Phillips and Cloonan, 1987; Smith, 1988). These trends and developments are described in Chapter 13, and the skills needed to function in the home health care field are described in Chapter 14.

OTHER CONTEMPORARY TRENDS

Nursing Shortage

Inevitably the inequity in nursing salaries was noticed by the public. Starting in 1985 enrollments in nursing schools started to decline. This decline was predicted and studied by the Cooperative Institutional Research Program (CIRP) of the American Council on Education. Each year CIRP surveys a sample of beginning students from approximately 550 colleges and universities. Included are questions about their intended majors. The number of freshmen choosing nursing started to decline in 1984. The talent pool for nursing had been drawn primarily from women, and women started selecting law, business, medicine, science, and engineering in patterns similar to those exhibited by men students (Green, 1987). By 1985 the predicted shortage of students was felt in all collegiate programs, but the shortfall was most marked in the baccalaureate programs. The American Association of Colleges of Nursing reported a 28% decline in enrollment in baccalaureate nursing programs from 1983 to 1988 (AACN, 1988).

With a total of approximately 2 million registered nurses, 1.6 million of whom are employed, that shortfall in enrollments should not yet be a significant figure (Secretary's Commission, 1988). However, hospitals and agencies nationally were reporting serious nursing shortages. In 1987 Otis Bowen, secretary of health and human services, appointed a commission to study the problem. After examining all available evidence, the commission concluded that there is a shortage of nurses but stated it was not caused by the enrollment declines in the schools. Instead, the demand for the services of registered nurses has increased. In addition to the factors already discussed in this chapter, the PPS for Medicare reimbursement and the shorter hospital stays have actually increased the market for registered nurses. Home health care and nursing homes are demanding more nurses, and the shortened hospital stays decrease the time needed to accomplish all essential services including client education and discharge planning (Secretary's Commission, 1988).

Budgets are tight, and hospitals are substituting registered nurses for a variety of other workers. This is because the registered nurse role is extremely versatile. Linda Aiken has written about this elastic use of nurses that becomes problematic when there is a shortage. She calls registered nursing the elastic profession. She notes that whenever salaries for registered nurses are low, those nurses are used in place of nursing aides and practical nurses. In addition, they can perform certain aspects of the roles of secretaries, laboratory technicians, pharmacists, physical therapists, physicians, and social workers. Consequently hospitals often substitute this one general all-purpose worker in place of hiring several specialized professionals. This pattern lessens when the relative salaries of registered nurses increase (Aiken, 1982, 1983; Aiken and Mullinex, 1987).

Following this reasoning, a shift in hospital employment practices should take place as salaries for registered nurses increase. That pattern can actually be seen now. The salary increase should be more substantial than in the past cycles because of the increased job market in home health care nursing. However, there might also be a narrowing of the nursing functions to focus more on complex nursing responsibilities. Not all nurses are happy about this possibility. Some prefer not to work with practical nurses and nursing aides, and they are willing to carry extra responsibility and do without a variety of other professionals. Unfortunately, reasonable salaries for registered nurses are linked to a more complex health care delivery team.

Hospital Reorganization

Besides discharging clients early and hiring more registered nurses, hospitals are responding to inflation and government efforts to curb costs with a variety of other efforts. Some are attempting to diversify their services to counter dwindling inpatient income. They are setting up home health care agencies or emphasizing the outpatient centers, even setting up units that have been dubbed by terms such as "surgicenter," where complex treatment procedures are performed and the client is then sent home. Diversifying in this fashion is called vertical integration (Freund and Mitchell, 1985). Other hospitals are dealing with their problems by horizontal integration. They are forming chains with other hospitals, or they are breaking one hospital into two corporations—one for profit and one not for profit. This type of corporate restructuring allows the hospital to reassign assets to different legal and taxable entities. The nonprofit arm does not have to pay taxes on the philanthropic contributions it receives or on the money it brings in for client care. It is also eligible to issue tax-exempt bonds. The profit arm of the corporation can attract much needed capital investors (Batchelor, 1985).

The investor-owned hospitals seem to be doing well in the current cost-cutting climate. The big growth spurt for corporations that manage hospitals for a profit started with the inflationary period after 1965. Investor-owned hospitals supply 11% of the hospital beds. Net revenues earned in 1981 by the five largest hospital management companies (Hospital Corporation of America, Humana, American Medical International, National Medical Enterprises, and Lifemark) were $5.48 billion. The investor-owned hospitals are making further gains in this cost-cutting climate because they are already aware of costs and have developed economical management systems (Mark, 1984).

Preferred Provider Organizations

The inflation in the cost of health care is also leading industry to take another look at health insurance costs. These costs were for a time ignored because of the tax advantage attached to them. Contributions to employee health plans were considered a legitimate business expense, so employers could count contributions to health plans against their tax bill, and contributions were not considered taxable income for employees. Consequently employees were often more pleased to get health care benefits than an increase in salary. However, at current cost levels health insurance is becoming a significant burden to American industry despite the tax advantage. Industries are therefore seeking out preferred provider organizations (PPOs). PPOs negotiate contracts to provide health care services at a discount to specified groups such as employees of one firm or the members of a pension fund (Rice and others, 1985). Early PPOs were set up by physicians, hospitals, or insurance companies; now the sponsorship also includes hospital chains (Gabel and others, 1986). PPOs will probably expand the role of nurse practitioners because they use alternative approaches to health care delivery to save money. They are expected to expand significantly, particularly if the tax system is changed to view health insurance that is provided by employers as taxable income (Bloch and Pupp, 1985).

Community Nursing Centers

For the past several years, bills to establish community nursing centers have been introduced in the Senate by Senator Daniel K. Inouye. He envisions nurse-managed centers that would provide preventive health care, health teaching, treatment for episodic illnesses, and assistance to clients with self-management of chronic illnesses. Clients needing secondary and tertiary care would be referred as needed. Although the nursing center bills seem to be gaining support in both houses of Congress, they have not been passed yet.

There is, however, evidence that the nursing center concept is growing in acceptance as nurse-managed primary health care centers are being started throughout the country. A clinic established by nursing faculty members at the University of Texas in Galveston, Texas, provides health assessment, immunizations, teaching, and referrals for children from poverty neighborhoods (Nugent and others, 1988). In Atlanta a team of two nurse practitioners runs a clinic for homeless people financed by the state. They see more than 5800 clients a year, treating them for skin problems, trauma, and respiratory problems while constantly teaching health. The two nurse practitioners find that many of their homeless clients desperately need referrals to mental health facilities (Pearson, 1988). A Buffalo clinic, sponsored by a Division of Nursing grant, employs both a nurse practitioner and a community health nurse. It operates in the city mission where homeless men and families are seen.

HEALTH CARE DELIVERY SYSTEMS IN OTHER COUNTRIES

To put the American health care delivery system in perspective, a brief description of systems in selected other industrialized countries is presented.

United Kingdom

The British are covered by the National Health Insurance program. It was legislated in steps, with workers being given limited coverage in 1880. Benefits were increased and the plan was extended in 1911 so that most of the blue-collar work force was covered for basic medical services. The National Health Insurance Act of 1948 came at a time when the Labour party was strong and the sentiment for social programs was supportive. Coverage was extended to all British residents with no individual fees for service (Sidel and Sidel, 1977).

The system includes three components. General practitioners work on a capitation basis giving primary care. These services cover 90% of illness. Hospital care by specialist physicians, nurses, and other members of the health care team are paid on a salary basis. Local health department nurses and other workers are also salaried. The health departments have traditionally focused their work on preventive care but have recently started adding a primary care component.

Probably the key element in the system is the panel physicians. Until recently they worked alone, but now about half are organized into group practices. Each client chooses or is assigned a panel physician, and the client enters the system through that physician who makes referrals to hospitals when they are needed. The average panel in Great Britain in 1975 was 2300 persons per physician, which meant a long work week and short client visits. There are significant differences between the high incomes of hospital specialists and those of local general practitioners (Roemer and Axelrod, 1977).

The system provides almost universal coverage, and it is well liked by the public. The panel physicians are less satisfied because of their heavy work schedule and relatively low salaries compared with those of specialists. Separation of the general practitioners from the specialists also lessens the intellectual stimulation provided by seeing seriously ill clients and working with colleagues who have advanced educations. Salaries of nurses and other health workers are low compared with American standards, with a much lower percentage of the gross national product being spent on health care than in the United States (Sidel and Sidel, 1977).

Recently the large American hospital chains, including Hospital Corporation of America, Humana, National Medical Enterprises, and American Medical International, have expanded into foreign markets. The conservative government of Margaret Thatcher has been particularly receptive to this growth in the United Kingdom, seeing it not only as a way to replace outdated hospitals but as private sector competition to the National Health Service (Berliner and Regan, 1987). Milton Roemer, who is a staunch supporter of national health insurance, wrote an editorial in the *American Journal of Public Health* indicating his distress with this development and arguing that it provides luxury health care to affluent Britains, hospital profits go to the United States, and public concern for needed improvements is being diverted, since the U.S. hospitals provide a separate alternative for the rich (Roemer, 1987).

Germany

The German health care delivery system was established by Prince Otto von Bismarck in 1883. It mandated that individuals join a sickness fund that contracted for the necessary care. There are now about 200 such funds operating in West Germany, covering about 87% of the population. Within the group, clients can choose their own general practitioners and are referred to specialists only when needed. Physicians are paid on a fee-for-service basis, with fee levels being negotiated by the sickness funds and the local association of physicians. Hospitals are run by local government, and their staffs are salaried. Surveys of those enrolled in sickness funds have indicated that 90% would remain if the funds were voluntary instead of compulsory.

Although satisfaction with the system is high, it is not without problems. To get reimbursement, physicians with few patients tend to require more visits per client than busy physicians. A 1966 study found that physicians who saw 2500 to 3000 clients per calendar quarter provided 5.06 services per person, whereas those seeing 1000 to 1500 clients provided 6.24 services per person, and those seeing fewer than 1000 clients provided 8.0 services per person. From this it would seem that at least some of those extra visits to practitioners with small client loads may have been motivated by a desire to keep up income or that physicians with large client loads saw clients too seldom. From the provider's point of view, the greatest complaint is the amount of paperwork required to obtain reimbursement. From the government point of view, the system is expensive to operate unless there is rigid fee control (Roemer, 1969).

Union of Soviet Socialist Republics

The Union of Soviet Socialist Republics (U.S.S.R.) nationalized health care in 1917 as a part of the Russian Revolution. A series of epidemics, a shortage of health workers, and the general disorganization related to both World War I and World War II slowed full implementation of the system. However, as the Soviet Union industrialized and grew more prosperous, funds were made available to train more health workers.

The health care delivery system is governmentally operated, centrally planned, and integrated into the overall planning of the economy. This integration allows use of the health care delivery system to serve other economic goals. For example, in line with the efforts to industrialize, workers have been made an important focus of the system. Occupational health and safety is well developed. Clinics and even hospitals are located at work sites so that health care is immediately available to workers. On the less positive side, this total integration of the health care delivery system and government has led to the charge that the mental health system is at times used as a political tool for restraining people who have unpopular ideas (Sidel and Sidel, 1977).

Health workers at all levels are salaried, and health care is free to the entire population. Most primary care is given in polyclinics or health centers. There is a strong emphasis in the Soviet Union on improving the health of mothers and infants, and some of the polyclinics specialize in these aspects of care.

Although in the immediate postrevolutionary period it was hoped that physicians would become just another group of workers instead of maintaining their prerevolutionary high status, the economic system is still hierarchic with physicians at the top. Women constitute 70% of the physicians in the Soviet Union, but there is stratification along sex lines within the profession with most women working in the polyclinics and hospitals, whereas men fill the administrative, university, and medical specialty slots (Sidel and Sidel, 1977).

Nurses, feldshers, and pharmacists constitute the three groups of middle medical workers. The hospital nurses are supervised by ward physicians rather than by head nurses as in the United States. This further emphasizes the power of physicians and results in the nurses serving the physicians instead of the clients (Sidel and Sidel, 1977). Feldshers are an interesting carryover from the barber-surgeons of an earlier era. In rural areas they often work independently as primary care doctors. In urban areas they are supervised by physicians. Soviet health care planners seem to be ambivalent about feldshers. At times, as during World War II, the work of feldshers is highly praised, but at other times there is talk of phasing out the occupation. At the bottom of the hierarchy of health workers are the orderlies, attendants, and ambulance drivers who have minimal formal education.

Despite the fact that the Soviet Union spends significantly less on health care than the United States, the system is one of the most popular government services in the U.S.S.R., and even the personnel shortages and other pressures of World War II did not lead to dissatisfaction. For example, the Harvard Russian Research Center interviewed Soviet émigrés shortly after the war and found a remarkably high level of satisfaction with the physician-client relationship. Those refugees who eventually settled in the United States felt that one of the few advantages the Soviet Union had over the United States was their health care delivery system (Glasser, 1970).

Canada

Comprehensive, government-administered health insurance plans were set up in all the Canadian provinces in the late 1960s. These plans provide basic hospital care, nursing services, and medical care. The system is financed by a combination of provincial and federal funds. The provincial plans were in place first, and federal assistance was added later. This means that policy decisions about the administration of the systems are at the provincial level, and there are variations in coverage of such items as prescribed drugs, dental service, and optical care. When federal aid was first legislated, support was on the basis of the amount spent by the province. As the plan matured, a per capita reimbursement plan was used to make the available funding more comparable from one province to another (Cultural, Public, and Information Programs Bureau, 1983).

Although a visitor to the British Isles is covered for basic health care, there is a three-month waiting period to establish eligibility in the Canadian provinces. A few people still buy private health insurance to cover such additional services as dental care, private duty nursing, and prescribed drugs, but economic survival is possible without extra insurance.

The registered nurse and the registered nursing assistant are the two types of nurses in Canada. There are also personnel who are trained on the job, including orderlies, nurses' aides, practical nurses, and psychiatric nurses. Most registered nurses are prepared in diploma programs. The Canadian Nurses Association has resolved to move the educational system for registered nurses to the baccalaureate level by the turn of the century. Despite the fact that none of the provincial nurse practice acts have yet been amended to make this a law, collegiate nursing education is expanding rapidly.

Nurse practitioner programs were established in the early 1970s in many of the provinces, and government commissions reported favorably on their accomplishments (Abu-Saad, 1979; Sackett and others, 1974). However, the movement has failed to expand significantly in the current decade. Instead, departments of family medicine were expanded to increase the number of physicians in the community.

Despite the broad coverage of national health insurance, Canadian nurses say the Canada Health Act could be significantly strengthened if nursing were made more visible and if more health-oriented, preventive services were covered in addition to physician-oriented illness care. Nurses are, however, just starting to become politically visible, so it will probably take time to achieve these goals (Dick, 1983; Warrington-Turke, 1983).

Sweden

The Swedish system is in many ways similar to the American system. Economically it is pluralistic with costs being borne by the state, employers, and consumers. It is an expensive system with a high percentage of the gross national product being spent on health care (Sidel and Sidel, 1977). Health care personnel are relatively plentiful. Physicians are divided as they are in Britain into an ambulatory group and hospital specialists (Glasser, 1970). The health care delivery system functions as an organic whole with local communities directing the day-to-day care, yet the services are well coordinated at the regional and national level without any sense of government domination (Abu-Saad, 1979).

Sweden has a particularly strong occupational health system with joint union-management safety committees functioning in the work place. Many members of the committees have finished a 40-hour course in worker health and safety. The local committees have the power to hire and fire the occupational health professionals, as well as the power to stop the production process if they perceive a hazard to the health of the workers. In an editorial in the *American Journal of Public Health,* Ray Elling compares this situation with the one in the United States: "In the United States workers are still struggling for the right to know and have not raised the right to refuse nor the right to stop hazardous production seriously" (Elling, 1988).

Before 1966 Swedish nursing education took place in three-year programs. It was then cut to five semesters, and a shorter practical nurse course was also developed. Advanced nursing education beyond the basic two and one half years is used to prepare educators, administrators, and specialists such as midwives and community health nurses. Community health nursing is particularly strong in Sweden. It is in fact the major focus of the primary health care delivery system (Abu-Saad, 1979). Clients come to the community health centers to see a variety of health team workers, but often it is for a nurse visit (Sidel and Sidel, 1977). Probably because of the greater use of nurses and the more rational organization of the health care delivery system, preventive health care is more common in Sweden and the poor are probably better cared for than anyplace else in the world. Because of these factors, including some of the similarities to the U.S. health care delivery system, as well as the differences, Sweden consistently has a low infant mortality rate.

Some experts believe that infant mortality rates are indeed a good index of the well-being of a society, as well as its health care delivery system. Table 9-1 lists the 1980 infant mortality rates from the lowest ones to the U.S. rate. As can be

TABLE 9-1 Infant Mortality in 1980 in Selected Countries (Death Rate per 1000 Live Births)

Country	Rate
Iceland	5.4
Sweden	6.7
Japan	7.4
Finland	7.7
Switzerland	8.5
Netherlands	8.7
Denmark	8.8
Norway	8.8
Fiji	9.9
France	10.0
Canada	10.9
Australia	11.0
Spain	11.1
Ireland	11.2
Luxembourg	11.5
Singapore	11.7
Lichtenstein	11.8
England, Scotland, and Wales	11.8
United States	12.6

noted in the table, although the United States spends the highest percentage of gross national product and the most dollars on health care, the infant mortality rate is some distance from the optimum level when compared with the other industrialized countries. All of the countries described in this review fared better with the exception of the U.S.S.R., which has a more socialized, less well-financed, and much less sophisticated health care delivery system. The infant mortality rate in the U.S.S.R. was 27.2 per 1000 live births in 1980 (United Nations, 1981).

SUMMARY

Although the American health care delivery system is expensive, it is not so well thought out or so well coordinated as many. It makes less effective use of nurses than do the systems of some other countries, and it distributes resources unequally, placing an emphasis on the highly specialized tertiary care services such as organ transplants rather than the application of the knowledge that is at hand to prevent illness. There is less concern for the poor. Thus the infant mortality rate in United States in 1985 fell to 10.6 per 1000 live births but the rate for white infants was 9.3, whereas the rate for black infants was 18.2. When income alone is used as a variable, the figures are comparable. The high death rates for disadvantaged babies pulls down the overall American statistics (US Bureau of Census, 1988).

After long years of political struggles the first national health insurance programs were passed in 1965. The Medicare program finances health care for the elderly, and Medicaid provides care for disabled persons and welfare recipients. Implementation of these programs in 1966 marked the beginning of an inflationary period in health care. In addition to the two federal programs, this inflation was also caused by the increases in the numbers of hospital beds, increases in health care personnel, the treatment orientation of the system, the growth of high technology, demographic factors, and the increases in malpractice litigation.

The current era is marked by efforts to control health care costs. The PPS for Medicare is the first major step in this direction. It has shortened hospital stays and stimulated a growth in the home health care industry. It is probably also contributing to a growing shortage of nurses, although other factors are also involved in this development. Other current trends in health care delivery include the growth of PPOs and the development of community nursing centers.

When it is compared with other health care delivery systems the American system is good but not outstanding. It is expensive and sophisticated, but there are important gaps in its coverage including the poor and minority populations.

QUESTIONS FOR DISCUSSION

1. Explain why the costs of health care have escalated rapidly over the past three decades.
2. What is the difference between a diagnostic related group and a prospective payment system, and what is the function of each?
3. Describe three major trends taking place in the health delivery system.
4. Compare the health care systems of three different countries with those in the United States, and indicate the advantages and disadvantages of each.

REFERENCES

Abu-Saad H: Nursing: a world view, St Louis, 1979, CV Mosby Co.

Aiken L: The nurse labor market, Health Affairs 1:30, 1982.

Aiken LH: Nursing's future: public policies, private actions, Am J Nurs 83:1440, 1983.

Aiken LH and Mullinix CF: The nursing shortage: myth or reality, N Engl J Med 317:641, 1987.

American Association of Colleges of Nursing: Nursing shortage fact sheet, Washington, DC, 1988, The Association.

American Nurses' Association: Facts about nursing 84-85, Kansas City, Mo, 1985, The Association.

Barnes CD: A case study. In Bullough B, editor: The law and the expanding nursing role, ed 2, New York, 1980, Appleton & Lange.

Batchelor GJ: Corporate restructuring of nonprofit, tax-exempt hospitals, Nurs Econ 3:201, 1985.

Berliner HS and Regan C: Multinational operations of US for-profit chains: trends and implications, Am J Public Health 77:1280, 1987.

Blendon RJ: Health policy choices for the 1990s, Iss Sci Technol 2:65, 1986.

Bloch H and Pupp R: Supply, demand and rising health care costs, Nurs Econ 3:119, 1985.

Bodenheimer T, Cummings S, and Harding E: Capitalizing on illness: the health insurance industry. In Navarro V, editor: Health and medical care in the US: a critical analysis, Farmingdale, NY, 1977, Baywood Publishing Co.

Bullough B: Nurse practitioners: the new victims of the malpractice crisis, J Pediatr Health Care 1:331, 1987.

Bullough VL and Bullough B: Health care for other Americans, New York, 1982, Appleton & Lange.

Coleman JR and Smith DS: DRGs and the growth of home health care, Nurs Econ 2:391, 1984.

Corning PA: The evolution of Medicare: from idea to law, Research Report, No 29, Washington, DC, 1969, US Government Printing Office.

Cultural, Public, and Information Programs Bureau, Department of External Affairs: Canada: health and welfare, Reference Series 18, Ottawa, 1983, Department of External Affairs.

Davis C: Home care and its financial support: future directions and present policies. In Lewis EP, editor: Home health care: issues, trends and strategies. Report of a conference, July 8-10, 1987, Washington, DC, 1987, US Department of Health and Human Services, Health Resources and Service Administration, No HRP-0907168.

Davis CK: The federal role in changing health care financing. I. National programs and health financing problems, Nurs Econ 1:10, 1983.

Davis CK: The status of reimbursement policy and future projections. In Williams CA, editor: Nursing research and policy formation: the case of prospective payment. Papers of the 1983 scientific sessions, Kansas City, Mo, 1984, American Academy of Nursing.

Davis EJ: Home care—what's needed, Public Health Nurs 4:82, 1987.

Dick D: What's happening: getting our act together, Can Nurse 79:50, 1983.

Edwardson SR and O'Grady BV: The impact of prospective payment systems on nursing care in community settings. In Impact of DRG's on nursing: report of the Midwest Alliance in Nursing, Washington, DC, 1988, Department of Health and Human Services, Health Resources and Services Administration, Division of Nursing, HRSA 87-336(P).

Elling RH: Workers' health and safety (WHS) in cross-national perspective, Am J Public Health 78:769, 1988.

Freund CM and Mitchell J: Multi-institutional systems: the new arrangement, Nurs Econ 3:24, 1985.

Gabel J and others: The emergence and future of PPOs, J Health Polit Policy and Law 11:305, 1986.

Glasser WA: Paying the doctor: systems of remuneration and their effects, Baltimore, 1970, The Johns Hopkins University Press.

Graduate Medical Education National Advisory Committee: Summary Report, vols 1-7, HRA Publication No 81-651-657, Washington, DC, 1980, HRA Publications.

Green KC: The educational "pipeline" in nursing, J Prof Nurs July/Aug 3:247, 1987.

Griffith EI: The changing face of home health care, Public Health Nurs 4:1, 1987.

Harris MD: The impact of DRGs on nursing care in community settings. In Impact of DRG's on nursing: report of the Mid-Atlantic Regional Nursing Association, Washington, DC, 1988, Department of Health and Human Services, Health Resources and Services Administration, Division of Nursing, HRSA 87-339(P).

Joel LA: DRGs and RIMs: implications for nursing, Nurs Outlook 32:42, 1984.

Kalisch BJ and Kalisch PA: Politics of nursing, Philadelphia, 1982, JB Lippincott Co.

Kleffel D: The impact of hospital DRGs on nursing care in community health settings. In Impact of DRG's on nursing: report of the Western Institute of Nursing, Washington, DC, 1988, Department of Health and Human Services, Health Resources and Services Administration, Division of Nursing, HRSA 87-338(P).

League of Women Voters of New York State: The health care puzzle in New York State, New York, 1985, The League.

Lewis EP: Home health care: issues, trends and strategies, Washington, DC, 1987, US Department of Health and Human Services, Health Resources Administration, No HRP-0907168.

Mark BA: Investor-owned and nonprofit hospitals: a comparison, Nurs Econ 2:240, 1984.

Marmor TR, Wittman DA, and Heagy TC: The politics of medical inflation. In Marmor TR, editor: Political analysis and American medical care, Cambridge, Mass, 1983, Cambridge University Press.

McNutt DR: GMENAC: its manpower forecasting framework, Am J Public Health 71:1116, 1981.

Meyers AR: "Lumping it:" the hidden denominator of the medical malpractice crisis, Am J Public Health 77:1544, 1987.

Mitchell M and Dibble S: Acute care nursing: impact of DRGs. In Impact of the DRGs on nursing: report of the Western Institute of Nursing, Washington, DC, 1988, Department of Health and Human Services, Health Resources and Service Administration, Division of Nursing, HRSA 87-338(P).

Nugent KE and others: A model for providing health maintenance and promotion to children from low-income, ethnically diverse backgrounds, J Pediatr Health Care 2:175, 1988.

Pearson L: Profiles: providing health care to the homeless—another important role for NPs, Nurse Pract 13:38, 1988.

Phillips EK and Cloonan PA: DRG ripple effects on community health nursing, Public Health Nurs 4:84, 1987.

Reinhardt U: Physician productivity and demand for health manpower, Cambridge, Mass, 1975, Ballinger Publishing Co.

Remick H: Dilemmas of implementation: the case of nursing. In Remick R, editor: Comparable worth and wage discrimination: technical possibilities and political realities, Philadelphia, 1984, Temple University Press.

Rice T and others: The state of PPOs: results from a national survey, Health Aff 4:25, 1985.

Roemer MI: The organization of medical care under Social Security, Geneva, 1969, General International Labour Office.

Roemer MI: Foreign privatization of national health systems, Am J Public Health 77:1271, 1987.

Roemer MI and Axelrod SJA: A national health system and Social Security, Am J Public Health 67:462, 1977.

Rubenfeld MG and others: The nurse training act: yesterday, today, and . . ., Am J Nurs 81:1202, 1981.

Russel LB: Inflation and the federal role in health. In McKinlay JB, editor: Politics and health care: Milbank Reader 6, Cambridge, Mass, 1981, MIT Press.

Sackett DL and others: The Burlington randomized trial of the nurse practitioner, Ann Intern Med 80:1137, 1974.

Secretary's Commission on Nursing: Interim Report, Washington, DC, 1988, US Government Printing Office.

Shortell SM: The organization of health care. In Lee PR, Estes CL, and Ramsay N, editors: The nation's health, ed 2, San Francisco, 1984, Boyd & Fraser.

Sidel VW and Sidel R: A healthy state: an international perspective on the crisis in United States medical care, New York, 1977, Pantheon Books.

Smith JB: The impact of DRGs on nursing care in community settings. In Impact of DRGs on nursing: report of the Southern Regional Education Board, Washington, DC, 1988, Department of Health and Human Services, Health Resources and Services Administration, Division of Nursing, HRSA 87-337(P).

United Nations, Department of International Economic and Social Affairs: 1981 Statistical Yearbook, New York, 1983, United Nations.

US Bureau of the Census: Statistical abstract of the United States, 1988, ed 108, Washington DC, 1988, US Government Printing Office.

US Department of Health and Human Services, Health Care Financing Administration: 1983. HCFA background paper: technical facts on Medicare prospective payment system for hospitals, Washington, DC, 1983, US Government Printing Office.

US Department of Health and Human Services: Report on nursing: fifth report to the President and Congress on the status of health personnel in the United States, Washington, DC, 1986, US Department of Health and Human Services, NTIS Accession No. HRP-0906804.

Warrington-Turke K: The evolution of accountability in nursing in Canada, Can Nurs 79:34, 1983.

Whitney F: 1983. The GMENAC report: an opportunity for nursing. In Bullough B, Bullough V, and Soukup MC, editors: Nursing issues and nursing strategies for the eighties, New York, 1983, Springer Publishing Co.

Wing KR: Public health and the law: recent amendments to the Medicaid program; political implications, Am J Public Health 74:83, 1984.

BIBLIOGRAPHY

American Nurses' Association: Facts about nursing 82-83, Kansas City, Mo, 1983, The Association.

O'Grady BV: The practice of home health care: trends, issues, strategies. In Lewis EP, editor: Home health care: issues, trends and strategies. Report of a conference, July 8-10, 1987, Washington, DC, 1987, US Department of Health and Human Services, Health Resources and Service Administration, No HRP-0807168.

Roemer MI: An introduction to the US health care system, New York, 1982, Springer Publishing Co.

US Department of Health and Human Services, Health Care Financing Administration: Health Care Financing Rev 6:3, 1984.

CHAPTER

10

Social Change and Politics

Stephen Pendleton

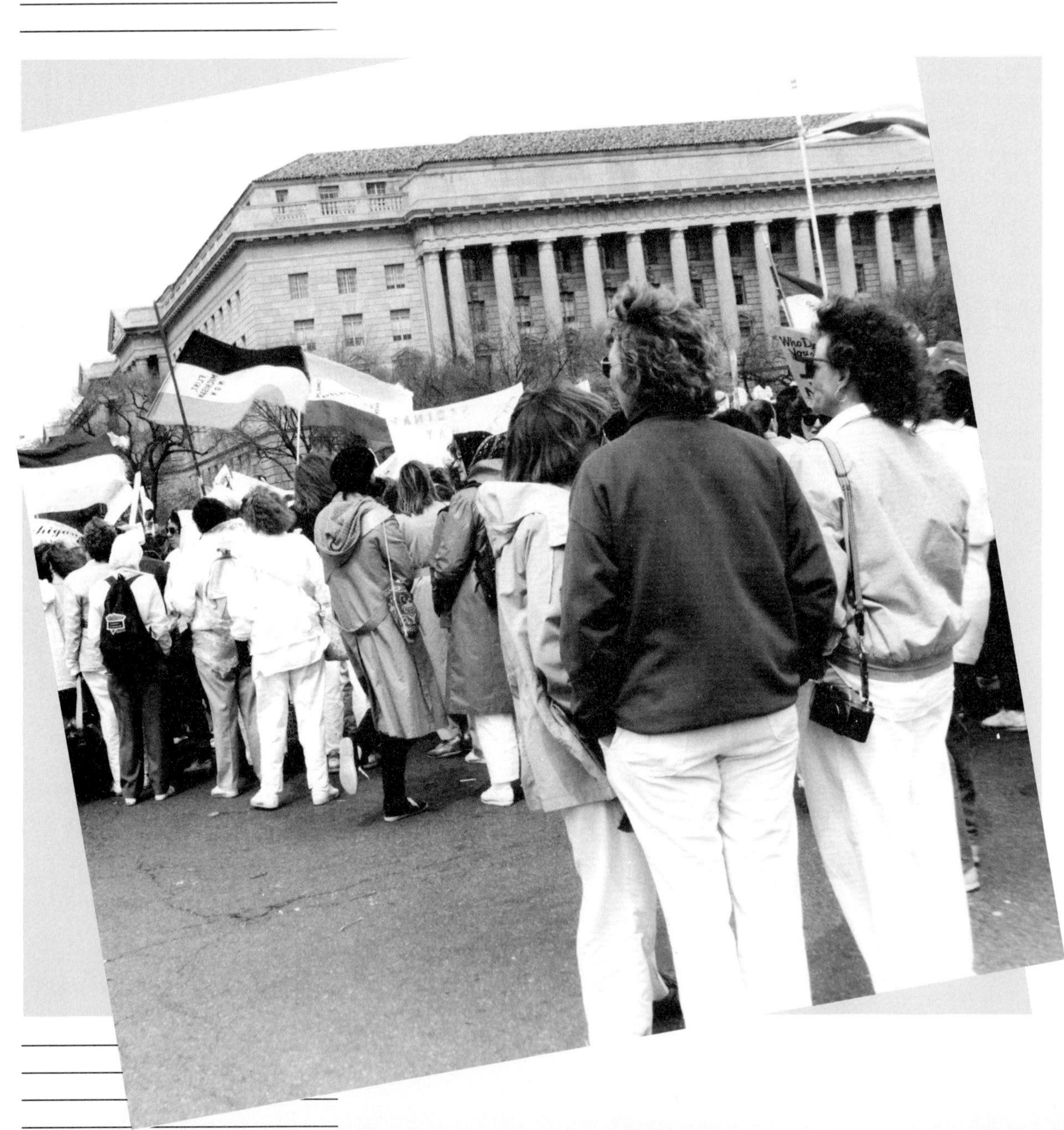

CHAPTER OUTLINE

OBJECTIVES

After completing this chapter, the reader should be able to:

1. Describe what is meant by social change.
2. Identify at least four theories of social change.
3. Distinguish between a task function and the socioemotional function of a group.
4. Explain the use of exchange theory and psychoanalytic theory in explaining the interaction of group members.
5. Illustrate why some legislators are effective in getting a bill introduced and passed.
6. Use Kurt Lewin's theory of driving and restraining forces to plan a political action.

NURSES IN THE COMMUNITY are often called to serve as change agents. The health and welfare of a community is dependent not only on nurses' giving advice and information to clients, but also on their trying to bring about change. This includes changes in client behavior that might cause problems and the elimination of conditions in the community that are harmful to client health and welfare. Sometimes the nurse can bring about change in the behavior of individuals simply by pointing out the consequences of their behavior, but usually some sort of group reinforcement or agitation is necessary. Alcoholism is a good example of this, since no matter what a nurse might say, few alcoholics can quit drinking without their families and group support.

In many cases the nurse must take a more active role and not only identify problems or refer clients, but also organize community groups and shape the policy agendas of community decision makers. This is particularly true when trying to deal with the problems of pollutants and toxins discussed in Chapter 6, but the same generalization applies to numerous other areas of community health nursing. Some nurses, such as Lillian Wald, who founded the Henry Street Settlement, and Margaret Sanger, who led the campaign for more effective contraceptives, were extremely effective in bringing about changes. Most nurses, however, lack the ability and skills of these two leaders, as well as the opportunities they had, but nurses can become more effective in the nursing role. That is the purpose of this chapter.

Essential to bringing change is some understanding of what social change is all about. For the purposes of this chapter social change can be defined as "change over time in one or more of three dimensions—social organization, culture or technology" (Stokes, 1984).

Each dimension impinges on the others, and all are interrelated. A good example is the industrial revolution of the last part of the eighteenth and first part of the nineteenth centuries in which changes in the means of production brought about by technology led to concentration of industry in urban areas and gave rise to a new social class with different values than its predecessor. By the end of the nineteenth century, western Europe and the United States had shifted from rural, agrarian areas to urbanized, industrial societies, and Western culture itself was transformed. An example of the change in the nature of the care of the sick brought about in the last part of the nineteenth century is the emergence of modern nursing and the expansion of the hospital care that it permitted. Similarly the current deinstitutional movement is changing both the role of nursing and that of the hospital.

SOCIAL CHANGE THEORIES

The why and how of social transformation have been the subject of heated debate for more than a century, with various competing groups trying to develop a theory to explain change. Some theories, such as those associated with Karl Marx, have led to mass movements designed to beget change. Other theories seemed to have had little acceptance. Four theories still seem to have many advocates, although some of them make adaptations of their own to these grand theories of social change. This chapter, however, is not the place to examine all the nuances of these theories but rather a place to discuss some of them in general terms to better understand the processes involved in social change.

Evolutionary Theory

One social change theory is based on Charles Darwin's theory of evolution. Darwin argued that species altered through natural selection; that is, accidental changes in instinctual behavior or physical capacity enable a species or part of a species to adapt and survive better. This biologic explanation was then applied to human society, and the result was what is known as social Darwinism. The key advocate of this theory of change emphasizing survival of the fittest was the nineteenth century philosopher, Herbert Spencer. He maintained that societal development was promoted through competition among humans, with the fittest individuals winning wealth, status, and power, and their offspring being most likely to survive (Stokes, 1984).

Spencer argued that this evolutionary process of social change was best left free from government interference, since government intrusion into social processes would have unintended consequences that ultimately might affect a society's ability to survive (Coser, 1971). This view today is best expressed by the Libertarian movement, which wants to exclude government from most areas of human activity and allow the greatest freedom possible for the fittest to develop. The evolutionary view is also supported by some political conservatives, although each group modifies Spencer's ideas (and Darwin's) to meet its own ideology.

Functionalist Theories

Functionalists see society as a set of interrelated, reinforcing subsystems such as the family, the economic system, the political system, and cultural subgroups. Some aspects of the theory are influential in the study of the family (see Chapter 12). Each of these systems serves a function in maintaining social order. The leading advocate of such ideas was the twentieth century American sociologist Talcott Parsons. He held that the natural condition of a society (or a social system) was an equilibrium or balance among the interdependent subsystems (Parsons, 1957). This means that a change in any part of a social system could generate changes in other parts causing an imbalance until the system managed to establish a new equilibrium. Inevitably, according to this system, subsystems are likely to change only incrementally along with the whole social system.

Critics of functionalism argue that the theory fails to account adequately for changes, since its main concerns are for stability and balance, and thus functionalism easily becomes a rationalization for the status quo. Whether this is completely true is debatable, but functionalist theories have often become a justification for a conservative view of social change in which any alteration in a social subsystem is somehow portrayed as a threat to the stability of the social system.

Conflict Theory

Conflict theorists believe that society is composed of competing groups struggling over the distribution of power, goods, and status. Social change is a product of this conflict, as some groups prevail and some are defeated, although occasionally stalemates occur (Denisoff and Wahrman, 1983). Karl Marx is the best-known conflict theorist. In simple terms, Marx believed that the struggle of social classes for political and economic dominance provided the pressure that changed society gradually and that social classes in turn evolved from the organization and control of production.

Marx maintained that society changed as classes struggled with one another over economic and political control, as well as cultural values. New classes would emerge from this and result in a change in the base of society and a concomitant change in its superstructure. Marx used as an example the challenge of the rising bourgeoisie, or middle class, to the old nobility and the subsequent and ultimate challenge of the proletariat to the bourgeoisie.

Many variations have been made in Marx's theory of conflict and social change, and many of them are associated with the community or countries that base their ideologies on Marx. Some theorists in the conflict school, however, have argued that conflict is ubiquitous in human society. All societies produce authority structures that divide power unevenly among their members, making conflict inevitable. This is Ralf Dahrendorf's theory. Coser has a slightly different explanation (Coser, 1971), as do others (Stokes, 1984). Conflict theory has also been used to study the family.

Driving and Restraining Forces

The social change theory used by Kurt Lewin focuses on driving and restraining forces. It is derived from a more social psychologic perspective than the previous theories discussed, and perhaps for this reason nurses have found it particularly attractive. Lewin conceptualized the behavior of people in groups as a dynamic balance between driving and restraining forces with change occurring when the equilibrium between the two forces breaks down. In this sense Lewin's theory incorporates some of the functionalist theory, as well as some of the conflict theory. What looks like a stable situation is an equilibrium brought about by a balance between opposing forces; driving and restraining forces create a balance (Lewin, 1958). It is illustrated in Fig. 10-1. Social change occurs when one of the restraining forces weakens or disappears, or when the driving forces are strengthened.

This short discussion of theories should make it clear that social change is not easy, but when it does take place, it affects many sections of society, bringing about what has popularly been called future shock (Toffler, 1970). This is particularly true in the health field where the technologic innovations and scientific breakthroughs that have prolonged life have left the Western world with an aging population for which society has not yet developed effective coping strategies. New technologies have also created conflict and brought about alienation by making many health care job skills valueless. In the process the nature of the roles of community health and home health care nurses has changed.

This leaves the nurse with the basic problem of whether to tinker with the system to help individuals adjust or agitate enough so that the system will make changes. Regardless of the path, and there are many in-between steps, most of the change is done in and through groups, since groups shape social life and individual behavior in a variety of ways. Groups are also more powerful than an individual in bringing about change.

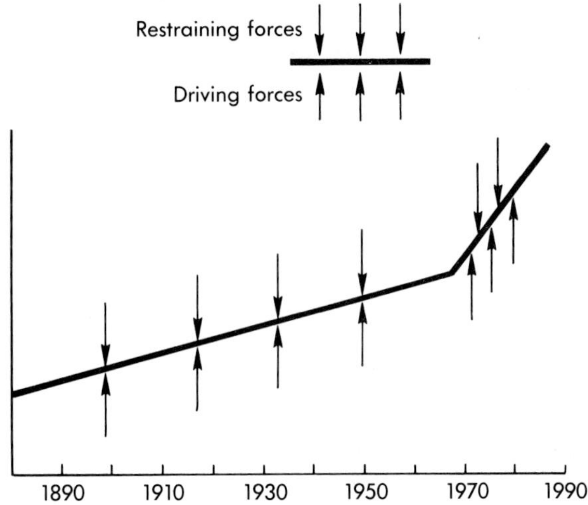

FIG. 10-1. Graph of changes in scope and function of nursing role during past 100 years as visualized using Lewin's theory.

Importance of Groups

The nineteenth century German social scientist, Georg Simmel (1858-1918), contended that human beings create their reality through the process of interaction with one another. Language, culture, and institutions, as well as the way the physical world is perceived, are all products of social interaction of individuals, or sociation (Coser, 1971).

Social interaction, or sociation, involves individuals communicating with one another and shaping one another's behavior and perception. To be a group, according to Simmel and others, members must share several attributes. Groups usually have a distinctive set of social relationships among the members, interdependence among group members, a feeling that the behavior of one member is relevant to other members, and a sense of membership, or a "we" feeling (Hess and others, 1985). Groups can range from family units to work groups to health care teams to students in a nursing class. Some theorists divide them into primary groups and secondary groups. Primary groups are small units where members have close, warm, intimate, and personal ties with one another and share goals and a common world view. This is different from secondary groups, which have fewer emotional ties among members and less intimate interaction that involves only certain aspects of the participants' lives (Coser, 1971).

Group activities in turn can be divided into at least two divisions—those that might be called *task functions* and those that are classified as *socioemotional functions.* Task function refers to what is called the oriented dimension, the purpose for which the group exists, whereas socioemotional functions refer to the interpersonal, social, and psychologic dimensions of the group, that is, the ways groups serve the social needs of their collective members and the psychologic needs of individual members.

An example could be a childbirth preparation group set up to train prospective parents in birthing techniques and prenatal care. While doing this group members build the confidence of the parents through participation and provide each of them with emotional support and the benefits of shared experiences. Such groups frequently take on a life of their own, and many childbirth preparation group members continue to meet and exchange ideas long after they have delivered the child for whom they attended the group. In this case the socioemotional functions of the group held individuals together after their task-oriented function was completed. Groups that maintain high cohesion tend to perform their task functions most effectively, and cohesion itself is a product of the socioemotional attachments of its members. Peer counseling groups, for example, are planned to make good use of the socioemotional ties that can accompany the task orientation in a small group.

Norms

The cohesion of a group and its ability to perform task functions are both shaped by the norms that evolve within the group. Group norms are the "shared standards for behavior, attitudes and perception that characterize all kinds of groups" (Sampson and Marthas, 1981). Norms can promote task functions by placing a high value on group accomplishment, and they can encourage behavior that serves socioemotional functions, thereby helping to maintain the group. Sometimes these two group functions can conflict as can the norms that promote them.

Norms also promote what has been called the social reality function (Sampson and Marthas, 1981). The assignment of such a task to a group assumes that the processes regarding what to define as factual and how to interpret such data are inherently social in nature (Baskin and Aronoff, 1980.) Group norms shape the processes whereby facts are defined and the possible meanings are interpreted, since it is clear that individuals often adjust what they see to fit what their groups have determined to exist (Steinbrunner, 1974).

Groups and group norms, in addition, structure the frame of reference used by members to develop meaning and interpretation in cases of great uncertainty. Groups are a valuable aid to individuals in reducing the uncertainty that often attends individual perception. Groups also foster resistance to interpretations or facts that do not fit the established consensus of the group, and in this case groupthink can lead to resistance to innovation. Groupthink occurs when members of a group so greatly value consensus that facts and interpretations that undermine consensus beliefs are ignored, suppressed, or denigrated (Janis, 1982). Groupthink is especially likely in highly cohesive groups, groups that might be the most efficient in accomplishing task functions if not the most effective. Groupthink is also likely when those who disagree are expelled. Groupthink is characteristic of dogmatic and rigid groups, but almost any group can fall prey to it, since most of us want to belong enough that we do not threaten our social groups.

Helping explain the interaction of group members is also a favorite focus for theory, and two of these, psychoanalytic theory and exchange theory, are often used in nursing. Sigmund Freud is the source of the psychoanalytic approach. He pointed out that when people interact, they do so on two levels, one conscious, explicit, and open to public view, the other unconscious, implicit, and hidden from public view. This is sometimes called the hidden agenda. Human interaction involves multiple meanings and intentions occurring on multiple levels, and the hidden agenda is often unrelated to the overt issue at hand. It is possible for groups to consider matters rationally and make rational decisions, but psychoanalytic theory suggests the intrusion of private, often unconscious, concerns into social interaction (Sampson and Marthas, 1981).

Exchange theory contends that individuals interact with one another to seek satisfaction. Interaction becomes a mutual exchange of actions that each participant finds more or less satisfying. If an interaction does not lead to adequate satisfaction, individuals often reduce their group activity or withdraw altogether. People tend to participate in interactions when what they receive is equal to or greater than what they contributed (Stokes, 1984).

This listing of theories about social change and group dynamics can be much extended, since we have only touched the surface of some of the theories involved. Knowing some of the theories, nevertheless, should prove useful to nurses in assessing community health needs, as well as the capacity of community groups to address the needs. The nurses' involvement with groups can be for limited, specific goals, related to particular therapeutic needs such as the prevention of substance abuse and child or spouse abuse or mainstreaming the handicapped, with limited therapeutic goals. Alternatively nurses may seek public policy–related outputs from both formal and informal groups such as insurance companies, government agencies, and legislatures, all of which can be lobbied to bring about policy changes. Groups can draw public attention to health problems such as the failure of many private insurance plans to provide adequate coverage for cancer, Alzheimer's disease, or other chronic illness.

USE OF THEORY TO INFLUENCE PUBLIC POLICY

Whether organizing or participating in informal or formal therapy groups, nurses should be able to use their understanding of both group principles and social change to promote narrowly or broadly conceived health goals.

Since so much of what nurses do in the community is associated with government at the local, state, or national level, much of the change they want to bring about involves a political process. Yet nurses as a group are somewhat innocent about politics. To be effective, however, nurses must know how to lobby effectively for what they want; and this includes involving other groups to bring about social change.

As a general rule lobbying for something is best done at the lowest level possible, since this is where the individual or small group can bring the greatest pressure. For most nursing causes this means the local level rather than the state or national level. If lobbying does move to the Congress and state legislatures, it is important to understand how these bodies function. They do most of their work through committees. Bills go first to committees where they are referred to subcommittees that may kill them or refer them back to the full committee with or without changes. The process through which a bill becomes law is shown in Fig. 10-2.

This means that to get a bill introduced, the

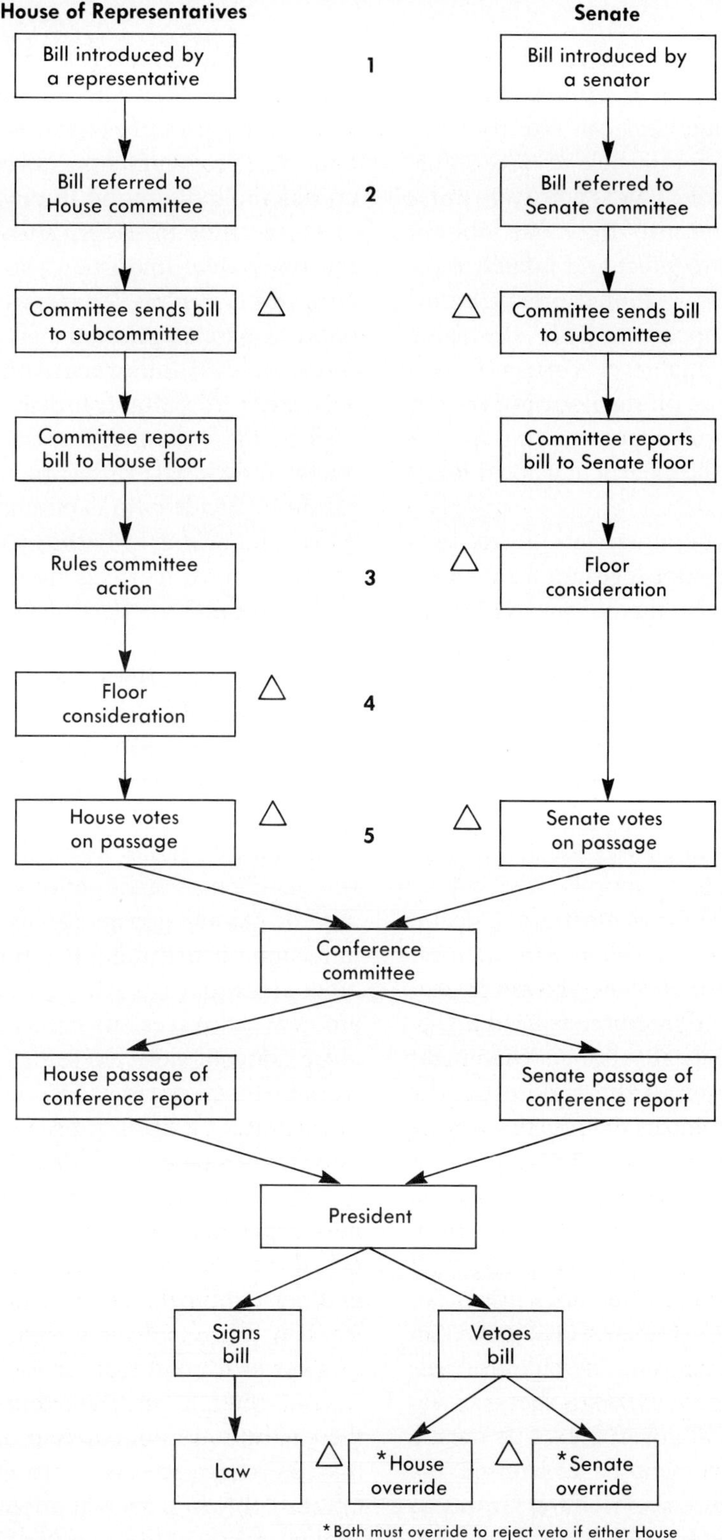

FIG. 10-2. Possible path a bill can take to become a law. Triangles indicate points where nurses (or others) can lobby a bill. President can also be lobbied.

proper committee chair or member must be contacted. The legislator from a group's area may not be on the committee that can effect change or may not have enough influence to have someone else introduce the bill. This is why state nurse organizations are important—the nurse lobbyist in the state capital can contact and influence the correct committee chair. National organizations are also extremely important, since the same thing is true at the national level. Once a bill has cleared committee and is on the floor for vote, it is important for the local or regional nurses' association to influence their particular local legislator.

As a general rule, federal legislation preempts state legislation just as state legislation preempts local legislation. Until the time of the New Deal under President Franklin D. Roosevelt (1933-1945), the federal government deferred to state governments in many policy areas on the assumption of "reserve powers"; that is, there were some areas of power that were reserved only for state governments. These reserve powers included police powers, as well as powers needed to provide for the health, safety, morals, and convenience of the citizens. This left most of the health care issues in the hands of either state or local governments. Since the mid-1930s, however, federal courts (the ultimate interpreters of the U.S. Constitution) have largely abandoned what might be called dual federalism, or the notion that the federal and state governments operate in separate distinct spheres, and the federal government today is involved in a wide range of state and local policies. States, however, are still banned from exercising exclusive federal powers.

This growth of federal power does not mean that state and local governments lack power in areas of concern to nurses, since much of the federal intervention has been through the granting of federal funds to local governments. It is here that the federal government has exercised the greatest control on health and welfare. Grants to state and local governments can be broken down into two large classifications—categoric grants that allocate money for specific programs and block grants that allocate funds for relatively broad categories of programs conducted by local and state governments. Local officials exercise considerable discretion in block grant programs.

At one time in American history, party organizations were important. Political parties built power by extending services to voters and through political patronage, or the giving of jobs or contracts to loyal followers. Although some of this still exists, the establishment of the civil service system, the widespread use of primaries, which allows individuals rather than the party organization to decide who is nominated for a political office, and particularly the increasing importance of media have lessened the power of the party organization. The effect of this has been to make many, if not most, contemporary candidates for office political entrepreneurs, that is, they set up their own campaign, raise their own campaign funds, and although they have a party affiliation, they rely less on party organization than their own organizations.

Since local candidates need and want groups to vote for them, campaign for them, and give them money, nursing groups can exercise considerable influence on a candidate's policy if they know how. This is particularly true with candidates who are new office seekers. Influencing incumbents is more difficult, since the same factors that tend to weaken party organization strengthen the value of incumbency, if only because name identification remains a key to getting elected. It is the need for name identification through radio, television, newspaper, and direct mail advertising that has raised the cost of campaigning and made it more and more difficult for challengers to succeed unless they can get adequate financial backing or the support of a number of special interest groups.

Even though most nursing organizations by their nature are nonpartisan, they must indicate that they have something to give to be effective in their lobbying. Several nonpartisan groups, including some of the more political nursing organizations, do endorsements for candidates from one or more parties who meet their criteria of being effective advocates of nursing legislation. Some groups, however, cannot endorse because by their nature they are educational and nonprofit. This is where individual nurses must come into play.

Since nurses are often divided in their opinions between various political philosophies, it is important that they become active in the campaigns of those candidates they agree with and support. This means giving money if possible, volunteering to do precinct work, or carrying out some of the other mundane tasks that must be done. When the active nursing lobbyist then goes to elected officials and asks for their support on a key nursing vote, the visibility of politically active nurses demonstrates that there is a constituency concerned about the way political decision makers act.

Organized groups must also pass resolutions, involve other groups in their lobbying efforts, and educate the public about what they want. The more allied groups that support their cause, the more successful nursing lobbies are.

Nurses, however, must be aware that they are not regarded by most legislators or government officials as disinterested parties. In fact, on the national scene, and to a lesser extent on the state scene, the so-called health lobby can be divided into two broad categories—groups for providers of health care and public interest groups. Health care providers' groups comprise health care professionals and institutions, including physicians, nurses, pharmacists, dentists, public health workers, as well as hospitals, nursing homes, and even medical supply manufacturers and pharmaceutical houses. Public interest groups include two different types of organizations—consumer groups and intergovernmental groups. Consumer groups attempt to represent the general interests of health service consumers, and these groups include organized labor, American Association of Retired Persons, Consumers Union, and similar groups. Intergovernmental groups include state and local officials, since governors, mayors, county officials, and legislators lobby the federal government not only for funds but also to influence social policy.

Public interest groups focus chiefly on representing the health policy interest of the general public. Intergovernmental groups are concerned with fiscal and general policy issues of state and local governments and sometimes claim that they also represent the public interest. Consumer groups organize health service users to monitor legislative and implementation activities.

The provider groups have a more complicated image. They are perceived as representing the special interests of the providers, since they seek policies that enhance the ability of health professionals and institutions to control health care delivery. Although provider groups work to secure the allocation of greater resources for providers, they often disagree among themselves how this should be done. In this situation, nursing can be particularly effective if it can win some of the so-called public interest groups to its own viewpoint.

Some of the success of special interest groups was summarized earlier in this book. Evidence of this is the increase in federal funds for health care. Between 1955 and 1983, health care expenditures increased their share of the gross national product (GNP) from 4.4% to 10.8%, and many expect that even with heroic efforts to hold costs in check, the U.S. government may ultimately spend 15% of GNP on health care (Mechanic, 1986). The great increase in resource allocation to health care owes much to the combination of forces behind the health care lobby, although in retrospect it seems that the major benefits of the system have gone to physicians represented by the American Medical Association (AMA) and hospitals represented by the American Hospital Association (AHA), primarily because of the preservation of the fee-for-service system. This is changing too, however, and it is to the credit of both the American Nurses Association (ANA) and the American Public Health Association (APHA) that they have somewhat different lobbying reputations from the AMA or the AHA.

The ANA and APHA have had their greatest influence on general public interest health issues. The APHA has concentrated its attention on general community health interests because it is a coalition of groups whose primary focus is public health, and it has usually been able to count on the ANA for support. Legislative and executive branch decision makers consider APHA to be an authoritative voice on public health concerns such as disease control, water supply, sanitation, and research priorities. The ANA has had its greatest influence on general health legislation.

Given this background on the national picture, it seems clear that the ANA is most effective as a part of a coalition. It also implies that nurses must organize. This emphasizes the importance of joining the ANA or the APHA or more specialized groups, since it seems clear that interests that are unorganized or poorly organized can have little effect on decision makers, regardless of the level of government at which they try to operate.

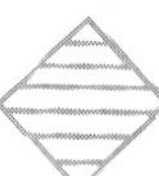

ANALYZING A POLITICAL ACTION TASK

1. What is the political change you want to make? (A new law, or changed regulations)
2. What is the target for political action? (The legislature, a board, or an administrator)
3. List the organizations, power blocks, or persons that fall into each of the following categories:

DRIVING FORCES	NEUTRAL FORCES	RESTRAINING FORCES

4. How can the restraining forces be neutralized?
5. How can the neutral forces be converted to driving forces?
6. How can the driving forces be supported and mobilized? (Coalition building, teaching, and rallying)

SIX-STEP POLITICAL PROCESS

Given an organization the actual political process can be carried out using a step-by-step plan. Here the various theories of social change help guide the process, but in actual lobbying, the social change theory of Kurt Lewin described earlier seems particularly helpful. The organization that is trying to achieve change in a specific area analyzes the positive, or driving, forces, the negative, or restraining, forces, and the neutral forces related to the issue. An example of this process is shown in the boxed material.

Carrying Out the Process

1. The right of nurse practitioners to prescribe drugs is the desired political change used as an example.

2. This change requires approval by the state legislature, so in this case the state government offices are the target of the lobby. Although sometimes it is possible to get the governor to request such changes from the legislature, or a group such as the state board of nurses might have power to issue such regulations on their own, in most states it requires lobbying the legislature to achieve a change in the law.

3. Writing prescriptions, however, is a change for which nurses require allies. Who are these allies? Perhaps nurses could gain support of organized groups of senior citizens on the grounds that giving nurses the right to prescribe drugs would give better and less expensive service to senior citizens. Nurses might also get some support from drug companies, organized labor, or other public interest groups. Those who would not support the change should be encouraged to remain neutral. Pharmacists might not support the change, but they may be willing to remain neutral if they are contacted and consulted. Probably leading the opposition would be the AMA.

4. How can the restraining forces be neutralized? Physicians might become less hostile and more neutral if compromises or limitations can

be negotiated. For example, the number or variety of drugs to be prescribed could be limited to specific categories. We know that most physicians rely on 20 or 30 drugs in their practice, and although the specified drugs should not be named, since the drug industry keeps changing and new drugs appear on the market, classes of drugs could be listed and periodically updated. Physician hostility might be further lessened if the board of nursing worked in conjunction with the board of medicine to periodically issue new lists of drugs.

5. Converting the neutral forces to driving forces is also important. Pharmacists are usually regarded as neutral forces on this issue; however, since pharmacists are eager to extend their own scope of practice, nurses might agree to support pharmacists' efforts in turn for support. Women's groups can be moved from neutral to driving forces if the issue can be shown to involve women's health care, better child care, or other issues with which women as a group are concerned.

6. The last step is the key—namely, the mobilizing of friends and allies to lobby for change. This involves effective publicity of the cause, rallying of support through parties or even demonstrations, and educating of the public and the legislators of the factors involved. If the restraining forces can be lessened and the driving forces can be increased, the nature of the political equilibrium that holds the forces in check will change, and ultimately some change will come about.

Change, however, does not come without demand for change and organized effort to bring it about. Nurses potentially have the power to bring about change in their work place, in the community, in their state, and even in the country if they can pull together and bring out their allies.

SUMMARY

A development that gradually alters the social organization, culture, or technology of a society or group is called social change. This process can be examined from a variety of theoretic vantage points including evolutionary theory, functionalist theory, conflict theories, and Lewin's format, which analyzes social change in terms of the driving and restraining forces that either speed or hinder change. The latter approach can be used to suggest ways to influence the political process. An understanding of group process and group norms can also facilitate effective political participation.

QUESTIONS FOR DISCUSSION

1. What is social change theory? Give three examples.
2. How does a knowledge of theory help nurses influence public policy?
3. Why are groups important in any theory of social change?
4. Take an example of a change you want to see achieved, and illustrate how you would proceed using the six-step political process.

REFERENCES

Baskin W and Aronoff CE: Interpersonal communication in organizations, Santa Monica, Calif, 1980, Goodyear.

Coser L: Masters of sociological thought, New York, 1971, Harcourt Brace Jovanovich Inc.

Denisoff RS and Wahrman R: Introduction to sociology, New York, 1983, Macmillan Publishing Co.

Hess BB and others: Sociology, ed 2, New York, 1985, Macmillan Publishing Co.

Janis I: Group think, ed 2, Boston, 1982, Houghton Mifflin Co.

Lewin K: Group decisions and social change. In Maccoby E, Newcomb T, and Hartley EL, editors: Readings in social psychology, New York, 1958, Holt, Rinehart & Winston Inc.

Mechanic D: From advocacy to allocation: the evolving American health care system, New York, 1986, Free Press.

Parsons T: The social system, Glencoe, Ill, 1957, Free Press.

Sampson EE and Marthas M: Group process for the health professions, ed 2, New York, 1981, John Wiley & Sons Inc.

Stokes R: Introduction to sociology, Dubuque, Iowa, 1984, Wm C Brown Group.

Toffler A: Future shock, New York, 1970, Random House Inc.

BIBLIOGRAPHY

Alinsky SD: Rules for radicals, New York, 1981, Random House Inc.

Benne KD and Birnbaum M: Principles of changing. In Bennis WG, Benne D, and Chinn R, editors: The planning of change, ed 2, New York, 1979, Holt, Rinehart & Winston Inc.

Bottomore T, editor: A dictionary of Marxist thought, Cambridge, Mass, 1983, Harvard University Press.

Bullough B, editor: The law and the expanding nursing role, ed 2, New York, 1980, Appleton & Lange.

Bullough V and Bullough B: History trends and politics, Norwalk, Conn, 1984, Appleton & Lange.

Cobb R and Elder C: Participation in American politics: the dynamics of agenda-building, Boston, 1972, Allyn & Bacon Inc.

Cox F and others: Strategies of community organizations, Itasca, Ill, 1979, FE Peacock.

Dolbeare KM: American public policy: a citizen's guide, New York, 1982, McGraw-Hill Inc.

Hrebenar RJ and Scott RK: Interest group politics in America, Englewood Cliffs, NJ, 1982, Prentice Hall.

Jones CO: An introduction to the study of public policy, ed 3, Monterey, Calif, 1984, Brooks/Cole Publishing Co.

Kingdon JW: Agendas, alternatives, and public policies, Boston, 1984, Little, Brown & Co Inc.

O'Connor J: The first crisis of the state, New York, 1973, St Martin's Press Inc.

Salisbury RH: An exchange theory of interest groups, Midwest J Political Science 13:1, 1969.

Sorauf FJ: Party politics in America, ed 2, Boston, 1972, Little, Brown & Co Inc.

Steinbrunner JD: The cybernetic theory of decision, Princeton, NJ, 1974, Princeton University Press.

Waitzkin H: A Marxist view of medicine. In McNall S, editor: Political economy: a critique of American society, Glenview, Ill, 1981, Scott, Foresman & Co.

Withorn A: Serving the people: social services and social change, New York, 1984, Columbia University Press.

Wolfe A: America's impasse: the rise and fall of the politics of growth, New York, 1981, Pantheon.

APPENDIX

NURSES' COALITION FOR LEGISLATIVE ACTION

American Academy of Nurse Practitioners
179 Princeton Boulevard
Lowell, MA 01851

American Assembly for Men in Nursing
c/o College of Nursing
Rush University
600 South Paulina, 474-H
Chicago, IL 60612

American Association of Colleges of Nursing
Suite 530, One Dupont Circle
Washington, DC 20036

American Association of Critical Care Nurses
One Civic Plaza
Newport Beach, CA 92660

American Association of Neuroscience Nurses
22 South Washington Street, Suite 203
Park Ridge, IL 60068

American Association of Nurse Anesthetists
216 Higgins Road
Park Ridge, IL 60068

American Association of Occupational Health Nurses, Inc.
3500 Piedmont Road, NE
Atlanta, GA 30305

American College of Nurse-Midwives
Suite 1120, 1522 K Street, NW
Washington, DC 20005

American Holistic Nurses' Association
P.O. Box 116
Telluride, CO 81435

American Nephrology Nurses' Association
North Woodbury Road, Box 56
Pitman, NJ 08071

American Nurses' Association
2420 Pershing Road
Kansas City, MO 64108

American Nurses' Association (Washington Office)
1101 14th Street, Suite 200
Washington, DC 20005

American Organization of Nurse Executives
840 North Lake Shore Drive
Chicago, IL 60611

American Public Health Association/Public Health Nursing Section
1015 15th Street, NW
Washington, DC 20005

American Society of Nursing Service Administrators
840 North Lake Shore Drive
Chicago, IL 60611

American Society of Ophthalmic Registered Nurses, Inc.
P.O. Box 3030
San Francisco, CA 94119

American Society of Plastic and Reconstructive Surgical Nurses, Inc.
North Woodbury Road, Box 56
Pitman, NJ 08071

American Society of Post-Anesthesia Nurses
2315 Westwood Avenue
Suite 1, P.O. Box 11083
Richmond, VA 23230

American Urological Association, Allied
6845 Lake Shore Drive
P.O. Box 9397
Raytown, MO 64133

Association for Practitioners in Infection Control
505 East Hawley Street
Mundelein, IL 60060

Association of Operating Room Nurses
10170 East Mississippi Avenue
Denver, CO 80231

Association of Rehabilitation Nurses
2506 Gross Point Road
Evanston, IL 60201

Dermatology Nurses Association
North Woodbury Road, Box 56
Pitman, NJ 08071

Emergency Nurses Association
666 North Lake Shore Drive, Suite 1131
Chicago, IL 60611

International Association for Enterostomal Therapy, Inc.
5000 Birch, P.O. Box 2690-175
Newport Beach, CA 9266-

Nurses' Association of the American College of Obstetrics and Gynecology
600 Maryland Avenue SW, Suite 200 East
Washington, DC 20024

National Association of Neonatal Nurses
35 Maria Drive, Suite 855
Petaluma, CA 94952

National Association of Orthopaedic Nurses, Inc.
North Woodbury Road, Box 56
Pitman, NJ 08071

National Association of Pediatric Nurse Associates and Practitioners
1000 Maplewood Drive, Suite 104
Maple Shade, NJ 08052

National Association of School Nurses, Inc.
P.O. Box 1300
Lamplighter Lane
Scarborough, ME 04074

National Black Nurses Association, Inc.
P.O. Box 18358
Boston, MA 02118

National Flight Nurses Association
Allegheny General Hospital
320 East North Avenue
Pittsburgh, PA 15212

National Intravenous Therapy Association
87 Blanchard Road
Cambridge, MA 02138

National League for Nursing
10 Columbus Circle
New York, NY 10019

National Nurses Society on Addictions
2506 Gross Point Road
Evanston, IL 60201

National Organization of Nurse Practitioner Faculties
Star Route, Box 150M
Corrales, NM 87048

Nurse Consultants Association, Inc.
P.O. Box 25875
Colorado Springs, CO 80936

Oncology Nursing Society
3111 Banksville Road
Pittsburgh, PA 15216

Society of Gastrointestinal Assistants, Inc.
1070 Sibley Tower
Rochester, NY 14604

The Washington Tripartite Group—a coalition of American Association of Colleges of Nursing, American Nurses' Association, and National League for Nursing—can be reached at the address of each individual group.

IN the hospital and other institutional settings the nursing process is applied to the individual client. In the community the unit of concern may still be the individual, but it is often the family or the whole community. When the focus is broadened in this way, the five-step nursing process is still used but there are some other differences in the nursing role.

When the overall community is the unit of concern, the assessment step is significant. The community assessment process requires the nurse to take into account such variables as age, sex, income level, type of occupations, educational level, and ethnic makeup of the population. Building on this foundation is an examination of the structure of the community including both official and unofficial sources of power, the types of groups that exist in the community (informal as well as formal), and the health history of the community. After gathering data on all these measures, the nurse can make a nursing diagnosis or draw up a problem list, setting priorities for planning intervention strategies. As in bedside nursing, after the planning and nursing intervention have taken place, it is necessary to evaluate the effectiveness of the measures that were taken. Unlike bedside client care, however, community health rarely cures the ills of the community, nor does the community die, but new problems emerge that require repetition of the process.

A knowledge of the theories of family structure and function, family interaction, and family development and an appreciation of the impact of the sociocultural variables on the family facilitates the nursing process when it is applied to the family. The nurse can then give guidance to and support the family, as well as individual family members.

Community background and family setting, however, are important not only to those nurses who go on to specialize in a community nursing area, but also to nurses who specialize in other areas. The client in a hospital setting is not just a person with an illness, but one who is part of a family of some kind and who comes from a particular segment of the community. Thus the content offered in this community nursing text represents another part of the circle of knowledge that is essential for all of nursing.

UNIT IV

The Client

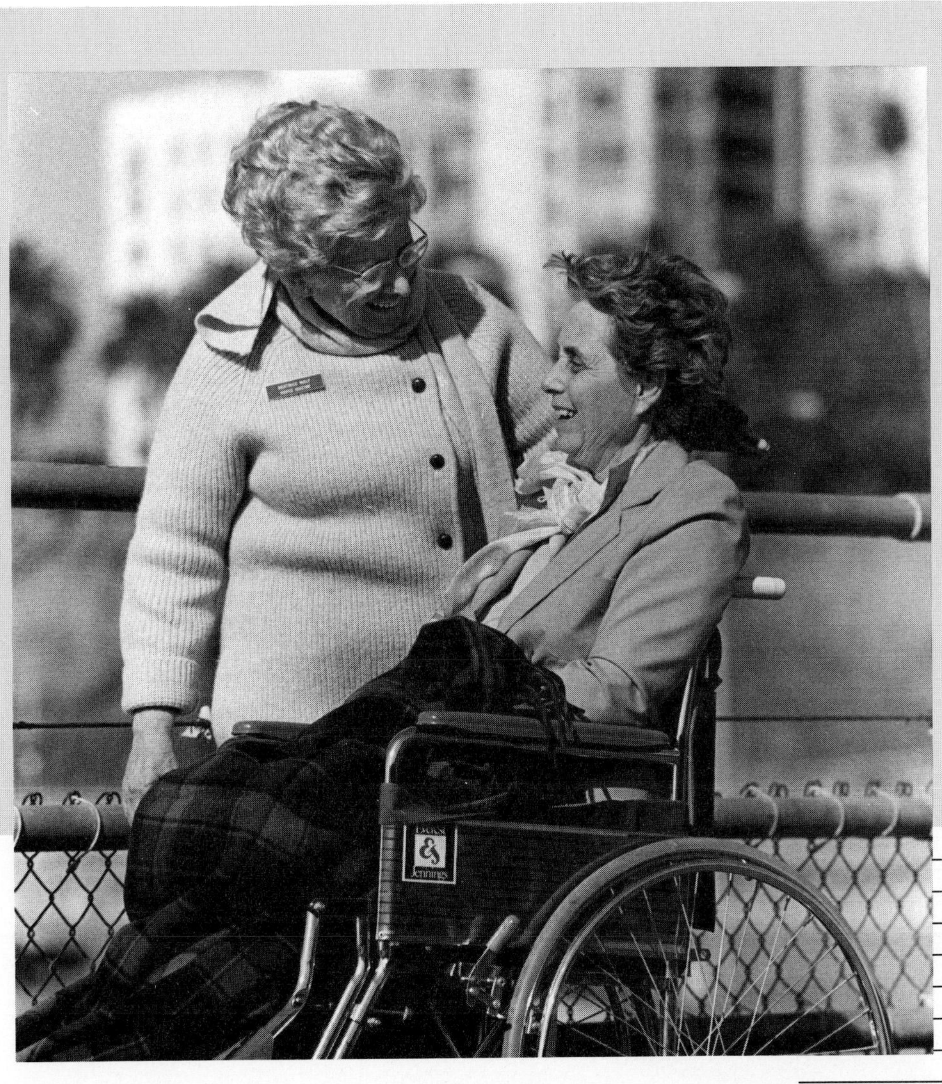

CHAPTER 11

Community as a Client

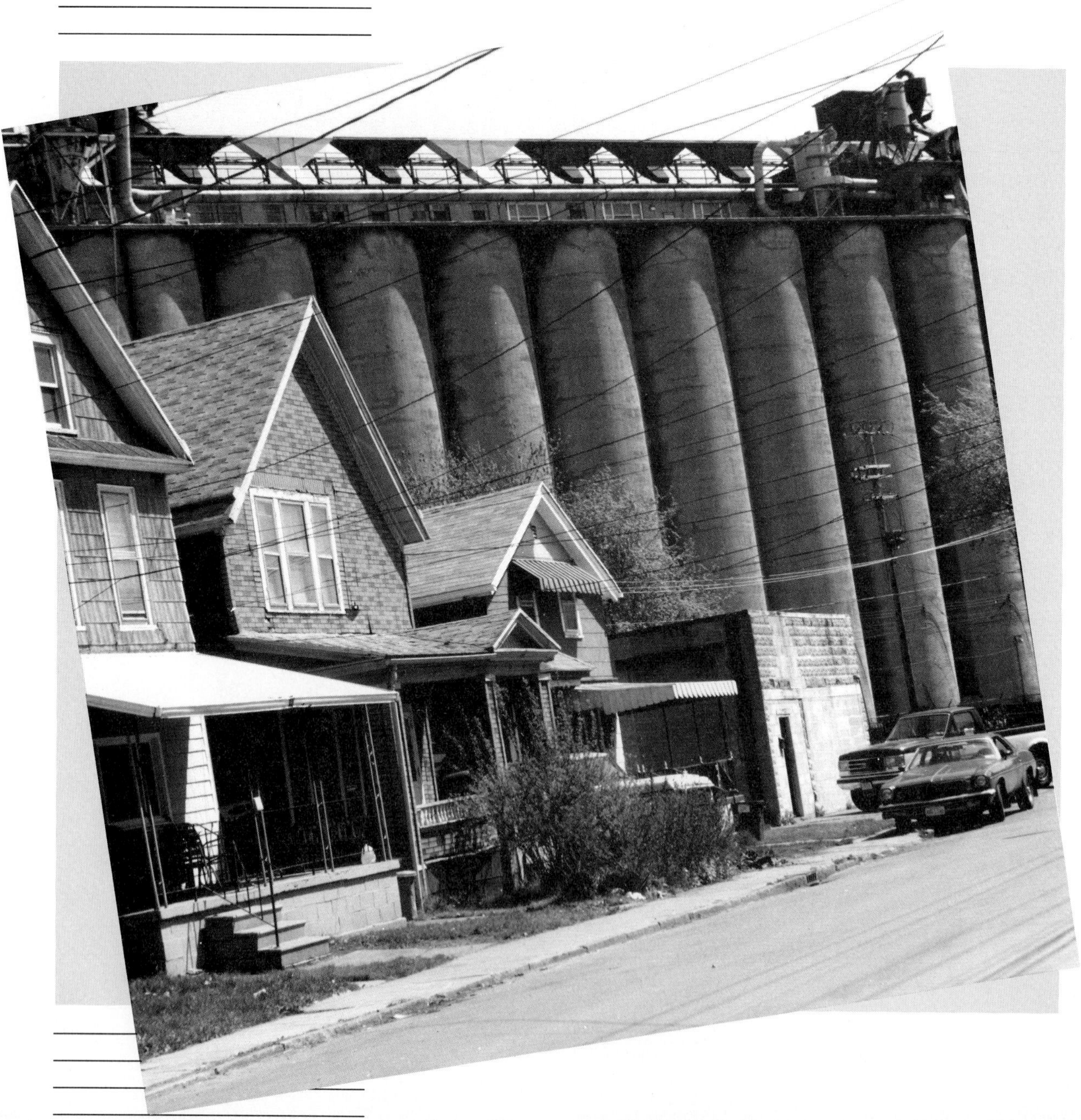

CHAPTER OUTLINE

Community Assessment
- Step 1: Define the community
- Step 2: Describe the people
- Step 3: Identify structures that organize the community
- Step 4: Identify health risk factors
- Step 5: Identify resources for dealing with risk factors

Community nursing diagnosis

Planning

Implementation

Evaluation

Case study 1: Community nursing process in the city
- Community assessment
- Community nursing diagnoses
- Planning and implementation
- Evaluation

Case study 2: Community nursing process in a student health center
- Community assessment
- Community nursing diagnosis
- Planning
- Implementation
- Evaluation

Summary

OBJECTIVES

After completing this chapter, the reader should be able to:

1. List the steps involved in a community assessment.
2. Understand the concept of the community nursing diagnosis and differentiate it from the nursing diagnosis of an individual client.
3. Describe the planning and implementation processes in the community.
4. Explain the difference between process and outcome evaluation procedures.
5. Apply the community nursing process in a variety of community settings.

A FOCUS ON the total community and its needs is probably the key attribute of community health nurses (ANA, 1985). To a certain extent this is also true of other community-based nurses, including those who give home health care, work in schools or industries, or provide primary health care services. The broader picture of health care is a heritage from the public health movement, which holds that health care policy should be based on the needs of the total population rather than the needs of a privileged few. Public health advocates argue that the first priority of society should be the prevention of broad-scale illness. For example, they hold that public money should be provided to immunize all children and carry out other broad-scale preventive measures rather than to finance expensive experiments with heart transplants for a few individuals.

At the community or institutional level, where most nurses work, national priorities are important, if only because every community health nurse wants to see all children appropriately immunized. However, local needs are also important. A local epidemic of cocaine addiction or environmental hazards from chemical waste gain the attention of the local health team.

The nursing process is the vehicle that translates this viewpoint into an operational system. The integration of the public health point of view into a nursing process format can be seen in the description of the nursing role that was drawn up in 1980 by the nursing section of the American Public Health Association (see box). Since that time, the nursing process has been expanded to include an additional step, that of nursing diagnosis. The five-step community nursing process is outlined in this chapter.

> COMMUNITY HEALTH NURSING PRACTICE
>
> Community health nursing practice is a systematic process by which:
>
> 1. the health and health care needs of a population are assessed in collaboration with other disciplines in order to identify sub-populations (aggregates), families, and individuals at increased risk of illness;
> 2. a plan for intervention is developed to meet these needs, which includes resources available and those activities that contribute to health and its recovery, the prevention of illness, disability, and premature death;
> 3. a health care plan is implemented effectively, efficiently, and equitably; and
> 4. an evaluation is made to determine the extent to which these activities have an impact on the health status of the populations.
>
> The plan of action is based on and is consistent with (1) community needs and expectations, (2) agency purpose, philosophy and objectives, (3) available resources, (4) the scientific knowledge available, (5) accepted criteria and standards of nursing practice, and (6) the client's (community, group, family, and/or individual) participation, cooperation, and understanding. Any plan of action must consider other services and organizations in the community and coordinate planning in order to make maximum use of these resources.

From American Public Health Association: The definition and role of public health nursing in the delivery of health care, Washington, DC, 1980, The Association.

COMMUNITY ASSESSMENT

Community assessment is a key element in the nursing process at this level when the community is thought of as the client. The goal is to identify groups of people who are at increased risk for illness, disability, or premature death and to find resources that can be used to cope with the risk factors or needs for service that are identified (Higgs and Gustafson, 1985; Shamansky and Pesznecker, 1981). The assessment is easier if the nurse comes to the task with a generalized knowledge of the field of community health and an understanding of epidemiologic research methods. This knowledge can be gained not only from reading texts, but also from the periodical literature in the field. The knowledge base sensitizes the observer to possible risk factors and possible resources. For example, nurses who are employed

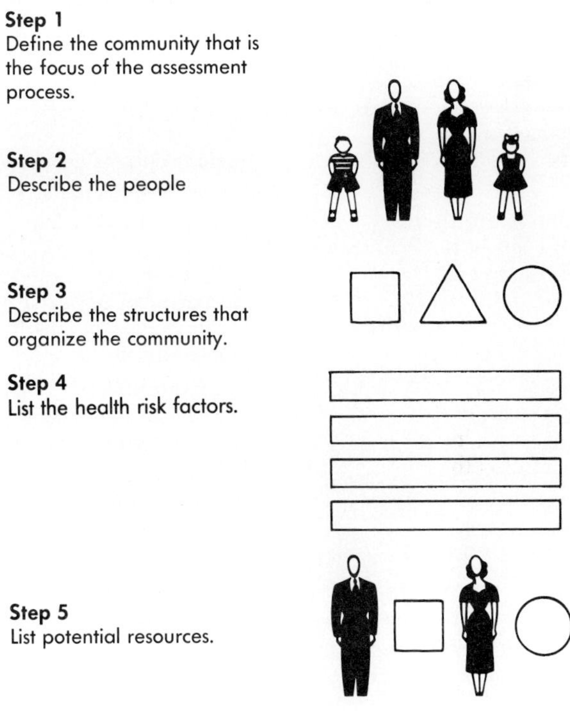

FIG. 11-1. Community assessment process.

in industrial plants should have a knowledge of the major hazards that are common to their industries. This alerts them to possible risk factors such as injuries from machines or chemicals, or high stress levels from noise, repetitive work, or high expectations for performance. If the community being studied has a high rate of unemployment, a knowledge of the stresses related to both unemployment and poverty is important. As the assessment process is carried out, the generalized knowledge base can be augmented by returning to the literature to learn more about the risk factors that emerge from the analysis. The community assessment process is shown in Fig. 11-1.

Step 1: Define the Community

The first step in the assessment process is to define what is being called a community. Community has many meanings. For example, it can refer to a city (Cleveland or Palmdale), a section of a city (the Near North Side of Chicago), a work force (asbestos workers), or a student body in a single school. All of these aggregates of people share characteristics that could make them a community, even though some of them do not share a contiguous living space. A nurse could be employed to manage the health problems of any of these communities, which makes them all appropriate units of concern (Muecke, 1984). However, the assessment model requires that nurses agree on a definition of the community parameters before other data are considered. Data are then gathered to describe the people in the community, the structures that organize the community, the major health care problems or risk factors present in the community, and the resources that can be used to deal with the problems. As much as possible the assessment should be done in a stepwise fashion because the first two elements (people and structures) provide clues to the last two elements (health risk factors and resources) (Cook, Baker, and Shamansky, 1984).

Step 2: Describe the People

Table 11-1 outlines the five categories of data that should be gathered about the people in the community—sex and age distribution, income levels, occupations, educational levels, and ethnic identities. Collectively these factors are called demographics. Demography is the study of populations, and these demographic elements help describe the population of the community.

The age and sex distribution of the community can be assessed using vital statistics, including birth and death records, institutional records, or census data. The U.S. census is done every 10 years, and census tracts are the local units used to cluster the data. In large cities a census tract includes several adjacent blocks, whereas a village or small town could be included in a single census tract. These units are usually small enough to reflect neighborhood characteristics. Census reports

TABLE 11-1 The People Community Assessment: Step 1

Categories of data related to people	Rationale for collecting data	Possible sources
Age and sex	Age and sex are variables in susceptibility to illness	Census data Senior citizens groups Observations
Income levels	Poverty is implicated in many health problems and serves as a deterrent to use of resources	Bureau of Labor Statistics Census data Department of Social Services Observations
Occupations	Work-related hazards Unemployment relates to poor health Type of work relates to income	City directory Bureau of Labor Statistics
Educational levels	Relates to income levels Low levels of education a barrier to use of resources	Census data Observations
Ethnic makeup of the community	Cultural patterns relate to acceptance of interventions Language can be a barrier to use of resources	Observations Question experts Census data

are available in major libraries in the government documents collection. If no library is at hand, reports can be ordered from the superintendent of documents in Washington, D.C., or they may be available in a city or county planning office (US Department of Commerce, 1980).

Using these data, it is possible to draw a population pyramid. This is a device for illustrating the age and sex distribution of an area. The pyramid is usually divided into five- or 10-year increments with males and females on either side. The term "pyramid" is used, since the largest concentration of persons is usually in the youngest age groups, and, as people die, the pyramid narrows. A broad-based pyramid suggests a large population of children. Fig. 11-2, *A* and *B* show two population pyramids. Fig. 11-2, *A* illustrates a central city population with a high concentration of children, a significant number of female heads of families, and a shortage of jobs for young men, many of whom have left the area. Fig. 11-2, *B* illustrates a suburban community that includes a senior citizen housing development. Notice the concentration of older women who have survived their male contemporaries. The first population pyramid offers clues to possible risk factors such as childhood diseases and teenage pregnancy, whereas the second suggests chronic diseases of the elderly and loneliness of widows who have survived their spouses.

The next three items in the assessment model (income, occupation, and education) are all elements in the social stratification system. The concept of stratification means the hierarchic ranking of people according to their wealth, power, or social class. Power is ordinarily defined as influence over or authority to make decisions for others. Wealth is usually defined and measured in terms of income, property, or other possessions. Social class refers to groups of people identified in terms of the other two major variables (wealth and power), as well as their prestige and

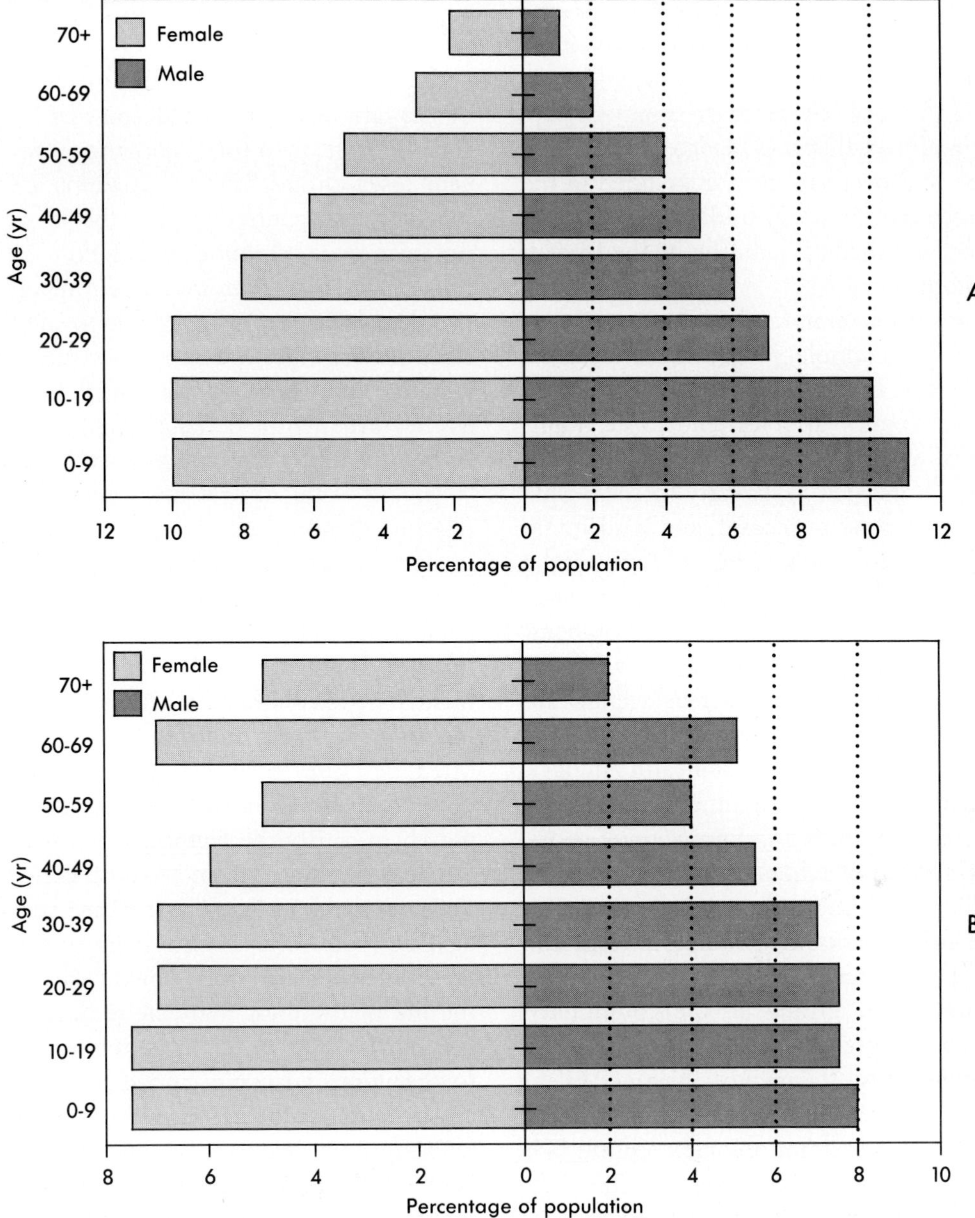

FIG. 11-2. Population pyramids. **A,** Central city census tract. **B,** Suburban census tract.

life-styles. Social class is currently measured by such indicators as reputation, occupation, education, and life-styles. Sometimes these demographic factors are linked, and the term "socioeconomic status" is used to describe them collectively (Bendix and Lipset, 1966; Lenski, 1955; McCord and McCord, 1977).

The three socioeconomic factors used in the community assessment model were selected because they are the variables most frequently used to assess socioeconomic status and because the data are often available from secondary sources. The telephone book, the city directory, and publications by the local chamber of commerce describe the major industries. Income and educational levels and occupations are included in the census report, and more up-to-date employment patterns are published periodically by the Bureau of Labor Statistics.

The three socioeconomic variables tend to intercorrelate. For example, low educational levels lead to poor jobs and low incomes. Moreover, all three socioeconomic variables tend to be implicated in health risk factors (Bullough and Bullough, 1982; Kane, 1985). Poverty forces people to economize on food purchases, and inadequate nutritional education leads people to leave out the nutrients that are important to good health. Poverty increases hazards in the living environment, such as lead paint and contamination with microorganisms, and crowding increases exposure to disease. Low education levels lead to lack of understanding of the dynamics of health and lack of sophistication with managing the health care delivery system. Laborers are exposed to more on-the-job hazards than white-collar workers. Because of the interrelationship of socioeconomic status and health risk factors, this part of the assessment is important.

The major ethnic groups in the community are identified because language may create communication barriers. If language barriers exist, cultural sensitivities would then need to be considered in plans for teaching and intervention (see Chapter 21).

If more demographic data are needed to supplement the data collected using secondary sources, the nurse can carry out an informal or formal study. The informal study can be carried out by walking through the community, talking to people, and observing clients. The formal study could use a survey design with interviews or questionnaires.

Step 3: Identify Structures That Organize the Community

Early theorists of urban life saw the central core of the city as disorganized and attributed many social problems to this disorganization. More recent research has found that slums are not particularly disorganized; rather the structures that organize poor neighborhoods tend to differ from those that organize more affluent neighborhoods (Suttles, 1968). It is important to identify those structures as clues to risk factors and as ideas for resources that can be used to deal with problems as they are identified. Table 11-2 lists categories of organizations that can be identified.

The government or official unit of power that has jurisdiction over the community should be identified. Often there is an overlap, with a city government being responsible for police and fire protection and hospitals and public health care services being provided by the county government. The telephone book is one source of information about these units, and the daily newspaper often describes their activities. If jurisdictional lines are unclear, a visit to the seat of government may help clarify the picture.

The community agents of social control include the police, the judicial system, the social service agencies, and the health department. Usually these agencies are more obvious participants in the life of the poor than the rich, and although they can be supportive, they often seem oppressive to the poor. To compound the problem, police and probation officers, social workers, and nurses who staff the agencies are usually middle-class people, so they have a different world view from their clients' (Bullough and Bullough, 1982). This creates barriers to communication and furthers feelings of oppression. The first step in dealing with these barriers is to know that they exist, and the second step is for the professional to try to understand the other world view. Again these agencies can be identified by using the telephone book or noting the buildings they occupy and

TABLE 11-2 The Community Structures Community Assessment: Step 2

Types of structures	Rationale for collecting the data	Possible sources
Type of government or management	Identify resources, power that can support or be a barrier	Visiting seat of government (City Hall) Administrative charts
Agents of social control	Resources, power, barriers	Telephone directory Asking people
Informal power structures	Power for change, barriers, communication links	Asking people Survey data
Voluntary structures	Resources and gaps in service	United Way listings Department of Social Services
Family structures	Resources and gaps in resources for unconnected people	Vital statistics Survey data Census data

observing their impact on the lives of the client population.

Identifying the informal power structure of a community is somewhat more difficult. At the upper end of the socioeconomic ladder, the informal power structure can be studied by listing the persons who are members of the boards of directors of the banks, the large businesses, and the voluntary organizations. Overlapping and clustering of power can be noted. Sometimes the powerful individuals are also formally clustered by membership in exclusive clubs, which until the 1988 Supreme Court decision excluded women and minorities. Members of this group are often the major informal, or backstage, decision makers about the allocation of community resources, with the more obvious government bodies making the formal, up-front decisions. At the other end of the socioeconomic spectrum, the power structure may include youth gangs or even a clustering of the customers of a neighborhood bar. The groups can be barriers or support groups for dealing with health risk factors, so an understanding of their role in the life of the community is important. However, keen observational skills are required to identify informal power structures.

The voluntary organizations in the community are more obvious. They include groups such as the Cerebral Palsy Association, the Red Cross, the Salvation Army, private health organizations, and the Boy Scouts or Girl Scouts. Usually these groups are linked by the United Way or the United Fund. They are important community resources. Churches are another important group of voluntary organizations that can be resources. Churches may also provide clues to the ethnic identity of people in the community.

Family structures are a crucial resource for dealing with client problems. Chapter 12 identifies the various family structures. The pattern of families may also provide clues to risk factors. For example, a community that includes many small nuclear families needs services for children.

Step 4: Identify Health Risk Factors

A list of the possible risk factors in the community can be made using vital statistics that show the leading causes of death, clinic records, and reports of communicable diseases (Ibrahim, 1985). Other risks can be derived from an understanding of the people in the community. These possible risk factors can be further defined using epidemiologic studies from the literature that provide information about the causal factors for disease. For example, if heart disease is a leading cause of death in the community, the Framingham epidemiologic study, which is described in Chapter 4, is useful because it identifies the risk factors for heart disease, including diets high in cholesterol, smoking, sedentary life-style, hypertension, and diabetes (Dawber, 1980). These factors then become community risk factors. Communicable diseases are particularly important in communities that include young children. If the workers in the community face specific environmental hazards, these should be listed.

Step 5: Identify Resources for Dealing with Risk Factors

Resources include the health department, churches, and other voluntary agencies. If social changes are needed to combat the risk factors, a knowledge of the workings of the community power structure and the communication patterns in the community is important.

COMMUNITY NURSING DIAGNOSIS

The community nursing diagnosis can be thought of as the last phase of the assessment process (Gebbie, 1982), although it also initiates the planning process. It integrates the concept of the nursing diagnosis, which is described in Chapter 3, with the epidemiologic research process, described in Chapter 4. The community nursing diagnosis is focused on the community instead of the individual (Muecke, 1984).

The nursing diagnostic process as it is described in Chapter 3 describes an actual or potential, acute or chronic health problem. It can be physiologic, psychologic, sociocultural, or spiritual. The nurse uses the diagnosis to summarize the data gathered in the assessment process.

The nursing diagnoses that have been outlined and accepted by the North American Nursing Diagnosis Association include three components—title, defining characteristics, and the etiologic and other related factors (Carpenito, 1983). A nursing diagnosis is different from a medical diagnosis or a client problem list because it narrows the acceptable diagnostic statements to those problems that fall under the purview of the nurse rather than the physician or other members of the health care team (Duncan, 1988). In the hospital setting the nursing diagnosis is sometimes shaped to complement the medical diagnosis so that the activities of the physician are supported and the client is monitored by the nurse.

The community nursing diagnosis has a different starting point. It uses the list of health risk factors and converts them to a nursing diagnosis. The nursing-medical boundary is less salient in the community, which has more overlapping roles than the hospital setting, but there is still need for the list to be narrowed to focus on the problems nurses need to address (Muecke, 1984). For example, poverty is a risk factor for disease, but it is not a nursing diagnosis because it is a problem society needs to focus on collectively. Nurses have no specialized duty in the realm of poverty; rather nurses share responsibilities with other citizens. This refining and winnowing narrows the risk factors to produce nursing diagnoses.

Sometimes a single diagnosis is used as a statement of priority, and the other risk factors are dealt with later. The process of settling on a single community diagnosis or a small group of priorities should be carried out in consultation with other members of the health care team so that responsibilities can be allocated collectively and expectations are shared among team members. The community nursing diagnosis emerges as a statement of priority for the planning process.

PLANNING

Planning involves the agency administrator, one or more nurses, and possibly other health care workers. The group process helps establish a consensus. The process includes a survey of the resources identified in the assessment phase, a discussion of the actual availability of the resources, and plans to gain access to them. If new activities and programs are to be launched, administrative support services need to be planned. At all times current technology should serve as a reality factor in planning. For example, if the AIDS epidemic was the focus of the planning, a broad-scale immunization plan is still premature. It is hoped that before this book is too old researchers will have developed a vaccine, but for now education to avoid exposure is a better plan.

IMPLEMENTATION

Implementation of the plan follows. If the plan is for a public information program, brochures could be designed and printed, media people would be consulted, and persons in the power structure would be contacted for support or at least to prevent them from becoming barriers. If a new service is to be established, funds need to be identified, and the health care team must have an organizational structure designed, equipment secured, protocols for service drafted, and the service provided. When the individualized services are provided, the goal is to implement the plan as identified in the community nursing diagnosis, but the day-to-day focus moves to the nursing process as it applies to the individual client.

EVALUATION

Evaluation is the process by which the impact of the program is assessed. Two kinds of measures can be used—those that look at processes and those that look at outcome. *Process measures* evaluate the program by counting the number of procedures that were carried out. For example, if the focus is on improving prenatal care, a process measure would be the number of prenatal clients seen before and after the program was under way. If the goal was to increase the number of persons vaccinated against rubella to decrease birth defects in the community, the process measure would be the number of people vaccinated. *Outcome measures* are the results of the program for clients. For example, the outcome measure for the rubella vaccination program might be the number of birth defects in the community per 1000 live births. Both process and outcome measures are important (ANA, 1985; Yura and Walsh, 1983).

Two somewhat fictionalized case studies are presented to illustrate the nursing process focused on the community as a client rather than the individual as a client. The first case study describes the work of a group of nurses employed in a health station in a small city (80,000) that is contiguous with a large metropolitan area. The second describes the nursing process in a college health center.

CASE STUDY 1: COMMUNITY NURSING PROCESS IN THE CITY

This city has long been known as a poverty area with many health and social problems. A major feature of the landscape is a large oil refinery located on the edge of the business district. The refinery provides employment for a group of local blue-collar workers, but the management contingent commutes to work from higher priced neighborhoods outside the city. The community health center is located on the south side of the city. The center is a county facility, but some funds come from reimbursements for services provided to Medicare and Medicaid clients. Because the city is known as one of the major trouble spots in the county, the county government has offered a grant to the health center staff if the group can submit a plan for effective use of the funds. The center supervisor, a community health nurse, meets with a committee of three other community health nurses and asks them to plan how to spend the proposed grant money and to carry out the project if it is funded. The group coordinates its activities with the center medical director, social worker, and the other nurses. They start the community nursing process with an assessment of the city.

Community Assessment

Definition of the Community

The community is an independent city of 80,000 persons located in a large metropolitan area.

The people

The city population is younger than the population of the metropolitan area, and it includes more young women than young men. A population pyramid illustrating the population in comparison with that of the large metropolitan population is shown in Figure 11-3, *A* and *B*.

Incomes are low with a median family income only 55% of that of the metropolitan area; 23% of the families are classified as living below the poverty line; 28% of the households are headed by women.

The oil refinery workers are the only well-paid group of blue-collar workers. Other industry is sparse, and business is hampered by the physical appearance of the area. Many people go outside the area to shop. The unemployment rate was 11.5% when the metropolitan rate was 5%.

Only 32% of the population has graduated from high school, although all but 3% have had some type of schooling in either the United States or Mexico.

Blacks constitute 74% of the population, whereas 21% of the population are of Spanish origin, primarily from Mexico. The black population tends to be Protestant, whereas the Mexican-Americans are Catholic (US Department of Commerce, 1980).

Structures

The city government is independent with a part-time mayor, but the high unemployment rate and low median income serve as a deterrent to tax collection. The police department is well organized and busy. A localized branch of the metropolitan drug organization occupies much of the police force's time, although the low educational level and low marriage rate leave a significant contingent of young males free for gang activities. The health department clinic is housed in a county-state satellite building that includes a social service office for families needing assistance, a Planned Parenthood satellite office, and an office of the Association for the Blind. The churches are well organized and strong.

A high-level, affluent, informal power structure is missing in the city, but white-collar businessmen and a few blue-collar workers have risen to power in city government and in branches of men's fraternal organizations such as Elks and Moose. Probably the major positive source of informal power is found in the churches. The drug sellers constitute a negative, informal, power source.

Health Risk Factors

1. Drug addiction, including cocaine, heroin, and marijuana
2. High rates of low birth weights
3. High unemployment levels
4. Low incidence of prenatal care
5. Low levels of immunization for childhood illnesses
6. High rates of unplanned pregnancies
7. Occupational hazards for the refinery workers including burns, chemical exposure, and injuries
8. Hepatitis B and AIDS, particularly among IV drug users
9. Poor nutrition
10. Lack of sophistication with the health care delivery system

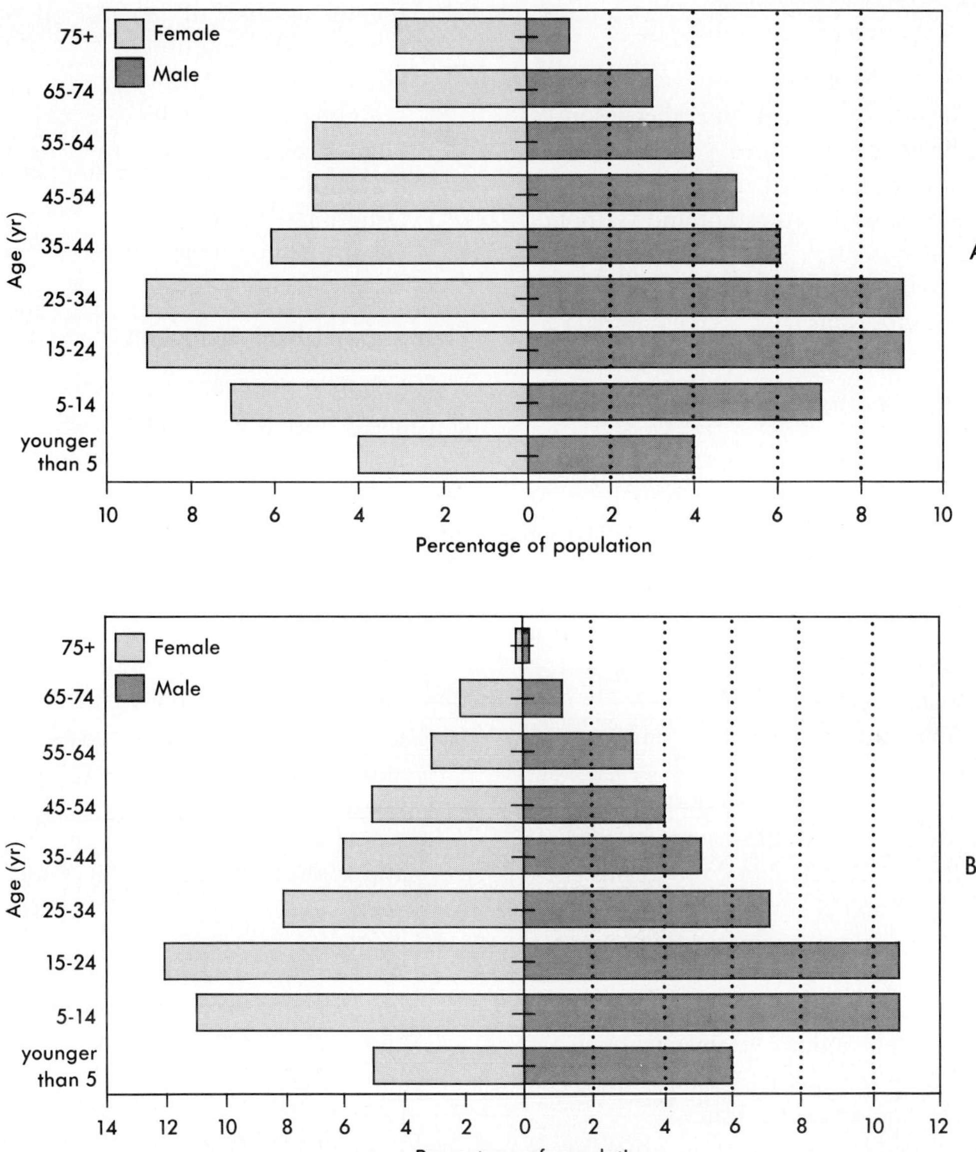

FIG. 11-3. Population pyramids. **A,** Metropolitan area. **B,** Small city.

11. Poor dental health
12. Injuries from gang activities
13. Depression related to unemployment and other stresses

Resources

1. County health department and other resources within the county structure
2. The local government of the city
3. The churches, both Protestant and Catholic
4. The school system
5. The voluntary, fraternal, business, and social service organizations

Community Nursing Diagnosis

After a discussion of the many health risk factors found in the community, the committee focused on two nursing diagnoses as a starting point for planning. Personnel restrictions precluded attempts to broaden the attack on the health problems in the community. Each of the agreed on nursing diagnoses clustered several risk factors and other social factors.

1. Community nursing diagnosis: High rate of infants with low birth weights
   Defining characteristics of the problem: Of the infants born in the last year, 18% had birth weights less than 2500 grams.
   Related factors:
   Low levels of participation in prenatal clinics
   Poor prenatal nutrition
   High rates of unplanned pregnancies
   School dropouts among young women
   High teenage pregnancy rates
   No identifiable sex education programs in the community
   Client population not sophisticated about health care delivery system
2. Community nursing diagnosis: Subgroup in the community addicted to cocaine, heroin, or marijuana
   Defining characteristic: A group of persons addicted to one or more of these substances
   Related factors:
   Identified cases of hepatitis B and AIDS among IV drug users
   High unemployment rates, particularly among young adults
   High school dropout rate in secondary school
   Drug-related crimes
   Deaths from overdoses

Planning and Implementation

Although both of these nursing diagnoses were considered important problems with serious implications for the welfare of the population of the city, the nursing committee decided to focus first on infants with low birth weights primarily because the data about the problem were more complete and the nursing expertise in the area was greater. The following plans were implemented:

1. The federal Women, Infants, and Children (WIC) program sponsored by the U.S. Department of Agriculture was investigated and an application was made for funds. This program provides supplemental food to women, infants, and children. The planning and application phase of this effort took one year, and the program was then implemented.
2. An educational program was planned and implemented with the help of the schools, churches, and Planned Parenthood. It featured an outreach discussion and teaching program focused on the following topics:
   Human sexuality
   Contraceptives
   Sexual decision making
   Coping with the health care delivery system
   Risk factors for low birth weight including youth, rubella, smoking, other substance abuse, and poor nutrition

3. A media campaign to advertise the services of the health center including its immunization programs, prenatal care, and contraception

Evaluation

Process criteria for evaluation included a judgment as to whether the WIC and the outreach programs actually were established and whether clients, particularly young women, participated in the program.

The major outcome criteria was a measurement of a trend over time showing a lower rate of infants born with low birth weights.

CASE STUDY 2: COMMUNITY NURSING PROCESS IN A STUDENT HEALTH CENTER

When Ms. C. Johnson, an experienced school and college health nurse, was hired as the administrator of the student health service at State College, she decided to institute the nursing process to improve the services of the center. She started the process with an assessment of the college student community.

Community Assessment

Definition of the Community

The community is a state college student body including 19,000 full- and part-time students; 30% of the group reside in dormitories on campus, and the remainder live off campus and commute.

The People

Men outnumber women, constituting 53% of the group. Most of the group (79%) are between the ages of 17 and 29, 14% are between 30 and 39 years old, and the remainder are older.

Median parental income in 1978 was $40,000, although 12% of the group came from families with incomes of less than $20,000; 30% of the student body receive no funds from parents or family members.

Occupations are for the most part temporary, part-time and low salaried, although there is a significant potential for future increases in income.

The educational level is high; all members of the population are high school graduates and 11% of the group have completed baccalaureate study and are enrolled in graduate programs.

The population of the college community is primarily white but 8% are black, 3% are Asian, 2% are Hispanic, and 1% are Native American. Foreign students make up 5% of the community with a concentration of students from the Far East and Africa.

Structures

The college administration is the official structure organizing the community. It divides the students into undergraduate and graduate contingents and divides them by departmental majors. The two student bodies (graduate and undergraduate) are organized into associations, which provide part of the funds for the student health center. The funds are secured by fees from the students.

The agents of social control include the faculty, the student body organizations, and the campus police. These agents are not perceived as oppressive by the community.

The student body itself is the major informal network. The voluntary structures include a variety of clubs, academic organizations, fraternities, sororities, and service organizations. The faculty could be called on as resources when needed. The family structures are in a period of transition, with some students focusing on their family of origin and others moving to form their own nuclear families.

Health Risk Factors

1. Respiratory and related infections
2. Urinary tract infections
3. Vaginitis
4. Poor life-style patterns, including the use of alcohol and drugs and smoking
5. Infectious mononucleosis
6. Poor nutrition
7. Sexually transmitted diseases including AIDS, venereal warts, gonorrhea, and chlamydia
8. Unplanned pregnancy
9. Stress and stress-related illness

Resources

1. Student health center
2. Private physicians and health care facilities outside the college
3. Voluntary campus organizations
4. Official university administration
5. Student organizations

Community Nursing Diagnoses

Several of the risk factors lend themselves well to conversion to nursing diagnoses. However, Ms. Johnson decided that for budgetary reasons only one community nursing diagnosis should be worked up at a time. "Poor nutritional status" was the diagnosis selected for the community. This was partly because it is a problem that nurses can tackle. In addition, the nurse practitioners and physicians who saw students in the student health center for treatment of episodic illnesses reported that students' nutritional status seemed to be worsening.

Community nursing diagnosis: Poor nutritional status

Defining characteristics: A significant number of persons with a daily diet that provides less than the recommended daily allowances of nutrients as published by the Food and Nutrition Board of the National Research Council (1980)

Related factors:
Obesity
Anorexia and bulimia
Societal pressure to be thin (particularly for women)
Popularity of fast foods
Acceptance of fad diets
Knowledge deficits regarding diet

Planning

The first step in planning to cope with this problem was to consult the literature to try to better understand the paradox of poor nutrition in a population characterized by a reasonable educational and income level. Alford and Bogle's work (1982) suggested that some of the observed problems were essentially carryovers from adolescent eating habits. Some of the young adults have not learned to cope with newfound freedom from parental guidance, and their busy schedules combining part-time work, study, and a social life led to dependence on fast foods. This was verified by empiric studies. Marrale and others (1986) analyzed diet diaries from a sample of 437 university students and rated only 25% of the reported diets as good. In addition, 54% of their sample reported that they were on a diet at the time of the study and their diets were particularly deficient in crucial nutrients. In another university sample, 4% of the women and 0.4% of the men, were found to have symptoms of bulimia (Zuckerman and others, 1986).

Using the information from the literature and the community assessment process, Ms. Johnson and the staff of the student health center decided they would not try to fight the dieting trend head-on. Rather, a consulting nutritionist was called in, and a series of diet workshops was planned. The workshops were scheduled with alternative day and evening schedules. The planned content included information about essential nutrients, risk factors in diet such as cholesterol and high salt, information about calories, and sample diets that were well balanced and safe. A special workshop for vegetarians was planned. Resources within the university were identified to publicize the plan.

Implementation

The plan was implemented with only a few changes as the program developed. Weighing in was added as a measure to gauge weight loss.

Evaluation

The process was evaluated by counting attendance at workshops. Outcome evaluation was more difficult because hard data were needed on the nutritional status of the population before and after the project. Before nurses started the project, a study of diets of a sample of the center clients who came in for episodic care was done. They were asked to fill out a diet diary recalling foods they ate the day before their current illness began. This same data collection process was repeated at the end of the project, and improvement was noted. The center nurse practitioners and physicians also kept a record of obesity—clients who weighed 20% more than their ideal weight or more—and the cases of anorexia and bulimia that came to their attention. There was a slight downward trend in these data although the findings were not statistically significant.

SUMMARY

To be effective, community health nurses must focus on the total community and its needs. One way to do this is to conceptualize the community itself as a client and then apply the nursing process, including a community assessment, a community nursing diagnosis, and the appropriate processes of planning, implementation, and evaluation. A knowledge of the research literature related to communities facilitates the nursing process at this level.

QUESTIONS FOR DISCUSSION

1. List the steps involved in a community assessment.
2. Compare and contrast a nursing diagnosis of an individual client with that of a community.
3. What is the difference between a process and outcome evaluation?
4. List and explain what kind of resources might be available for a nurse to turn to for support in a community.

REFERENCES

American Nurses' Association, Council of Community Health Nurses: A guide for community-based nursing services, Kansas City, MO, 1985, The Association.

American Public Health Association: The definition and role of public health nursing in the delivery of health care, Washington, DC, 1980, The Association.

Bendix R and Lipset SM: Class status and power: social stratification in comparative perspective, ed 2, New York, 1966, The Free Press.

Bullough V and Bullough B: Health care for the other Americans, New York, 1982, Appleton & Lange.

Carpenito LJ: Nursing diagnosis: application to clinical practice, New York, 1983, JB Lippincott Co.

Cook TH, Baker DJ, and Shamansky SL: Community assessment. In Schoolcraft V, editor: Nursing in the community, New York, 1984, John Wiley & Sons Inc.

Dawber TR: The Framingham study: the epidemiology of atherosclerotic disease, Cambridge, Mass, 1980, Harvard University Press and the Commonwealth Fund.

Duncan HA: Duncan's dictionary for nurses, ed 2, New York, 1988, Springer Publishing Co Inc.

Food and Nutrition Board, National Research Council: Recommended dietary allowances, ed 9, Washington, DC, 1980, National Academy of Sciences.

Gebbie K: Toward the theory development for nursing diagnoses classification. In Kim J and Moritz DA, editors: Classification of nursing diagnoses, New York, 1982, McGraw-Hill Inc.

Higgs Z and Gustafson DD: Community as a client: assessment and diagnosis, Philadelphia, 1985, FA Davis Co.

Ibrahim M: Epidemiology and health policy, Rockville, Md, 1985, Aspen Publishers Inc.

Kane, DV: Environmental hazards to young children, Phoenix, 1985, The Oryx Press.

Lenski G: Power and privileges: a theory of social stratification, New York, 1955, McGraw-Hill Inc.

Marrale JC, Shipman JH, and Rhodes ML: What some college students eat, Nutrition Today 21:16, 1986.

McCord W and McCord A: Power and equity: an introduction to social stratification, New York, 1977, Praeger Publishers.

Muecke M: 1984. Community health diagnosis in nursing, Public Health Nurse 1:23, 1984.

Shamansky SL and Pesznecker B: A community is . . . , Nurs Outlook 29:182, 1981.

Suttles GD: The social order of the slum: ethnicity and territory in the inner city, Chicago, 1968, University of Chicago Press.

United States Department of Commerce, Bureau of the Census: 1980 census of the population and housing—census tracts Los Angeles—Long Beach, California, Standard Metropolitan Statistical Area PHC80-2-226, Sections 1 through 4, Washington, DC, 1980, US Government Printing Office.

Yura H and Walsh M: The nursing process, East Norwalk, Conn, 1983, Appleton & Lange.

Zuckerman DM and others: The prevalence of bulimia among college students, Public Health 76:113, 1986.

BIBLIOGRAPHY

American Public Health Association, Public Health Nursing Section: Operational definition of public health nursing. In American Nurses' Association, Council of Community Health Nurses: A guide for community based nursing services, Kansas City, 1985, American Nurses' Association.

Anderson EI and McFarlane JM: Community as a client: application of the nursing process, Philadelphia, 1988, JB Lippincott, Co.

CHAPTER

12

Family Assessment: A Base for Nursing Practice

Cathleen Getty and
G. Winnifred Humphries

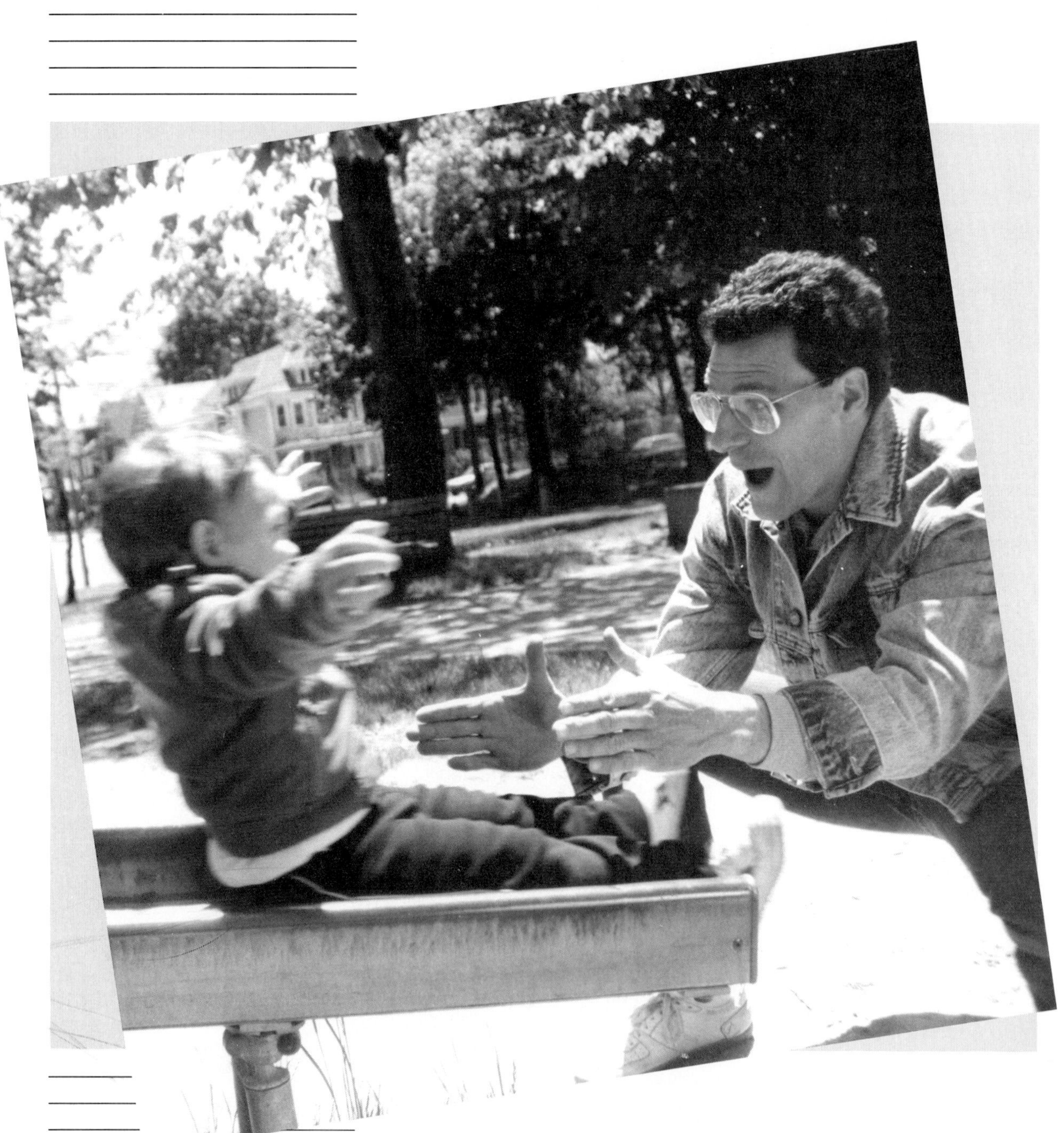

CHAPTER OUTLINE

OBJECTIVES

After completing this chapter, the reader should be able to:

1. Use a theoretic framework in developing a systematic approach to nursing assessment and intervention with families.
2. Understand critical family functions and their implications for the well-being of members and of society.
3. Discuss ways in which socioculturally based values and beliefs shape family functioning.
4. Understand how a family's life context affects its ability to carry out its functions.
5. Consider the interplay between a family's place in the life cycle and its health concerns.
6. Use the nursing process to foster a family's capacity to carry out its health care function.

As the locus of health care provision shifts from hospital to the client's home, nurses are called on to gain a broader perspective of contemporary family functioning, as well as to come to terms with the practice implications of this awareness. However, in the United States there is great emphasis placed on individuals—their right to control their destinies and their obligation to master their environments. Inevitably then, health care professionals are influenced by these deeply held values, and health care professionals' practice reflects this strong individualistic bias. This tends to narrow caregivers' perspectives, diverting them from a more comprehensive appraisal that would include the biosocial context within which each person is rooted. The family functions to provide for the physical, psychologic, and social needs of its members. In addition, it plays a crucial role in socializing members to the ways of society and in this mediating role thus links society and the individual. In carrying out these roles, it makes a powerful impact on its members and therefore merits our careful consideration.

When nurses address family issues, they tend to examine them against the backdrop of society's image of the ideal family, the *nuclear family*, which comprises a married couple and their children. This image persists despite the fact that varying structural forms have always existed in American society. For many, the nuclear family represents the most effective form for providing for the needs of its members. Others are critical of its capacity to do this work on its own, citing the frequent necessity for both parents to work, the burgeoning divorce rate, and the potential for isolation of such family groups from sources of social support. The debate over the relative effectiveness of the two-parent family has recently been overshadowed by concern about the growing number of single-parent families—in large part the outcome of the increase in divorces and in out-of-wedlock pregnancies. The question here is, "If two parents are unable to do the job, how can one do it?" This chapter does not presume to resolve these questions, but they are raised because they alert the reader to the complexity of the issues inherent in this subject matter as the functioning of families is examined.

THEORETIC FRAMEWORK

Currently there is a variety of conceptual frameworks and approaches that guide the study and analysis of family behavior in organized and logical ways: structural-functionalism, symbolic interactionism, the developmental (or life cycle) approach, and conflict theory. Although each of these approaches has something important to contribute to the understanding of families, none of them is sufficiently comprehensive to account for all dimensions of family life. For this reason the integration of several of these approaches within an ecosystems perspective is proposed. Such an amalgam is particularly helpful not only in coming to terms with the complexities of family life, but in planning and implementing appropriate nursing interventions with families. The major components of this approach are presented in Chapter 12.

Ecosystems Perspective

The term "ecosystem" is drawn from two approaches to understanding the functioning of living organisms. The first, ecology, is the branch of biology that deals with the relations between organisms (for our purposes, individuals) and their environments. The second, general systems theory, requires that these relationships be viewed as systems that operate in ways that are significant to all interacting participants. Synthesizing the two, an ecosystems approach is one that is concerned with the systemic relations of individuals and their environments. By analogy, then, the human ecosystem is one that involves not only the individual, but also that person's family and significant others, as well as all other relevant aspects of a family's social and physical environments.*

Every *system* (and systems may be as different in size and complexity as the individual, the fam- in size and complexity as the individual, the family, or a community agency) is made up of a series of interrelated elements. It is the interrelationships among these components or *subsystems* that bind systems into a whole. These are interactional systems, and, according to the theory, they continue to be functional only if they remain open to the impact of change in the other systems with which they interact. For example, change in one subsystem of a family is likely to be felt throughout all its constituent parts.

Conflict between parents has an impact on their children and on extended family members; illness or unhappiness in a child influences, to one degree or another, the lives of all other family members. This impact or influence is transmitted through messages that are communicated throughout the system. These messages are referred to as *feedback,* a form of interaction or provision of information that advises the system of the need to accommodate itself to the needs of its constituent subsystems, as well as to the environment. It is this process of accommodation that serves to bring the family system into balance, or *homeostasis.* The term implies a maintenance of the status quo, but in understanding families it is useful to conceive of these operations as dynamic and as providing a certain degree of stability for the system while also allowing for development and change (Watzlawick, 1967). For a system to function effectively, these processes require regulation, or governance. When applied to family systems, this governing function serves to regulate interactional processes with the aim of ensuring that systemic goals are achieved. Because the parents are the adults and serve as the family architects, in Satir's terms (1983), it is expected that they assume the executive or leadership role.

System interaction with environment is crucial to the ongoing life of open systems and has particular relevance for the study of human interaction. It is especially important in the examination of families in their milieux because the processes involved in the adaptation of one to the other require investigation to gain an understanding of the type and degree of mutual fit between the two. Not only do environments influence the lives of individuals, but people are also active, to one degree or another, in modifying their environments as they go about meeting their needs.

To the degree that environment and person are successful in operating in ways that meet their mutual needs, *reciprocity* is said to prevail. Where there is a disruption in the reciprocal processes both within the system and between the system and its environment, stress of one kind or another results. These strains, in turn, call into play *coping* efforts directed toward stress reduction, as well as toward goal achievement and problem solving. The family tests and reshapes its coping strategies, gradually developing patterns that become characteristic over time. This is *goal-oriented behavior* involving not only past experience but also some anticipation of the future in combination with a capacity for spontaneous change when warranted (Germain and Gitterman, 1980). For example, depression of a community's economy may result in high unemployment rates with concomitant strains for affected families. When a father who is the primary provider loses his job, that family not only suffers the loss of economic resources, but is likely to be affected by role changes as well. The father, at least temporarily, experiences the stress associated with loss of an important role in the family, while the mother may be called on to assume the role of primary economic provider. If, with the help of the children, the father can take on functions earlier allocated to the mother, and if the mother in turn is reasonably successful in locating sufficiently remunerative work and in dealing with these role changes, the family may be viewed as having coped successfully. Their mode of coping may, in fact, bring about adaptive

*E.H. Auerswald (1968) was the first to identify and advocate an ecologic systems approach to the study of human interaction.

changes in their interactional patterns, with the father relating more closely to the children and the mother finding gratification in her changed role.

At the same time, the community is reciprocally influenced in that the family remains economically independent and self-sufficient. It is important to note, however, that there are likely to be differences in the coping of families, depending on their social circumstances. Cultural background clearly affects a family's functioning in crucial ways. Values, customs, norms, and prescriptions regarding sex and gender roles, childrearing patterns, attitudes toward aging, illness, and the maintenance of health, and the necessity to seek help all deeply influence a family's behavior and its capacity for and style of coping. Other important influences derive from social class status; that is, the economic circumstances, occupational and educational characteristics, and often the physical environment and place of residence of families exert a marked influence on the degree to which they have the internal and external resources to accomplish their goals, aspirations, and functions.

Structural-Functional Perspective

The structural-functional approach has grown out of a social systems perspective and, as the name implies, is concerned with the analysis of the structure and functioning of social units and their component parts. A family's *structure* refers to its organization—the patterned ways in which members are related to and interact with one another, as well as the family's reciprocal relationships with other systems in the society (Eschleman, 1981). The relationship of this approach to the ecosystems perspective is evident here, in that structural-functionalism views the family unit as embedded in its social milieu.

Structural patterns vary within and among cultures. A nuclear family (mother, father, and children) has a different structural form from that of an extended family (mother, father, and children living with two or more generations of kin), and this can give rise to important differences in lifestyles. The ways in which they organize the work of the household, rear the children, and provide social and economic support, for instance, are likely to be quite different. On the other hand, a particular type of family organization is likely to have predictable consequences despite its cultural context. For example, families headed by single parents have similar structural arrangements—a sole adult in the parent role—and because of this it can be anticipated that they face similar difficulties in functioning. The family is short of adult members, and unless outsiders can be drawn in to perform adult work, the shortage is likely to result in a unit with overtaxed resources and unmet needs.

Function is a concept complementary to that of structure (Eschleman, 1981). Systems perform certain expected or required activities, or functions, and such activity is intimately related to the system's structure. Within the structural-functional perspective, *family function* refers to the tasks the family performs for the society, other social systems and institutions, and its members, as well as tasks performed to ensure its own maintenance.

Children are nurtured and reared in culturally sanctioned ways to prepare them for adult work and family and citizen roles within society. Additionally, the family is expected to meet the emotional needs of the adult members. The structural-functionalists' concern with order is readily apparent in the preceding material. They are particularly interested in the balance and stability of systems and therefore emphasize those processes and functions that further the harmony of the system.

Most prominent among those who use a structural-functional approach in clinical work with families is Salvador Minuchin (Minuchin, 1974; Minuchin and Fishman, 1981), who has applied systems and structural concepts to assessing and intervening in family problems. In the previous section, it is noted that systems have constituent parts called subsystems and that the relationships between these components bind the system into a functioning whole. When the system under scrutiny is a family, the individual members alone or in combinations such as the parents or the siblings may be viewed as family subsystems.

The *structure,* or characteristic patterns of interaction within the family, is central to Minuchin's analysis. Because such behavior recurs regularly among family members, it can be assumed that over time the family has developed a set of prescriptions, or *rules,* for how interactions should be conducted. In fact, a complex set of rules that guides all dimensions of family life evolves from societal values and belief systems and the family's ethnic heritage and social class, as well as the personal idiosyncrasies of the members. As previously indicated, the governing system of the family works to foster the observance of these rules.

For Minuchin, the nature of the *boundary* separating the family from its environment, as well as the boundaries that demarcate one subsystem from another, are also of key importance. He makes the point that boundaries are determined by the rules defining who participates and how (Minuchin, 1974). When these structural rules are clear, each family subsystem understands who is part of a transaction, who is not, and what roles those who are participating are to assume in relation to each other and the outside world (Aponte and Van Deusen, 1981). Boundaries therefore operate to maintain the differentiation between systems. Where they are not clear, members of subsystems are vulnerable to outside interference as in the classic situation of the grandparent who meddles in the affairs of both parent and child subsystems. Situations like this, in which boundaries are seriously weakened and made more permeable make it difficult for family members to experience a sense of autonomy or individual competence. On the other hand, where boundaries are too rigidly defined, interaction between subsystems is decreased and constricted. Members are then emotionally separated from each other by rigid boundaries that make it unlikely for the distress of one system to evoke a response in another. For example, parents may be so deeply invested in their marital relationship that the children are excluded and interaction between parents and children is restricted and insufficient to their needs.

It is evident, then, that the degree of clarity of boundaries can provide a useful guide for evaluating family functioning. For the family to perform its tasks, boundaries must be flexible to provide an adequate exchange of resources with the environment while retaining the identity of the family as an autonomous unit. Boundaries must also be regulated in such a way as to allow for the individuation of members, all perceiving themselves as separate from the others, yet as integral parts of the family.

Social Role

Social roles, the more or less characteristic sets of behavior expected of the occupant of a particular social position (Merton, 1957), provide us with an illustration of the patterning of behavior in families. For example, society provides certain prescriptions as to how persons occupying the role of mother should behave, and because of this it is possible to predict certain similarities in maternal functioning across families. Although the dominant thrust in a society may be embodied in one set of prescriptions, for example, expectations that a "proper" mother assumes the primary nurturant function in families, remaining at home and available for her child's needs, a subculture might hold varying expectations that allow for creative or economically rewarding work outside the home. An additional perspective is useful in accounting for the variations in role behavior. Symbolic interactionist theorists emphasize that individuals interpret the influences of the environment in subjectively meaningful ways, defining a role in terms that are compatible with their own perception of what is appropriate. For instance, a woman may view herself as only one of many (husband, extended family, friends, and day-care staff) who are responsible for the nurturing of her children.

Interactions are likely to be harmonious when family members have similar expectations for how each ought to behave in relation to one another. Where expectations are incompatible, *role conflict* is likely to follow. When family members experience stress in relation to fulfilling the obligations of a role, for example, where they are vague, contradictory, or overwhelming, they are likely to suffer from *role strain.*

A variety of factors figure in society's shaping of family role expectations. Among these are age, ordinal position in the family, and gender. Although these variables certainly affect social interaction, society attaches additional meaning to them that goes beyond and at times alters their original significance in profound ways. To illustrate, gender, a biologic trait, is used as the determinant for *sex role*—to differentiate between what is considered "appropriate" for male and female behavior. As implied previously, women may be constrained in their roles as women, wives, and mothers on the basis of gender-linked prescriptions and, of course, men may experience constrictions as well.

For a family to fulfill its obligations to society and to its own members, it needs to provide in some way for the carrying out of essential functions. The roles associated with these functions may be specified in a variety of ways. The following are among the most important: nurturing, sexual, economic provider, stress management, leadership, child socialization and care, home maintenance, kin and community relations, and health care. Although these roles are often associated with persons holding particular positions in family constellations (father or mother, for example), it is important to recognize that roles are not always allocated in the same way. For instance, although in North America it is usually assumed that husbands take responsibility for home maintenance tasks outside the house and wives for those on the inside, the reverse or some combination of the two may be equally or more effective for a particular family. Roles may also be shared among members as when both parents and older children take responsibility for the socialization and care of a younger child.

Crucial to an evaluation of role performance are issues having to do with the assigned individual's capacity and skills for carrying out the associated tasks. If, in the foregoing example, children caring for the younger child are sufficiently mature and skilled and they receive enough support and guidance from parents who are also competent in their participation in the role, it is probable that strains will be minimal and the outcome congruent with the needs of all.

Power Allocation and Decision Making

Because the resources available to any social system are variable and limited, their distribution assumes critical importance. As a result, those who control the distribution have access to crucial sources of power and can strongly influence the operations and outcomes of the system. Clearly, placement in the social structure greatly influences the types and amounts of *external resources* to which a family has access. This has a bearing on the problems the family must face, on their ability to manage them, and ultimately on their valuing of themselves. Certain groups have always been penalized in this regard in our society, ethnicity and racial origin serving as major determinants of social position and therefore of access to the sources of societal power.

Not only do external resources figure in the family's coping capacity, but internal resources, such as availability of members and their personal and interactional competence, also play a major role. It is the power structure of the family that determines the control and distribution of these assets. Power and authority relations, like other family operations, develop in response to the values and traditions of the society, as well as to the belief systems and aspirations of the members themselves. Patterns of male dominance have prevailed in society and within its institutions. This had led to gender-based inequities in the family power structure, males having had greater power and control over the more consequential aspects of family life (Nelson and Taylor, 1981). In whatever way power and authority are apportioned in a family, their allocation inevitably affects decision making. Those with greater power dominate the process, taking the lead on issues that "really count" (as in the exercise of a parental role) and permitting other members a role in selected areas (as when a dominant parent determines that a child is competent in a particular area or when a dominant mate views a partner as qualified to exercise the requisite judgment).

Although major structural changes ensuring equality of men and women have not been fully realized, the women's movement has had a leavening influence, reflected in a more egalitarian power structure in some families. However, where inequities continue to be great, less powerful members are more dependent and less autonomous because their options to test out and develop their risk-taking and problem-solving abilities are restricted by those with more power. Conflict is inevitable under the circumstances, although it may not necessarily be expressed openly.

Family Life Cycle Perspective

Developmental theorists account for change in family systems by conceptualizing a series of inevitable stages in the family life cycle. This approach assumes that these stages are universal and come about as this social unit works toward meeting the maturational needs of its members and the functional requirements of the society. Although the stages are not always specified in precisely the same way, there is general agreement that they evolve in response to sets of experiences common to the life history of all families. They are therefore closely tied to the tasks confronting the family as it copes with the developmental requirements of the children. Because of this inherent bias, these approaches are limited in their capacity to elucidate the life cycle experiences of families with variant forms. For example, the tasks confronting childless couples and multigenerational, extended families are not well elaborated by life cycle theorists. In addition, they imply that families are not truly families unless the parents are heterosexual and married.

Despite these deficits in the established theories, life cycle considerations need to be included in any comprehensive assessment as they help us locate a family in its life cycle position and anticipate its circumstances during the particular phase of its life work. The family's place in the life cycle can serve to sensitize us to stage-related health concerns as well.

As previously mentioned, several developmental models are cited in the literature. Duvall's model (1977), the one most frequently used, comprises eight stages extending from the formation of the family to the retirement and old age of the parents. However, another developmental model, advanced by McGoldrick and Carter (1982), has particular merit because it provides for a transitional phase during which the young adult is separating from the family of origin and has not yet married. Further, it delineates the primary focus of the work ("key principles" in the model) that must be accomplished for the family to make a smooth transition into the ensuing stage and spells out the related tasks. This section expands this model, incorporating some of the work of Duvall, to account for subphases in the experiences of the family with young children and during later life. As Friedman (1981) does, this section provides for consideration of stage-related health concerns (Table 12-1).

To illustrate the utility of the preceding model, let us take as an example the family of a working couple, both in their early fifties, whose children are now adults with families of their own. The

TABLE 12-1 The Stages of the Family Life Cycle and Related Health Concerns*

Family life cycle stage	Emotional process of transition: key principles	Stage-related family tasks	Stage-related family health concerns
1. Between families: the unattached young adult	Accepting parent-offspring separation	Differentiation of self in relation to family Development of intimate peer relationships Establishment of self in work	Adequate nutrition and exercise in light of single life-style Drug and alcohol abuse Management of sexual expression and functioning including birth control, abortion, and sexually transmitted diseases Management of work-related and interpersonal stress
2. The joining of families through marriage: the newly married couple	Commitment to new system	Formation of marital system Realignment of relationships with extended family and to include spouse	Management of stress related to marital role adjustment Family planning Planning of pregnancy and birth
3. The family with young children Early childbearing families Families with preschool children Families with school children	Accepting new generation of members into the system	Adjusting marital system to make space for a child or children Taking on parenting roles Realignment of relationships with extended family to include parenting and grandparenting roles Realignment and extension of relationships with community to include educational and child-care resources	Well baby and child-care including immunizations Management of acute and chronic child health problems Environmental safety Understanding of children's needs and abilities based on developmental levels Management of role strain associated with expansion of family system
4. The family with adolescents	Increasing flexibility of family boundaries to include children's independence	Shifting of parent-child relationships to permit adolescents to move in and out of system Refocus on midlife marital and career issues Beginning shift toward concerns for older generation	Intensified interest on marital pair in health promotion and management of risk factors Management of tensions arising from adolescents' increasing pressure toward individuation and autonomy Heightened risk of adolescent substance abuse, automobile accidents, and other accidents

TABLE 12-1 The Stages of the Family Life Cycle and Related Health Concerns—cont'd.

Family life cycle stage	Emotional process of transition: key principles	Stage-related family tasks	Stage-related family health concerns
5. Launching children and moving on	Accepting a multitude of exits from and entries into the family system	Renegotiation of marital system as a dyad Development of adult-to-adult relationships between grown children and their parents Realignment of relationships to include in-laws and grandchildren Dealing with disabilities and death of parents (grandparents)	Management of stress arising from "reshaping" of family Dealing with young adult separation from family Management of impact of aging grandparents—provision of assistance and care, coping with their death Dealing with emerging chronic health problems of marital pair
6. The family in later life Families of middle years Families in retirement and old age	Accepting the shifting of generational roles	Maintaining own or couple functioning and interests in face of physiologic decline; exploration of new familial and social role options Support for a more central role for the adult children Making room in the system for the wisdom and experience of the elderly; supporting the older generation without overfunctioning for them Dealing with loss of spouse, siblings, and other peers, and preparation for own death. Life review and integration	Promotion and maintenance of health Deterioration of physical or mental health or both, coping with loss of function, provision of assistance and care Management of stress generated by changing role relationships within marital dyad and among parents and children

*Modified from McGoldrick M and Carter CA: The family life cycle in normal family processes, New York, 1982, The Guilford Press. Selected subphases drawn from Duvall EM: Marriage and family development, New York, 1977, JB Lippincott Co.

family, having recently adapted to the children's leaving home, is now likely to be involved in redefining relationships to allow the children to assume adult status with their parents and parental status with their own offspring. Concurrently, the parents are working to accept the changed status of their children, as well as their own new grandparenting roles. In addition to the foregoing, one or both of the parental partners may be assuming some level of responsibility for their aging parents (now great-grandparents) while meeting the demands of home and work.

This family, moving toward resolution of the launching phase, is likely to be confronted with a set of stage-related health concerns. Actually, several stages and their respective health concerns can be identified in the family just described. The middle-aged members may well be facing the chronic health problems that commonly surface among persons in this age-group, stresses in connection with their changing roles, as well as the increasing infirmity and approaching death of their own parents. At the same time, the adult children are likely to be confronting issues associated with their childbearing status.

Health Care Function

The family's management of health concerns like the ones previously mentioned is greatly influenced by its beliefs about health and illness. Although these are certainly shaped by the dominant society, they are also affected by social class and ethnic and other cultural reference groups. Because of these divergent influences, it cannot be assumed that families define health and illness in the same way or that their patterns of responding to them are alike (Tripp-Reimer, 1984). For instance, some may typically define members as healthy until an illness interferes with their ability to work, whereas others take a more anticipatory view, identifying a condition as an illness long before it interferes with their functioning.

Further, there are important implications here for family role relationships during health and illness. Sets of expectations guide the behavior of the members who are ill, as well as that of the persons who are responsible for family health maintenance and nursing the sick. For example, one mother may be expected to carry out her usual round of tasks during a relatively severe illness, whereas another, in comparable circumstances, is encouraged to recuperate while others take on her work. In one family an elderly grandparent's care is seen as most effectively carried out by the "skilled personnel" of a nursing home. In another, members feel obligated to "care for their own." Whatever the relationship patterns, families are called on to alter their characteristic styles of coping to deal with health-related crises.

Assessment issues focus on the family's sensitivity to the health needs of its members and on its ability both to determine when care is needed and to provide it. Nurses may inadvertently work in such a way as to constrain families in their attempts to deal with their health care problems, operating on the premise that only scientific practices are appropriate and acceptable. It is essential that the nurse respect and support the family's efforts where their approach has beneficial consequences or is at least neutral in its effect. However, when their treatment efforts or inattention to problems has an apparently or potentially negative impact, it is imperative that the professional endeavor to influence the family to alter their behavior. For this interaction to be effective, the alternative approach must be translated so that it has meaning within the family's frame of reference. For instance, a father who presents himself as a man whose wife and children count on him to "bring home the bacon" may be unwilling to obtain a medical examination despite sporadic chest pain and shortness of breath. Although he is not responsive to health teaching and the nurse knows that his inaction is not a result of his lack of understanding of his symptoms, she may feel that she must try to convince him to seek medical advice. In view of the fact that he appears deeply invested in the role of family provider, the nurse should be well advised to reframe the discussion by moving from a focus that stresses "convincing by educating" to one that engages him at the level of his probable concern about the potential implications of the symptoms for his self-image and role performance. This is likely to alter the nature of the interaction, making it a mutual enterprise as opposed to the earlier approach that might well have become increasingly adversarial.

BASE FOR CLINICAL ACTION

The preceding theoretic perspectives play a central role in the structuring of this chapter's approach to assessment and intervention with families. Our orientation is rooted in the following set of propositions regarding the family and its functioning:

1. The family is a dynamic social system that acts to:
   - Sustain and nurture its members
   - Provide for the maturation and development of the individual, fostering health, autonomy, and competence
   - Socialize its members into roles that are responsive to the requirements of the society and to the needs and aspirations of the family itself
2. The family is not only embedded in its environment, it is also interactive with its environment, and, in consequence, a family's capacity to carry out its functions is heavily dependent on its reciprocal relationship with the environment.
3. The family's success in performing its tasks is also contingent on the family's capacity to regulate the interaction of family members so that the crucial roles are assigned and performed.
4. Individuals require a role in the family structure that provides for autonomy in the meeting of their own needs.
5. The family's ability to manage stress deriving from its internal and external transactions has considerable import for the physical and psychologic well-being of family members and for its continuing integrity as a complete unit.
6. Community health nurses, as agents of societal institutions, can foster the family's capacity for carrying out its functions.

Two fundamental questions remain. First, what is a family? Eschleman (1981) defines family broadly as "a kinship-structural group of persons related by blood, marriage, or adoption, usually related to the marital unit and including the rights and duties of parenthood." This chapter contends, however, that any group of persons living together should be assessed in terms of the degree to which they *serve* as families for their members. Finally, what is a normal, healthy family? Any evaluation of normality implies that the family in question has been judged against a set of standards. These criteria, an arbitrary means of describing the typical, tend to be applied as though they represented the correct way of being. Nonetheless, the making of judgments is inevitable because it is part and parcel of daily living. Although it is impossible to be value free, it is possible to operate in such a way as to recognize the biases inherent in our judgment, refraining from too stringent an application of standards without consideration of the values and goals of the family in question. Therefore, this chapter avoids these labels as much as possible and emphasizes evaluation of a family's functioning, stressing its ability to perform its tasks and not making rigid assumptions as to how this can best be accomplished.

ASSESSMENT PROCESS

All of us make judgments constantly, with or without a reliable information base or a rational framework for its interpretation. However, it is essential that nurses, as responsible professionals, develop a basis for more conscious and fewer biased decisions that are grounded in information gained from a planned approach to data collection.

The preceding theoretic propositions serve this purpose, providing a framework for the assessment of families. Using data obtained during the assessment process, the nurse makes nursing diagnoses (judgments), formulates a plan of action, and intervenes on this basis. Often diagnoses and plans are tentative in nature and require confirmation through further assessment and evaluation, a process that is elucidated later in this chapter. In the section that follows, several aspects of family life crucial to an understanding of family functioning are delineated. However, before doing so, several issues regarding the assessment process per se should be discussed.

Under what conditions is a family assessment appropriate? Some degree of family assessment is always necessary when the family itself has been defined as the client. When an individual is the client, an appraisal of the family network is called for to discern its composition, as well as the degree to which it both stresses and supports the person.

How comprehensive should the exploration be? Should every dimension of family life be examined with every family? This is clearly impractical in light of the competing demands for a nurse's time and attention. Practicality, however, is only one aspect of the question. *Relevance* is the key determinant of what should be explored and probed. If, for example, it is necessary for a nurse to visit a family because of the parents' refusal of immunization for their preschool child, it is likely that the nurse would first move to explore their level of knowledge, and this is entirely appropriate. However, without some understanding of the family's cultural values, the nurse is not likely to have sufficient information to adequately diagnose the problem or to plan interventions that are congruent with the family's health beliefs. On the other hand, it is not likely that a full exploration of other aspects of family life, such as the marital relationship, is necessary in this instance. Certain facets of the relationship *are* likely to be germane and therefore likely to require examination—in particular, the couple's interactional patterns with regard to power allocation and decision making. Unless there are clues to the contrary, probing of additional areas would probably be unproductive. The aim is not merely to collect data but to obtain information sufficient to the understanding and management of the family's problem(s).

How can one best make use of an assessment guide? An assessment schema is designed to orient the assessor toward a comprehensive examination of the client situation. All too often, however, it is used in a nondiscriminating fashion and slavishly followed rather than being tailored to the actual circumstances with which the professional is faced. This may come about because either professionals equate "complete" detail with excellence in practice, or, distressed by lack of structure in interacting with clients, they feel more secure if the outline controls the interview.

Despite the potential for such misapplication, a guide *does* serve to direct and focus our attention, helping organize our thinking along lines deriving from a theoretic perspective. With these cautionary notes in mind, the boxed material that follows is a general guide for the assessment of families, whatever their form and structure. It is apparent that the assessment dimensions of the guide are rooted in the three major theoretic frameworks that were already delineated in this chapter.

CLINICAL APPLICATION

The following section presents a case study describing the experience of a community health nurse with a client family, and then the nurse's assessment of the family is organized and presented according to the guide provided earlier.

Rivera Family

Carlos and Rosa Rivera, a young Puerto Rican couple, have recently brought their first baby home from the county hospital. The local public health nursing department was notified and asked to visit the family. The infant, Luis, was born with a ventricular septal defect that caused him to be kept in the hospital for several weeks following his mother's discharge, and the couple has been told that he requires surgery to correct the prob-

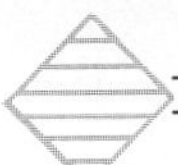

FAMILY ASSESSMENT GUIDE

DEMOGRAPHIC DATA

Family name:
Address:
Telephone:
Presenting Problem:
Family form and composition: Identify family form, listing family members and others living in household.

	Name	*Age*	*Sex*	*Relationship to family*	*Occupation*	*Education*
1.						
2.						
3.						
4.						
5.						
6.						

FAMILY LIFE CONTEXT

This dimension calls for an examination and assessment of the environmental context within which a family functions. In accomplishing this, the characteristics of systems with which the family interacts are identified and the nature of the interaction is evaluated. The significance of sociocultural influences must also be taken into account. With these data as background, sources of both stress and support become more apparent.

1. Characteristics of housing. (Consider, for example, condition of structure, adequacy of space and furnishings, and safety.)
2. Characteristics of neighborhood. (Consider condition, availability of resources, and safety.)
3. Degree and type of interaction with systems in community. (Using the ecosystems map provided in Fig. 12-1, identify the significant community systems with which the family interacts, indicating the characteristics of these ties.)
4. Social support network. (Again using the map, specify the family's ties with relatives, friends, neighbors, and others who play an important role in the family's life.)
5. Delineation of problems. (Identify any problems emerging from this portion of the assessment. Do any family members share this view of the situation? Indicate any internal or external resources available for responding to the difficulties.)

FAMILY STRUCTURE AND FUNCTION

Here the major patterns and characteristics of family interrelationships are identified and assessed. A central feature is the analysis of the family's ability to accomplish its functions through its role structure and role relationships.

1. Role relationships and functions. Examine the positions and roles of each family member, considering the degree of competence, conflict, and strain associated with the performance of each. Consider the roles listed below.
   - Nurturing—Who is responsible for attending to the emotional needs of members? Is each member receiving attention sufficient to needs?
   - Sexual—Do adult members indicate that there are problems with their sexual relationships? If so, what is their nature? If there are children, are the adults sensitive to their psychosexual development, providing education and guidance as needed?
   - Economic provider—Who is responsible for securing income? Is it adequate for family needs?
   - Stress management—Who is responsible for alleviating tension? Is the responsible member effective in keeping stress at a manageable level?
   - Leadership—Who performs the leadership tasks? Do they provide sufficient organization and structure to ensure that family roles and tasks are carried out?

Continued.

FAMILY ASSESSMENT GUIDE—cont'd.

Child socialization and care—Who is responsible for the education and discipline of the children and for monitoring their safety and general well-being? Is there evidence that the children's physical, social, and emotional development is adequately fostered?

Home maintenance—Who is allocated this role? Are these functions carried out in such a way as to keep the home safe and comfortable, in keeping with the family's resources?

Kin and community relations—Who initiates and maintains communications and ties with relatives, friends, and community institutions? To what degree are these efforts effective in ensuring that the family receives needed social support and resources?

2. Power dimensions. Assess the family power structure and its decision-making process.

   Power structure—How is power allocated? Is it shared or does one member dominate? Is there adequate adult leadership with regard to the family's carrying out of its tasks?

   Decision-making process—Who decides what and how? Are decisions effected in such a way that the essential functions of family life are facilitated?

3. Delineation of problems. Specify any problems emerging from this portion of the assessment. Do any family members share this view of the situation? Identify any internal or external resources available for responding to the difficulties.

FAMILY DEVELOPMENTAL STAGE

Identify the family's position in its life cycle and the developmental stage of each member. Assess its ability to recognize and respond to the stage-related needs of individual members, specifying the external and internal resources that serve to support or inhibit its functioning in this regard. The form shown in Fig. 12-2 is useful for organizing these data.

HEALTH CARE FUNCTION

Identify the family's current health and illness concerns and their beliefs about appropriate management, and indicate the resources available to them.

1. Health concerns and problems. What does the family believe to be its current health and illness concerns? What do you, the nurse, identify as the family's current health and illness problems? How do you account for any differences in these assessments?
2. Management of health concerns and problems. What does the family see as appropriate care and treatment? Who do you believe should provide it? In what ways is this similar to or different from your thinking?
3. Family resources. What resources does the family need to manage its health problems? To what extent are the necessary external and internal resources accessible?

FINAL SUMMARY

On the basis of your assessment of the five preceding dimensions, list the identified problems, including your own evaluation of the family's readiness and ability to deal with them at this time. What resources do they require to cope with the problems? Are the resources readily available? If not, how might they be secured? What role can the nurse assume in facilitating the family's coping efforts with regard to each problem?

lem sometime after his first birthday. He is now two months old.

Sara Cooper, the assigned community health nurse, is familiar with the Riveras' neighborhood. It is part of a working-class community of small houses, many of which are lived in by their owners. Originally the neighborhood was largely Italian, but it is now primarily Puerto Rican. A Roman Catholic church with its associated elementary school, as well as shops and other small

ECO-MAP
Name
Date
Social welfare
Work
Health care
Church
Extended family
Family or household
Recreation
Recreation
Extended family
Friends
School
Fill in connections where they exist.
Indicate nature of connections with a descriptive word or by drawing different kinds of lines;
for strong, for tenuous, for stressful.
Draw arrows along lines to signify flow of energy, resources, etc.
Identify significant people and fill in empty circles as needed.

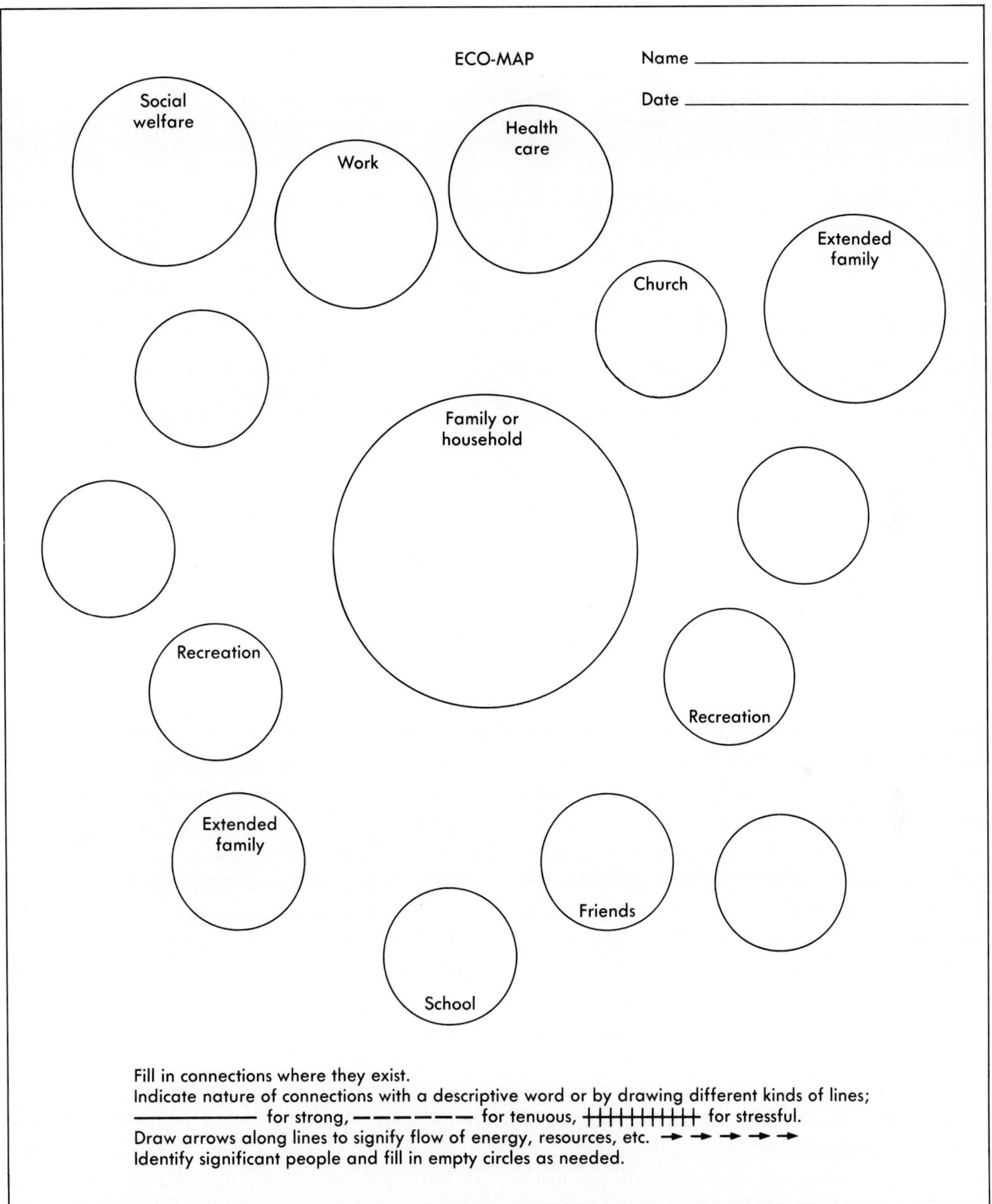

FIG. 12-1. Eco-Map. Diagrammatic assessment of family relationship. (From Hartman A: In Compton BR and Galaway B, editors: Social work processes, Homewood, Ill, 1984, Dorsey Press.)

Unit	Life cycle stage	Stage-related tasks	Problems in task performance	Resources available or needed
Family				
Member 1				
Member 2				
Member 3				
Member 4				
Member 5				

FIG. 12-2. Life cycle form.

businesses, are scattered throughout the district. A neighborhood health center has been in operation for the last year and provides well baby services for those who wish to use them.

Sara finds the Riveras living with Rosa's parents, Mr. and Mrs. Santos, in a two-story family dwelling, their grocery business occupying most of the first floor. Rosa is at home with the baby, her mother, and her maternal grandmother, Mrs. Morales. On preliminary examination, Luis appears to have good color and Rosa reports that he is sleeping well and slowly gaining weight. However, Mrs. Santos breaks in to say that her daughter is still clumsy about handling the baby and that she and Rosa have agreed that she (Mrs. Santos) would take major responsibility for Luis while Rosa does most of the housework and begins looking for a job.

During the remainder of the visit the nurse discusses their routines with regard to the baby's care, learns that Luis is scheduled for a checkup at the health center that same week, and also secures the following information about the family. Carlos, 20, and Rosa, 18, are currently living with Rosa's parents because they are financially unable to live independently. There is also some indication that this is quite agreeable to Mrs. Santos, who pointedly states that Rosa is "her baby" and that all three of her other children are "married and gone." She says this despite the fact that the two boys, Felipe, 25, and Tomas, 23, live nearby as does Linda, 21, and all visit back and forth. The sixth member of the Santos' current household, Mrs. Morales, 80, Mrs. Santos's mother, has lived there since her husband's death in Puerto Rico a year ago. She has diabetes for which she receives insulin daily and has been told that it is important for her to observe appropriate dietary restrictions although she is resistant to doing so. However, the problem of most concern to Mrs. Santos is the fact that her mother "doesn't want to do anything or take care of herself anymore." She still tends to attribute this to her mother's response to losing her husband and to moving to a totally new environment. Sara, however, observes that Mrs. Morales looks frail and that she seems withdrawn and quite confused.

Even though the nurse recognizes that Mrs. Santos plays a pivotal role in this household, in which there is a deteriorating older member, as well as a fragile infant in need of attention, she decides that before she can complete her assessment, more information is required about Carlos, Rosa, and their plans for themselves as a family unit. She therefore arranges to visit again on Carlos' day off and at a time when Mrs. Santos has indicated that she normally substitutes for her husband when he takes an afternoon break from the shop.

During this next home visit, Sara takes the opportunity to meet Mr. Santos who has come upstairs to the family quarters for a quick snack while his wife is downstairs. She then joins Carlos and Rosa in the living room where they are sitting with the baby. While the nurse examines Luis, Rosa reports on the visit to the health center where she was encouraged by the physician's findings and pleased to have been told that obviously the baby had been receiving good care. Carlos was quiet during this interchange, responding only to direct questions.

Because Sara is interested in learning more about the Riveras and their life together as a couple, she redirects the discussion. Rosa takes the lead and the following information emerges. Her parents, who had been small shop owners in Puerto Rico, emigrated to America before she was born. The family had lived with her mother's sister Teresa, who had been in the United States for several years, until they had sufficient funds for a down payment on their current residence and business.

With some prompting from Sara, Carlos reveals that he left Puerto Rico with his parents when he was 14. He found that adjustment from a small Spanish-speaking Puerto Rican town to a large cosmopolitan mainland city difficult but managed to complete the tenth grade before he left school to find irregular work in whatever the market for unskilled laborers could offer. Most recently he has been employed as a laborer in construction, but previously he had worked part-time delivering groceries for Mr. Santos. During this period, he had met Rosa and they began dating.

Rosa, a bright and conscientious student, had completed the first semester of the 12th grade when she learned that she was pregnant. With encouragement and assistance from some of her teachers, she was able to complete the school year and secure her diploma shortly before her eighteenth birthday and the baby's birth. Both families were distressed about the pregnancy and exerted considerable pressure for the couple to marry as soon as possible. This is what Carlos and Rosa themselves wanted, and the marriage took place four months before the baby's birth. Despite the earlier tensions, Mr. and Mrs. Santos were fond of Carlos, believing him to be "a good worker" who would do his best to be a good husband and father. For his part, Carlos respected the Santoses, admiring their reliability in business and their devotion to each other. Things went quite well until Luis' birth.

At this point in the interview, the nurse notes that both Carlos and Rosa seem reticent about revealing more about their concerns. When she comments on this, Carlos bursts out that he does not want *his* son to have surgery. He believes that Luis' heart problem is "God's will" and that if he is to recover he will do so with God's help and the family's care. Rosa admits, tearfully, that she has also felt this way at times, fearing that the baby's defect represents a punishment for his having been conceived out of wedlock. On the other hand, she believes that the doctor "knows his business" and points out that he has told her that this kind of surgery is now much more common and much more successful than it has been in the

TABLE 12-2 Rivera Family Framing Composition

Name	Age	Sex	Relationship to family	Occupation	Education
Geraldo Santos	52	Male	Head of extended family, married to Inez; Rosa's father	Owner of small grocery	Not known
Inez Santos	49	Female	Married to Geraldo; Rosa's mother	Housewife and part-time clerk in family grocery store	Not known
Rosa Rivera	18	Female	Married to Carlos; Luis' mother	Housewife	High school graduate
Carlos Rivera	20	Male	Married to Rosa; Luis' father; son-in-law to Mr. and Mrs. Santos	Construction worker	10th grade
Luis Rivera	2 mo	Male	Newborn son of Carlos and Rosa		
Imelda Morales	80	Female	Inez's mother	Unemployed; occupational history not known	Not known

past. As a result, although she is still concerned about the surgery, she is currently much more worried about her mother's ability to continue to help her as her grandmother, Mrs. Morales, is needing more and more attention and care. Sara responds to the couple's distress by acknowledging their concerns. She recognizes that Carlos is not likely to be immediately responsive to a plan focused on medical intervention. Sara does, however, see reason to believe that, with some help, he is likely to be ready to invest in planning that centers on the provision of good family care for Luis. With this in mind she schedules a meeting for the very near future so that she can discuss with them ways of dealing with their concerns.

Later the nurse thinks about the family's situation within the context of their social class and ethnicity and prepares the following assessment summary.

Assessment of Rivera Family

Demographic Data

Family name: Rivera, Carlos, Rosa, and Luis
Address: 2530 Elm Street
Telephone: 562-5670

Presenting problem: Luis, newborn son of Carlos and Rosa Rivera, has been diagnosed as having a congenital ventricular septal defect that requires careful monitoring.

Family form and composition: The Riveras are part of an extended Puerto Rican–American family. The members of the family are listed in Table 12-2.

Family Life Context

The Riveras, Carlos and Rosa, a young, recently married couple, and Luis, their newborn son, live with Rosa's parents, the Santoses, in a working-class neighborhood on the north side of the city. Both are members of immigrant families, and with the exception of Mrs. Morales, the maternal grandmother, all are bilingual, speaking Spanish and English.

1. *Characteristics of housing.* The Santos' two-story home is well maintained. The family store is on the first floor along with a small apartment in which Mrs. Morales resides. The main living quarters, which include three bedrooms, are upstairs. In view of this, space appears adequate for the family's

needs at this time—the Riveras have their own bedroom and there is one for Luis as well, although he now sleeps in his crib in his parents' room.

2. *Characteristics of the neighborhood.* The neighborhood is an old one showing signs of both slow deterioration and recent urban renewal. Although the health center, small businesses, church, and school are within walking distance, private or public transportation is needed to reach hospitals and other public service institutions.
3. *Degree and type of interaction with systems in community.* Rosa and her mother bring the baby to the neighborhood health center, and the Santoses have a Puerto Rican family physician, Dr. Miranda, whom they see when they are sick. Although there are religious objects in the home, the families' degree of active affiliation with the church is not known.
4. *Social support network.* The Riveras rely heavily on Rosa's parents for support. Although other Santos family members reside in the neighborhood, and Carlos' parents live in the city, the characteristics of these relationships are not yet known. The same is true for any relationships Carlos and Rosa may have with peers.
5. *Delineation of problems*
   a. *Space.* Although there is sufficient room for all household members, some change in the allocation of space may prove useful. The Rivera couple might benefit from an opportunity for increased separateness from the rest of the household, while Mrs. Morales, whose mental alertness is diminished, can be monitored more easily if she is relocated in the main living quarters.
   b. *Social support.* The members of the immediate household rely heavily on one another for support, and it appears that Mrs. Santos will have increasing responsibility for the care of her mother. Therefore it seems important to determine whether she is willing and able to get help in managing this responsibility from her sister, Mrs. Santiago, and her other children.

Family Structure and Function

Only a beginning assessment has been done in this area. Some preliminary findings follow.

1. *Role relationships and functions* (Fig. 12-3)
   a. *Nurturing.* Mrs. Santos appears to assume this role with all members of the household (perhaps of the extended family?), although Rosa is struggling with taking on a nuturing role in relation to her son.
   b. *Sexual.* There has not been reason to explore this area thus far; however, Mr. and Mrs. Santos appear to accept the Riveras' sexual relationship now that it is legitimized by their marriage. There is no firsthand information from Carlos and Rosa themselves.
   c. *Economic provider.* Mr. Santos and, to a lesser extent, his wife perform this role for the larger household. Carlos has taken on the role of economic provider in relation to his wife and baby, although his earnings are insufficient for their needs at this time.
   d. *Stress management.* Although it is possible that other members of the household and of the extended family play a role in this regard, it would appear that Mrs. Santos takes major responsibility here with her efforts to balance the stresses of caring for her aging mother, relieving her husband's pressures in the store and caring for her infant grandson. It *does* seem that Rosa is also struggling with taking on some aspects of the role in that she is currently concerned with finding ways through which the pressures of Luis' and Mrs. Morales' care can be managed. She may also play a buffering role for Carlos in relation to health care

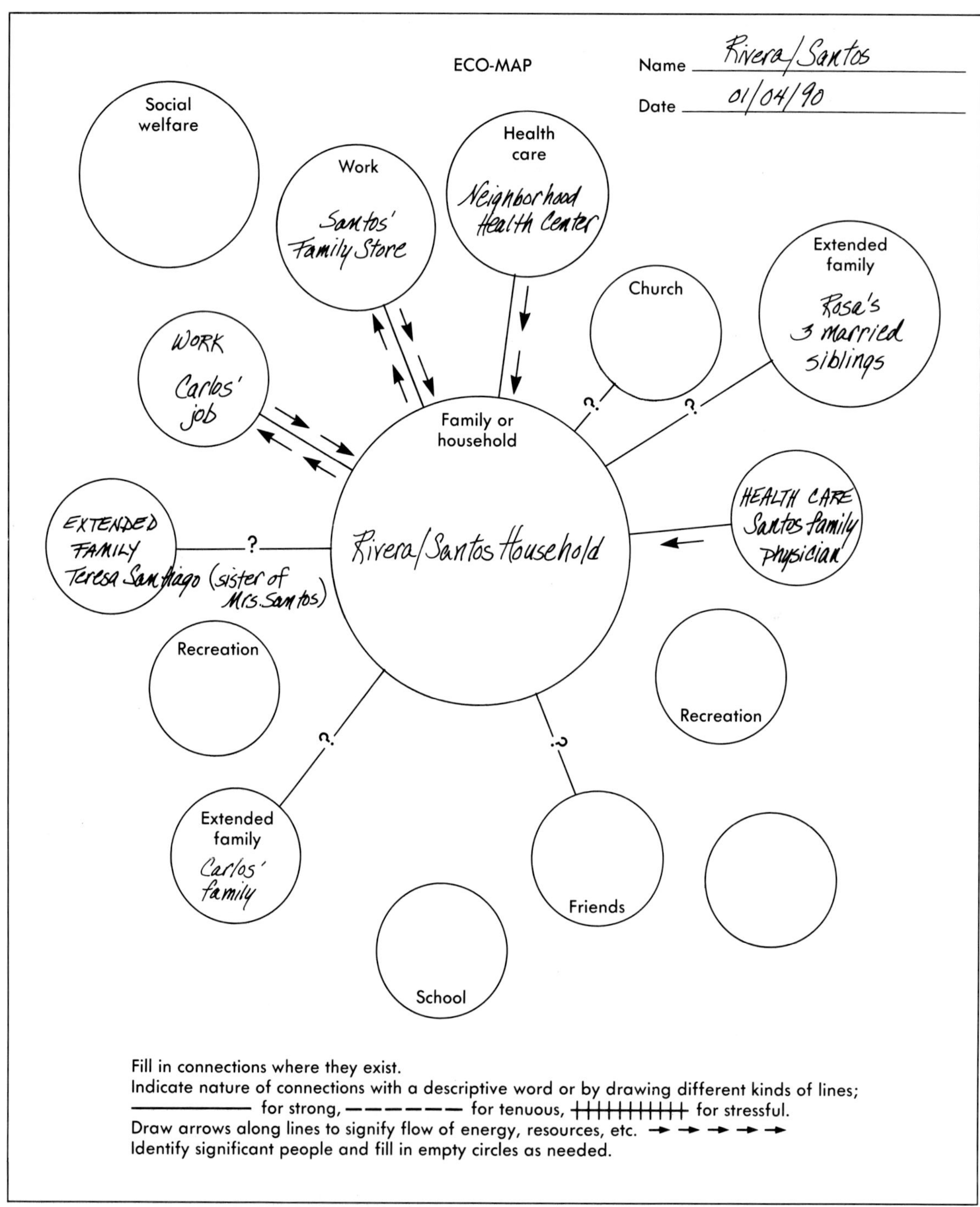

FIG. 12-3. Eco-Map of Rivera/Santos family.

personnel. It is important to note, however, that although there may be some issues as to how the stress management role is allocated, the family appears to be working at dealing with issues as they arise.

e. *Leadership.* Leadership tasks currently appear to be primarily carried out by Mrs. Santos although Mr. Santos may participate in ways that are not yet apparent. It is the Santoses who pressured for the marriage and made room for the young family in their home. In addition, Mrs. Santos clearly plays a leadership role where Luis' care is concerned. There is evidence, however, that Rosa is worrying about how she might take on more responsibility, and Carlos is obviously concerned about exerting more influence with regard to the baby's care.

f. *Child socialization and care.* All members of the household appear responsive to Luis socially and emotionally. They do such things as watch him, talk to him, and listen for his cries. It is, however, Mrs. Santos who takes primary responsibility for feeding and bathing him, tending to him at night if Rosa calls for help. Rosa shares the role to a certain extent under her mother's supervision. It would appear that Luis' development is being adequately fostered at this time.

g. *Home maintenance.* Housekeeping tasks are shared by Mrs. Santos and Rosa. The house is clean and comfortable, and there are no apparent safety hazards. The store is also clean and tidy, the exterior of the building is well maintained, and the lawn in the small backyard is regularly mowed. It seems likely that Mr. Santos and Carlos carry out the associated tasks.

h. *Kin and community relations.* In-depth data are lacking in this area. However, there is some evidence that Mrs. Santos is instrumental in maintaining ties with relatives. The family moved in with her sister when they first arrived. It is Mrs. Santos who does such things as make room in her home for her aging mother and care for her.

2. *Power dimensions*

   a. *Power structure.* Information regarding power allocation is incomplete, especially in the case of Mr. Santos, whose role is not at all clear. It is evident, however, that Mrs. Santos exerts considerable influence in household relationships. The Riveras, still largely accepting of their dependent status, have comparatively little power in the family.

   b. *Decision-making process.* Many aspects of the family decision-making processes are not known at this time, but it is clear that Mrs. Santos plays a strong role in decisions regarding Luis. At the same time, there is some question as to the degree of decision-making autonomy of Carlos and Rosa with regard to their own lives and that of their baby. It appears that the decisions essential to the maintenance of the family are attended to but that there may be some lurking tensions regarding how much the Riveras are free (or want to be free) to control their own lives.

3. *Delineation of problems.* See "Final Summary" at the end of this section.

Family Developmental Stage

This extended family is experiencing, concurrently, multiple life cycle phases: the Riveras, newly married (five months), are now in their early childbearing years, whereas the Santoses, having "launched" most of their children, are in transition to the later stages of family life. Pertinent life cycle data are summarized in the life cycle chart (Table 12-3).

TABLE 12-3 Life Cycle Chart

Unit	Life cycle stage	Stage-related tasks	Problems in task performance	Resources available as needed
Family	1. Early childbearing (accepting new generation of members into the system)	Adjusting marital system to make space for child(ren) Taking on parenting roles Realignment of relationships with extended family to include parenting and grandparenting roles Realignment and extension of relationship with the community to include educational and child care resources	The extended family arrangement both contributes to and hinders task performance: 1. The Riveras are assisted in parenting, but they do not take on sufficient responsibility to become competent. 2. Mrs. Santos helps with parenting others, but this is an additional responsibility when she is becoming increasingly taxed by caring for her mother. 3. The Santoses remain invested in their last child, and this may keep them from reinvesting in one another.	Two kinds of resources seem needed here: (1) Guidance in reallocation of roles and tasks. The Riveras need assistance in becoming more comfortable in assuming greater responsibility for Luis' care. Mrs. Santos needs assistance in giving up her parenting of Luis and assuming a less-involved, grandparent role. (2) Support. Mrs. Santos needs help in caring for her mother. Extended family members may be recruited for this work.
	2. End of launching (accepting a multitude of exits from and entries into the family system)	Renegotiation of marital system as a dyad Development of adult-to-adult relationships between grown children and their parents Realignment of relationships to include in-laws and grandchildren Dealing with disabilities and death of parents (grandparents)		
Rosa Rivera, 18	Late adolescence	Development of self-identity Preliminary work on: Differentiation of self in relation to family or origin Development of intimate peer relationships Establishment of self in work	Although still a teenager, Rosa has been thrust into adult roles, first wife and soon after mother—the latter requiring even greater maturity because of her infant's health problem. As a result, she has not completed tasks of adolescence and young adulthood. In addition, she is experiencing difficulty in taking on a parenting role.	Rosa needs guidance in: 1. Assuming and becoming more skillful in parenting tasks (Mrs. Santos may help in this), 2. Attending to her new marital relationship, 3. Developing or reinvesting in family and friend relations, and 4. Developing or reinvesting in work and other interests. A family service agency may help in this.
Carlos Rivera, 20	Young adulthood	Differentiation of self in relation to family of origin Development of intimate peer relationships Establishment of self in work	At 20, Carlos is involved in three life cycle stages. Although he has apparently differentiated himself from his own parents and has established himself in work, he and Rosa have not had time to develop their marital relationship before becoming parents.	Carlos needs support in: 1. Assuming an active role in the general and health care of his son, 2. Attending to his marriage, and 3. Evaluating the adequacy of his family and friendship ties. Rosa can play an active role here.

Inez Santos, 49	Mid-life	Refocus on and evaluate mid-life marital and career issues	There is some evidence to suggest that because of her heavy investment in family, Mrs. Santos is not able to give sufficient attention to tasks that will better prepare her for later life—that is, redefinition and reinvestment in her marital relationship, as well as clarification of her future life work.	Mrs. Santos does not define her heavy investment in family as problematic. Rather, it appears congruent with her values and definition of her family role. Should she acknowledge strain, the nurse could help her consider: 1. Developing or renewing friendships (the church may figure in here), 2. Reinvesting in her marital relationship, and 3. Developing or reinvesting in work and recreational interests.
Geraldo Santos, 52	Mid-life	As above	Mr. Santos appears to be heavily invested in his work. Although this is likely to provide a focus for his life from now to retirement, it may keep him from sufficient investment in his marital relationship and in family concerns, thus contributing to his wife's stress and leaving him poorly prepared for life after retirement.	It is unlikely that Mr. Santos defines his investment in work as an area needing change. Any moves on his wife's part to alter her role behavior and their relationship are likely to prompt changes on his part.
Luis	Infancy	Physiologic, psychologic, and social development, including bonding with parents	Luis' parents and grandparents are providing sufficient nurturance to allow him to master his developmental tasks. He might be hindered somewhat in this by his cardiac condition, however.	The family has adequate resources at this time to provide this infant with the necessary nurturance and care.
Imelda Morales, 80	Later life	Maintaining own functioning and interests in face of physiologic decline; exploration of new familial and social role options Dealing with loss of spouse, siblings, and other peers, and preparation for own death. Life review and integration	Physiologic and psychosocial factors have caused deterioration of Mrs. Morales' ability to carry out her social roles.	Mrs. Morales needs a physical and psychosocial assessment for diagnosis and treatment of her condition. The nurse can play an important facilitative role here in helping the family recognize her needs in this regard and in ensuring appropriate referral and follow-through.

Health Care Function

1. Health concerns and problems. The Santoses and the Riveras are concerned about Luis' health, his current care, the recommended surgery, and its outcome. Rosa and her mother are clearly concerned about the grandmother's deteriorating physical and emotional health, and it is likely that Mr. Santos and Carlos are also concerned to some degree or another. The family does not appear to define Luis as actively "ill" currently but appropriately view him as vulnerable and at greater risk of becoming ill than are other infants his age. It is not yet clear whether they define Mrs. Morales' condition as an illness.

   The nurse concurs with them in their identification of these as areas of concern but differs in that she believes Mrs. Morales to be ill and in need of a medical evaluation and treatment. She is also concerned with several other areas that the family has not defined as problematic per se. They have to do with tensions arising from family role relationships—the strain and conflict associated with Carlos' and Rosa's taking on their parenting roles, as well as the strain and overload associated with Mrs. Santos' multiple nurturing and caretaking roles.

   Because the changes in Mrs. Morales' behavior have come about following her husband's death and her move to the United States, the family has viewed them as normal responses to these major life events. Her increasing incapacitation is attributed to the normal aging process—"she's been through a lot and is getting old."

   As their current role behavior has grown out of their preferred patterns of interaction, it is valued as "how things are done"—parents are supposed to come to the aid of their children.
2. Management of health concerns and problems. The family understands and accepts that Luis' condition requires regular, careful monitoring and accepts the health center's role in this. Rosa and Mrs. Santos are ready to consider surgical intervention; Carlos is not.

   Although they have not identified Mrs. Morales as ill and therefore in need of care it is likely that they would consider a referral to Dr. Miranda, their family physician. (The health center might be acceptable to them as well. A geriatric nurse practitioner is available, and several staff members speak Spanish and could serve as interpreters for Mrs. Morales.)
3. Family resources. As previously noted, the family has adequate internal and external resources available to them to deal with their health concerns. The issue at this point is to help them identify the need for the most appropriate care.

Final Summary

It appears that there are several areas of actual or potential difficulty here. The issue of who is responsible for Luis' welfare and care is central. Mrs. Santos is ready to take it on, perhaps partly out of her need to keep her own "baby," Rosa, close to her. At the same time, it seems inevitable that she will be increasingly pulled in her own mother's direction should Mrs. Morales deteriorate further. Rosa is fearful about taking responsibility for her baby, yet she is also distressed about the growing burden on her mother. This may be true for Carlos also. In addition, Carlos has given evidence of health and illness beliefs that need to be dealt with if Luis is to receive needed medical treatment. A related issue is whether the Riveras are ready for more autonomy, and if so whether this might best be accomplished gradually through their continuing to live with Rosa's parents or whether they will do better if they move away from the family home. The nurse is inclined to favor their moving out but recognizes that she may be culturally biased in this respect, since this is what she would do. Therefore she is ready to consider that their remaining more intimately tied to the family may better meet their needs at this time in view of Rosa's fears, their inexperience as parents, and because of their precarious financial situation.

Although no one in the family has presented the problems in precisely these terms, it would seem that at least Mrs. Santos, Rosa, and Carlos are aware of the tensions or latent tensions associated with planning for the baby and with assumption of responsibility for his care. It is also likely that these three, as well as Mr. Santos, are all, at some level, concerned with issues relating to financial independence for the Riveras, as well as with the degree to which they should assume responsibility for their own lives as a family. Whether they would agree about solutions to these problems is another matter.

Currently it seems that, in their own ways, the Santoses and the Riveras are all working to deal with their problems and that they have found some solutions that are serving them reasonably well. Despite some strains, all members of the household (with the possible exception of Mrs. Morales) seem well-disposed toward one another and they seem motivated to deal with the difficulties. They appear ready to make use of the community health nurse as a resource in coping with the problems. It is also possible that family life education will be useful for Rosa and Carlos, and certainly support and guidance should be offered to them, as well as to Mrs. Santos who plays a pivotal role in the current management of the problem and who will be greatly affected by any changes the younger couple may make.

INTERVENTION

A careful assessment of family needs, capacities, and resources paves the way for the identification of problems and relevant goals for intervention. The knowledge and expertise of the nurse must be brought to bear in goal setting and planning interventive strategies. However, if the therapeutic enterprise is to have a successful outcome, it is essential that goals be formulated on the basis of client needs, definition of problems, and beliefs about what constitutes the appropriate remedy. It may also be tempting for nurses to assume a "lone ranger" stance in relation to intervention, believing that all responsibility for effecting change rests on their shoulders, when in fact the family is more likely to invest in implementing and maintaining the changes if it is involved in the actual process. By the same token, the nurse may look to external sources, failing to recognize internal assets that may be mobilized to serve the family both in its present difficulties and in times of future need.

Concurrently, nurses need to determine both what they have to offer in light of their role, knowledge, and expertise, and whether the goals call for interventions that go beyond their role and capacities. As with individual clients, a variety of roles and functions may be appropriate for use by the community health nurse in work with families. Among them are the following:

1. *Support.* Responsiveness to client distress and need that conveys the message that the professional can be counted on for help and concern.
2. *Education and guidance.* Provision of information and counsel that takes into account the client's knowledge, capabilities, and psychologic readiness.
3. *Role modeling.* Assumption of a stance or type of behavior that demonstrates a way of managing new or problematic behavior.
4. *Monitoring.* Careful review and evaluation of client circumstances and functioning to determine whether further intervention is needed.
5. *Facilitating.* Fostering the client's ability to make use of capacities and resources.
6. *Advocacy.* Acting in the client's behalf to ensure the provision of needed goods and services.
7. *Referral.* Linking client and appropriate service provider.

Referral is called for when nurses determine that clients require help beyond what the nurses can provide. The process involves more than merely supplying a name and address because a variety of factors may get in the way of a productive outcome. For example, the nurse may view a particular agency as entirely appropriate to a family's needs, whereas the family may see it as inaccessible or threatening. On the other hand, the family may follow through with the recommendation but be poorly received by agency personnel. The likelihood of success in the completion of a referral is contingent on the nurse's determination that the family concurs with the necessity and appropriateness of the referral. It is of course also dependent on the receptivity of the *responding* agency or agent, and it therefore behooves the nurse to ensure either that a satisfactory connection is made or that an alternative plan is instituted.

A further issue is involved here. Nurses have come to rely on other disciplines, not always recognizing or valuing the special expertise of other nurses. It is important that nurses broaden their perspective to include members of their own profession among those whom they define as competent practitioners. For example, couples in need of marital counseling may be referred, quite appropriately, to psychologists, social workers, or psychiatrists. However, clinical specialists in psychiatric and mental health nursing also practice in this field and should be considered when referrals are contemplated.

As noted earlier, evaluation is the last crucial component of the nursing process. This may imply that it is undertaken only after a nursing plan has been implemented, but in reality it is integral to the ongoing process. The adequacy of an assessment may be questioned as additional facts come to light. Goals may be revised and interventive plans and strategies may be redesigned in response to newly emerging evidence. It is of course essential to institute an *overall* evaluation of the family's situation and of the nurse's work with them to assess the effectiveness of the total process.

PLAN OF INTERVENTION WITH THE SANTOS AND RIVERA FAMILIES

On the basis of the problems in her assessment of the Santos and Rivera families, Sara Cooper developed the plan of intervention summarized in Table 12-4.

With this beginning plan in hand, Sara is in a position to shape her interactions with the Santos and Rivera families. All of it may of course be subject to modification depending on how accurately the assessment mirrors the actual situation and on the degree to which it has captured the family's readiness and ability to move toward the identified goals.

TABLE 12-4 Plan of Intervention for the Santos and Rivera Families

Problem area	Goals	Interventive strategies	Evaluation
Health and care of Luis			
Anxiety and underinvolvement of Rosa and Carlos	Rosa and Carlos take on more responsibility for Luis.	1. Discuss Rosa's uncertainties, resolving them where possible. 2. Concurrently, support Mrs. Santos in "teaching" Rosa (Carlos if he is receptive) to give daily care to Luis. 3. Model care of baby for Rosa if Mrs. Santos's teaching is insufficient. 4. Provide education and guidance for Carlos with respect to Luis' medical condition and the need for surgery as this draws closer. (Consider suggesting he accompany Rosa and Luis to the health center.)	1. Monitor the degree to which Rosa (and Carlos) are able to take on more of Luis' care. 2. Assess the degree to which Mrs. Santos allows Rosa to assume more of Luis' care. 3. Continue to evaluate the causes for Carlos' resistance to surgical intervention.
Overinvolvement of Mrs. Santos in Luis' care	Mrs. Santos gradually decreases her direct care of Luis.	5. Facilitate Mrs. Santos's gradual pulling back from involvement with Luis by acknowledging and commending her skills in teaching her daughter how to mother.	
		6. Monitor Luis' development, providing education and guidance to the family in this regard.	4. Assess Luis' health development and growth.
Lack of competence of Carlos and Rosa in parenting role	Rosa and Carlos become more effective in their parenting. Rosa and Carlos experience more gratification in their parenting.	Refer to strategies 1 to 4 and 6. 7. Facilitate Rosa's and Carlos' gaining pleasure in their parenting by modeling pleasurable interactions with the baby.	5. Assess the degree to which parenting provides gratification for them.

Continued.

TABLE 12-4 Plan of Intervention for the Santos and Rivera Families—cont'd.

Problem area	Goals	Interventive strategies	Evaluation
Lack of autonomy of Carlos and Rosa as individuals and as a couple	Carlos and Rosa gain some independence.	8. In the course of working with the couple, gradually elicit their thoughts and feelings regarding their goals and aspirations for themselves. 9. Develop objectives with them for increasing their independence should they wish to do so. (Consider, for example, their move to the downstairs apartment.) 10. Refer them for financial family life counseling, if needed and acceptable.	6. Evaluate whether it is appropriate at this time to develop interventions designed to assist Carlos and Rosa in developing greater autonomy.
Mrs. Santos' overinvestment in her parenting role	Mrs. Santos pulls back from her parenting role and begins to invest more in marriage, work, and friends.	Refer to strategies 2 and 5. 11. Support Mrs. Santos in identifying ways of gaining gratification in interactions with her husband, friends, and family.	7. Assess Mrs. Santos' readiness to decrease her investment in her children and reinvest in her marital relationship and outside interests.
Health and care of Mrs. Morales Deterioration in Mrs. Morales' physical and mental condition Increasing caretaking demands on Mrs. Santos	Mrs. Morales receives medical evaluation and recommended treatment. Mrs. Santos receives necessary support in caring for Mrs. Morales.	12. Help the family to identify Mrs. Morales' need for diagnosis and treatment. 13. Link family with appropriate health care provider. 14. Assist family in identifying what additional help is needed, as well as the sources that might provide support. (Consider such things as help from relatives and moving Mrs. Morales upstairs.) 15. Refer family to community resources if necessary.	8. Evaluate the family's readiness to define Mrs. Morales as in need of medical care. 9. Monitor Mrs. Morales' referral to ensure she receives appropriate screening and treatment. 10. Assess the family's readiness to identify that they need help in caring for Mrs. Morales. 11. Monitor to ensure that needed assistance is secured.

SUMMARY

Work with families is most effective when it derives from a thoughtful, theoretically based assessment that encompasses the total unit, and from a plan for intervention that is generally consonant with the family's perception of what is needed and what they themselves can achieve. In this way the nurse and family become partners in a collaborative enterprise.

QUESTIONS FOR DISCUSSION

1. What is the difference between a nuclear and an extended family?
2. Describe three theories of family interaction.
3. What are the developmental tasks faced by a family?
4. Give some examples of a nurse's role in anticipatory guidance and support of family functions.

REFERENCES

Aponte HJ and Van Deusen JM: Structural family relationships. In Gurman AS and Kniskern DP, editors: Handbook of family therapy, New York, 1981, Brunner/Mazel Inc.

Auerswald EH: Interdisciplinary versus ecological approach, Family Process 7:202, 1968.

Duvall EM: Marriage and family development, ed 5, Philadelphia, 1977, JB Lippincott Co.

Eschleman JR: The family: an introduction, ed 3, Boston, 1981, Allyn & Bacon Inc.

Friedman MM: Family nursing—theory and assessment, New York, 1981, Appleton & Lange.

Germain CB and Gitterman A: The life model of social work practice, New York, 1980, Columbia University Press.

McGoldrick M and Carter EA: The family life cycle. In Walsh F, editor: Normal family processes, New York, 1982, The Guilford Press.

Merton RK: Social theory and social structure, New York, 1957, The Free Press.

Minuchin S: Families and family therapy, Cambridge, Mass, 1974, Harvard University Press.

Minuchin S and Fishman HC: Family therapy technique, Cambridge, Mass, 1981, Harvard University Press.

Monrroy LS: Nursing care of Raza/Latina patients. In Orque MS, Bloch B, and Monrroy LS, editors: Ethnic nursing care: a multicultural approach, St Louis, 1983, CV Mosby Co.

Nelson M and Taylor P: Power relationships in marriage: the fine print in the oral tradition. In Getty C and Humphreys W, editors: Understanding the family-stress and change in American family life, New York, 1981, Appleton & Lange.

Satir V: Conjoint family therapy, ed 3, Palo Alto, Calif, 1983, Science & Behavior Books, 1983.

Tripp-Reimer T: Reconceptualizing the construct of health: integrating emic and etic perspectives, Res Nurs Health 7:101, 1984.

Watzlawick P, Beavin JH, and Jackson DD: Pragmatics of human communication, New York, 1967, WW Norton & Co.

THE origins of the home health care movement were in the nineteenth century when the early visiting nursing services were established. Home nursing continued as a small but important nursing role during most of the twentieth century. However, it was overshadowed by the more preventive care–oriented public health or community health nursing role. Now the pendulum has swung back, and the direct-care role of the home health care nurse is again being emphasized.

These changes started when Medicare and Medicaid were first implemented in 1965, but the movement escalated rapidly after 1983 when the payment mechanism for the federal government programs changed to a capitation plan. Hospitals were motivated to discharge clients much earlier, so there was a sudden, dramatic need for home health care. In addition, a concurrent movement in mental hospitals deinstitutionalized large numbers of clients. With this increased demand for services, new providers entered the field, including large corporations, and small companies run by nurses and others. Hospitals also extended their focus to include the care and supervision of clients confined to their homes.

The current emphasis on home health care includes another new feature. High technology is important in the care of many clients. This creates new challenges for nurses who are involved in either the direct care of clients or the case management of clients in their homes. The chapters in this section are designed to explain the changing nature of home health care and present an overview of the technology that is involved in that care.

Home Nursing

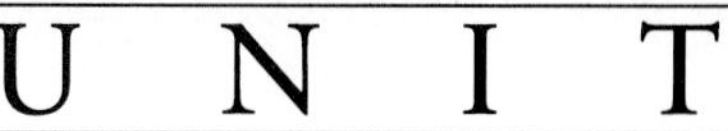

UNIT V

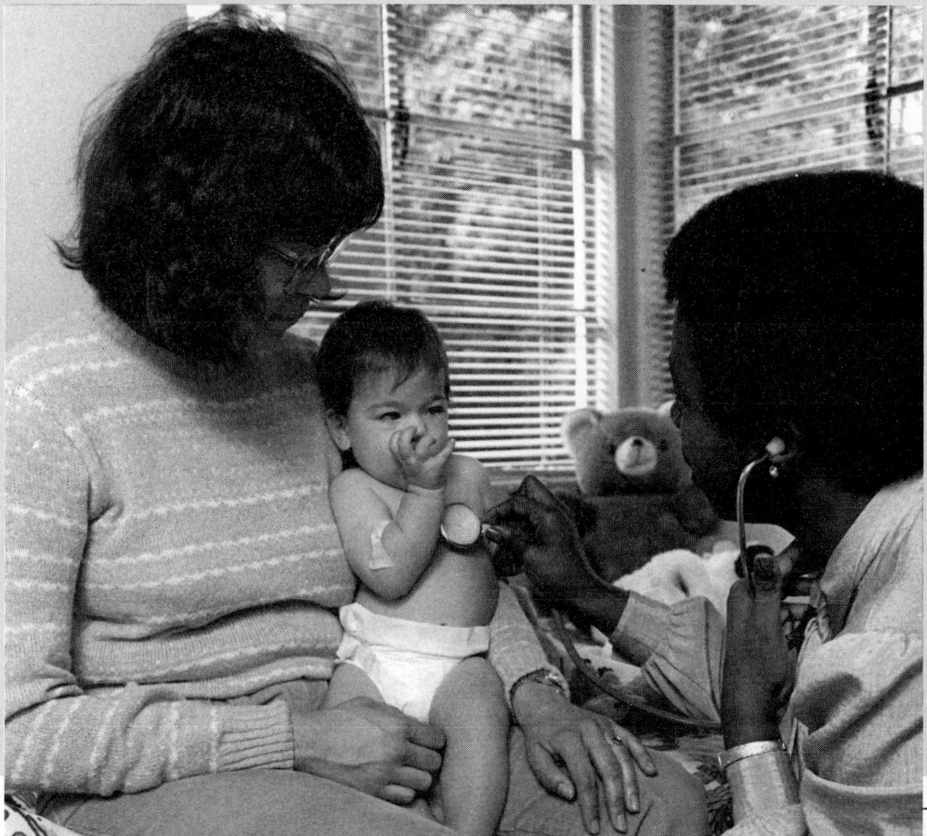

CHAPTER

13

Home Health Care Nursing: The Changing Picture

G. Lorain Brault

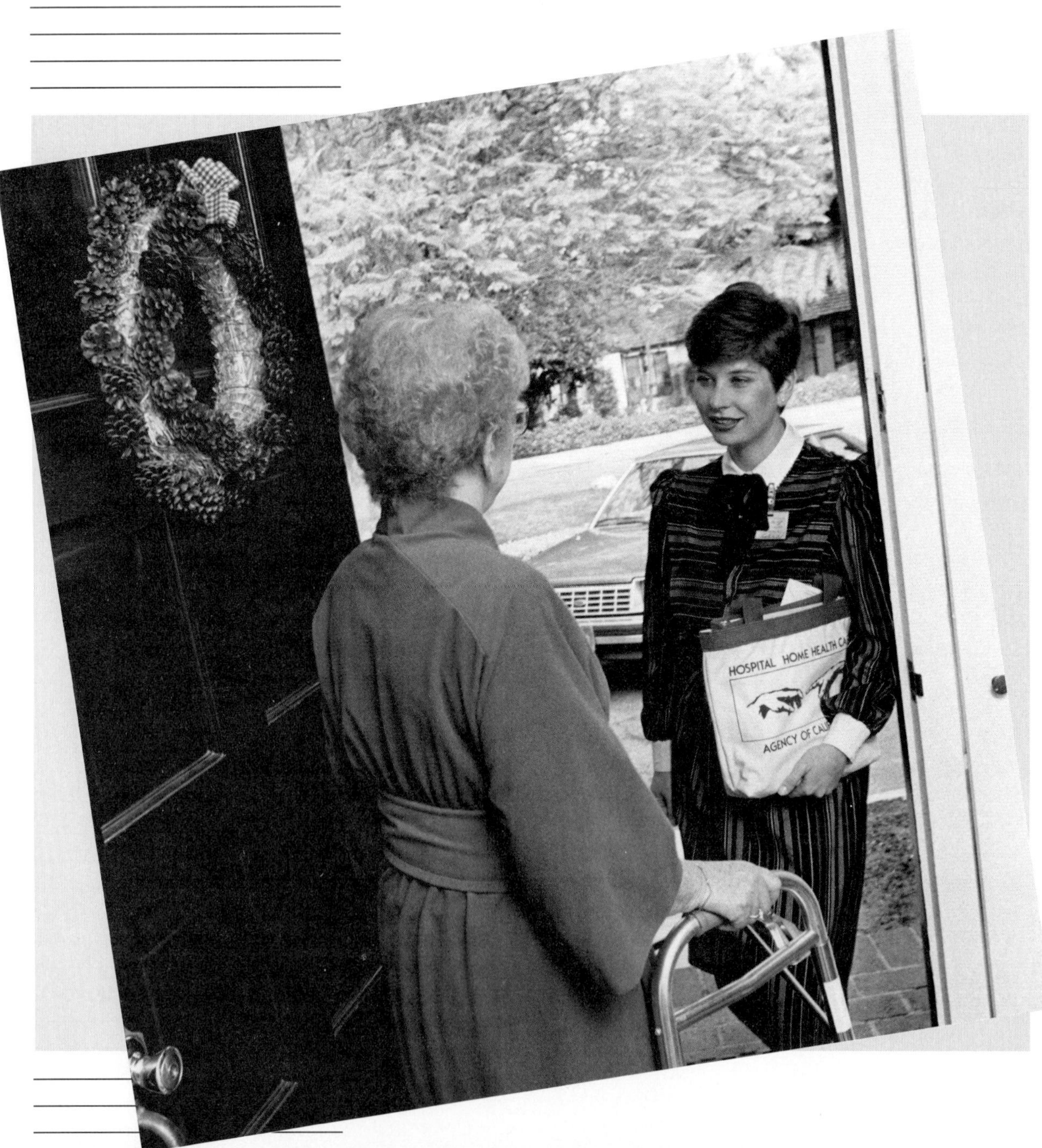

CHAPTER OUTLINE

Historical perspective
- Visiting nurse services
- Other historical influences
- Medicare

Causal factors in the development of home health care
- Legislation
- Escalating hospital costs
- Demographic influences
- Changing nature of home health care
- Technology and the growth of home health care

Home health care in operation
- Traditional services and the home health care team
- Hospice as a component of home health care
- Private service component of home health care
- Durable medical and respiratory equipment

Payment for home health care
- High technology service
- Federal government sources
- Medical insurance
- Private client payment
- Charity contributions
- Client eligibility criteria

Regulations and quality in home health care

Role of the nurse in home health care
- Staff nurse
- Clinical specialist and nurse practitioner
- Supervision
- Administration

Future of home health care
- Growth projections
- Providers of home health care
- Future role of the visiting nurse service
- Changes in government reimbursement
- Human immunodeficiency epidemic
- Future trends in home health care

Summary

OBJECTIVES

After completing this chapter, the reader should be able to:

1. Discuss the growth of home health care and its relationship to federal legislation.
2. Develop a rationale to support the standard: "The home health agency administrator should be a nurse."
3. Define the full scope of services available for home health clients and discuss the payment sources for each major service.
4. Evaluate the role home health and hospice service might play in the future of community health care with particular attention to U.S. demographic changes and the human immunodeficiency virus (HIV) epidemic.

HOME HEALTH CARE is an emerging community health care segment that has received a great deal of publicity and government attention during the 1980s. The growth of home health care has been extraordinary since 1972, with a particularly rapid growth spurt after the 1983 Medicare amendments. During the years 1983 to 1985, the number of home health agencies grew 47%. Since then growth has been slower, but it has continued. With that growth came increased government expenditures for home health care. However, the estimated $2.5 billion the government spent in 1988 on Medicare home health care represents only 3% of Medicare expenditures.

Home health care is defined as the provision of multidisciplinary health care to the sick, disabled, and injured in their place of residence (NLN, 1976). This home health care differs from the definition of community health care given by the American Public Health Association—a synthesis of nursing and public health practice applied to the promotion and preservation of the health of the population (APHA, 1980). Public health nursing has evolved primarily as a wellness model, whereas home health care has evolved as a medical-based model. Home health has emerged as the largest employer of nurses within the community-based nursing roles described earlier in the book. Despite the medical model, which includes nursing practice that is dependent on the physician, home health nursing includes clear independent roles and responsibilities for primary, secondary, and tertiary prevention for clients and families in the home setting (Orem, 1985).

There are several ways in which home health agencies are classified. One classification used is freestanding versus hospital based. Another classification is by type of operation and organization.

Common types of operation and organization include voluntary, official, facility based, private nonprofit, and proprietary. The primary example of a voluntary agency is the visiting nurse service. The visiting nurse service is governed by a board of directors from a local community and often provides service that is paid for by charitable funds, as well as by medical insurance or the client directly. An official agency is one governed by an official organization such as the public health department. Facility-based organizations can be governed by hospitals, rehabilitation facilities, or skilled nursing facilities. Private, nonprofit organizations and proprietary organizations are generally governed by their owners; however, proprietary agencies are profit-making organizations.

HISTORICAL PERSPECTIVE

Visiting Nurse Services

The history of home health care in the United States began with the visiting nurse service approximately 100 years ago. As has been discussed elsewhere in the text, the American movement, which began in 1885, was inspired by the work of William Rathbone in England. Pioneering district nursing programs in Buffalo, Philadelphia, and Boston developed independently and employed nurses to treat and instruct the sick in the home under physicians' orders.

In 1885, the Visiting Nurse Society of Buffalo was formally organized, followed in 1887 by the Visiting Nurse Society of Philadelphia and in 1888 by the Instructive District Nursing Association in Boston. All three organizations were originally supervised by nonnurses, but by 1900 the organizations had hired nurses to supervise the nursing staff.

The district nursing service in New York, organized to care for the sick poor in their homes, was the first service formed by nurses. Lillian Wald and Mary Brewster established the service in 1893 under the auspices of the Board of Health and coined the term "public health nurse" (Tinkham and Voorhies, 1977).

By 1900 there were 20 agencies similar to the visiting nurse services providing home care to the poor. By 1910, there were 1902 agencies that provided home nursing services (Dock, 1922).

TABLE 13-1 Medicare Reimbursement and Use for Home Health

Calendar year	Reimbursement (in millions of dollars)	Clients (in millions)	Average charge per visit (dollars)
1977	371	597	25
1981	860	1080	36
1985	2100	1450	54
1988 (estimated)	2516	1375	63

Health Care Standards and Quality Bureau, Health Care Financing Administration. Reported by National Association for Home Care, verbal communication, April 1988.

These agencies had grown in large cities and small towns with no apparent uniformity in their organization. They were financed by charities, public boards, churches, and voluntary boards. Some of the agencies charged clients set fees for service, charged fees based on ability to pay, or provided service at no charge.

Other Historical Influences

Another important development, as indicated earlier, took place in 1909, when Metropolitan Life included home nursing as a covered service in New York and gradually extended the coverage to many other communities. By 1920 home nursing service was being covered by a large number of other health insurance carriers (Mundinger, 1983).

The first hospital-based home health program began in 1946 when Montefiore Hospital in New York developed its "hospital without walls." This was the first multidisciplinary team approach and the first program to use homemaker paraprofessionals (Mundinger, 1983).

Medicare

In 1966, Title XVIII of the Social Security Act was implemented. This was a program of health insurance for the aged and disabled that became known as Medicare. This legislation probably had the most significant impact on the development of home health care in the United States (Table 13-1). Suddenly funding for home health care shifted from the private and charitable sectors to the third-party payment modes, with Medicare as the primary source of reimbursement. This legislation not only changed the method of payment, but also altered the types of services offered and dictated the types of agencies eligible for payment for services rendered to Medicare enrollees.

CAUSAL FACTORS IN THE DEVELOPMENT OF HOME HEALTH CARE

Legislation

Title XVIII of the Social Security Act, or Medicare, has two major components—Part A, which was intended to cover hospitalization and some hospital-related home and home health nursing services, and Part B, which pays for physicians, outpatient therapy, and other home health care services. Part B is considered a supplemental insurance to Part A and requires that enrollees pay a fee for coverage. When it was enacted in July 1966, Part A home health services required that the client had been previously hospitalized to be eligible for home health benefits. There was also a 100-visit limit to the Medicare home health benefit and a copayment required for Part B home health care services.

The Medicare legislation authorized the secretary of health, education and welfare to establish

TABLE 13-2 Growth of Medicare Certified Agencies

Type of agency	1982*	1983*	1984*	1985*	1986†	1987†	1988†
Voluntary	517	520	525	514	510	496	489
Combined	59	58	59	59	62	55	52
Official	1211	1230	1226	1224	1192	1073	1021
Rehabilitation facility–based	16	19	22	20	17	12	10
Hospital facility–based	507	579	894	1277	1350	1439	1454
Skilled nursing facility–based	32	136	175	129	117	97	102
Proprietary	628	997	1596	1943	1918	1846	1789
Private nonprofit	619	674	756	832	824	766	735
Others	50	45	21	4	4	1	1
TOTAL	3639	4258	5274	5983	5996	5785	5653

*Modified from Health Care Standards and Quality Bureau, Health Care Financing Administration: Growth of Medicare certified agencies, Home Health Line 10:51, 1985.
†Modified from Health Care Standards and Quality Bureau, Health Care Financing Administration: Growth of Medicare certified agencies, Home Health Line 13:436, 1988.

and administer the Medicare program. That department later became the Department of Health and Human Services (DHHS). Today the regulation of Medicare is handled by the Health Care Financing Administration (HCFA) within the DHHS.

There have been amendments to the original legislation every one or two years since 1966. It is important to note that a number of those amendments have significantly modified the direction of home health care.

In 1972 there were changes that deleted the copayment for Part B home health care benefit and required the setting of cost limits. These limits required Medicare to pay the cost of the service, the charge for the service, or the calculated cost limit—whichever was the smallest amount. This amendment also authorized homemaker demonstration projects for the first time.

In 1977 the Medicare and Medicaid antifraud and antiabuse amendment was legislated. It required disclosure of the ownership of the health care agency and uniform cost reporting and allowed HCFA to assign regional intermediaries to process Medicare home health care billings.

The Omnibus Reconciliation Act of 1980 brought the most significant changes in the direction of the home health care industry. It eliminated the three-day period hospitalization requirement for billing, as well as the requirement for a deductible payment. These changes allowed the home health benefit to become an alternative to instead of an extension of hospitalization. This same act allowed much wider participation for proprietary agencies in Medicare reimbursed home health care. Table 13-2 demonstrates the growth of Medicare-certified home health agencies from 1982 to 1987. It should be noted that the proprietary agencies began an increased growth curve after the passage of this legislation.

The Tax Equity and Fiscal Responsibility Act (TEFRA) of 1982 provided a prospective pricing system for hospitals. This system used diagnosis-related groups (DRGs) to set payments for Medicare hospital stays. The hospital is paid a fixed rate based on the client's diagnosis, regardless of the length of hospital stay, and therefore there is an economic incentive to shorten the length of hospital stay. Hospitals recognized the important role home health care could play in providing clinical supervision for those clients who might leave the hospital one or perhaps two days sooner than they would have before the DRG prospective pricing system was implemented. Table 13-2 also demonstrates the growth of hospital-based programs since TEFRA was passed.

A 1983 amendment authorized the study of prospective pricing systems for home health care. However, the implementation of demonstration projects for home health care have been delayed.

In 1985, legislation was passed that had the net effect of reducing home health care expenditures for Medicare (Rak, 1985). An upper limit was placed on the reimbursement levels per visit. Currently no home health care visit can be reimbursed for more than 112% of the average per 1985 visit cost.

The Omnibus Budget Reconciliation Act of 1987 contained new requirements for the review of home care quality. It clarified beneficiary rights and expanded the training requirements for nonlicensed home health care providers. It also established a toll-free hotline for complaints regarding home health care providers.

The Medicare Catastrophic Act of 1988 expanded the visits that could be reimbursed to cover home visits made seven days per week for 38 days. It also added an intravenous drug therapy benefit and eliminated the 210 day limit for hospice Medicare service.

TABLE 13-3 Cost to Medicare by Type of Service

Type of service	Medicare cost (dollars)
Home care admission	819
Skilled nursing admission	1710
Hospital admission	3675

Modified from Health Care Financing Administration: Building a long-term care policy: home care data and implications, Publication No 98-484, Washington, DC, 1985, US Government Printing Office.

Escalating Hospital Costs

Hospital costs had been escalating at rates greater than the cost of living index for a number of years. For several years before the passage of the 1982 Tax Equity and Fiscal Responsibility Act, hospital costs were rising at rates exceeding 11% per year. In the fiscal year ending September 1983, the growth of the medical care component of the consumer price index rose only 7.5%. In the fiscal year ending September 1984 the medical care component grew 6.1% (Gallivan, 1984). Although the growth of medical care expenses has decreased, health care in the United States still represents $320 billion, or 10.5% of the gross national product. Approximately 40% of health care dollars are received by hospitals.

Costs per hospital stay are still exceeding $3000 (Hospital Trust, 1985). Table 13-3 reviews the cost per stay among the various types of care covered by Medicare.

This high cost of hospitalization has prompted not only the federal government but private insurance companies, industry (which often bears the cost of high health insurance), and the consumer to look for alternatives to hospitalization or ways to decrease the length of hospital stays. This trend has contributed to the growth of the ambulatory care industry and the home health care industry.

Demographic Influences

The growing segment of the population older than age 65 has already had an impact on the growth of home health care and still represents the majority of the home health care client population. Figure 13-1 illustrates the projected growth of the aged population. Although the population in general increased 9% during the last

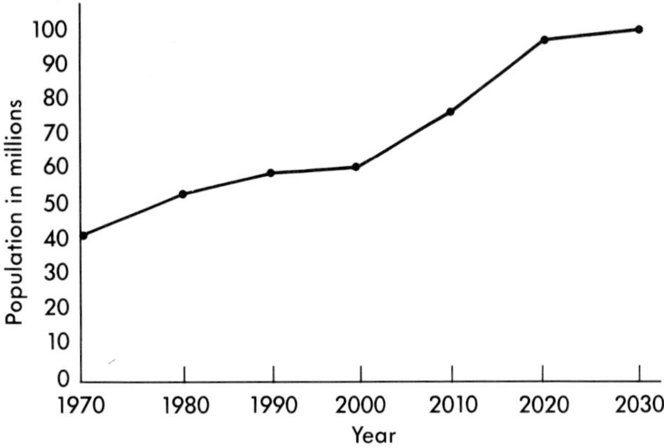

FIG. 13-1. Population growth for persons aged 55 years and older. (Modified from US Department of Commerce, Bureau of Census.)

10 years, the population older than age 85 increased by more than 50% (Halmandaris, 1985).

The elderly population is growing and becoming a more knowledgeable consumer group. There is no question that the elderly and their families prefer home health care to a nursing home. This was validated in a public opinion survey completed in 1985 that found that 72% of respondents preferred home care to a nursing home (Cetron, 1985). More elderly couples are living independently but require assistance when their spouse becomes temporarily ill and homebound.

Changing Nature of Home Health Care

Home health care has developed many faces during the last 15 years. The most common term used to describe home health care until the early 1980s was "fragmented." The traditional agencies provide medical treatments in the home. Staffs include nursing personnel with fewer services being provided by rehabilitation therapists. The traditional agency also provides home health aides when ordered by physicians. Until the legislative changes discussed earlier in this chapter, these agencies were primarily voluntary and official agencies. They received payments from Medicare and insurance companies, client private payments, and charitable donations for service to those unable to pay.

Another home care service segment comprises those proprietary agencies providing home health services not paid for by Medicare, such as private duty nursing in the home and homemaking services. These services are paid for primarily directly by the client, although some private duty nursing is paid for by medical insurance. Still another fragment of home health care service is the durable medical equipment (DME) companies. These companies provide beds, wheelchairs, walkers, and other medical equipment needed by the client in the home and were paid by insurance companies, Medicare Part B, and private clients. Some of the DME companies also provided respiratory and oxygen equipment in the home, but other companies were set up to supply only respiratory equipment and oxygen for the home.

The newest entrants in the already confused home health care business are the companies who supply only enteral and parenteral nutrition service, intravenous therapy service, or both, which are primarily paid for by Medicare Part B and medical insurance.

Table 13-2 noted that there were in excess of 5700 Medicare-certified providers of home health care, but when the whole spectrum of businesses is examined (including the medical equipment dealers that provide home care), estimates of the total number of providers exceed 10,000 (SMG-Louden, 1986).

With the large number of providers and the fragmentation of service, competition among home health care providers is growing as well. The growth of the facility-based programs have begun to erode the client base of the freestanding agencies. DME and private duty-homemaker companies have also begun providing the traditional services that were once the province of the voluntary and official agencies. Finally, the proprietary agencies with their significant growth and marketing emphasis were probably the first group

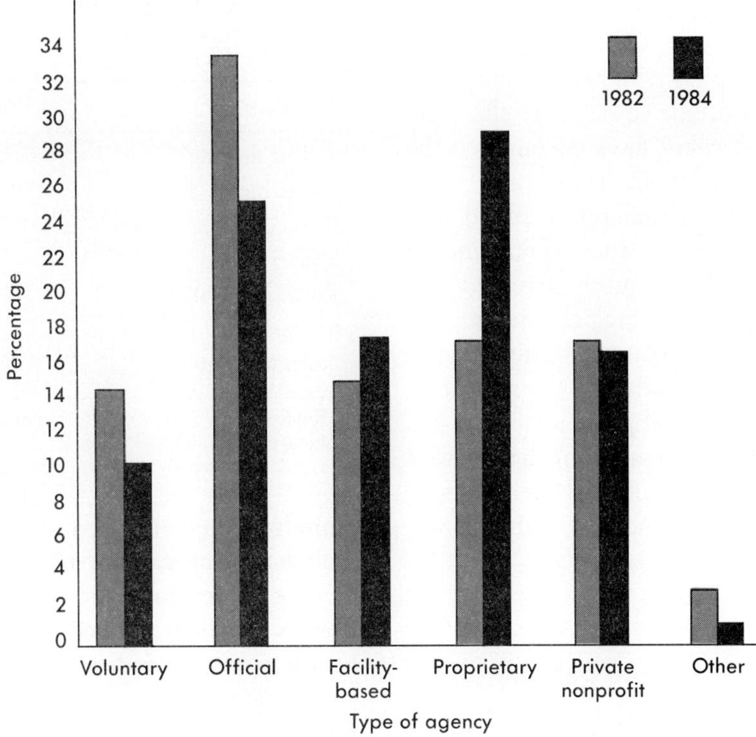

FIG. 13-2. Changes in types of agencies between 1982 and 1984. (Modified from SMG-Louden: Home care market atlas, United States, Chicago, 1986, SMG-Louden Ventures.)

to recognize that the market could best be served by providing *comprehensive* home health care services. The recent changes, including the growth and decline of various types of agencies, can be seen in Fig. 13-2.

Providing comprehensive services, which means traditional services, DME, respiratory equipment, and private duty and homemaker services, as well as intravenous and nutritional therapy, is changing that fragmentation in the industry. Although the proprietary agencies may have begun the trend, they are by no means alone. The facility-based, nonprofit and voluntary agencies have quickly recognized that to increase or maintain their market share, they must provide comprehensive service for the consumer.

Home health care by definition has changed from a periodic visit by a nurse or therapist to encompass an entire line of services and products provided to the client in the home.

Technology and the Growth of Home Health Care

The final causal factor in the growth of home health care is the recent emphasis on high technology services in the home. High technology service in home care today includes such therapeutic activities as parenteral nutrition, intravenous therapy, chemotherapy, home ventilator management, apnea and cardiac monitoring, and high-risk pediatric home care.

This high-technology home care segment has been encouraged primarily by the nature of the client who requires home health care rather than by true technologic advances. The technology is borrowed from the acute care setting and adapted to the home environment. Clients who are discharged from the hospital with more acute needs and physicians who decide to delay or eliminate hospitalization for a client have encouraged the technologic advances in home health care.

Not only has the high technology added new services, medical supplies, and equipment to home care, it may also require increased frequency of visits. The shift to high technology service and equipment has demanded that new or at least reoriented skills be added to the repertoire of the nursing staff providing the service to the home health care client. Many home health care agencies have begun hiring clinical specialists or even specialty teams to provide the high technology service (Weinstein, 1984).

TABLE 13-4 Services by Discipline Offered by Home Health Agencies

Discipline	Offered by agencies (%)
Skilled nursing	98
Home health aide	93
Physical therapy	80
Speech therapy	64
Medical social service	53
Occupational therapy	50
Nutritional guidance	23

Modified from SMG-Louden: Home care market atlas, Chicago, 1985, SMG-Louden.

HOME HEALTH CARE IN OPERATION

Traditional Services and the Home Health Care Team

Regardless of the auspices of the agency, whether voluntary, hospital-based, or any other type of agency, a core of services are generally provided by any home health care agency following a physician-approved plan of treatment. These basic services include skilled nursing, home health aide service, physical therapy, occupational therapy, speech pathology, and medical social service. These services may be provided by full-time or part-time staff of the agency or by independent professional contractors. Table 13-4 illustrates the percentage of agencies offering the various types of basic services. It should be noted that more than 80% of agencies provide skilled nursing and home health aide and physical therapy services.

Skilled nursing care includes assessment, treatment, client and family education, evaluation, and coordination of all client services by registered nurses. Skilled nursing uses the nursing process, which includes assessment, nursing diagnosis, planning, intervention, and evaluation when providing nursing care. A physician-approved plan of care is developed to direct the home health client's medical regimen, however, the home health nurse has independent responsibilities for providing necessary primary, secondary, and tertiary prevention for clients. Certain levels of skilled nursing care may be provided by the licensed practical nurse or the vocational nurse under the supervision of a registered nurse.

Home health aide service is provided under the supervision of a registered nurse or in some situations a therapist. The home health aide assists clients with activities, therapeutic exercises, and limited homemaking duties such as meal preparation.

Physical therapy is provided to evaluate the client's neuromuscular and functional abilities and to initiate treatment to relieve pain, develop or restore function, or to prevent disability. It is an excellent example of tertiary prevention in home health service.

Occupational therapy is provided to help clients develop or maintain the ability to perform ADLs. This may include adapting the environment to make daily activities easier.

Speech pathologists provide therapy for clients who have developmental or organic origin communication disorders. These disorders may relate

TABLE 13-5 Medicare Hospice Program Data

Month/year	Number of facilities	Number of admissions	Dollars (in millions of dollars)
9/84	119	2,098	3.5
9/85	233	14,874	33.8
10/86	279	34,865	102.2
10/87	417	91,475	278.3

Modified from Background material and data on programs within the jurisdiction of the Committee on Ways and Means, Home Health Line 13:177, 1988.

to the areas of speech, language, or hearing, as well as swallowing disorders, which are often a sequela of cerebrovascular accidents.

Social service is provided to assist clients in coping with illness-related social, mental, emotional, or financial problems. This service may be in the form of direct counseling or referral to appropriate community referral sources.

In addition to the basic services, there are other types of activities that may be provided in the traditional home health agency, such as nutritional counseling and providing medical supplies, laboratory services, home-delivered meals, transportation, and volunteer visitors.

Hospice as a Component of Home Health Care

A hospice specializes in the care of the terminally ill. Although there are freestanding and facility-based hospices, many are associated with home care programs. They are commonly associated with visiting nurse services and agencies under the auspices of religious organizations. These programs vary in nature but are usually designed to help the client and the family cope with the last few months of life. Emphasis is placed on symptom control and maintaining the family unit. Although inpatient acute care does occur, there is an effort to keep the client in the home or the freestanding hospice environment. Before 1983, most hospice care was paid for by charitable organizations, grants, or demonstration project money. Recently there has been an increase in medical health insurance coverage, and Medicare began reimbursing hospice care in 1983 under strict guidelines using a daily rate formula. Table 13-5 demonstrates the dramatic growth of Medicare-certified hospice programs showing an increase of nearly 350% in the first four years of the program. Even with that level of growth, there are still only 480 Medicare-certified hospices out of an estimated 1700 hospices in the United States (Rak, 1988).

In addition to the Medicare certification process, hospices can elect to be accredited. The Joint Commission for Accreditation of Health Organizations (JCAHO), the hospital accrediting body, began providing accreditation for freestanding and affiliated hospice programs. In April 1988 JCAHO reported that 355 hospice programs throughout the United States have been accredited under their stringent standards.

Private Service Component of Home Health Care

The private service component is defined as private duty nursing, homemaker services, or companion services that are provided in the home. These are the services that are not covered by Medicare and are paid for primarily by clients and families. In the case of private duty nursing, there are certain circumstances when the service may be paid for by medical insurance benefits.

Private duty nursing is performed by registered and licensed practical-vocational nurses and may be under the direction of a physician or may be provided at the request of a spouse or family member. It may be scheduled on an hourly basis, shift basis, or even a daily basis.

Homemaker service includes light housekeeping, meal preparation, personal care, and child care. These activities are usually performed one to three times per week on a two- to four-hour basis.

Companion service, sometimes called "sitter" service, is generally requested when a family member must leave a frail or confused elderly client alone for a period ranging from a few hours a week to a 24-hour day.

There are a number of services that are variations of the companion or homemaker service, including live-in service, sleep-in service, or respite care. Respite care is usually homemaker-companion service rendered for a weekend or vacation period for families with homebound elderly.

Durable Medical and Respiratory Equipment

Durable medical and respiratory equipment has been provided by equipment rental companies for many years but since the late 1970s has been incorporated by some of the service companies. This was particularly true with some of the proprietary and facility-based companies that decided to expand their home health care service line. Durable medical equipment includes such items as hospital beds, wheelchairs, walkers, canes, commodes, and other medical equipment used in the home. Respiratory equipment includes such items as home oxygen, intermittent positive pressure breathing equipment, and ventilators. There has been a recent trend in the home health industry to identify durable medical and respiratory equipment used in the home setting as home medical equipment (HME). HME is generally covered by Medicare Part B and in some circumstances by Medicare Part A and medical insurance benefits. Changes in Medicare reimbursement for HME in 1989 had the effect of decreasing the amount paid by the government programs for equipment in the home setting.

PAYMENT FOR HOME HEALTH CARE

High Technology Service

As discussed earlier in the chapter, high technology services commonly include intravenous and parenteral nutrition therapy, chemotherapy, ventilator management, apnea and cardiac monitoring, and high-risk pediatric home care. These services require upgraded skills for the home care registered nurse and the public health nurse. In addition, these services require that skilled nursing coverage be provided by the agency 24 hours per day. The home health care nurse must not only perform these treatments, but also be able to teach many of the complex skills to the client and the family of the client, since these treatments must be provided frequently. High technology services are frequently covered by medical insurance benefits, or Part A or Part B of Medicare.

Federal Government Sources

There are four government payers for home health care; they include Title XVIII (Medicare), Title XIX (Medicaid), and Title XX (grant-in-aid) of the Social Security Act, and Title III of the Older Americans Act (OAA).

Medicare legislation and amendments have already been discussed at length earlier in this chapter. Medicaid (known as MediCal in California) was enacted in 1965 and enabled states to provide medical service to low-income people. Its cost is shared by the state and federal government based on a per capita formula. Medicaid provides services for disabled, blind, and elderly persons and families with dependent children. Medicaid, like Medicare, requires physician certification but limits the home health care services covered. However, the homemaker or choreworker services are still not part of the benefit, and the payment rates for Medicaid are substantially lower than Medicare. Home health care services represent approximately 1% of the yearly Medicaid expenditures (Spiegel, 1983).

Title XX, grant-in-aid, was enacted in 1974. The legislation allowed states a great degree of discretion in providing programs of social and health-related programs directed toward more efficient functioning of the family or individual in the home setting. It included homemaker and choreworker services, home management, and home health aide service. Title XX eligibility requires that clients have low incomes with needs for specific social service or are members of certain designated client groups. States are given latitude with regard to payment for these services. Many of the services are provided free to the client or may be on a sliding scale based on ability to pay. Funding for the Title XX services is shared by the state and federal governments on a 25% to 75% basis. There have been federal expenditure ceilings set at $3.3 billion for 1985 and the following years. Home-based services represent a substantial portion of the Title XX expenditures (Spiegel, 1983).

Title III of the OAA was enacted in 1965 and provided several programs that related to home health services for persons older than 60 years. The programs are designed to help the elderly maintain an independent life-style. Home health components include the skilled services of nurses, therapists, home health aides, and homemakers, as well as health education, home-delivered meals, and home repairs. Additional services may include training of individuals to monitor health status and meals in congregate settings. Area Agencies on Aging coordinate funding, so services vary from state to state and area to area. The estimated expenditure for the program in 1985 was $670 million (Rak, 1985).

Medical Insurance

Private medical insurance companies are now covering home health care services. According to a 1987 report by the Bureau of Labor Statistics, the number of firms that had home health coverage rose from 37% in 1983 to 66% in 1986. It was also found that coverage for hospice care has been increasing since 1984.

Coverage for home health services varies significantly from company to company and often includes more than one type of coverage. The coverage may be major medical coverage for a post-hospitalization period; it may be a part of the basic benefit; or it may be a home health care rider. Most of the home health service plans include coverage for basic skilled nursing, therapy, home health aide service, equipment, and medical supplies. Plans are more variable on the coverage for high technology home health services. The plans require medical certification of need for service and may require copayments from clients. The copayment may be 80%/20% arrangement with 20% paid by the client. A number of insurance plans cover private duty nursing by registered or practical nurses but almost never cover any kind of homemaker or choreworker service.

In 1985 it was reported that 90% of Blue Cross and Blue Shield plans provide some type of home health benefit and a smaller number cover hospice care. It was also found that 47 of the 55 Blue Cross and Blue Shield plans actually contracted with a variety of types of home health agencies to provide home health service for their beneficiaries (Management Rounds, 1985).

Private Client Payment

There has also been growth in the number of clients requesting service that is not covered by any third-party payment source. The services, which are routinely of the homemaker-companion variety, are used in conjunction with covered services or may be arranged for individually. These services are paid for by the individual client or family.

Charity Contributions

In addition to the government funding certain services for the indigent and elderly, there are charitable organizations such as United Way and religious groups that provide funds to home health agencies and hospices. There are also private contributors who support fund-raising for home health agencies to help provide home health service for clients in need of service. These are clients who cannot pay for home health care or who "fall through the cracks" of the eligibility criteria for various government-funded services.

Charitable funds are usually provided for the voluntary and religious or other nonprofit agencies. Other agencies, not eligible for charitable contributions, often include a limited number of free visits or sliding scale visits in their yearly budget because of the nature of the home health care client and industry.

Client Eligibility Criteria

Since a large portion of the home health service is provided to the Medicare-qualified population, this section focuses on Medicare eligibility and compares other payers to the Medicare criteria.

The client must meet three requirements to qualify for Medicare home health benefits. The clients must require *intermittent skilled care,* the client must be *homebound,* and there must be a *medical necessity.*

The skilled care requirement has been expanded from the direct hands-on care provided by nurses to include client instruction when it is relevant to the acute diagnoses. The Medicare definition of skilled care is much more limiting than a usual nursing practice definition. Although assessment and evaluation are part of the process of a home skilled care visit, those skills must be coupled with the hands-on treatments and teaching to meet the skilled care definition of Medicare. Additionally, Title XVIII states that "illness prevention, health promotion, and maintenance care are disallowed even though of a highly professional nature" (Mundinger, 1983).

Intermittent is defined by the Medicare Home Health Agency Manual (HFCA, 1980) as being performed at least once every 60 days on a predictable basis. Although that is the literal definition, services are commonly provided once, twice, or three times per week. Since the more acute cases have been discharged to home care, it is possible to see daily or even twice daily treatments being approved by Medicare for a limited period and still meeting the intermittent criterion. The duration of the intermittent visit is not clearly defined by Medicare but has frequently been interpreted to mean four hours or less per day and less than seven days per week.

Homebound persons are not necessarily confined to bed but, according to the Medicare Home Health Agency Manual, have "a normal inability to leave home and consequently, leaving their homes would require a considerable taxing effort" (HCFA, 1980). This criterion has been generally interpreted to mean that clients require assistive devices and special transportation to leave home. It has been more tightly interpreted to mean clients can leave home only to receive medical care. By any definition, this homebound criterion significantly limits the number of clients who qualify for home care. There have been numerous efforts over the last several years to delete this eligibility criterion, but they have been unsuccessful (Committee on Aging, 1984).

The third eligibility criterion is medical necessity. This is not a qualitative requirement, nor is it related to the client's condition as were the previous eligibility requirements. It simply requires that the physician establish a medical plan of treatment, and that the plan be signed by the physician and reviewed with the home care professional staff periodically. This criterion requires that all services that are provided for the appropriately defined homebound client and that meet the skilled care requirement are under the direct order of a physician.

REGULATIONS AND QUALITY IN HOME HEALTH CARE

The home health industry has inconsistent regulation of its services. There are licensing laws that vary from state to state and exist in less than one half of the states. There are accrediting bodies that develop standards and accredit some segments of home health service. There is a certification process for agencies that want Part A Medicare and Medicaid payment sources.

Of the 10,000 or more providers of various types of home health services, some 5600 have obtained *Medicare certification*. This is a process that involves the preparation of standard documents, as well as an on-site visit to ensure that all Medicare standards are met by the agency. After the initial certification, there are generally yearly visits to ensure that adherence to standards and regulations is being maintained. The Medicare certification criteria are the only federal standards that exist for home health services, and this certification process is performed only for those agencies that desire Medicare-Medicaid payment. In 1986 the Sixth Omnibus Reconciliation Act extended the peer review system (PRO), which was mandated for hospitals, to include review of home health agency complaints. In 1987, the Omnibus Budget Reconciliation Act devoted a section to home care quality, however, the only substantive change in regulation was the mandating of a prescribed training program for nonlicensed staff who met minimum standards. It also established a hotline for complaints and questions about home health agencies.

Some states also require licensing of home health agencies. In general, licensing laws are similar to Medicare certification and both applications and on-site visits are performed at the same time as the Medicare certification. There are providers of some services to non-Medicare clients in the home who are neither licensed nor certified by the above methods.

There are three professional groups who accredit home health agencies. There is the voluntary accreditation that is performed jointly by the National League for Nursing and the American Public Health Association (NLN/APHA, 1976). Once this accreditation is achieved, it is granted for five years. In 1987, a new subsidiary of the NLN, called the Community Health Accrediting Program (CHAP), was formed and began a more comprehensive program of home health accreditation.

The second accrediting body is the Joint Commission on Accreditation of Health Organization (JCAHO). This accreditation is mandatory only for hospital-based home health programs if the hospital is seeking the accreditation. JCAHO also accredits hospice programs. In 1988 JCAHO issued new comprehensive standards for all types of home health service (JCAHO, 1988).

It should be noted that until 1989 none of these professional groups provided accreditation for the full scope of services or providers and that all the accrediting programs are still voluntary and expensive for the home health provider.

A third voluntary accrediting body is the National Home Caring Council, which accredits only the Homemaker and Home Health Aide services. This accreditation covers only the nonprofessional services.

In terms of quality control on an internal basis, there are two mandated committees that are required in the Medicare-certified agency. These committees include physicians, nurses, therapists, and community members. One committee, the utilization review committee, reviews medical records for appropriateness of the care provided. In addition, there is the professional advisory group, which reviews specific administrative and personnel policies, scope and coordination of services, and the yearly budget. This group then makes recommendations to the director of the agency. Beyond these requirements, agencies may or may not have additional quality control measures.

Quality assurance standards have been developed by the American Nurses' Association but have not been widely disseminated (ANA, 1986). There are also quality assurance models that have been developed and published for home health agencies, examples of which are the Florida Association of Home Health Agencies Quality Assurance Program and the Pennsylvania Assembly Quality Assurance Project (Spiegel, 1983). However, there is a widespread agreement that quality control and outcome measurements for quality assurance in home health care need to be promulgated and more fully used by home health programs.

ROLE OF THE NURSE IN HOME HEALTH CARE

Staff Nurse

There are a multitude of roles for the nurse in the home health setting, from the staff nurse who provides direct care for the client and family to the administrator of the home health agency.

The educational preparation for the role of home health care nurse should be a baccalaureate (NLN, 1976). The home health care nurse must apply the nursing process in the community setting and practice with a minimum of supervision. There is a need for more independent judgment and decision making than in most other types of community health nursing practice or institutional nursing practice. The home health care nurse requires skills from both episodic (cure) and distributive (care) models of practice. Home health practice, like all community-based nursing practice, requires skills in relating to many age groups and cultures with varying socioeconomic levels. Home health nurses must also be skilled in health maintenance and all levels of prevention. Finally, the home health nurse should be able to apply conceptual models that provide a focus for developing organized, systematic, and holistic approaches to provision of nursing service to the client and family. In meeting all of these requirements, the home health nurse needs to apply knowledge from natural sciences, social sciences, and humanities, as well as from nursing education (Gallagher, 1981).

Although the baccalaureate is the *ideal* educational preparation for the staff nurse in home health care, it is not always the level of preparation found in home health agencies at the staff level. Whether this is because of the shortage or maldistribution of baccalaureate nurses or by choice of the agencies, the outcome is that all levels of educational preparation are found in home health staff nursing practice.

Certainly, education is not the only criterion of quality service in home health care practice. Since the staff nurse provides direct physical care, as well as teaching and health promotion, it is critical that the nurse have strong technical and assessment skills. In this era of high technology care in the home, the staff nurse's skills to be broader in clinical scope than the community health nurse of the past. Nurses need to be as proficient in intravenous therapy techniques and problem solving as they are in nursing diagnostic skills and health education and promotion. The direct care giver must be able to adapt technical skills acquired in episodic practice to the less controlled environment of the home and family.

In addition to the role of direct care giver, the staff nurse in home health care may also be assigned the role of case manager. The case manager coordinates all services provided for any client and supervises any nonprofessional staff providing service to the client. The case manager generally coordinates interdisciplinary assessment, diagnosis, planning, intervention, and evaluation for their caseload of clients.

Clinical Specialist and Nurse Practitioner

The home health agency setting provides an ideal opportunity for the advanced nursing clinician to serve in a staff nursing and expert consultant role. Home health agencies, which carry large specialty case loads, may use oncologic, respiratory, maternal-child, and medical-surgical clinical specialists.

These specialists, prepared at the master's degree level in nursing, are used as direct care givers for the most complex clients within their specialty. The clinical specialist also consults with other staff nurses on clients within the specialty. The educator function of the specialists is used in program development and in service education for staff members and the community.

The geriatric, pediatric, family, and adult nurse practitioners (NPs) may also be used effectively in the home health agency. Although NPs' preparation is often at the master's degree level, they may also be prepared in a certificate program. NPs have advanced assessment, diagnostic, and management skills and serve as care givers for clients with diverse diagnoses and complex needs for care and education.

The enterostomal therapist (ET), who is a registered nurse with advanced training and certification, is frequently used in the home health agency. The ET may be a staff nurse or a nurse who independently contracts with the home health agency to provide ostomy and decubitus care and consultation.

Supervision

The size of the home health agency determines both the types and the number of supervisory roles for nurses within the agency. In larger agencies there may be a number of team leader-coordinator positions, whereas in a small agency this position may or may not exist. The team leader position is generally filled by a baccalaureate nurse. The team leader generally assumes both supervisory and case manager responsibilities. The number of cases is generally reduced along with the number of visits so that a portion of the team leader's time is spent in team supervision. The team leader should be able to apply theoretic concepts as a basis for practice decision and to assist other team members in evaluating client and family responses to the home health care team's interventions. The team leader often has the responsibility for scheduling and coordinating client service.

The supervisor in an agency may supervise the entire professional staff of a small agency or a group of team leaders in a larger agency. The person in this position is routinely responsible for supervision of clinical practice, providing orientation and evaluation of staff, and may also include responsibility for hiring and dismissing personnel. An overall statement of responsibility usually includes the carrying out of the qualitative and quantitative goals for clinical practice within the agency. The supervisor within the home health agency is more frequently a baccalaureate prepared nurse with a public health nurse (PHN) credential and home health or community health experience.

Administration

The director of nursing position, often expanded to the director of professional services, is the highest home health position that must be filled by a registered nurse according to Medicare regulations. Actually Medicare regulations are less stringent than many state regulations, only *preferring* that the nursing director is a PHN with experience. In practice, many states mandate or strongly recommend that the director of nursing position be filled by the baccalaureate PHN with community or home health experience or both. There are a few states that recommend that the nurse be prepared at the master's degree level to hold the director of nursing position. The ANA standard for home health care does require a professional nurse with a master's degree (ANA,

1986). The position is responsible for administration and direction of all client care activities and personnel activities and is charged with fostering the professional growth of the clinical staff.

The administrator, also known as executive director or president in some agencies, is responsible for the overall direction and administrative activities of any agency. This position has often been filled by a nurse, although no regulatory agency or standard of practice mandates a nurse as head of a home health agency. The ANA standards state a preference that the chief executive of the home health agency be a nurse (ANA, 1986). If nurses wish to continue to serve in this key role for decision making and direction within home health care, it will be necessary for them to become as well versed in administrative and business practices as they are in nursing theory and practice. As home health has begun to mature in the health care industry, it is not uncommon to see home health agencies being managed by administrators with business, public administration, health care, or hospital administration degrees, experience, or both.

TABLE 13-6 Growth of Medicare Certified Home Health Agencies

Year	Number of agencies	Percent change
1980*	2962	—
1982*	3639	22.8
1984*	5337	46.6
1986*	5994	12.3
1988†	5653	−5.6

*From SMG-Louden: Home Care Market Atlas, Chicago, 1985, SMG-Louden.
†From Health Care Standards and Quality Bureau, Health Care Financing Administration: Home Health Line 13:436, 1988.

TABLE 13-7 Projected Growth of Home Health Products and Services in the United States (expressed in millions of dollars)

Item	1983	1988	1995*
Total home health expenditures	6,307.2	12,207	24,850
Services	3,302.9	6,799	14,222
Durable medical equipment	1,007.0	1,755	2,650
Home health care supplies	1,997.3	3,653	7,980

Modified from Business Trend Analysts, Predicasts Industry Studies Division: US home health care markets, Commack, New York, 1984, Business Trend Analysts.
*Projected.

FUTURE OF HOME HEALTH CARE

Growth Projections

The growth of home care is demonstrated earlier in this chapter. A review of Table 13-2 demonstrates growth by type of agency. Experts predict that the number of home health care agencies will continue to grow through 1990, as shown in Table 13-6, but at a slower rate than the 1984 growth rate, which exceeded 46% in one year.

The number of Medicare-certified agencies reached a high of 5994 agencies in August 1986. Since that time the number of Medicare-certified agencies has declined a modest 6%. This slowing of growth and modest decline in number of agencies was due in part to consolidation of agencies in the industry. The slowing of growth was also due to Medicare Part A retroactive denials of payment, which forced some agencies out of the Medicare portion of home health care in 1987. The largest contribution to the decline was the proprietary providers. Hospital-based providers continued to grow even as the industry growth slowed.

In a recent study of home health care markets, dollars spent on home health care products and services doubled between 1983 and 1988 and are predicted to more than double again between 1988 and 1995 as demonstrated in Table 13-7.

Providers of Home Health Care

In the 1970s and early 1980s, there was a significant difference in the services provided by various types of home health care providers. Future providers of home health care, whether voluntary, proprietary, or facility-based, will probably be more alike. Balinsky and Shamus (1985) discuss the emergence of a new entity in home health care. They suggest that both major types of home care agencies, proprietary and voluntary, have evolved from their historical perspectives and are now capitalizing on each other's strengths.

The home health agency of the future will require all the caring skills and social consciousness of the voluntary agencies while developing the marketing and business skills demonstrated in the past by the proprietary agencies. The provider of the future will need to provide a broad range of services and health care products to a more informed consumer.

Both the voluntary and the proprietary freestanding community agencies already find themselves in direct competition for referrals with the hospital-based home health care providers. A 1985 study by the National Research Corporation indicated that more than one half of all hospitals offer some form of home health care service (Jensen, 1985). Home care needs are growing every year; however, there may still be a limit to the number of agencies that can provide efficient and cost-effective home health care in any community. This limitation may encourage the merging of freestanding and facility-based programs into larger home health care programs. Smaller agencies are more vulnerable to the problems created by dealing with the government payers. This may encourage mergers and purchases among home health care providers.

Future Role of the Visiting Nurse Service

The voluntary visiting nurse associations (VNAs) who pioneered home health care have demonstrated no growth in the number of agencies during the past 10 years. Although the VNAs still enjoy a large portion of the home health visits, they have been declining in dominance over the past 10 years. In a recent article a VNA advocate said, "VNAs have two choices. They must either prove themselves as efficient, effective providers of home care while continuing to develop innovative programs in the preventive health arena, or they must relinquish home care to others" (MacKenzie, 1985). In an effort to maintain its position in home care, the Visiting Nurse Association of America has recently been formed with goals for marketing, business systems, fundraising, and enhancing effectiveness. In April 1988 the organization reported a membership of more than 80 affiliate members. The role of VNAs as the dominant home health provider is being challenged, and its future role, after 100 years of service, will probably be decided in the next decade.

Changes in Government Reimbursement

Just as hospitals have had to readjust to the prospective payment system that Medicare mandated in 1982, home health care will be facing new and demanding changes in Medicare payment systems. Demonstration projects to test a number of new payment systems for home health care were to go into effect in 1989. The demonstration projects were temporarily delayed but will undoubtedly be completed and reviewed, and a new system of payment for Medicare home care will be mandated within the next few years. Whatever decision is made, the goal is to make payments prospective in nature and to decrease the amount being paid for home health care.

Another recent government action has allowed Medicare beneficiaries to sign up for health maintenance organizations (HMOs) instead of selecting the traditional Medicare program. The copayments and deductible payments are generally waived under these circumstances and the HMO receives 95% of the usual cost borne by the Medicare program. This shift to the HMO provider of health care also makes demands on home health care agencies. Home health care agencies will find themselves marketing services to HMOs who will pay for Medicare clients in HMOs. The HMOs may require home health care agencies to develop a capitation arrangement instead of the current fee for service payment arrangements. These changes in methods of payment and efforts to decrease the government dollars being expended for health care in general, and home care in particular, require flexibility and efficiency from future home health care providers.

Human Immunodeficiency Virus Epidemic

The disease that experts predict will consume huge amounts of health care dollars is named the human immunodeficiency virus (HIV) epidemic. The estimated number of cases of the HIV infection in the United States, based on data available, is between 1 million and 1.5 million (Report of the Presidential Commission, 1988). The role that home health and hospice programs play in providing posthospital care, alternate care, and support for dying HIV-infected clients is being defined. There is strong support from government, the health care industry, and the HIV-infected clients indicating that home health and hospice care may prove the most compassionate and cost-effective treatment in the HIV epidemic (Doste, 1987).

Future Trends in Home Health Care

The future of home health care is bright; substantial growth is projected for products, services, and number of agencies through the 1990s. The population older than 65 years, which will continue to use home health services, will soon be a large and powerful group of consumers. Technology is making more and more types of services available in the home. Naisbitt's theory of high technology–high touch, which suggests that for each level of technology introduced into society there is a corresponding human response, can reach its most sophisticated levels in home health care and hospice (Bartkowski and Swandby, 1985).

One significant blot on the horizon is the dependence of home health care on government programs to pay for a substantial portion of the home health care bill. Although there is a support from public and congressional groups for home health care expansion, this decade will not go down in history as one that supported social and medical programs. Current expansion and future expansion is probably dependent on the private sector, particularly the private insurance and HMO providers.

Home health care from birth to death will be the goal of future home health care. To achieve that goal, home health care agencies must continue to find baccalaureate nurses with strong community-based nursing background and high technology skills for home health care.

The nursing shortage that exists and is predicted to continue into the 1990s poses challenges to home health specifically and to the whole spectrum of community-based nursing providers in general. Home health nursing is an attractive field with both autonomy and control over practice and should fare well in the competition to attract nurses.

The nurses who do select home health as their career are faced with the same challenges as the home health care industry. Nurses are forced to change and adapt to continue to maintain control of client care and professional staff in home health care.

SUMMARY

The home health care component of the community-based nursing role has grown dramatically in the last decade. The government health cost containment agenda, along with significant demographic and epidemiologic factors, suggests that the growth will continue, although at a somewhat slower rate. Home health service will continue to serve as an extension of acute care, particularly in the elderly population; however, the greater growth is likely to be in home health as an alternative to hospitalization.

Insurance companies and HMOs are expanding their coverage to encompass home health and hospice. The government, on the other hand, is attempting to decrease its expenditures on health care in general. These trends along with the HIV epidemic suggest that home health will increase the amount of service to younger populations.

The community-based model for the baccalaureate nurse with knowledge of nursing theory and the nursing process, as well as practice in community-based settings, remains the ideal nursing practitioner for home health care.

QUESTIONS FOR DISCUSSION

1. Illustrate the influence of federal legislation on the growth of home health care.
2. What are the government agencies involved in the payment for home health care?
3. Should the administrator of a home health care agency be a nurse? Why or why not?
4. Why is hospice care a component of home health care?
5. Explain why the increasing number of AIDS cases will increase the demand for home health care.

REFERENCES

American Nurses' Association: Standards of practice for home health care, Kansas City, 1986, The Association.

American Public Health Association: The definition and role of public health nursing in the delivery of health care, Washington, DC, 1980, The Association.

Balinsky W and Shamus JN: Proprietary and voluntary home care agency evolution: the emergence of a new entity, Home Health Care Services 2:5, 1985.

Cetron M: Public opinion of home care: a survey report summary, Caring 10:12, 1985.

Dock LL: The history of public health nursing, Public Health Nurse 14:524, 1922.

Doste T: Going home to die; developing home health services for AIDS patients, Hospitals 61:55, 1987.

Gallagher BM: Nursing role in home health care. In Jarvis L, editor: Community health nursing, Philadelphia, 1981, FA Davis Co.

Gallivan M: Cost control's impact pervades '84 news, Hospitals 58:35, 1984.

Halmandaris VJ: The future of home care in America, Caring 85:4, 1985.

Health Care Financing Administration: Home health agency manual, Pub No 11, Washington, DC, 1980. US Department of Health and Human Services.

Hospital Research and Education Trust: Economic Trends 1:11, 1985.

Jensen J: Third annual national study of administrators by National Research Corporation, Modern Health Care 15:76, 1985.

Joint Commission on Accreditation of Health Organizations: Home care standards, Chicago, 1988, The Commission.

MacKenzie JA: Order out of chaos: changes in community and home care, Nursing and Health Care 6:37, 1985.

Management Rounds: Most Blue Cross/Blue Shield plans cover home care, Hospitals 59:64, 1985.

Mundinger MO: Home care controversy: too little, too late, too costly, Rockville, Md, 1983, Aspen Publishers Inc.

National League for Nursing: Accreditation of home health agencies and community health nursing services, Pub No 21-1622, New York, 1976, The League.

National League for Nursing: Baccalaureate education in nursing: key to a professional career in nursing, Pub No 15-1311, New York, 1977, The League.

Orem DE: Nursing concepts of practice, New York, 1985, McGraw-Hill Inc.

Rak K, editor: Home health line, vol X, Washington, DC, 1985, Home Health Line.

Rak K, editor: Home health line, vol XIII, Washington, DC, 1988, Home Health Line.

Report of the Presidential Commission on the Human Immunodeficiency Virus Epidemic, Pub No 0-214701:QL3, Washington, DC, 1988, US Government Printing Office.

SMG-Louden: Home care market atlas United States, Chicago, 1986, SMG-Louden Ventures.

Spiegel AD: Home health care, Owings Mills, Md, 1983, National Health Publishing.

Subcommittee on Health and Long Term Care, House Select Committee on Aging: Building a long-term care policy: home care data and implications, Pub No 98-484, Washington, DC, 1984, US Government Printing Office.

Tinkham CW and Voorhies EF: Community health nursing: evolution and process, New York, 1977, Appleton & Lange.

Weinstein SM: Special teams in home care, Am J Nurs 84:343, 1984.

BIBLIOGRAPHY

Bartowski JJ and Swandby JM: Charting nursing's course through megatrends, Nursing and Health Care 85:374, 1985.

Department of Health and Human Services: 1988. Secretary's Commission on Nursing: Interim Report, Washington, DC, 1988, The Department.

National Association for Home Care: 1985. Report No 139, Washington, DC, 1985, The Association.

CHAPTER 14

High Technology in Home Health Care

Mary Ann Ludwig

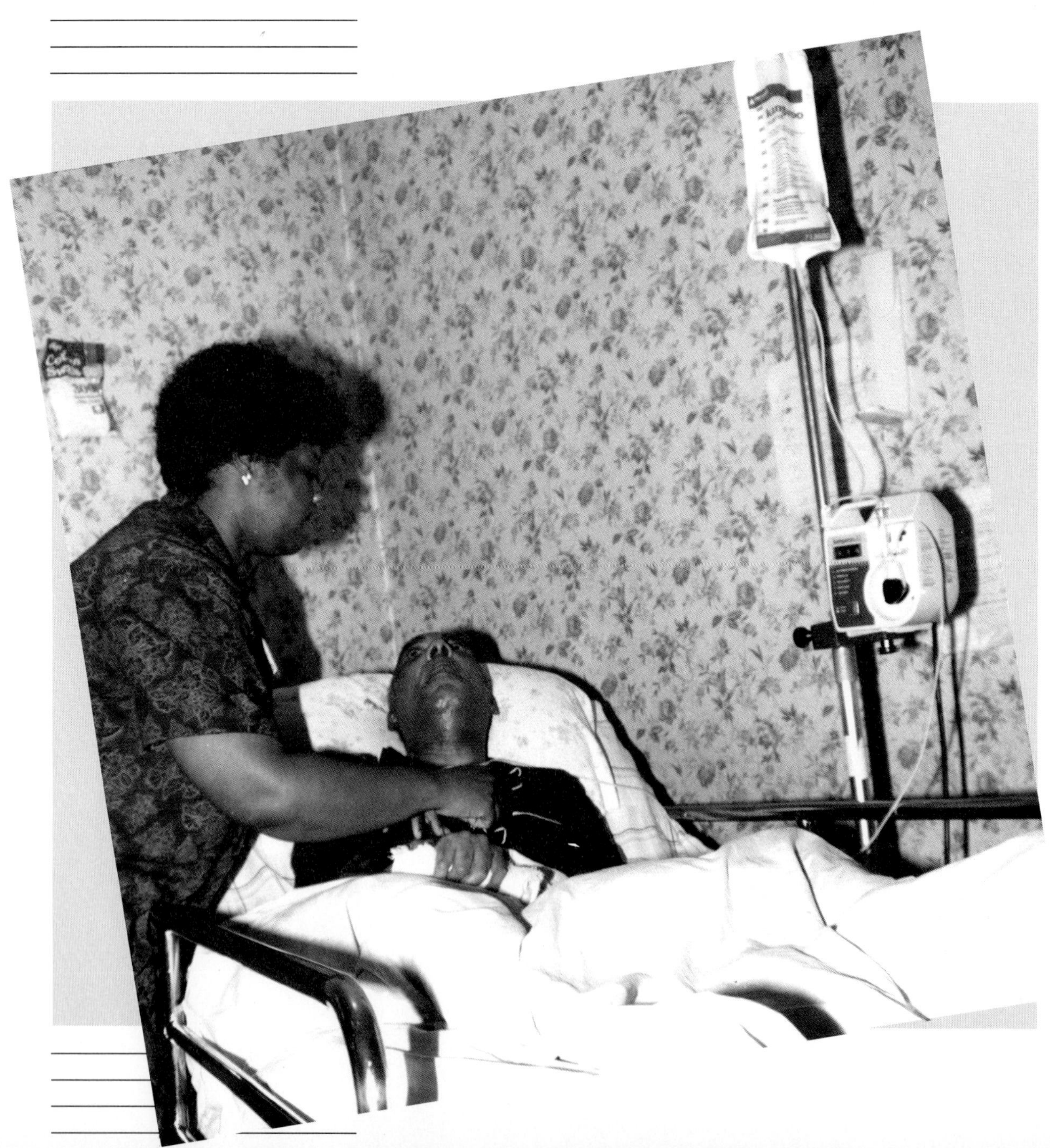

CHAPTER OUTLINE

Assessing readiness for high technology home care
- Medical stability
- Role of the family
- Home environment
- Financial resources
- Teaching considerations

Home health agency

Provider roles
- Vendor nurse
- Case manager

Complex therapies in the home
- Infusion therapies
- Infusion delivery systems
- General nursing responsibilities
- Teaching guidelines
- Antibiotic therapy
- Parenteral nutritional therapy
- Chemotherapy in the home
- Pain management

Phototherapy

Apnea monitoring

Enteral therapy

Mechanical ventilation
- Noninvasive negative pressure ventilatory support
- Invasive positive pressure ventilators
- General considerations
- Education for client, family, and caretaker

Summary

Appendix: Protocols for procedures performed in the home

OBJECTIVES

After completing this chapter, the reader should be able to:

1. Describe high technology home care.
2. Identify a variety of new roles for nurses working in the home setting.
3. Assess clients for eligibility for high technology home care.
4. Plan care for clients requiring complex therapies in the home setting.
5. Develop teaching plans for clients and families requiring high technology therapy in the home setting.

As indicated in Chapter 1 there has been a recent resurgence of home health care nursing. The goal of this nursing role is to deliver individualized services to clients and families in their homes. A further refinement of this role includes the delivery of high technology care in the home. According to Haddad (1987) the use of complex technology under the supervision of a physician and registered nurse distinguishes high technology home care from supportive, custodial home care. Advances in technology related to health care have led to a growing number of clients who depend on a medical regimen requiring complex equipment and skilled nursing intervention in the home setting. Examples of this high technology include use of ventilators, renal dialysis, home intravenous therapy, parenteral and enteral nutritional support, pain management, chemotherapy, phototherapy, and apnea monitoring in the home environment.

Along with advances in technology, changes within the health care system and in society have also contributed to the increased demand for home health care incorporating the use of high technology. The factors that have greatly influenced this change are the move by Medicare to a prospective reimbursement system and the advent of diagnosis related groups (DRGs). These factors have motivated hospitals to discharge clients sooner, leading to increased demands for home health care services, particularly for Medicare clients.

This state of affairs provides a challenge for nurses working in the home setting. They must not only provide supportive and custodial care to meet the needs of clients and families, but must also incorporate acute-care techniques in the home setting. This blending of skills provides a challenge to nurses working in the home health care field. The role of the nurse involved in high technology care centers on organizing and coordinating care. Responsibilities generally include gathering an accurate health history, assessing the client's physical and psychosocial needs, planning care, delivering relevant high technology nursing care, evaluating that care, communicating with other health team members, and educating the client and family in relation to care. Because of the sophistication of the technology now being used in the home setting, nurses with backgrounds in critical care nursing in either the intensive care unit or the cardiac care unit are being recruited to join the home health care team.

ASSESSING READINESS FOR HIGH TECHNOLOGY HOME CARE

As indicated by Haddad (1987), criteria to identify candidates for high-technology home care generally include medical stability, the desire for home care, the home environment, and the client's financial resources.

Medical Stability

The medically stable client must be ready to be managed without the need for constant physician involvement. For example, if clients are discharged from the hospital with a home care plan of antibiotic therapy, they must be past the acute phase of an infection; the white blood cell count and sedimentation rate may still be elevated, but their cultures are usually negative. If a wound is involved, it must be resolving itself. Clients' home pain management should be carefully adjusted in the hospital setting to a level that keeps them as comfortable as possible without being lethargic or in periodic pain. This careful adjusting of level of medication continues in the home setting as necessary under the physician's orders. Clients receiving hyperalimentation–parenteral nutritional therapy should be cycled and ready to withstand infusions. Usually they should be ready to receive the prescribed amount of fluid over a period of approximately 12 to 16 hours rather than a 24-hour period. Depending on desire of the individual or the family, clients may receive infusions through the night so that they have some freedom during the day or, if bedridden, may receive infusions during the day when a caretaker can monitor the client more easily.

Role of the Family

The desire for home care as expressed by the client must be examined carefully. For home care to succeed it is important that the family also expresses this desire and is willing and able to meet the needs of the client. Without strong support from significant others, high technology home care can be stressful and disruptive to a household. If family members are pushed into taking the client home early, they may be resentful and feel unable or unwilling to perform care as needed. On the other hand, the family may wish to bring the client home, but the client may feel more secure in the acute-care setting. Some clients do not wish to be a burden to the family or feel uncomfortable having family or friends performing personal care and are embarrassed, ill at ease, and anxious. Therefore it is essential to the success of high technology home care that both client and family are in agreement. If both the client and the family truly express a desire for high technology home care, the nurse must determine if they exhibit a readiness and ability to learn and understand concepts, side effects of treatment, danger signals, and what to do when problems occur. If the client and the family do not exhibit the level of intelligence required or are still adjusting to the impact of the illness or injury, the nurse may find they have an inability to retain information, lessened ability to follow logical progressions, and an inability to make comparisons and decisions concerning aspects of the disease or treatment. One of the most useful teaching approaches under these circumstances is to deal with issues concretely as they occur. Actually clients exhibiting these behaviors are poor candidates for high technology home care, since when sophisticated equipment and complex treatment regimens are integral to care, it is neither feasible nor advisable to deal with problems concretely as they occur. Clients and family must be prepared in advance to identify problems and know how to deal with them alone or when and how to quickly get the appropriate assistance. Secondly, compliance to the treatment regimen may also be jeopardized if the client or family has a history of substance abuse. This area must be carefully evaluated.

It is also essential to know if the client has a good support system. Are family members available and able to provide care? In lieu of family, does the client have friends or neighbors willing to assist with care on a regular basis? Is someone available on an occasional basis to provide relief for the regular caretaker? Without a good support system, high technology home care is in jeopardy.

Home Environment

When determining whether the home environment is suitable for high technology home care, one generally considers factors related to home safety, sanitation, heating and cooking capabilities, and physical barriers that may be hazardous to implementing care.

With these general factors there are several variables specific to high technology home care that must be addressed. They include desirable location of electrical outlets for installation of equipment, electrical wiring, space for storage of supplies, refrigeration capabilities for storage of perishable supplies, and location of the home.

Equipment such as ventilators, monitors, infusion or enteral therapy monitors, portable phototherapy units, and other necessary items are generally installed in the client's bedroom. If the bedroom is small or crowded with furniture and does not allow for good maneuverability of the client and easy access by caretakers, another room must be chosen. For example, the client's bed may be moved by the family into the living room or dining room as a temporary measure and the equipment can be installed there.

Location of electrical outlets must also be considered when positioning the equipment in relation to the bed or chair the client will use when various treatments are carried out. It is important that the equipment not be plugged into outlets already carrying such things as lights, televisions, or heaters. The fuse box should also be checked, and the family should know how to change fuses or trip circuit breakers.

One area of the home should be designated for storage of disposable supplies such as dressings, tubing, needles, catheters, and gloves. This area must be clean and accessible to the family and the caretaker while carrying out treatment.

Perishable supplies such as medications or nutritional solutions may need to be refrigerated. The client must have access to an adequate refrigerator for these supplies. Occasionally the family may make arrangements to borrow, buy, or rent a small refrigerator for storage of the client's supplies.

Location of the client's home is also an important factor in determining suitability. If the home is an urban high crime area, it may be difficult to find employees to enter the neighborhood on a 24-hour basis. Proximity to health care facilities should also be considered. Delivery of medications, supplies, and equipment and availability of the hospital or physician must also be considered (Haddad, 1987).

Financial Resources

Financial planning must also be considered. Although clients' financial statuses should not affect their right to high technology home care, it must be considered. It is necessary to know what reimbursement sources clients have available to them. These resources include private insurance, Medicare, and Medicaid. If clients do not have sufficient coverage, it must be determined whether they are financially able to pay for home care.

Teaching Considerations

Because clients or their families perform health care procedures in the absence of the nurse, client and family teaching must be an ongoing and integral component of high technology home care. The first step in the teaching process generally begins with discussion between the physician, hospital staff, and vendor or vendor nurse about the learning needs of the client and family at the time when eligibility for high technology home care is determined. To be eligible for high technology home care, the client, a family member, or a significant other must be able to learn and be willing to assume responsibility for care. Factors that may interfere with the teaching process include the developmental and educational level of the learner, cultural and language barriers, emotional involvement, and level of anxiety. All these factors must be considered and accounted for in the teaching plan. Once it is decided that the client will go home on the high technology program, the staff nurse, vendor nurse, and the home health agency case manager (see later section on roles) begin the educational process with the client and family in the hospital setting. Follow-up instruction is continued by the case manager in the home setting after discharge.

When developing teaching plans, home health care providers need to take into account the following general guidelines, which are based on the teaching principles discussed in Chapter 5:

1. Just as client and family involvement facilitates the assessment and planning process, including them in designing the teaching sessions increases the probability of learning.
2. Active participation enhances learning, and therefore learners need to learn by doing—handling equipment, returning demonstrations, and freely discussing feelings and attitudes toward performing care and treatments.

3. Careful selections of terms and wording of instructions to match the developmental and educational levels and cultural and ethnic origins are important considerations. If a language barrier exists, an interpreter may be needed, since written instructions should be in the client's and family's language.
4. To avoid overwhelming the client and family with too much information and too many facts and details, content to be learned should be broken down into small, manageable segments that allow clients to progress at their own rates.
5. Clients and family must be rewarded with praise and encouragement for learning. Positive reinforcement must be planned and must be perceived as a reward by the client.
6. Teaching sessions should not be rushed. Each session should be scheduled to accommodate the client, the family, and the attention span of the individual learner.
7. Whenever possible, environmental distractions, including noise, clutter, and interruptions, should be eliminated.
8. It is essential that the nurse be respected as a credible source by the client and family.
9. Learners must be aware of how important the lessons are. They must realize the importance of good hand washing and carefully timed treatments or medication administration and the need for good record keeping.
10. The anxiety level of the learners must be carefully assessed, and measures must be taken to help the client and family overcome feelings of helplessness, fear, and anxiety. Developing a good rapport between the learner and instructor can help alleviate anxiety and increase confidence in the learner.

Content to be taught is determined by the physical and mental condition of the client and the type and number of treatments and medications ordered. Therefore teaching content varies from client to client. Even though teaching must be planned to meet unique needs of each individual, consistency is encouraged wherever possible. Use of protocols related to specific treatments helps ensure that all caretakers function in a consistent manner and thus avoid confusion for the client and decrease the chance of errors and omissions.

Along with these general considerations that can be applied to all client and family teaching, whether in the hospital or home setting, the use of high technology in the home presents several issues that must be addressed by community health nurses. These issues include anxiety, fear, importance of schedules, good record keeping, and contingency plans.

Anxiety

The goal of the teaching plan is to make clients and their families as independent as possible. Once clients leave the security and support of the hospital, their anxiety levels generally increase. The family and client now must assume responsibility for care and treatments that were routinely performed by qualified health care workers. Clients and their families are alone in the home, attempting to give care and treatments that may be unfamiliar to them. The community health nurse must support them through this critical period to help them gain confidence in their own ability to handle the situation. All care and treatments must be demonstrated, and clients or caretakers should gradually be incorporated in the care under the direction of the nurse until they feel they are able to function on their own. How long this takes is determined by the learner's ability, background, self-confidence, and desire to become independent.

Fear

The anxiety felt by the client and family is often the result of fear. This fear stems from many sources. Many individuals are afraid of causing the client pain while carrying out treatments. They must be given good explanations regarding the necessity and value of the activities, how they relate to the client's well-being and comfort, and the best way to do things to avoid causing discomfort. Individuals are also afraid of doing something wrong. To help overcome this they need careful instructions, both verbal and written. As the caretakers grow more confident in their abilities, it is hoped this fear will be alleviated.

Another source of fear revolves around the use of needles and machines. This fear is real and stems perhaps from fear of the unknown, bad experiences with injections, lack of experience handling equipment, and lack of understanding how the equipment works. The nurse must spend time both demonstrating how to use the equipment involved and allowing the client and caretakers time to handle the materials, practice drawing up medications, and set up and handle the equipment until they become more comfortable and self-confident. Written materials should be left regarding operation of all equipment, procedures to follow, and most important, what to do when things go wrong.

Contingency Plans

Contingency plans are specific steps to follow when things go wrong. These plans should be developed by the nurse and family working together.

Caretakers and clients should be aware of signs and symptoms that indicate a change in the client's condition and should know a number to call and whom to contact to get help and advice when necessary.

Caretakers or clients should also be taught basic maintenance of equipment. This includes how to change bulbs and fuses, how to flush infusion lines, what alarms on the equipment mean, and what to do if they go off. They must also be able to recognize malfunctions and have a number to call for assistance and advice. It is also helpful if a nearby neighbor or other family member is on standby to help, give support, or relieve the caretaker when problems arise.

Schedules and Records

Because much of the client care is carried out by the client or caretaker in the absence of the nurse, it is essential that schedules be faithfully adhered to and records be carefully kept. The client or caretaker must be familiar with the schedule of treatments and the importance of adhering to this schedule. This schedule should be arrived at through consultation with all involved to be most efficient for the nurse, the least disruptive to the family, and the most beneficial to the client.

Caretakers must also be aware of the importance of careful recording of all procedures, client observations, medications, intake and output, and response to care. Whenever possible, flow sheets should be reviewed carefully with the client or caretaker. It is important that they be aware that careful record keeping facilitates good communication between the client or caretaker, the nurse, and all other members of the health care team.

In summary, planning is an essential step in caring for the high technology home care client. Goals of planning must be mutually agreed on by all clients, caretakers, and health care team members. The focus is generally on providing as much independence for the client and family as possible. Planning for consistency between health care workers and caretakers is facilitated by the use of protocols. Plans are most effective when clients and families are integral members of the planning team. Planning for the education of the client, family, and caretakers must be comprehensive and based on individual needs of all concerned.

If all the above criteria are met, follow-up nursing service is arranged with a local home health care agency to manage the case.

HOME HEALTH AGENCY

Home health agencies may be a government agency, such as the local public health department, or a private agency. Requests for services are screened to determine whether the agency can meet a client's needs. Criteria for admission to an agency are unique to each agency but generally address similar issues. First and foremost the agency must have qualified personnel to provide the type and amount of services needed. Since the advent of high technology home care, agencies have been motivated to hire nurses with backgrounds in critical care and form teams of highly skilled individuals to be assigned to clients with acute-care needs. Second, the client must be under the care of a physician who writes a plan of treatment for home care and is available for emergencies. If clients do not meet criteria for admission by a particular agency, they are generally referred to other agencies or facilities that can provide services needed. Once appropriateness for admission is established by an agency staff member during a home or hospital assessment visit, the case is turned over to a case manager.

PROVIDER ROLES

The major roles for nurses in the exciting new field of high technology home care are vendor nurse and case manager, each role having its own unique responsibilities and range of skills.

Vendor Nurse

The vendor nurse is employed by a company that provides drugs, supplies, equipment, or services to clients in their homes. Individual vendors may have a contract with specific hospitals, or the vendor may have contracts with specific home health care agencies. Health care reimbursement agencies may require that vendors be certified. Vendors offer 24-hour service and are responsible for delivery and inventory of supplies and installation and maintenance of equipment. Generally a vendor nurse in the employ of a vendor agency assesses a client and family in the hospital to determine whether they constitute an appropriate client for home care. If on assessment the client meets the necessary criteria, the vendor nurse begins teaching the client and family about the equipment and procedures while the client is still in the hospital. This is usually followed by a visit to assess the home environment to arrange for delivery of supplies, proper storage of materials, and installation of equipment.

Case Manager

A second role for the nurse in the delivery of high technology home care is that of a case manager directing a multidisciplinary team. As indicated in Chapter 2, the concept of the case manager developed in social work rather than nursing. However, it is now emerging as an important nursing role. Clients with complex health care needs may be assigned to case managers with the appropriate, highly specialized skills. These case managers oversee the care of a caseload of clients to coordinate services to them. Responsibilities of the case manager are diverse and comprehensive.

Case managers coordinate all services provided to clients by the home agency, including informal support, and use other community resources to carry out the agency's plan of care. They work with other health, social, and community organizations. They consult with the client's physician, social worker, and discharge planner. They are responsible for maintaining current clinical records, conducting case reviews, and completing required specific client records and reports as needed. They plan, integrate, and coordinate the services of the home health aides who in turn relay information necessary for service integration. Case managers are also responsible for ensuring that physicians are notified regarding significant changes in a client's status, and they carry out all specialized nursing interventions and teaching as needed (Visiting Nursing Association of Buffalo, 1985).

Assessment by the Case Manager

Once it is determined by the vendor or vendor nurse that a client is a candidate for high technology home care, the case manager assigned to the client by the home health agency also assesses the client and family to develop the plan of care. The information gathered is also used to identify the type of technical skills required and the number of nurses, aides, and therapists needed to meet the client's particular needs. The client and family should be included in the assessment and planning of care as much as possible to alleviate anxiety and give them as much control of the care as possible. Examples of assessment forms used for physical and environmental assessment are shown in Figs. 14-1 and 14-2. Assessment forms vary in depth and detail from agency to agency but generally address the same areas of concern, using a systematic approach to data collection. If the client is confused or incompetent, the nurse must rely on the family to complete the assessment.

Once all assessment data are gathered, they are analyzed to develop a prioritized problem list including the client's actual and potential problems. This is written in the form of a nursing diagnosis. In some agencies the subjective, objective, assessment, plan (SOAP) format is used.

Planning for High Technology Home Care

The goal of high technology home care is to help the client and family achieve as much independence as possible until resolution of the case through return to wellness, readmission to the acute-care facility, or death. Care objectives are developed that reflect the needs of the individual client and family, and interventions are designed to meet these objectives. Evaluation is based on predetermined outcome criteria related to the overall goal and each objective. The case manager develops and coordinates the care plan. Based on needs, appropriate referrals are made to other team members including social workers, physical therapists, occupational therapists, nutritionists, and home health or personal aides. Fig. 14-3 shows an interdisciplinary referral form.

Fig. 14-4 is an activity worksheet that is developed for ancillary personnel. The case manager goes over these activities with the home health or personal aide. All procedures are demonstrated and the ancillary personnel, the client, or the caretaker returns the demonstration in the presence of the case manager. All activities of the interdisciplinary team are coordinated by the case manager who in turn is responsible for all record keeping and communication with the physician and vendor.

Case managers may function as primary nurses or coordinators of a team. The team of nurses who care for clients with high technology needs may then facilitate the 24-hour care needed by these clients through weekly or daily team conferences. At these conferences the case managers review all high technology clients, noting progress and unmet needs. To ensure continuity of care, accurate and complete recording and charting must be carried out to provide information to all team members regarding clients' progress, changes in status, treatments and skilled care given, and teaching to family and clients accomplished. Fig. 14-5 shows an example of nursing

Text continued on p. 311.

VNA
VISITING NURSING ASSOCIATION OF BUFFALO, NEW YORK, INC.

NURSING REVIEW OF SYSTEMS

KEY:
Imp. = Impaired
N/A = Not Applicable

☐ INITIAL EVALUATION
☐ REACTIVATION
☐ ANNUAL UPDATE

BLOOD PRESSURE:			TEMP.:		PULSE:		RESP.	HT.:
Left Arm	Right Arm	Sitting ☐ Standing ☐ Lying ☐		Oral ☐ Axillary ☐ Rectal ☐	Apical	Radial		WT.:

	Yes	No	N/A
SKIN:			
Temp. Imp.			
Color Imp.			
Turgor Imp.			
Integrity Imp.			
VISION:			
Acuity Imp.			
Tearing			
Glasses			
HEARING:			
Acuity Imp.			
Discharge			
Aid			
MOUTH:			
Membranes Imp.			
Chewing Imp.			
Dentures			
NOSE/THROAT:			
Discharge			
Swallowing Imp.			
Trach./Laryn.			
SPEECH:			
Response Imp.			
Appropriate			
Comprehen. Imp.			
RESPIRATORY:			
Dyspnea @ Rest			
Dyspnea on Exert.			
Orthopnea			
Cough			
Sputum			
Lung Sounds: LUL			
LLL			
RUL			
RLL			
RML			
CARDIOVASCULAR:			
Pain			
Numbness - Feet			
Leg Cramps			
Pedal Pulses Imp.			
LLE Color Imp.			
RLE Color Imp.			
LLE Temp. Imp.			
RLE Temp. Imp.			
Edema			

	Yes	No	N/A
GASTROINTESTINAL:			
Masses			
Tenderness			
Bowel Sounds Imp.			
Ascites			
NUTRITION:			
Appetite Imp.			
Nutrition Imp.			
Hydration Imp.			
Fluids Balance Imp.			
ELIMINATION:			
Bowel Habits Imp.			
Bowel Control Imp.			
Diversion			
URINARY:			
Clear Urine			
Concentrated Urine			
Frequency			
Pain/Burning			
Control Imp.			
Nocturia			
Diversion			
REPRODUCTIVE:			
Breasts Imp.			
Vaginal Discharge			
Prostate Imp.			
NEUROLOGICAL:			
Affect Imp.			
Numbness - Hands			
Motivation Imp.			
Coordination Imp.			
S. T. Indicated			
P. T. Indicated			
O.T. Indicated			
M.S.W. Indicated			
HHA Indicated			

Fluid Restriction: ______

Special Diet: ______

ASSISTIVE DEVICES (LIST):

	GOOD	FAIR	POOR	UNAB[LE]
MUSCULOSKELETAL:				
ROM: RUE				
RLE				
LUE				
LLE				
Bed Mobility				
Transfer Ability				
Sitting Balance				
Standing Balance				
Ambulation				
ADL ABILITIES:				
A.M. Hygiene				
Bathing				
Dressing				
Feeding				
Meal Prep.				
Shopping				
Housework				
Laundry				
Telephoning				
Sleeping				

COMMENTS:

______ CARE PROVIDER SIGNATURE   ______ DATE

031083

FIG. 14-1. Assessment form. (Courtesy Visiting Nurse Association of Buffalo, NY.)

VNA
VISITING NURSING ASSOCIATION

ENVIRONMENTAL EVALUATION

PAGE 1 OF 2

AWARENESS OF DIAGNOSIS	PATIENT		FAMILY		MARITAL STATUS	S	M	S	D	W	ALLERGIES:
	Y	N	Y	N							

PRIMARY LANGUAGE	RELIGION	LITERATE		OCCUPATION
		Y	N	

HEALTH/COMMUNITY RESOURCES	ADDRESS AND/OR CONTACT PERSON	PHONE
Other Physicians		
Pharmacy		
Community Resources		

SIGNIFICANT OTHERS: Lives Alone [Y] [N]

NAME	LIVES IN		SEX		AGE	RELATIONSHIP	PERTINENT INFORMATION (HEALTH, PHONE, ETC.)
	Y	N	M	F			
	Y	N	M	F			
	Y	N	M	F			
	Y	N	M	F			
	Y	N	M	F			
	Y	N	M	F			

NEXT OF KIN	EMERGENCY CONTACT
Name	Name
Address	Address
Phone Relationship	Phone Relationship

DISRUPTIVE INFLUENCES

DIRECTIONS TO HOME

ENTRY DATA

FIG. 14-2. Environmental evaluation form. (Courtesy Visiting Nurse Association of Buffalo, NY.)

VNA
VISITING NURSING ASSOCIATION

ENVIRONMENTAL EVALUATION

PAGE 2 OF 2

CARE OF PATIENT		TRANSPORTATION ☐ Available ☐ Unavailable	
Name of Care Giver ______		TYPE NEEDED:	☐ Auto
Capability of Care Giver	☐ Good ☐ Fair ☐ Poor	☐ W/C Ambulance	☐ Ambulance
Adequacy of Care	☐ Good ☐ Fair ☐ Poor	☐ Taxi	☐ Other

HEALTH HISTORY

☐ No significant health history.
☐ Past history unclear as provided by patient/family.

MEDICAL HISTORY	DATE	SURGICAL HISTORY	DATE

SOCIO-ECONOMIC DATA

Housing	☐ Adequate	☐ Inadequate	Income	☐ Adequate	☐ Inadequate
Sanitation	☐ Adequate	☐ Inadequate	Home Relationships	☐ Functional	☐ Impaired
Neighborhood Resources	☐ Adequate	☐ Inadequate			

MENTAL/BEHAVIORAL

Alert:	☐ Always	☐ Sometimes	☐ Never
Confused:	☐ Always	☐ Sometimes	☐ Never
Judgement:	☐ Good	☐ Fair	☐ Poor
Acceptance of Illness:	☐ Good	☐ Fair	☐ Poor
Acceptance of Limitations:	☐ Good	☐ Fair	☐ Poor
Motivation:	☐ Good	☐ Fair	☐ Poor

ADDITIONAL COMMENTS

LONG TERM NURSING GOALS	DATE

PROGNOSIS TO GOALS: ☐ Good ☐ Fair ☐ Poor ☐ Guarded

ESTIMATED LENGTH OF SERVICE:
☐ Less Than 2 Months
☐ 2 - 4 Months
☐ 4 - 6 Months
☐ More Than 6 Months

"Patient Bill of Rights" and emergency medical information provided/reviewed with patient/family on ______ .
date

______ CARE PROVIDER SIGNATURE ______ DATE

Fig. 14-2, cont'd. For legend see opposite page.

REFERRAL TAKEN BY ________ DATE __/__/__ TIME ____ AM PM

Visiting Nursing Association of Buffalo, New York, Inc.
(716) 874-5400

VNA

PATIENT'S REFERRAL AND TREATMENT PLAN

EFFECTIVE FROM	TO	DATE	REFERRED BY
			INSTITUTION
			DISTRICT / CT
REQUEST FOR: ( ) INITIAL ( ) CONFIRMING TELORDERS ( ) RECERTIFICATION ( ) DISCHARGE REPORT			HOSPITAL
			ADMISSION DATE / DISCHARGE DATE

PATIENT	PATIENT NAME LAST/FIRST/MIDDLE		BIRTHDATE	SEX
	HOME ADDRESS NUMBER AND STREET / CITY / STATE / ZIP		PHONE	
	DISCHARGE ADDRESS (IF DIFFERENT THAN ABOVE)		DISCHARGE PHONE	
GUARANTOR	RESPONSIBLE PERSON NAME LAST / FIRST / MIDDLE	RELATIONSHIP	PHONE	
	RESPONSIBLE PERSON ADDRESS		SOCIAL SECURITY NUMBER	
INS	REFERRAL NUMBER / MEDICARE NO / MEDICAID NO	BLUE CROSS/SHIELD NO	OTHER INSURANCE NO	
PHYSICIAN	PRIMARY MD NAME / ADDRESS		PHONE	
	SECONDARY MD NAME / ADDRESS		PHONE	
DIAGNOSIS	PRIMARY DIAGNOSIS		DIAGNOSIS KNOWN BY ☐ PATIENT ☐ FAMILY	
	SECONDARY DIAGNOSIS		PROGNOSIS	
	OTHER DIAGNOSIS		PROGNOSIS KNOWN BY ☐ PATIENT ☐ FAMILY	
SURGERY	PRESENT SURGERY	DATE OF SURGERY	EST. LENGTH SERVICE	
	PAST SURGERY	DATE OF SURGERY	FREQUENCY OF VISITS	

THERAPEUTIC GOALS

( ) REGAIN OR RETAIN FUNCTIONAL INDEPENDENCE ( ) PREVENT INSTITUTIONALIZATION ( ) CONTROL DISEASE AND PREVENT UNTOWARD EFFECTS

( ) PROVIDE SUPPORT CARE IN TERM. STATE OF ILLNESS ( ) PROMOTE WOUND HEALING AND PREVENT COMPLICATIONS ( ) OTHER (SPECIFY)

ACTIVITY	SELF	HELP	TOTAL HELP	IMPAIRMENTS AREA	NO	YES	PARTIAL	TOTAL	HOMEBOUND STATUS
AMBULATION				SIGHT					AMB W/ASSIST
TRANSFER				HEARING					AMB W/DEVICE
EATING				SPEECH					W/C BOUND
TOILETING				PARALYSIS					BED BOUND
BATHING				DECUBITIS					BLINDNESS
DRESSING				PROSTHESIS					END. TO PHYS LIM
COLOSTOMY				INCONTINENCE					AGOROPHOBIA
BEDBOUND MOBILITY				CONFUSION					OTHER:
WEIGHT BEARING STATUS									
									MED SUPPLIES:

BP	T	P	R	HT	WT	CATH. CHANGED
						SIZE ____ ☐ SIL. ☐ TEF. ☐ OTHER ☐ 5cc ☐ 30cc

DIET:

ALLERGIES:

MEDICATIONS AND TREATMENT

ACTIVITIES PERMITTED: ________

SERVICES REQUESTED: ( ) NURSING ( ) PT ( ) OT ( ) ST ( ) MSW ( ) HHHA ( ) OTHER

I certify that the above services are required. Patient is essentially homebound.

________ CARE PROVIDER SIGNATURE __/__/__ DATE ________ PHYSICIAN SIGNATURE __/__/__ DATE

FIG. 14-3. Client's referral and treatment form. (Courtesy Visiting Nurse Association of Buffalo, NY.)

Activity Worksheet

VISITING NURSING ASSOCIATION OF BUFFALO, NEW YORK
111 Great Arrow Avenue Buffalo, New York 14216
832-5400

Date: ____________ Staff Nurse: ____________ Div: ____________

Patient: ____________ Aide: ____________

Address: ____________ Tel. No: ____________

Emergency Contact: Name ____________ Relationship ____________ Phone ____________

Date Aide Placed: ____________

Days	Mon.	Tues.	Wed.	Thurs.	Fri.
Hours					

Estimated Length of Aide Service: ____________

****

Personal Care Activities

( ) Assist with bath including routing cleaning and filing of nails, care of teeth & mouth, shampooing and combing of hair
( ) Message bony prominences
( ) Special skin care (explain):
( ) Turning and positioning in bed
( ) Assist with transferring and ambulation
( ) Take vital signs (TPR), wt. and record
( ) Give bedpan, assist to bathroom, or give incontinent care
( ) Measure and record output or test urine
( ) Cleanse and change urinary drainage system and tubing
( ) Assist patient with care of colostomy bag & equipment
( ) Push fluids and record
( ) Assist patient in dressing and ADL
( ) ROM (active & passive)
( ) Assist with therapeutic excercises (must be demonstrated by nurse or therapist
( ) Reinforce sterile dressing
( ) Application of non-sterile dry dressing for non-involved wound
( ) Use of heat and cold (must be demonstrated by nurse/therapist
( ) Other (specify)-
____

GOALS: ____________
____
____

Housekeeping Activities

( ) Prepare and serve meals according to instructions
( ) Making and changing bed (occupied or unoccupied)
( ) Dusting and vacuuming the rooms the patient uses
( ) Dishwashing
( ) Tidying Kitchen
( ) Tidying Bedroom
( ) Tidying Bathroom
( ) Listing needed supplies
( ) Patient's personal laundry; may include necessary ironing and mending
( ) Send linen to laundry
( ) Perform other essential errands. (specify)-

(Special Observations and Precautions):
____
____
____
____
____
____
____
____
____

Form B017383 Rev. 1-1-87

FIG. 14-4. Activity worksheet for ancillary personnel. (Courtesy Visiting Nurse Association of Buffalo, NY.)

VNA
VISITING NURSING ASSOCIATION OF WESTERN NEW YORK, INC

NURSING
PROGRESS NOTES

KEY:
Imp. = Impaired
N/A = Not Applicable

☐ Conference/Telephone call ☐ Initial visit (see Review of Systems) ☐ Scheduled visit
☐ Unscheduled visit (explain) ________

BP	LYING	SITTING	STANDING	TEMP.:	PULSE: Apical	Radial	RESP.:	
(L)				Oral ☐				HT.:
(R)				Axillary ☐ Rectal ☐				WT.:

	YES	NO	N/A
SKIN:			
Color Imp.			
Turgor Imp.			
Integrity Imp.			
RESPIRATORY:			
Dyspnea @ Rest			
Dyspnea on Exert.			
Orthopnea			
Cough			
Sputum			
Lung Sounds Imp.			
CARDIOVASCULAR:			
Pain			
Pedal Pulses Imp.			
Edema			
Endurance Imp.			

	YES	NO	N/A
GASTROINTESTINAL:			
Bowel Sounds Imp.			
Ascites			
ELIMINATION:			
Bowel Habits Imp.			
Bowel Control Imp.			
URINARY:			
Clear Urine			
Concentrated Urine			
Frequency			
Pain/Burning			
Control Imp.			
Nocturia			
NEUROLOGICAL:			
Numbness - Hands			
Coordination Imp.			

MUSCULOSKELETAL:	GOOD	FAIR	POOR	UNABLE
ROM: RUE				
RLE				
LUE				
LLE				
Bed Mobility				
Transfer Abil.				
Sitting Bal.				
Standing Bal.				
Ambulation				

MULTIDISCIPLINARY SERVICES:
P.T. Active ☐ YES ☐ NO
O.T. Active ☐ YES ☐ NO
S.T. Active ☐ YES ☐ NO
M.S.W. Active ☐ YES ☐ NO
H.H.A. Active ☐ YES ☐ NO

Nursing diagnosis that necessitates visit: ________

Nursing procedures related to nursing diagnosis: ________

Patient/family response to nursing procedures: ________

Plan: Revisit (date) ________ to ________

☐ Telephone call: ________

☐ Conference: ________

Date ________ Time ________ Nurse's Signature ________

036683 Rev. 10/87

FIG. 14-5. Nursing progress notes. (Courtesy Visiting Nurse Association of Buffalo, NY.)

progress notes. If clients or families are carrying out treatments in the home, they must also carefully record all activities and the client's response to those treatments. To ensure continuity of care and quality assurance at all times, most agencies have developed protocols to follow when carrying out procedures and standard operating policies to direct all aspects of client care.

Protocols

Protocols are essentially descriptions of steps to be taken in carrying out a specific task. Needs for new protocols are identified based on need of client, vendor, and community. A high technology caregiver or a committee of high technology care team members writes the new policy or protocol. Steps in the procedure may be designed to meet specifications of new equipment to be supplied by the vendor or treatments ordered by the physician caring for the client. The new protocol is then generally reviewed by the medical advisory board of the home health agency. Advisory boards may be made up differently from agency to agency, but usually they contain individuals with a variety of backgrounds. For example, the board may consist of a physician, a pharmacist, a nurse, and a social worker. If standard policies and protocols are used to carry out client care, some sense of continuity is retained when members of the team must deal with the client and the case manager is not on duty.

As in the assessment phase, success of the plan of care is facilitated best if the client and family are consulted and considered. Haddad (1987) discusses the importance of the human factor and the high-touch quality of the home environment that gives high technology home care a unique advantage over hospital care. According to Haddad, the core characteristics of high-touch care are honesty, openness, and willingness. In the case of high technology clients, it should also include acceptance, touch, humor, listening, and spiritual support. Considering all these characteristics that must also meet the complex physical and technical needs of these individuals when planning care presents a challenge to the nurse in the high technology home care field. It calls for interaction with the family and client on a personal level. The pressures of time, numbers of clients, and cost-effectiveness may well hinder the nurse trying to plan comprehensive care. Developing a good rapport with the client and family and including them in the planning of care with the goal of independence always in mind should be the primary focus.

COMPLEX THERAPIES IN THE HOME

A variety of high technology therapies are available for treatment of the client in the home. This section addresses infusion therapies, enteral therapy, phototherapy, apnea monitoring, and mechanical ventilation.

Infusion Therapies

The process of introducing a liquid substance such as a drug, hydration fluid, nutritive substance, blood and blood product, or electrolyte solution into the body through a vein rather than the alimentary canal for therapeutic purposes is known as infusion therapy.

General Considerations

Infusion therapies were first used in the home as early as 1963. At this time infusion therapies were limited to hyperalimentation, hemodialysis, peritoneal dialysis, and chemotherapy. Currently, use of infusion therapies has been extended to include cancer pain management, hemophilia care, management of congestive heart failure, and antibiotic therapy. Management of infusion therapy for the client in the home requires a nursing staff skilled in physical assessment, problem finding and solving, management of complex equipment, and drug preparation and administration.

Generally a client who is to receive infusion therapy at home must have a capable person in the home during infusion, have received an educational program in the specific therapy from the vendor nurse or hospital staff while in the hospital setting, have arrangements made for follow-up care and reinforcement teaching by a case manager from the designated home health agency, and have resources available for activating emergency treatment, including a telephone and a number to call for 24-hour support service.

Another essential prerequisite for home infusion therapy is the maintenance of trouble-free venous access to prevent complications and subsequent rehospitalization. Therefore great care must be taken in selecting and placing either a peripheral line or a central venous catheter. This is usually done before the client is discharged from the hospital.

Choice of Site

Peripheral Venous Lines

The selection of a site should be based on client needs, convenience of the nursing staff, and length of peripheral venous lines therapy. A peripheral venous line in one of the extremities with a heparin lock is indicated for short-term therapy in clients at risk for central venous catheterization or who do not have central venous access. Factors limiting use of peripheral lines include repeated venipuncture, frequent changing of the intravenous needle site (every two to three days), solution concentration, flow rate, pain, sclerosis of the particular vein, and frequent clotting or blockage. A peripheral line is contraindicated if the client has peripheral vascular disease (Kasmer, 1984a).

Peripheral lines are often used for short-term intravenous antibiotic therapy for infective or inflammatory diseases such as osteomyelitis, endocarditis, cellulitis, wound infections, pneumonias, and septic arthritis. An intravenous cannula is placed directly in the client's forearm while the client is still in the hospital or on initial visit to the home after discharge. The site is protected by either a gauze or a transparent dressing. The antibiotic is injected directly into the bloodstream using either a gravity infusion system or an infusion pump. Peripheral lines are flushed after each dose of medication and at least daily when not in use (see Appendix).

Central Venous Lines

Assessment criteria for identifying a client as a potential candidate for an indwelling central venous catheter include frequency of need for venous access, length of treatment, mode of administration, venous integrity, and client preference (Goodman and Wickham, 1984).

If a client requires long-term treatment involving multiple procedures, such as intravenous chemotherapy, antibiotics, and hyperalimentation or total parenteral nutrition, simultaneously, it is more practical to insert a venous access device in a central line.

Venous Access Devices

A central catheter is inserted into the cephalic vein and threaded through the superior vena cava to the entrance of the right atrium during fluoroscopy with the client under local or general anesthesia (Fig. 14-6). The ends of the catheter are secured with a suture at the point of entry into the cephalic vein and at the exit site. The visible portion of the catheter is taped to the chest to prevent unnecessary tension (Kasmer, 1984b).

There are many venous access devices in common use, each having specific indications and features. Examples include the Broviac, Hickman, and Groshong catheters and implanted infusion parts such as the Medi-Port.

Broviac Catheter

The Broviac catheter was the first central venous catheter to be developed. It is a single-lumen

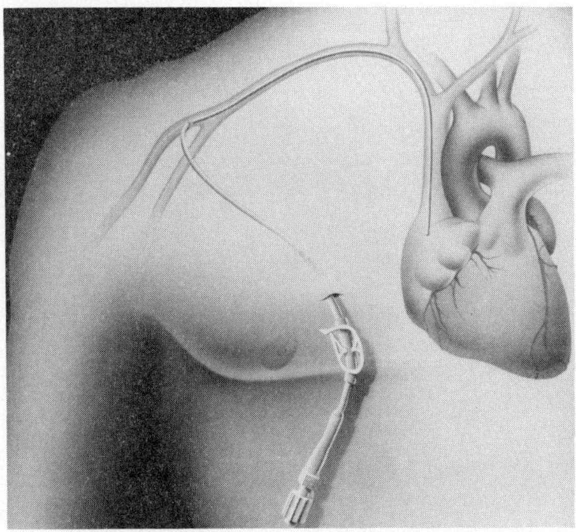

FIG. 14-6. Central venous catheter inserted into cephalic vein and threaded through superior vena cava to entrance of right atrium. (Courtesy CORMED, Inc.)

catheter, and it is used for administering concentrated, large-volume infusions such as total parenteral nutrition (Kasmer, 1984b). Because it is a single-lumen catheter, it is not practical for clients requiring complex care involving simultaneous hyperalimentation and infusions of perhaps antibiotics and pain medications. The newer venous access devices have multiple lumens and are more versatile.

Hickman Catheter

The Hickman catheter is a large-gauge Silastic or polymeric silicone rubber catheter with a Dacron felt cuff and is inserted in the superior vena cava outside the right atrium. This catheter can be obtained with either single, double, or triple lumens or entrance ways that differ in size and are color coded. Silastic catheters clot infrequently when flushed daily with a heparin solution (see Appendix). It is tunneled under the skin below the cutdown site and the catheter exit site (Fig. 14-6). A pressure dressing or single transparent dressing is placed over the exit site, and a separate small dressing is placed over the upper incision (see Appendix). The Dacron felt cuff is positioned in the tunnel to allow for the formations of fibrous adhesions around the cuff. After the fibrous tissue grows around the cuff, the risk of dislodgment is reduced. The risks of infection from skin flora are reduced because the cuff creates a barrier to infection.

The Hickman catheter is used extensively for venous access to clients who require long-term therapy such as intermittent transfusions, antibiotics, chemotherapy, pain management therapy, and frequent blood samples. It also used for clients who require administration of long-term parenteral nutrition solutions.

Groshong Catheter

The Groshong central venous catheter is also intended for long-term central venous access in adults and children for therapies similar to those cited for the Hickman catheter. It consists of a thin-walled translucent silicone rubber catheter with a radioscopic stripe and a pocketed two-way slit valve adjacent to a rounded, closed tip. This tip is placed in the right atrium of the heart via one of the large control veins. After tip placement the catheter is tunneled subcutaneously for several inches to the desired exit site as with the Hickman catheter. The Groshong catheter has a Dacron cuff like the Hickman catheter that serves the similar purpose of securing the catheter and reducing the potential for infection. This catheter has a much smaller outside diameter than many other long-term catheters and is less visible under clothing.

The major difference between the Hickman catheter and the Groshong catheter is the function of the Groshong's two-way valve. This valve opens outward during infusion and inward during blood withdrawal and closes automatically when not in use. Because of hydrostatic pressure once the catheter is in a vein and filled with any isotonic

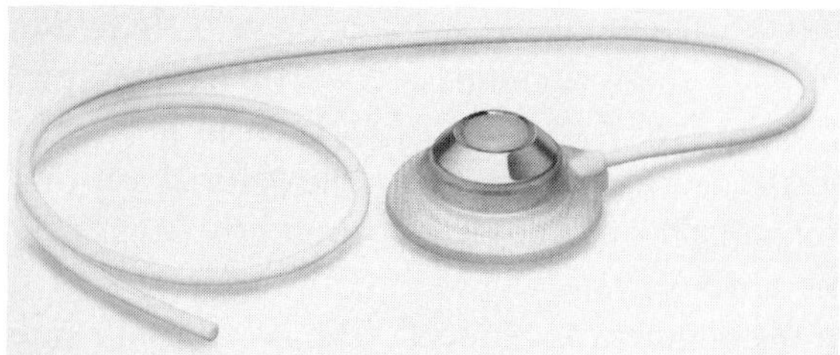

FIG. 14-7. Medi-Port—an implantable vascular access device. (Courtesy CORMED, Inc.)

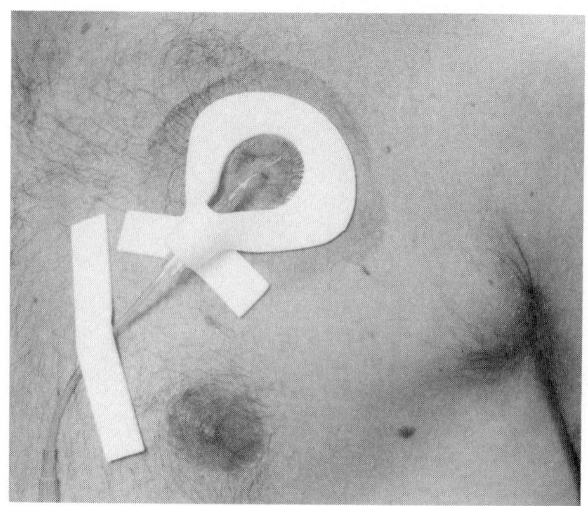

FIG. 14-8. Post Port-Gard—a self-adhesive device with transparent membrane for dressing site and securing needles into vascular access ports. (Courtesy CORMED, Inc.)

fluid, venous blood pressure is normally not sufficient to spontaneously open the valve inward and allow blood to back up into the lumen and clot the catheter. This feature eliminates the need for heparin irrigations or heparin locks to maintain catheter patency when not infusing fluids or withdrawing blood samples. All that is needed after infusion is irrigation with an isotonic fluid such as normal saline to clear the line. When not in use the catheter should be irrigated once every seven days. These features make the Groshong catheter safer and easier to use by health care workers, clients, and families involved in high technology home care.

Implantable Vascular Access Devices

Implantable vascular access devices are drug and fluid administration systems consisting of a self-sealing silicone septum encased in a port made of metal or plastic and attached to a silicone catheter (Winters, 1984). An example of this type of venous access device is a Medi-Port (Fig. 14-7). It provides vascular access in continual intermittent outpatient delivery of fluids and medications. The Medi-Port is used for injection of bolus intravenous therapy, infusion of continuous intravenous therapy, infusion of blood products, drawing of blood samples, and infusion of intermittent therapy such as pain medication or intravenous therapy. The implantable access device must be both implanted and removed during surgery. The Medi-Port requires little care and maintenance. Site care is minimal, and the catheter requires flushing only once a month when not in use. The Medi-Port is cosmetically appealing, since the port is implanted in the subcutaneous tissue and long-term placement of the specific needle (a Huber needle, which is a right-angle needle) for continuous infusions does not alter a client's mobility. This needle is inserted in the port and taped to the skin over the device and covered with a dressing over the entire site (Fig. 14-8).

These catheters may be placed in a vein for systemic drug and fluid therapy or in a specific artery for regional drug therapy. They are not indicated for home total parenteral nutrition because of fear of breakdown in the subcutaneous tissue over the port with daily needle punctures, the increased cost of the equipment, and the additional cost of surgical removal. Ports are also not placed for long-term antibiotic therapy for similar reasons. The Hickman catheter and the Groshong catheter are more appropriate choices.

Infusion Delivery Systems

Three types of delivery systems are commonly used for home care. They include gravity infusion, the infusion pump, and ambulatory infusion devices.

Gravity Infusion

Gravity infusion is the simplest and least expensive system. All that is used is an administrative set with a flow clamp that can be adjusted to control the number of drops per minute from the intravenous bag into the tubing. This must be monitored closely because there are no safety features to ensure that the rate does not change or the infusion does not run dry, allowing air to enter the line. This system is often used to administer antibiotics with a short infusion time. One disadvantage to using this method is that clients cannot ambulate during the infusion but must lie in bed or sit in a chair.

Infusion Pump

The infusion pump is useful in situations where a sustained flow rate is required. There are two different styles of infusion pumps—an infusion controller and a mechanical peristaltic or piston action pump. An infusion pump is propelled by gravity, and the flow rate is monitored constantly by a photoelectric eye. It is used predominantly for a peripheral venous access site. An example of this pump is an IVAC. These pumps are useful where a slow flow rate is needed for a long time or where therapy is being carried out without nursing supervision. A true infusion pump or peristaltic piston action pump forces the infusion through the intravenous tubing at a constant rate. These pumps are used for solutions such as hyperalimentation and infuse solutions at a high flow rate. A central line is usually a better choice for a high infusion rate. An example of this type of pump is an IMED. Both types of these pumps have safety features such as an emergency shutoff that stops the infusion when a problem occurs and sets off auditory or visual alarms that warn the client or caretaker. Safety features include air detection and signals for completion of infusion and occlusion of lines.

Ambulatory Infusion Devices

Ambulatory infusion devices are generally small and lightweight. They can be worn on a belt or carried in a shoulder holster. They allow the client to be completely mobile while receiving an infusion. There are two general types—syringe and peristaltic.

The syringe type of infusion device may be carried or hung on a pole. A 20 to 50 ml syringe is loaded with infusion material and placed in the pump. The pump automatically depresses the plunger of the syringe at a set rate. The drawbacks to the syringe type of infusion device are that they can delivery only small amounts of infusion at a time, they are expensive, and they have few safety features. They are usually used with peripheral lines.

The peristaltic type of infusion device has a reservoir bag with attached tubing that is threaded through the pump. These pumps may be used with a central venous catheter, and they may also be used peripherally. The pumps are capable of intermittent infusion and can be set to start and stop infusions over a 24-hour period. Thus the client can have almost complete freedom of movement all day.

There is a fairly wide variety of infusion delivery systems, each having its own advantages and disadvantages. Choice must be determined by type of infusion and unique needs of the client.

General Nursing Responsibilities

The nurse working with a client undergoing infusion therapy in the home setting is responsible for conducting ongoing assessment of the client's overall condition, preventing infection, maintaining patency of the catheter or line, educating the client or caretaker in relation to understanding all aspects of treatment, and creating a supportive environment for the client and the family as they adapt to the home treatment.

Ongoing assessment of the client consists of gathering data such as vital signs, changes in condition, response to treatment, energy level, sleeping patterns, appetite, mental status, and emotional state. The nurse also needs to assess the family in terms of coping mechanisms, anxiety level, and general ability to handle the situation, including ability to carry out the therapy and problems related to maintenance of the equipment.

The prevention of infection is of prime importance when caring for a client receiving infusion therapy through a peripheral or central line. The client or caretaker and nurse must use good handwashing and dressing change techniques. The client must be assessed for signs and symptoms of infection, including fever, shakes, chills, and lethargy. The catheter exit site must be assessed for purulent drainage, redness, edema, ulceration, tenderness, discomfort, or pain. If any of these are present, the nurse should notify the physician.

Along with prevention of infection, the nurse must guard against catheter malfunction. Catheter malfunction involves any of the mechanical problems that occur when caring for a client with an infusion line, particularly a central venous line. To help prevent catheter malfunction, the client or caretaker and nurse must be careful not to apply direct tension to the catheter or even force anything through the catheter.

Site dressing and tubing should be changed using an aseptic technique per physician's orders. The catheter cap should be discarded and replaced with a new sterile one when it is removed. If the catheter is not in use, the cap should be routinely replaced as indicated by the agency policy. Special padded clamps should be used to protect the tubing. The line should be flushed with an instillation of heparin after use for intermittent infusion of blood products or medications or withdrawal of blood. When not being used, the line should be flushed following manufacturer's directions for specific types of venous access devices and policy of agency.

The physician should be notified if catheter malfunctions are suspected, including obstruction, pain, leaking, or dislodgment. If the catheter appears to be occluded, no attempt to flush should be made and the physician should be notified. If the catheter is severed or cut, it should be immediately clamped with a padded hemostat on an intact portion of the catheter as close to the chest as possible and a physician should be notified. Clients should go to the emergency room at a hospital if they are unable to reach the physician or nurse. Severed or cut lines can be repaired by the nurse (see Fig. 13-16 for protocol). If the catheter becomes dislodged, pressure should be applied to the incision and exit site using a sterile gauze pad for 10 minutes and a physician should be notified.

Teaching Guidelines

The nurse should instruct the client and caretaker regarding the following:

1. Insertion of the catheter—purpose, site
2. Care of catheter
3. Prevention of infection
    a. Proper handwashing technique
    b. Signs and symptoms of infection
    c. Dressing change and cap replacement
4. Heparin flush procedures specific to type of venous access desired
5. Importance of patency
6. Emergency measures
7. Procedure to follow when instilling infusion

Antibiotic Therapy

Studies in antibiotic home care suggest a substantial savings to the client without affecting the quality of care (Poretz, 1982; Williams and others, 1982). Besides being cost effective, home antibiotic therapy has the added advantage of allowing clients to return to their homes and a more normal life-style while undergoing treatment.

Indications for Home Parenteral Antibiotic Therapy

Clients undergoing prolonged therapy for osteomyelitis, infectious endocarditis, septic arthritis and diuresis, infected prosthetic joints, and primary bacteremia are candidates for home care. Clients requiring repeated therapy for urinary tract infections, diabetic foot infections, cystic fibrosis, and neoplastic disorders can also benefit. Clients requiring short-term therapy for cellulitis, wound infections, pelvic inflammatory disease, mastoiditis, sinusitis, and pneumonia are also considered (Kasmer, 1984a).

Once it is determined that a client is a candidate for antibiotic home care, generally an intravenous cannula is placed in the client's forearm with a heparin lock in place. If there is need for multiple therapy, parenteral nutrition, frequent blood samples, or pain medication, a central venous line may be used instead.

Client Education

The client or caretaker to administer antibiotic therapy in the home is taught about the following:

1. The prescribed medication, its side effects, and the signs and symptoms to report to the nurse or physician
2. Preparation of solutions if the medication is not a premixed preparation
3. How to administer the medication, including how to use the infusion device, how to disconnect it at completion of infusion, and how to administer heparin to flush the line afterwards
4. Intravenous cannula care including obstruction, dislodgment, severing, or cutting of tubing and emergency measures
5. Injection site inspection and signs and symptoms of infection
6. Maintenance of daily records

Parenteral Nutritional Therapy

Parenteral nutrition is a complex form of infusion therapy that supplies the body with the total caloric and nutritional needs via a central intravenous route. Home parenteral nutrition was begun by Scribner and his colleagues in 1970 (Scribner, 1970). Research has demonstrated that home therapy for the client on home parenteral therapy results in a cost difference as high as 73%.

Indications for Use of Parenteral Nutritional Therapy

Parenteral nutritional therapy is prescribed for the client who is unable to take food orally. Diagnoses include Crohn's disease, short bowel syndrome in the child, cancer of the digestive tract, and several congenital anomalies.

Once a client is determined to be a candidate for home care, a catheter is placed surgically in the cephalic vein in the right atrium of the heart. Parenteral nutrition is usually given only via the central venous route using Hickman catheters, Groshong catheters, or implantable ports. An electromechanical infusion pump is used to control the rate of infusion. Blood is drawn on a routine basis by the nurse to monitor and assess the adequacy of the nutrient formula. Levels are reported to the physician, and the formula is adjusted accordingly.

Client Education

The client or caretaker recommended for home parenteral nutrition is taught the following:

1. Preparation of solution, if necessary, and proper handling, storage, and refrigeration of these solutions. These solutions may include amino acid solutions that contain pro-

tein, high-concentration dextrose injections for calories, intravenous fat emulsions or lipids for calories and essential fatty acids, electrolyte injections for balanced electrolyte intake, and vitamin injections to meet daily vitamin requirements
2. Use of the electromechanical infusion device or pump during infusion. Safe administrations of parenteral nutrition, including initiation and disconnection of therapy and pump functioning (see Appendix)
3. Care of the catheter between infusions
4. Maintenance of daily records of fluid intake and output, body weight, and urine glucose tests
5. Recognition and treatment of side effects and complications
6. What to report to the nurse and physician and when to call for assistance

Chemotherapy in the Home

The use of chemotherapy or antineoplastic agents has become a common mode of treatment for clients with cancer. Chemotherapy is used as a cure or a means of controlling advanced or recurrent disease, resulting in increased survival and improved quality of life for individuals with cancer (Goodman, 1984). Most chemotherapy programs are administered while the client is hospitalized or require the client to go to outpatient ambulatory settings. However, chemotherapy can be given effectively to homebound clients under the orders and direction of a physician.

Chemotherapeutic agents can be infused by a peripheral line. Clients requiring long-term intensive chemotherapy as treatment for solid tumors, acute leukemia, or bone marrow transplantation may require intravenous chemotherapy, antibiotics, blood products, parenteral nutrition, and pain management concurrently. In such cases a central venous line with a venous access device is appropriate. The central venous line is also used with vesicants, chemotherapy agents that cause local tissue irritation, and sloughing. Examples of these drugs are nitrogen mustard, vincristine, vinblastine, mitomycin, and doxorubicin, which are infused through a central venous line to prevent inadvertent subcutaneous infiltration.

Once a client is determined to be a candidate for home care, the infusion device is implanted and the first few chemotherapy doses are administered in the hospital or outpatient setting to detect and treat any problems or hypersensitivities that may occur. If no complications are evident, preparation for home care begins. Chemotherapy may be administered in intermittent or 24-hour continuous infusions using a pump-type infusion device that may be ambulatory, depending on client condition and preference. The drug may be infused over 24 hours to provide a continuous flow of medication, which maximizes therapeutic effect and reduces toxic side effects such as hair loss, nausea, and vomiting.

The nurse draws blood on a regular basis to monitor the blood count for side effects and blood levels of the chemotherapeutic agents. Chemotherapy should be withheld if the platelet count is less than 100,000 per cubic millimeter and white blood cell count is less than 4000 per cubic millimeter. The client needs safety supplies such as goggles, masks, gowns, gloves, impervious bags, and chemical safety containers to dispose of used equipment and medication containers.

Client Education

All procedures must be demonstrated to the client or caretaker who must be able to return the demonstration. The client or caretaker should be taught about the following:

1. The prescribed drug and its side effects including nausea, vomiting, hair loss, and lethargy
2. How to administer the drug and use the infusion device selected, including how to set up the infusion, disconnect when completed, and properly dispose of chemotherapy waste

products and equipment. These materials are placed in chemical safety containers usually provided by the vendor or home health agency and are collected by the nurse and transported to an institutional incinerator for disposal, usually at a local hospital. This is determined by agency policy.

3. How to flush the line following infusion as determined by type of venous access device used
4. Care of the catheter between infusions
5. How to change the catheter dressing
6. Maintenance of daily drug records
7. Signs and symptoms to be reported to the nurse and physician, including site appearance and signs and symptoms of injection

Pain Management

Indications for Use

Pain control allows the client with severe or chronic pain to move more freely, enhances the quality of life through improved mental and physical outlook, and enables the client to return to the home setting. The management of severe pain present in some clients with malignant neoplasms presents a challenge to the health care provider. Initially severe pain may be managed using analgesics by mouth. Once clients are no longer receiving adequate pain relief using these medications orally, if they have extreme nausea related to chemotherapy or palliative radiation treatment, another approach is needed. These complications are usually managed by switching to the parenteral route of administration. Home management of pain has proved cost effective and allows clients to remain in their homes during the terminal stages of illness.

Epidural catheters, central lines, and subcutaneous and peripheral sites may all be used for administration of analgesics using an infusion pump. The client may use a piston action pump like the IMED, if bedridden, or an ambulatory pump, if the client can move around. Another choice is a continuous subcutaneous infusion using an insulin pump. Insulin pumps can be used for analgesics and have several advantages—they bypass the oral-rectal route, therefore increasing tolerance to the medication, provide continuous infusion, which actually allows for a decrease in total dose, and are easy to administer in an ambulatory setting. Choice of pump is also influenced by the amount of medication needed. Children and adults who need small doses need a pump that is able to deliver small doses accurately. Clients with cancers that have spread to large areas of bone may have enormous analgesic needs, and thus require a pump that can accommodate frequent upward dosage adjustments (Klein, 1986). Once a client has been identified as a candidate for home care, site and method of administration are determined. The drug of choice is generally morphine (Klein, 1986). While the client is still in the hospital, the chosen method of infusion is begun and the dose of medication is adjusted to meet the needs of individual clients and their level of pain.

Clients need to be observed for continued pain control and also for unwanted side effects such as pronounced sedation, hallucinations, respiratory depression, or disorientation, which may require a decrease in the morphine rate (Klein, 1986). Generally client or caretaker education is begun in the hospital before discharge. Clients may be managed in the home for a long period. The first week or so they may require daily monitoring by the nurse from the home health agency. Once the client is stabilized and the family gains confidence, they may be assessed and monitored by the nurse on a weekly basis. Generally the condition of the client on home pain management deteriorates, and as the level of pain increases, the dosage level must be adjusted accordingly. Initially the client may require 5 to 10 mg of morphine per hour, and this may gradually need to be increased to as high as 150 to 200 mg per hour (Klein, 1986). At each visit the nurse needs to assess the client for vital signs, cardiopulmonary status, decreased neurologic status and level of sensorium, response to pain management, skin integrity, nutritional status, and bowel and bladder elimination. The site of catheter insertion must also be assessed for complications. The nurse should report any changes in sensorium, increased temperature, decreased urinary output, numbness or tingling, constipation, nausea or vomiting, itching or rash, increased pain, decreased sensorium, or shallow respirations less than 12 per minute (Jernigan, 1986).

Client Education

As in all types of infusion therapy, all procedures must be demonstrated to the client or caretaker. They in turn must be able to return the demonstration. The client and caretaker should be taught about the following:

1. The prescribed medication and its side effects. Symptoms to watch for include respiratory depression, central nervous system depression, ranging from drowsiness to coma, mood changes, euphoria, restlessness, bradycardia, orthostatic hypotension, nausea, vomiting, and constipation.
2. How to administer the drug and use the infusion device selected
3. How to flush the line following infusion as determined by thc type of line selected and care of the catheter between infusions
4. How to change the catheter dressing
5. Maintenance of daily records
6. Signs and symptoms to be reported to the nurse and physician, including site appearances and symptoms of infection

PHOTOTHERAPY

Phototherapy is the treatment of jaundice by exposure to light. Jaundice is a yellow pigmentation of the skin, conjunctiva, mucous membranes, and body fluids caused by bile deposits that result from excess bilirubin in the blood. Jaundice is a common problem affecting 50% of normal-term infants during the first week of life (Nelson, 1985). The normal full-term fetus has a hematocrit value of 50% to 65% in utero. The fetus needs this excess of red blood cells to carry oxygen during the prenatal period. Once babies begin breathing on their own after birth, this need disappears. Within a few days the excess red blood cells are destroyed and not replaced. Bilirubin is formed as the end product of the breakdown of the red blood cells and is removed from the bloodstream by specialized liver cells that conjugate the bilirubin and render it water soluble. This water-soluble, or conjugated, bilirubin is excreted through bile in the stool. The liver in a newborn is immature, and it takes approximately three to seven days to become effective. During this period the bilirubin level builds up and usually peaks at 12 mg around the third day of life. As the liver matures, the level drops. If the liver is not maturing at the expected rate or if the baby is not feeding well or passing stools to eliminate the bile, the level may continue to rise. A level of 20 mg is considered dangerous and can cause kernicterus or brain damage. Research and clinical observation indicate that there is a relationship between breast-feeding and jaundice (Locklin 1987). Breast milk jaundice occasionally occurs between the fifth and seventh day of life in a newborn. It is thought that certain women produce an enzyme in their milk that inhibits conjugation of bilirubin, so the blood level in the infant increases beyond the physiologic level. Breast-feeding may have to be discontinued for about 24 hours to allow the bilirubin levels to fall. If breast-feeding is discontinued, the mother should be encouraged to express or pump her milk to decrease her discomfort and maintain the supply of milk. The situation is ordinarily temporary, and it is not a contraindication to continued breast-feeding. A less common type of jaundice associated

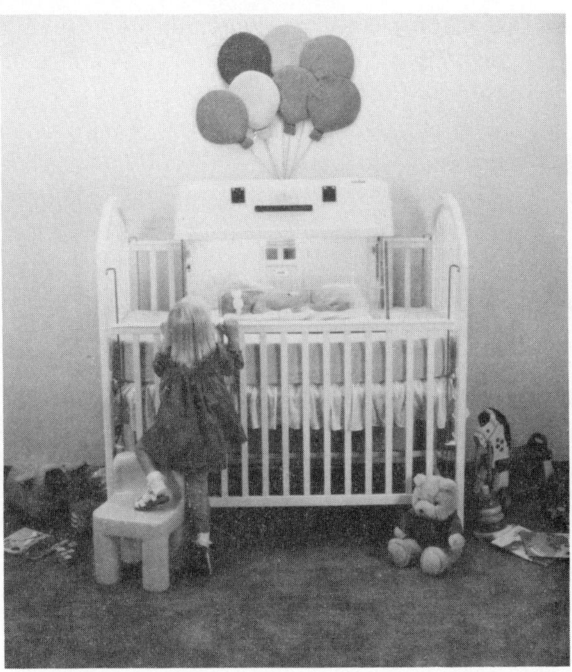

FIG. 14-9. Phototherapy in home setting. (Courtesy Rocky Mountain Medical Corp.)

with breast-feeding occurs in the first three days after delivery. It is caused by dehydration, so the remedy is more frequent feedings to hydrate the infant and to encourage the passage of meconium (Locklin, 1987).

Phototherapy has proved effective in reducing or preventing increased bilirubin levels in the newborn when it is related to this natural process. It has been used routinely in the hospital setting, generally prolonging the length of stay for the jaundiced newborn. Portable phototherapy units are now being used in the home to provide an alternative (Fig. 14-9). Family discharge with continued phototherapy is an option available; it allows the mother and baby to leave the hospital together, thus maintaining continuous bonding.

Generally, if the infant is to receive phototherapy at home, a good support system is needed to help the new mother care for herself and her baby and carry out the added responsibility of phototherapy. The baby and mother must be in stable medical condition. The home environment must have adequate wiring for the phototherapy equipment and heating and ventilation appropriate to the particular climate and time of year to provide a warm, draft-free environment for the baby.

Once it has been determined that the infant is a candidate for home phototherapy, a vendor is contacted to supply the needed equipment. The equipment includes the portable phototherapy unit, rectal thermometer, ophthalmic drops as ordered, eye covers to protect eyes from the light, and Velcro straps or paper tape to secure eye covers. The vendor or the nurse hired by the vendor assesses the client and family in the hospital setting, demonstrates the equipment to be used, and begins family teaching. The vendor also delivers and sets up the equipment in the home setting. A home health agency nurse may also assess the client in the hospital before discharge. After the client is discharged from the hospital, the case manager or nurse from the designated home health agency makes the initial visit to the home. A careful assessment is carried out including a history of the pregnancy, labor, and delivery. It must be determined whether the child is breast-fed or formula-fed; if the child is breast-fed, it must be determined whether the mother wants to continue. It is necessary to know how long phototherapy was used in the hospital, when the bilirubin level was last measured, and the pattern of the bilirubin levels. Physician orders must be reviewed, and the mother and support persons must be assessed to determine their understanding of the procedure.

The baby must be assessed, preferably with the clothes off and in bright natural light, to determine the extent of jaundice. Vital signs are taken and the baby is weighed and assessed for signs of dehydration, which include dry skin, decreased skin turgor, dry mucous membranes, depressed fontanelle, and decreased urine output.

Nursing Responsibilities

The nurse's responsibilities include the following:

1. Carrying out initial assessment as discussed previously
2. Collecting and setting up equipment
3. Explaining procedure to the caretaker (see Mother or Caretaker Education section)
4. Explaining use of a flow sheet for recording daily information and recording bile level and temperature (Fig. 14-10)
5. Setting up portable phototherapy unit following manufacturer's directions, checking lights to be sure bulbs are all working, and changing if necessary
6. Drawing blood for bilirubin level checks by either heel stick or venipuncture (as ordered) (see Appendix). Because light degrades the bilirubin level and gives a false value, turn off lights and use a covered specimen tube. Deliver to laboratory or agency to be analyzed.
7. Administering phototherapy by undressing babies, covering their eyes, placing them in the phototherapy unit, positioning them with blanket rolls, and turning on lights
8. Making sure the mother expresses and stores her milk when breast-feeding is interrupted during phototherapy to ensure she will continue to produce breast milk if she wishes to continue breast-feeding after the baby's jaundice is resolved.
9. Checking information on the caretaker's flow sheet and recording the bilirubin level during the daily visit. The baby is weighed and observed for changes in sclera, skin, feedings, stools, urine, and level of physical activity and alertness. The nurse discusses with the family any concerns or problems that have arisen since the last visit. The visit ends with the nurse drawing a blood sample. Drawing of the sample should be left until last because the baby generally cries and the procedure may be anxiety provoking for the mother or caretaker. The sample is delivered to a laboratory for bilirubin analysis.
10. Reporting bilirubin levels to the physician daily and contacting the vendor and closing the case when levels reach normal limits and the physician writes discharge orders

Client Education

All procedures should be clearly demonstrated, and wherever possible the caretaker should return the demonstration for the nurse. The caretaker or mother should be taught the following:

1. How to take and record the baby's temperatures either axillary or rectal as ordered
2. How to maintain daily records (Fig. 14-10). This record should include the temperature, type, and amount of feeding, appearance of eyes, number of wet diapers, and number and description of bowel movements.
3. How to cleanse the baby's eyes and instill eye drops if ordered. Eyes should be closed and then covered with eye pads that are secured in place with either paper tape or a Velcro strap. Eye covers should be snug but not so tight that they cause molding of the head. Eye covers should be checked often to prevent slippage, exposure of eyes to light, or occlusion of nostrils.
4. To remove all the baby's clothing including the diaper to ensure that the maximum amount of skin possible is exposed to the light and to place an open diaper under the baby and cover the testes when a male baby is in the supine position
5. How to turn phototherapy unit on and position the baby at the proper distance following the manufacturer's directions
6. To feed the infant every two to four hours and offer water between feedings to ensure adequate hydration. At feeding time the

24-hour phototherapy flow sheet	Date ______ Bili Level ______					
Time						
Temperature						
Intake: Type						
Amount						
Appearance of eyes (drainage, redness)						
Number of wet diapers						
Number of bowel movements						
Description						

FIG. 14-10. Flow sheet for caretaker of baby undergoing phototherapy.

infant should be taken out of the unit, the eye covers removed, and the eyes checked for redness and drainage. Uncovering the eyes during feeding allows for eye contact with the mother to encourage bonding and providing visual stimulation. The infant's temperature should be taken at this time to monitor for hypothermia or hyperthermia. All information related to condition of eyes, temperature, and feeding should be carefully recorded on the flow sheet.

7. After each feeding the baby should have eye covers replaced and be repositioned in the unit with blanket rolls to allow for maximum exposure. (Turn from right side to left side and onto abdomen—avoid supine position after feedings)
8. To monitor and record changes in number and description of bowel movements and urination, since phototherapy may increase water loss and cause dehydration
9. To cleanse the infant's skin carefully after each bowel movement, since skin may become excoriated from loose, green, bile stools.
10. To call the home health agency nurse if

there are any concerns, including temperatures less than 36.6°C (97.9° F) or more than 37.2° C (99.0° F) rectally, decreased urine output (normal is 8 to 10 wet diapers per day), depressed fontanelle, lethargy, poor sucking reflex, spasticity, and opisthotonos

APNEA MONITORING

Apnea is defined by the National Institutes of Health as "cessation of respiratory air flow." The respiratory pause may be central or diaphragmatic (no respiratory effort), obstructive (usually caused by upper airway obstruction), or mixed. Short (15 seconds) central apnea can be normal at all ages. Monitors have been developed to measure normal and abnormal physiologic processes such as breathing patterns. Infants who are monitored are classified as premature infants with apnea, bradycardia, or a heart rate of less than 80 beats per minute, children in families in which a sibling has died of sudden infant death syndrome (SIDS), and infants who experienced a so-called near-miss episode—they stopped breathing but were discovered in time by parents or hospital staff (Sheridan, 1985).

Apnea in the premature baby is believed to be related to overall immaturity. Premature infants also have trouble coordinating breathing with eating and may become cyanotic or have a drop in heart rate during feeds. In the past such infants were generally hospitalized until breathing was established. In response to financial pressures for early discharge, the decision is often made to send the baby home with an apnea monitor. Subsequent siblings who have died of SIDS have more irregular breathing patterns than children in normal control groups, and the risk of death from SIDS is increased up to fourfold (Sheridan, 1985). Depending on family preference, it is often decided to monitor subsequent siblings. If parents do decide on monitoring their baby, the preparation and education of the family can begin before the birth of the baby.

Parents of babies who have suffered a near-miss episode usually feel emotionally devastated and frightened. They are usually relieved to know they can monitor their child at home. Given their emotional state and anxiety level, they are poor candidates to learn all they need to know about apnea, the use of the monitor, and emergency measures. They need support and careful preparation to take their child home on the monitor.

Once it is determined that a baby is going home with an apnea monitor, arrangements are made to procure the appropriate equipment and supplies and to educate the family. Some hospitals have their own home monitoring service and provide all aspects of the care. Other hospitals depend on vendors and home health agencies to provide the equipment, education, and follow-up care.

Generally family education is carried out in the hospital before the baby to be monitored is discharged. Parents are required to demonstrate their ability to use the monitor and carry out cardiopulmonary resuscitation (CPR) before the baby is allowed to go home.

The nurse working with the family needs to consider why the baby is being monitored for apnea and provide support for the unique needs of the family based on this. To prepare the family for discharge, the nurse needs to know how long the monitor is expected to be used and if it is to be used continuously or just during sleep. The nurse should assess the baby for general health, observe for anomalies, and note the rate, rhythm, and character of respirations and any episodes of periodic breathing.

Procedure

1. Collect and set up equipment including the monitor provided by the vendor or hospital, electrodes and gel (if needed for the type of monitor used), lead wires, electrode belt, and flow sheet for the crib side (Fig. 14-11).

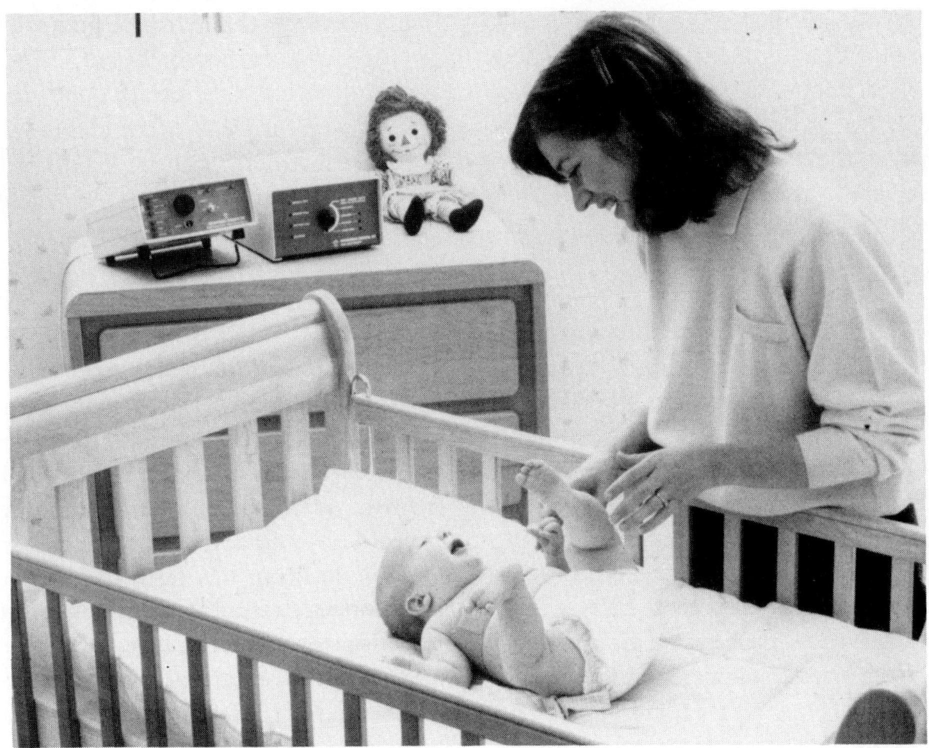

FIG. 14-11. Apnea monitoring of infant in home setting. (Courtesy Aequitron Medical, Inc.)

2. Position the monitor on a level surface next to the baby's crib and secure it from falling. The monitor should not be placed on top of another electric appliance such as a heater, a television, or a radio.
3. Connect the power cord and attach lead wires to the electrodes and the electrodes to the monitoring belt.
4. The belt should be wrapped snugly around the infant's chest at the point of greatest chest movement at the right and left midaxillary line and ¾ inch, or 2 cm, below the axillae.
5. The lead wires are connected to the cable according to color code, and the cable is then connected to the jack on the back of the monitor.
6. The sensitivity knob should be set to maximum; the alarm delay is set to the recommended time.
7. Turn on monitor. Alarms sound until sensitivity knobs are adjusted. Reset apnea and bradycardia alarms according to the manufacturer's specifications. Then adjust sensitivity controls so that indicator lights blink with each breath and heartbeat (auscultate the heart rate to be sure).

The family must be assessed for their understanding of all procedures to be followed at home.

Nursing Responsibilities

The nurse's responsibilities include the following:

1. Carrying out the assessment as described above
2. Educating the family regarding all procedures to be followed at home
3. Providing emergency phone numbers for

emergency medical care, nurse, physician, and supplier of equipment. If the family does not have a phone, a plan must be devised regarding how to get help in an emergency.
4. Supporting the family based on needs related to reason for home monitoring

Client Education

All procedures should be clearly demonstrated by the nurse, and the caretaker should return the demonstration. The caretaker or mother should be taught the following:

1. How to take pulse and respirations
2. CPR (usually before the baby is discharged from the hospital). A flow sheet outlining CPR procedures should be given to parents and hung on the wall over the baby's crib.
3. Using emergency procedures if apnea or bradycardia alarms sound, including the following:
   a. Checking the infant's respirations and skin color
   b. Readjusting sensitivity controls or electrodes if infant breathing and color are good
   c. Waiting 10 seconds to see if the infant starts to breathe spontaneously if the infant is not breathing but the skin is pink (if the infant does not begin to breathe, gently shake the baby or slap the bottom of the feet; if the baby still does not begin to breathe, start CPR)
   d. Trying to stimulate the infant by gently shaking or slapping the bottom of the feet if the baby is not breathing and is dusky or blue (if the baby does not begin to breathe, start CPR)
4. How to keep a cribside record of all alarm incidences on a flow sheet. This record should include time, length of apnea, infant's skin color, heart rate, stimulation measures taken, and medications given.
5. To report all incidences to a physician
6. To check the alarm periodically by disconnecting the sensor plug. The alarm should sound after the preset timer delay.
7. To be sure that other children in the home are instructed not to turn off or tamper with the monitor

ENTERAL THERAPY

Enteral nutrition involves the administration of liquified foods or formulas containing all necessary and adequate amounts of calories and nutrients to sustain life. It may be used as a supplement or as complete nutritional support for the client who is unable to take food orally. Home enteral nutrition has been used for clients with swallowing dysfunction or upper intestinal obstruction for many decades (Howard and others, 1986). Some indications for use in both adult and pediatric clients include anorexia and weight loss associated with chronic illness, pancreatic insufficiency, short bowel syndrome, gastrointestinal reflex, protracted diarrhea, malnutrition, Crohn's disease, neurologic disease with associated inability to swallow, anorexia nervosa, cystic fibrosis associated with malnutrition, cancer, and stroke.

Enteral therapy is the infusion of nutrient solutions into a client's gastrointestinal tract through a tube. The nutrient solution is then instilled into the digestive tract using a feeding bag and an administration set or an electromechanical pump such as a kangaroo pump (see Appendix), which controls the rate at which the solution is pumped. The feeding may be intermittent or continuous, or occasionally a bolus feeding is ordered. Bolus feedings are given using the barrel of an irrigation syringe or a funnel attached to the feeding tube. Choice of administration depends on tube location and client tolerance.

Enteral feedings may be administered through tubes placed in a variety of sites in the intestinal tract including nasogastric, nasoduodenal, and nasojejunal or through surgical placement of a tube in an opening, or ostomy, such as an esophagostomy, gastrostomy, or jejunostomy, and then guided into the intestinal tract. Home enteral nutritional feeding programs are less expensive and have fewer complications than home parenteral nutrition programs, and they are easier for the client and family to manage (Walsh, 1987).

Formula to be used for enteral feedings may be a home-blended or commercially prepared product. Generally a home-blended formula is cheaper and may be considered if the client or family is willing and able to prepare the formula. In addition, home-prepared formulas contain dietary fiber that may prevent constipation, and the formula can be individually adapted to meet needs of clients with specific problems such as diabetes or congestive heart failure (Bayer, 1983). Commercial formulas are stored in a dry place at room temperature. Once opened, formulas must be used immediately and any unused portion should be refrigerated in a clean, airtight container. They may be kept as long as indicated by the manufacturer and then discarded. Home-blended formulas should be tightly sealed, dated, refrigerated, and kept for no longer than 24 hours.

There are a number of problems associated with home enteral therapy including mechanical, physical, and psychosocial concerns. Mechanical problems are generally related to operation of the electromechanical pump. Tube blockage caused by food or medication and breakage or displacement may also occur. There may be leaking around the tube because the catheter balloon has become deflated or has slipped away from the intestinal wall or because the feeding tube is too small for the stoma.

Physical problems may be related to irritation around the stoma or tube. Although some erythema or drainage may be normal, gastric leaking or dampness may lead to increased redness, tissue breakdown, and bleeding. Excessive epithelial tissue may build up and interfere with care. The client may experience vomiting, diarrhea, or both for a variety of reasons including migration of the tube into the duodenum or jejunum, causing "dumping," which results in liquid stool, and blocking or irritation of the pylorus by the gastrostomy tube, which may cause vomiting. Vomiting may also result from too large or too rapid a feeding.

Psychosocial problems related to enteral feeding are related to receiving food in an unfamiliar manner and at unconventional times—even while sleeping. According to Maloney (1980), clients associate tube feeding with the feeling of thirst, the deprivation of tasting food, and an unsatisfied appetite for food. Simple comfort measures can be incorporated into care plans to assist these clients. The clients should rinse their mouth frequently with water or mouthwash, and frequent and thorough oral hygiene should be carried out. If permitted, a favorite food can be chewed, tasted, and spit out. Chewing ice chips or an occasional hard candy if permitted may meet the need for oral stimulation (Bayer, 1983).

Disturbance of body image is often associated with a feeding tube. Clients may be uncomfortable if the family or others see the enterostomy tube. Dependence on the tube or mechanical device can produce anxiety. Not eating with the family or being involved in the preparation of meals and the pleasure associated with meals and eating are contrary to values of society (Bayer, 1983). The client getting enteral therapy needs help and reassurances to cope with all these psychosocial problems.

Once it is determined that a client and family are candidates for enteral home care, it must be decided whether commercially prepared formula will be used or the client and family will be responsible for formula preparation. A type of feeding administration that will meet the client's needs and that can be handled by the client and family most easily must be selected. If home enteral therapy is to be carried out over a long period, as in the case of a chronically ill individual or a young child with a congenital defect such as short bowel syndrome, the infusion pump and supplies may be purchased by the family or rented with the rental payments credited toward the purchase. In a review by Howard and others (1986), clients on home enteral therapy are separated into short-term (clients with a malignancy) and long-term clients (clients with a benign long-term condition such as short bowel syndrome). Home enteral support service might be structured differently for each group. Short-term clients may be better served by more circumscribed nutritional support fluids and electrolytes only, with fewer potential metabolic implications and less in-hospital learning time. They may require more home nursing visits and a close link to a hospice program. Long-term clients, on the other hand, require all nutrients and, once established at home, may require more limited nursing support and encouragement to achieve maximum independence with as much social and physical rehabilitation as possible.

In a consumer survey of 172 home enteral clients (Howard and others, 1986), the four most desired features were pharmacy-mixed solutions, home delivery of supplies by a vendor, reimbursement management by a home care service, and a nurse available for a home visit at the time of discharge and round-the-clock emergency service to discuss problems and replace equipment.

The trend today is to work through a vendor who assesses the client and begins teaching in the hospital setting. The vendor also assesses the home setting, delivers supplies, and sets up equipment before the client is discharged from the hospital. The client and family are then usually followed by a home health agency case manager until services are no longer needed—the client and family are independent or the client is readmitted or dies.

Nursing Responsibilities

Nursing responsibilities vary depending on the type of enteral feeding procedure used. Initially the client is assessed for general condition including vital signs, status of disease process, and condition of site of tube insertion. If the feeding involves inserting a nasogastric tube before each feeding, the nurse must assess whether the client or the family is capable of inserting it. If they are not able, a plan must be devised to handle insertion and changing of the tube by the nurse until the client or family is ready to take over. The nurse determines the client or family understanding of all procedures and their ability to carry them out appropriately. The nurse also assesses the ongoing condition of the client including changes in condition and feeding response to initial and subsequent feeds, noting food allergies, nutritional problems, and indications of intolerance to feeding, including abdominal distention, nausea, vomiting, flatulence, and bowel changes.

The nurse is responsible for demonstrating all procedures to the family and for carrying out complex procedures when necessary, such as replacing gastrostomy tubes or inserting or changing nasogastric tubes if the client or family cannot. The nurse monitors the client's progress and reports to the physician as necessary.

Lastly, the nurse must work toward creation of a supportive environment for the client and the family as they adapt to the home treatment.

Client Education

Client or caretaker education is an essential area to be addressed by the nurse.

The content to be mastered before beginning home enteral feedings includes the following:

1. Feeding tube management, including insertion of the tube (if applicable), checking for proper placement, irrigation, and maintenance of the tube. Nasal tubes should be marked and taped to prevent them from slipping too far in or out of the enteral tract. The skin around the tubes should be cleansed daily and as needed with mild soap and water or antiseptic solution. Dressings should be changed daily at least. Any red-

ness, drainage, foul odor, tenderness, or excessive bleeding at the site of the feeding tube should be reported to the nurse.
2. Formula handling, including preparation of formula (if applicable), storage, length of time formula can remain at room temperature once it is prepared or the container is opened, and how to add medications and electrolytes as ordered
3. Feeding administration, including pump operation or gavage techniques
4. Recognizing and handling problems, including measurement of gastric residual, dealing with diarrhea or vomiting and symptoms of pulmonary aspiration. Clients and family should be taught to discontinue the feeding immediately if they have any respiratory difficulty, nausea, or vomiting and notify the nurse or home health agency.
5. Measuring intake and output every eight hours, weighing the client daily, and recording this information appropriately
6. Emergency telephone numbers of agency, nurse, physician, and vendor for help on a 24-hour basis

MECHANICAL VENTILATION

Mechanical ventilation can be defined as the inspiration and expiration of air from the lungs through use of a mechanical device that may be hand operated or machine driven. According to Sivak (1985), the need for mechanical ventilation may arise as a result of failure of the respiratory system caused by failure of either the lung parenchyma (the essential parts of an organ concerned with its function) or muscles. The symptoms of failure of the lung parenchyma range from acute tachypnea to chronic dyspnea at rest as a result of hypoxemia. Failure of the respiratory muscles is caused by hypercarbia and associated hypoxemia and ranges from an acute respiratory arrest to dyspnea. Therapeutic intervention through the use of mechanical ventilation is based on the disease process causing respiratory failure. The disease processes include fibrosis, pneumonia, retained secretions, bronchospasm or emphysema, and pulmonary edema of cardiac or noncardiac origin. The failure of respiratory muscles can occur from a decreased drive to breathe, stiffness and weakness of the chest wall as a result of cerebral degenerations, chest wall defects, respiratory muscle failure, neuromacular disease, and diaphragmatic dysfunction or fatigue of the muscles. Sivak (1983) classified clients who are dependent on mechanical ventilation into two categories—those who can be weaned completely or partially from mechanical ventilation and require rehabilitative care and those who become irreversibly ventilator dependent and require custodial care.

Initially the client requiring mechanical ventilation may be managed in an intensive care unit and as the condition stabilizes can move to some form of long-term institutional setting. To decrease the costs of care and improve the quality of life, many clients from either the rehabilitative or the custodial classification may be candidates for home care.

Care of the ventilator-dependent individual in the home dates back to the 1940s and 1950s and began as a result of the epidemics of poliomyelitis prevalent at that time. Because of an unprecedented number of polio clients with respiratory paralysis, respirator centers were established with the assistance of the March of Dimes. Many of those clients who survived required full- or part-time mechanical ventilation, and this resulted in a need for home care programs. When the polio vaccine was developed, the epidemics ceased and the need for specialized respiratory home health care providers diminished. Today, as a result of advances in technology, survival rates of victims of trauma and individuals with neuromuscular diseases have increased. Contemporary intensive care nurseries equipped with sophisticated technology and advanced nursing care preserve the lives of increasing numbers of high-risk infants born with a wide variety of conditions or problems related to prematurity, congenital anomalies, or both. Although these children initially survive, they frequently remain dependent on advanced life support technology and require costly long-term rehabilitative or custodial care. Therefore, because of the growing number of clients who remain dependent on mechanical ventilation indefinitely or for long periods, there is an increased interest in home care programs.

Equipment used by clients on mechanical ventilation falls into two general categories—noninvasive, negative pressure ventilatory support and invasive positive pressure ventilators.

Noninvasive Negative Pressure Ventilatory Support

Clients with neuromuscular disease or spinal injuries, where decreased lung compliance is not a problem, are candidates for noninvasive negative pressure ventilatory support. External negative pressure ventilators operate on the principle of the iron lung. They function in a manner similar to a vacuum cleaner, creating negative pressure and causing a sucking action on the chest. Lightweight portable ventilators are available that encompass the chest rather than the whole body as did the older tank type (iron lung). Other negative pressure devices include the rocking bed and the exsufflator, or pneumobelt.

The portable negative pressure ventilators are small and easy to operate and can be used without a tracheostomy or endotracheal tube. They do not cause pooling of blood in the extremities as the other tank ventilators do. They are used most frequently by clients who have fairly compliant lungs and the ability to control their secretions.

Invasive Positive Pressure Ventilators

Positive pressure ventilators are used in conjunction with either a tracheostomy or endotracheal tube and are usually used for clients with some form of respiratory obstructive disease or paralysis. According to Fischer (1985), a backup portable ventilator is required for emergencies and for clients who are ambulatory or wheelchair bound. These ventilators are powered with an automobile battery and can be mounted on the back of a wheelchair or on a cart with wheels (Fig. 14-12).

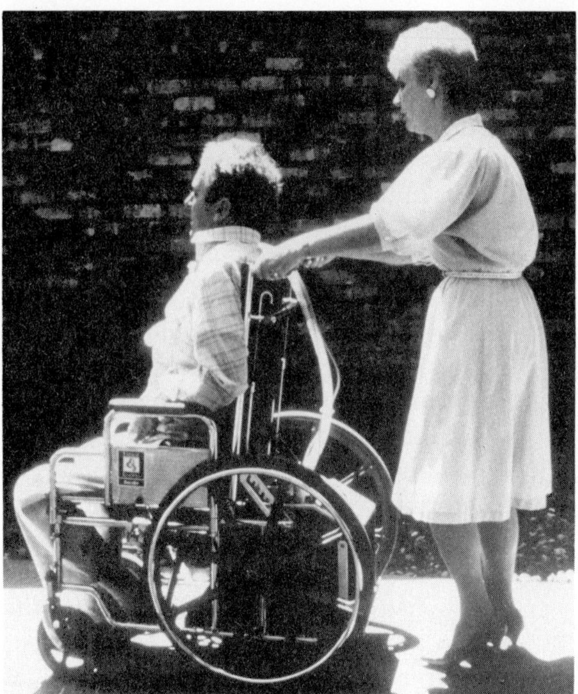

FIG. 14-12. Mechanical ventilator mounted on back of wheelchair. (Courtesy Aequitron Medical, Inc.)

General Considerations

Determination of a candidate for home care cannot be decided by the physician, client, or family alone but is rather a decision that must be made based on input from all parties involved. According to Shreiner Dnar, and Kettrick (1987), the process may be facilitated through an education process that helps the family understand the caregiving responsibilities and provides thorough explanations of the advantages, disadvantages, risks, and benefits for clients, whether they be children or adults, and the family. Initiation of a home care ventilator program requires a team effort including the physician, nursing staff, social worker, respiratory therapist, physical therapist, vendor, vendor nurse, home health care nurse manager, family or caretaker, and client.

The criteria for eligibility for mechanical ventilation in the home are consistent with criteria for all high technology home care. The family and client must want home care and be willing to accept the responsibility. It is more important to determine how self-motivated the client is than whether one family member can give care. If other family members, friends, or the community can provide respite care, full-time nursing can be obtained if needed. Lastly, the family or client must have the intelligence, manual dexterity, and hand-eye coordination needed to carry out respiratory treatments and techniques. The client must be medically stable. According to Shreiner, Dnar, and Kettrick (1987), "medical stability denotes the presence of a stable airway, oxygen requirements that do not fluctuate under baseline conditions, ventilatory support that insures arterial PCO_2 and PO_2 levels that are within safe physiological limits," and (in the case of the child) the ability to maintain a nutritional intake adequate to support growth and development.

It must be determined whether the client has adequate financial support. Expenses for a home ventilator program vary depending on the type of equipment needed, whether it is purchased or rented, whether full- or part-time nursing care is needed, and the length of time the client requires care.

Lastly the home environment must be assessed for the best location for the client and equipment. This varies depending on whether clients need full-time or periodic ventilatory support and whether they are ambulatory, wheelchair bound, or bedridden. The ventilator must be close to water and power supplies, and, where necessary, appropriate electrical wiring and outlets must be installed. If the client requires a wheelchair, it must be determined whether there is wheelchair access to the home and through the doorway to the bedroom and bathroom and whether stairs are present. The wheelchair needs a platform on the back for a portable ventilator. The home must be assessed for cleanliness and the presence of air pollution, especially smokers in the family. The family must notify the electric company and fire department that a ventilator-dependent individual is in the home.

Once it is determined that a client meets the criteria for home health care, a lengthy period of preparation is begun. Arrangements are made for a vendor to provide equipment and supplies and where indicated install them appropriately in the home.

A home health agency is contacted to provide follow-up care and 24-hour support service as needed. According to Fischer (1985), the first few days and weeks after discharge are critical. The success of the program rests on the availability and reliability of support personnel during this time. Frequent follow-up visits by the nurse case manager are usually needed to identify and deal with real and potential problems during this critical period. As the self-confidence of the family grows, members gradually need less support. The case manager is generally responsible for coordinating all aspects of care, assessing the client's condition, including drawing blood to periodically determine blood gas levels, reporting to the physician, assessing and reinforcing client and family teaching, adjusting the plan of care as needed, providing emotional support to the client and family, and acting as a source for referral and consultation.

The family, caretaker, or client begins a lengthy educational program that involves the efforts of all members of the team. Once it is determined they are ready, it is recommended that the family or caretaker actually care for the client for a 24-

hour period in the agency setting, demonstrating the ability to handle the equipment and all treatments and nursing care. It may also help ease the transition to home care if the client is sent home on a weekend pass to ease into the situation more gradually.

Education for Client, Family, and Caretaker

Care of the ventilator-dependent client is complex and varied.

Education before transfer to a home program is extensive and must be tailored to meet the needs of the particular client, the disease process, and the resources and support available. This education must begin in the agency before discharge to the home.

The family, caretaker, or client should be taught the following:

1. How to assess the client's condition, including changes in sputum, breathing pattern, and vital signs, signs of infection, and problems with the tracheostomy tube
2. How to record the daily condition of the client and when or what to report
3. How to maintain and troubleshoot the ventilator and oxygen equipment, including oxygen safety and precautions
4. To perform postural drainage and suctioning when necessary
5. How to care for the artificial airway (tracheostomy or laryngectomy where appropriate)
6. How to perform CPR
7. General nursing care of clients based on whether they are ambulatory, wheelchair bound, or bedridden. This would include hygiene measures, proper positioning, care of skin to prevent breakdown over pressure areas and range of motion exercises to prevent contractures, nutritional support, and in the case of a child promotion of well child maintenance and adequate growth, development, and education. Anyone who is ill, particularly anyone with an upper respiratory infection, should not come in contact with the client. Irritants, including smoke, pollen, or aerosol spray, should be removed from the air. An air conditioner may be helpful.
8. Emergency measures and contingency plans, including the following:
   a. Knowing phone numbers to call for 24-hour support and emergency medical assistance
   b. Placing the client on the backup ventilator before making adjustments if a problem occurs with the ventilator and notifying the vendor if the problem cannot be corrected
   c. Knowing how to manually inflate the lungs using an Ambu bag if both ventilators malfunction
   d. Checking circuit breakers and fuses in the home and how to change fuses where indicated
   e. Using the ventilator's internal battery in case of a power failure. Most home ventilators have an internal battery that will maintain function for about one hour. The power company should be notified and informed of the need for immediate attention. The client should use the backup portable ventilator and the oxygen supply should also be transferred to the portable equipment.
   f. Knowing how to respond to low and high pressure alarms on equipment following instructions of the vendor. If the problem cannot be corrected, a manual resuscitator with prescribed oxygen flow should be used and the vendor should be notified.
   g. In case of cardiac arrest, notifying emergency medical service and physician or home health nurse. While waiting for help, the client should be disconnected from the ventilator and CPR should be

initiated. When help arrives, the client is usually transported to the hospital.

h. If the client loses consciousness, notifying the emergency medical service and the physician or home health nurse. Vital signs should be monitored, and the client should be transported to the hospital if necessary.

i. If the client has seizures but has no history of seizures, notifying emergency medical service and carrying out general seizure precautions, disconnecting the ventilator, initiating manual resuscitation using the Ambu bag, and transporting to the hospital. If there is a history of seizures, treat as prescribed by the physician.

SUMMARY

Advances in technology and changes within the health care system and in society have contributed to the increased demand for home health care incorporating the use of high technology. The goal of high technology home care is primarily to help the child and family achieve as much independence as possible until resolution of the case through return to wellness, readmission to the acute care facility, or death. This state of affairs provides a challenge for nurses working in the home setting and has led to the development of a variety of new roles for nurses, each having its own unique responsibilities and requiring a wide range of skills.

Factors to consider when identifying candidates for high technology home care generally include medical stability, the desire for home care by client and family, the home environment, and the client's financial resources.

One approach used by home health agencies for the organization of high technology home care is to provide a multidisciplinary team approach under the direction of a nurse acting as a case manager. The case manager usually has a background in critical care and oversees the care of a caseload of clients. The role of the nurse involved in high technology care centers on organizing and coordinating care. Responsibilities generally include gathering an accurate health history, assessing the client's physical and psychosocial needs, planning care, delivering relevant nursing care of a high technology nature in the home setting, evaluating care, communicating with other health team members, educating the client and family in relation to care, and creating a supportive home environment as the client and family adapt to the treatment program.

A variety of high technology therapies are currently available for treatment of the client in the home. These therapies include infusion therapies such as antibiotic therapy, chemotherapy, pain management and parenteral nutritional therapy, enteral therapy, phototherapy, apnea monitoring, and mechanical ventilation.

QUESTIONS FOR DISCUSSION

1. What is a vendor nurse?
2. What is the difference between high technology home care and supportive custodial care?
3. What factors need to be taken into account in developing a teaching plan for home health care?
4. List three high technology therapies, and explain the procedures involved.
5. What is the role of the family caretaker in home health care?

REFERENCES

Bayer LM and others: Tube feeding at home, Am J Nurs 83:1321, 1983.

Fischer A: Long term management of the ventilator patient in the home, Cleve Clin Q 52:3, 1985.

Goodman MS and Wickham R: Venous access devices: an overview, Oncol Nurs Forum 11:16, 1984.

Haddad AM: High tech home care: a practical guide, Rockville, Md, 1987, Aspen Publishers Inc.

Howard L and others: A review of the current national status of home parenteral and enteral nutrition from the provider and consumer perspective, J Parent Enter Nutr 10:416, 1986.

Jernigan DK: Home management of epidural catheters for pain control, Caring 5:85, 1986.

Kasmer RJ, Hoisington LM, and Yukniewicy S: Home antibiotic therapy. I. An overview of program design, Home Healthcare Nurse 5:12, 1984a.

Kasmer RJ, Hoisington LM, and Yukniewicy S: Home antibiotic therapy. II. Drug preparation and administration considerations, Home Healthcare Nurse 5:19, 1984b.

Klein S: Continuous morphine infusion therapy in the home setting, Rx Home Care p. 59, June 1986.

Locklin MA: Assessing jaundice in full-term newborns, Pediatr Nurs 13:15, 1987.

Maloney M and Farrell M: Treatment of severe weight loss in anorexia nervosa with hyperalimentation and psychotherapy, Am J Psychiatry 137:310, 1980.

Nelson J: Textbook of pediatrics, New York, 1985, Vaughn & McKay.

Poretz D and others: Intravenous antibiotic therapy in an outpatient setting, JAMA 248:336, 1982.

Scribner BH and others: Long term total parenteral nutrition: the concept of an artificial gut, JAMA 212:457, 1970.

Sheridan MS: Things that go beep in the night: home monitoring for apnea, Health Soc Work 9:63, 1985.

Shreiner MS, Dnar MD, and Kettrick RG: Pediatric home mechanical ventilation, Pediatr Clin North Am 34(1):47, 1987.

Sivak ED: Long term management of the ventilator-dependent patient—preparation for home care, Cleve Clin Q 52:307, 1985.

Visiting Nursing Association of Buffalo: Policy manual, Buffalo, NY, 1985, The Association.

Walsh J, Persons C, and Wieck L: Manual of home health care nursing, Philadelphia, 1987, JB Lippincott Co.

Williams D and others: Outpatient intravenous antibiotics experience with 65 patients, Am J Intrav Ther Clin Nutr 14:33, 1982.

Winters V: Implantable vascular access devices, Oncol Nurs Forum 11:25, 1984.

BIBLIOGRAPHY

Andrews MM and Neilson DW: Technology dependent children in the home, Pediatr Nurs 14:111, 1988.

Barfoot KR: Home care of the child receiving nutritional support: a global approach, NITA 9:226, 1986.

Beckert BH: Removing the mysteries of parenteral nutrition, Pediatr Nurs 13:1, 1987.

Broaten D and others: Breast milk jaundice, J Obstet Gynecol Neonatal Nurs 14:220, 1985.

Carlsen KR: IV antibiotics: nursing considerations in the administration of the initial dose, NITA 9:62, 1986.

Dortch E and Spottiswoode P: New light in phototherapy: home use, Neonatal Network 4:30, 1986.

Fischer A: Long term management of the ventilator patient in the home, Cleve Clin Q 52:3, 1985.

Frates RC Jr and others: Outcome of home mechanical ventilation in children, J Pediatr 106:850, 1985.

Frey AM: Taking the confusion out of multiple infusion, NITA 9:460, 1986.

Hughes CB: A totally implantable central venous system for chemotherapy administration, NITA 8:513, 1985.

Hughes CB: Infantile apnea and home monitoring, Washington, DC, 1986, National Institutes of Health Consensus Development Conference.

Kanei I: Hickman catheters: your guide to trouble free use, Can Nurse 78:25, 1982.

Korthan M: Home total parenteral nutrition complications, NITA 8:231, 1985.

Maisil JM: Neonatal jaundice. In Avery GB, editor: Neonatology: pathophysiology of the newborn, ed 2, Philadelphia: 1981, JB Lippincott Co.

McConnell EA: Ten problems with nasogastric tubes and how to solve them, Nursing 19:78, 1979.

Moore MC and Green HL: Tube feeding of infants and children, Pediatr Clin North Am 32:401, 1985.

Poarblerg J and Balint JP: Gastrostomy tubes: practical guidelines for home care, Pediatr Nurs 11:99, 1985.

Rowland TW and others: Infant home apnea monitoring: a five year assessment, Clin Pediatr 26:383, 1987.

Shehan AM and Fitzgerald RJ: Home parenteral nutrition in childhood, Ir Med J 79:253, 1986.

Steiger E and others: Total parenteral nutrition and fluid/ electrolyte therapy in the home: nine years' experience, Cleve Clin Q 52:317, 1985.

Steiger E, Sattler L, and Wotsika L: Cost of a parenteral nutrition program, JAMA 244:2303, 1980.

Taylor MB: The effect of DRGs in home health care, Nurs Outlook 33:288, 1985.

Vargas JH and others: Long term home parenteral nutrition in pediatrics: ten years of experience in 102 patients, J Pediatr Gastroenterol Nutr 6:24, 1987.

Wagner JL, Fox H, and Power EJ: Technology-dependent children: hospital v. home care; a technical memorandum from the Office of Technology Assessment, U.S. Congress, Washington, DC, Philadelphia, 1988, JB Lippincott Co.

Walliser L: Enteral home therapy: a patient with complex needs, Home Health Care Professional 1:6, 1984.

Wildblood R, Strego A, and Strego PL: The how-to's of home IV therapy, Pediatr Nurs 13:42, 1987.

Wilkes G, Vannicola P, and Starck P: Long term venous access, Am J Nurs 85:793, 1985.

APPENDIX Protocols for Procedures Performed in the Home*

I. Insertion of butterfly or winged needle
  A. Definition
    1. Insertion of "butterfly" or winged needle
    2. Using a small-lumen, short-bevel metal needle with plastic wings
  B. Purpose
    1. For short-term therapy
    2. To administer IV push medications
    3. To obtain blood samples
  C. Equipment
    1. Alcohol swabs, betadine swabs, betadine ointment, or IV start kit
    2. 2 inch × 3 inch gauze pads or transparent dressing
    3. Winged infusion needle
    4. IV solution
    5. IV administration set
    6. Arm board
    7. Tape
  D. Procedure
    1. Explain the procedure to the client.
    2. Wash hands.
    3. Prepare IV solution and administration set. Expel the air from the administration set.
    4. Select the site for venipuncture and prepare the skin. (Refer to procedure "Preparation of Skin for Venipuncture.")
    5. Once the skin is prepared and the prepping solution is allowed to air dry, apply the tourniquet approximately 4 inches above the selected site. (If possible, place the tourniquet above the antecubital fossa to ensure adequate venous distention.)
    6. Remove the protective cover from the winged infusion needle, and hold the bevel upward.
    7. Anchor the client's skin firmly using caution not to contaminate the prepared site. Enter the vein with the bevel upward.
    8. Verify entry into the vein with a "flashback" of blood in the needle tubing. Care should be taken not to puncture the posterior wall of the vein.
    9. Slowly advance the needle, angling upward, a few centimeters. Allow blood to backflow and fill the tubing to expel the air.
    10. Remove tourniquet.
    11. Insert the IV tubing into the hub of the winged infusion needle tubing. Establish the fluid flow.
    12. Tape the winged infusion needle securely in place.
    13. Apply dressing. (Refer to procedure "Transparent or Gauze Dressing: Peripheral Catheter.")
    14. If the needle is to remain in place, label the dressing with the size and length of the winged infusion needle, the date of insertion, and your initials. This provides an accurate record of the care the client received.
    15. Document the procedure in the client's chart including the length and site of insertion and needle size.

    NOTE: No more than two attempts should be made. If successful cannulation is not secured with two attempts, the senior IV nurse or client service manager should be consulted.

II. Insertion of intravenous catheter
  A. Definition
    1. Insertion of a catheter into a vein to administer IV fluids or medication
  B. Purpose
    1. Used in short or long-term therapy
    2. Used when it is essential to maintain uninterrupted drug delivery
  C. Equipment
    1. Alcohol swab, betadine swabs, betadine ointment, or IV start kit
    2. 2 inch × 2 inch gauze pads or transparent dressing
    3. IV catheter
    4. Tape
  D. Procedure
    1. Explain the procedure to the client.
    2. Wash hands.
    3. Prepare IV solution and administration set or IV medication. Expel the air from the administration set.
    4. Select the site for the infusion and prepare the skin. (Refer to procedure "Preparation of Skin for Venipuncture.")

* Courtesy Visiting Nursing Association of Western New York, Inc, Buffalo, NY.

5. Once the skin is prepared and the prepping solution is allowed to air dry, apply the tourniquet.
6. Remove the catheter from the protective cover and hold the catheter with bevel upward. Be sure the catheter is seated securely on the introducing needle. If the catheter is over the needle bevel, it is not possible to perform a proper venipuncture.
7. Anchor the client's skin firmly using caution not to contaminate the prepared site.
8. Verify entry into the vein with a "flashback" of blood in the flash chamber.
9. Once the needle is in the vein, carefully introduce approximately ⅛ inch farther to ensure that entry of the catheter is into the lumen of the vein. If only the bevel of the needle, and not an adequate amount of the catheter, is in the vein, it may not be possible to "thread" the catheter of the needle into the vein.
10. Apply dressing. (Refer to procedure "Transparent or Gauze Dressing: Central Catheter.")

    NOTE: No more than three attempts should be made. If successful cannulation is not secured with three attempts, the senior IV nurse or client service manager should be consulted.

III. Transparent or gauze dressing change: peripheral catheter

A. Purpose
1. Prevention of infection of IV insertion site

B. Equipment
1. 2 inch × 2 inch sterile gauze dressings or transparent dressing
2. 1 inch tape
3. Three alcohol swabs
4. Three betadine swabs
5. Betadine ointment (omit with transparent dressing)
6. Waste receptacle

C. Procedure
1. Peripheral catheter dressings are to be changed if soiled, loosened, or wet. Otherwise, they may be left in place until site rotation is necessary (every 48 to 72 hours).
2. Choose a clean, uncluttered work area.
3. Place waste receptacle on floor near client.
4. Assemble all equipment.
5. Wash hands thoroughly.
6. Prepare work area. Open dressing and supplies using aseptic technique.
7. Remove old dressing with special care not to pull on the catheter.
8. Observe the catheter site for redness, swelling, or drainage. If these are present, remove catheter.
9. Clean the area surrounding the catheter with alcohol swabs. Start at the catheter exit site and cleanse in a circular motion, moving from the inside to the outside. Clean an area approximately 2 inches in diameter.
10. Apply betadine ointment (omit with transparent dressing).
11. Apply either sterile gauze dressing or transparent dressing.
    a. Open sterile dressing package and remove dressing. Place dressing over catheter exit site. Tape dressing on all four sides, providing an occlusive dressing.
    b. Open transparent dressing package, remove the protective backing, and place dressing over the catheter site. Remove protective border of transparent dressing once dressing is securely in place.
12. Document procedure.

IV. Administration of IV medication using minibag (via peripheral line)

A. Purpose
1. Administration of an IV medication using a small volume, sealed, parenteral administration system
2. Administration of an IV medication that has been premixed and diluted, via peripheral line

B. Equipment
1. IV solution (medication)
2. Administration tubing
3. IV pole
4. Povidone-iodine swab or alcohol swab
5. Needle disposal box
6. Tape
7. Saline flush
8. 2 inch × 2 inch gauze sponge
9. Towel

C. Procedure
1. Remove medication solution from refrigerator or freezer at time designated by pharmacist. Solution should be administered at room temperature.
2. Clean work area. Prepare the area as needed to protect the client's clothing and environment.
3. Assemble equipment.
4. Wash hands thoroughly.

5. Remove administration tubing from box and inspect tubing to ensure tubing and spike are intact. Straighten tubing and secure new needle on end of tubing.
6. Close the roller clamp to prevent inadvertent fluid flow through the tubing.
7. "Spike" the administration port with the tubing.
8. Invert the IV bag and suspend the bag and tubing from the IV pole at least 30 to 36 inches above the level of the client's heart while infusing. (An alternative to gravity infusion is the use of an electronic infusion device that regulates flow accurately.)
9. Squeeze the drip chamber to partially fill it (one third to one half full). If the drip chamber fills completely, it is not possible to see the drops drip. If this happens, crimp tubing at the bottom of the drip chamber. Invert the bag and gently squeeze the drip chamber until some fluid has returned to the bag.
10. Open the roller clamp to fill the tubing and needle with medication solution.
11. Check for patency of IV cannula by cleansing injection cap with povidone-iodine and slowly inject 1 ml of normal saline; observe catheter site for infiltration. If resistance is felt, do not push with force. Try to aspirate if unable to flush.
12. If heparin lock is patent, clean the rubber diaphragm with a povidone-iodine wipe. Remove the protective cap, and insert the needle into the diaphragm.
13. Secure with tape to prevent contamination caused by pistoning suction.
14. Regulate the clamp to allow solution to flow at specified rate.
15. When the solution bag is empty, close the roller clamp and remove the needle from the rubber diaphragm.
16. Heparinize the catheter following the instructions for "Heparinization: Peripheral Catheter."
17. Dispose of needle and other nondurable equipment.

    NOTE: Alcohol swabs may be substituted for povidone-iodine in this procedure.

V. Heparinization: peripheral catheter (heparin lock)
   A. Definition
      1. Instillation of heparin into a peripheral catheter
   B. Purpose
      1. To prevent clotting of blood within the catheter
   C. Equipment
      1. Heparin (dosage to be prescribed by physician)
      2. 5 ml syringe with 22 gauge needle, 5/8 inch length
      3. Alcohol swab
   D. Procedure
      1. Assemble supplies.
      2. Wash hands thoroughly with soap and water.
      3. Wipe heparin vial with alcohol and allow to dry.
      4. Draw up prescribed heparin dosage into syringe.
      5. Clear all air from syringe.
      6. Clean injection port with alcohol and allow to dry.
      7. Insert the needle of the heparin syringe into the injection port.
      8. Instill the heparin solution into the catheter. Withdraw needle.
      9. Document the procedure including amount of heparin instilled.

         NOTE: The heparinization procedure is done after each dose of medication and at least daily when no fluids are being infused.

VI. Heparinization: central catheter
   A. Definition
      1. Instillation of heparin into a central catheter
   B. Purpose
      1. To prevent clotting of blood within the catheter
   C. Equipment
      1. Heparin (dosage to be prescribed by physician)*
      2. 5 ml syringe with 22 gauge needle, 5/8 inch length
      3. Alcohol swabs
      4. Tape
   D. Procedure
      1. Assemble supplies.
      2. Wash hands thoroughly with soap and water.
      3. Remove tape holding catheter to dressing and allow catheter to uncoil.
      4. Wipe heparin vial with alcohol and allow to dry.

5. Draw up prescribed heparin dose into syringe.
6. Clear all air from syringe.
7. Wipe injection port of catheter with alcohol and allow to dry.
8. Open clamp on the catheter if present.
9. Insert the needle of the heparin syringe into the injection port.
10. Instill the heparin solution into the catheter.
11. To prevent backflow and clotting, while 5 ml of solution remains in the syringe begin to withdraw the needle while continuing to maintain pressure on the plunger until all heparin is instilled and syringe is withdrawn.
12. If clamp is present, change position of the clamp to prevent wear on the catheter. Close the clamp completely.
13. Retape catheter to the dressing with cap pointed up.
14. Document procedure including amount of heparin solution instilled.
    NOTE: Normal dosage of heparin at 100U per milliliter range from 250U to 500U (2.5 milliliters to 5.0 milliliters). Dosages varying from this should be verified with physician before administration.

VII. Transparent or gauze dressing change: central catheter
   A. Purpose
      1. Prevention of infection of catheter exit site
   B. Equipment
      1. Sterile gauze dressings (4 inch × 4 inch or 2 inch × 2 inch) or transparent dressing
      2. 1-inch tape
      3. Three alcohol swabsticks
      4. Three betadine swabsticks
      5. Betadine ointment (omit with transparent dressing)
      6. Waste receptacle
   C. Procedure
      1. Change central catheter dressings as ordered by the physician.
      2. Choose a clean, uncluttered work area.
      3. Place waste receptacle on floor near client.
      4. Assemble all equipment.
      5. Wash hands thoroughly.
      6. Prepare work area. Open dressing and supplies using aseptic technique.
      7. Remove old dressing with special care not to pull on the catheter.
      8. Observe the catheter site for redness, swelling, or drainage.
      9. Clean the area surrounding the catheter with alcohol swabsticks. Start at the catheter exit site and cleanse in a circular motion, moving from the inside to the outside. Clean an area approximately 2 inches in diameter. Repeat this procedure once.
      10. Using iodine swabstick, follow the same procedure as with the alcohol twice. Allow to dry for two minutes using a prepackaged iodine swabstick, cleanse down catheter from exit site approximately 2 inches toward cap.
      11. Use remaining alcohol swabstick. Cleanse area as in step 9 removing excess iodine.
      12. Apply betadine ointment (omit with transparent dressing).
      13. Apply either sterile gauze dressing or transparent dressing.
          a. Open sterile dressing package and remove dressings. Place two dressings over catheter exit site. Tape dressing on all four sides, providing an occlusive dressing.
          b. Open transparent dressing package, remove the protective backing, and place dressing over the catheter site. Remove protective border of transparent dressing once dressing is securely in place.
      14. Coil catheter over dressing and tape catheter to the chest with cap pointing upward.
      15. Document procedure.

VIII. Administration of parenteral nutrition (hyperalimentation)
   A. Purpose
      1. To provide adequate nutrition to sustain life and maintain normal growth and development
      2. To provide nutrition via parenteral route
   B. Equipment
      1. Solution
      2. Infusion pump
      3. Tubing
      4. Filter
      5. Catheter clamp
      6. Alcohol and betadine swabs
      7. Tape
      8. Additives

C. Procedure
   1. Remove solution from refrigerator at least two hours before infusion. Protect from heat and direct sunlight. Check label for name and expiration date.
   2. Prepare clean work area.
   3. Assemble all necessary equipment.
   4. Wash hands.
   5. Prepare additives as prescribed and add to solution.
   6. Connect administration set and filter.
   7. Spike bag with administration set and open clamp to remove the air and prime the tubing. (Thread tubing through the pump per specific pump instructions.)
   8. Set the infusion rate per physician's orders. For cyclic hyperalimentation some physicians prefer initiating the infusion at a slow rate, as well as the usual slowing of the infusion before termination.
   9. Clamp the catheter.
      NOTE: Catheter containing valves, such as the Groshong catheter, should *not* be clamped.
   10. Remove catheter cap and cleanse opening with betadine swab; allow to air dry (not necessary if using needle method into the injection cap).
   11. Remove protective cap from the end of the administration set and connect tubing to the catheter.
   12. Unclamp catheter, if appropriate.
   13. Turn pump on.
   14. When infusion is completed (if cyclic), reclamp catheter (if appropriate), disconnect tubing from catheter, cleanse catheter opening with betadine, attach new catheter cap, and unclamp. (Refer to procedure "Central Line Injection Cap Change.")
   15. Heparinize per physician's orders. (Refer to procedure "Heparinization: Central Catheter.")

IX. Bilirubin monitoring via heel stick
   A. Definition
      1. Puncturing the heel of an infant to obtain blood sample
   B. Purpose
      1. To obtain a sample blood to determine the level of bilirubin in the blood
   C. Equipment
      1. Lancet
      2. Alcohol pad
      3. Blood tube (specific to lab or hospital)
      4. Bandage
      5. Warm washcloth
      6. Plastic bag or plastic wrap
      7. Sterile lubricant
   D. Procedure
      1. Wash hands.
      2. Explain procedure to parent or responsible person present.
      3. Assemble equipment.
      4. Select site for heel stick.
      5. Wrap foot in warm, wet washcloth to improve blood flow.
      6. Apply plastic bag or plastic wrap to maintain warmth and protect bed linen. Keep foot wrapped for several minutes.
      7. Remove wrapping.
      8. "Milk" leg and foot, working toward the heel.
      9. Wipe heel with alcohol pad.
      10. Apply a thin layer of sterile lubricant to heel before puncture to facilitate collection of blood.
      11. Puncture skin firmly with lancet.
          NOTE: More than one puncture may be necessary to obtain an adequate amount of blood.
      12. With collection tube in one hand, squeeze heel firmly with other hand, milking leg and foot when necessary; collect droplets of blood in tube. Continue this process until tube is filled to appropriate level as marked.
      13. Secure cap on blood tube and label appropriately.
      14. Transport blood sample to laboratory promptly, protecting sample from sunlight.

X. Administration of enteral feeding via kangaroo pump
   A. Purpose
      1. To provide supplemental nutrition
      2. To provide nutrition within or by way of the intestine
   B. Equipment
      1. Enteral formula
      2. Tap water
      3. 50 ml catheter tip syringe
      4. Kangaroo bag with tubing

C. Procedure

1. Prepare a clean working area.
2. Assemble all equipment.
3. Wash hands thoroughly.
4. Explain the procedure to the client.
5. Check the enteral formula's expiration date.
6. Prepare formula as per physician's orders for full strength, three fourths strength, or half strength.
7. Place the client in a sitting position or semisitting position. Height of bed should be elevated at least 30 degrees during the feeding and at least 30 to 60 minutes after feeding. This helps prevent aspiration of formula.
8. Before each feeding the feeding tube must be checked for correct placement and gastric residual volume must be ascertained. Note the amount of residual and reinstill the contents back into the stomach. Report to the physician if gastric residual is in excess of 100 ml.
9. Open the package of kangaroo tubing, and close the roller clamp on the tubing.
10. Add the prepared formula to the feeding bag and close the top. Usually no more than six to eight hours worth of formula is hung. Formula is usually administered at room temperature.
11. Hang the bag from the IV pole.
12. Remove the protective cover from the administration tubing.
13. Squeeze the drip chamber, and allow the fluid to flow until the tubing is free of air bubbles. Close the roller clamp, and place the protective cover over the end of the administration tubing.
14. Insert the drop chamber between the black electronic eyes, and reset the bottom of the drip chamber on the ledge below the drop sensor.
15. Thread the elasticized portion of the tubing counterclockwise around the rotor and snap the white plastic disk into slot opposite the drip chamber. Secure tube.
16. Take a 50 ml catheter tip syringe and draw an appropriate amount of water into the syringe (usually 15 to 20 ml).
17. Unclamp or uncap the feeding tube and irrigate the feeding tube with water.
18. Remove the protective cap from the kangaroo administration set, and plug the end of the tubing into the feeding tube using an adapter if needed.
19. Open the roller clamp.
20. Set the desired rate by pushing the rate regulator buttons.
21. Depress the "on" button.
22. Tape all connections.
23. Monitor the client's tolerance to the feeding.

EACH AGE-GROUP PROVIDES A DIFFERENT AND UNIQUE CHALLENGE to the nurse. This section focuses on special populations and the problems that are likely to be encountered by nurses who go into some phase of community nursing. In the case of infants and preschool children, nurses assess developmental capabilities, follow through on immunizations, and assist parents in understanding what is taking place in each phase of development. This is particularly true in the case of the firstborn in a family. Aspects of child development and care that seem extremely obvious to the veteran professional often cause anxiety and concern in new parents. Much of the job of the nurse is to explain what is happening to children and to help parents distinguish problems from normal developmental changes.

This same situation exists with the school-age child, but new problems begin to appear such as learning disabilities, behavior problems, special health needs, substance abuse, sexuality, and suicidal tendencies; few parents are equipped to handle these issues. Adulthood presents new problems. Health hazards in the work place are particularly troublesome and require different skills for those nurses who work in these areas. This same age-group begins to have children of their own. Women's health care during pregnancy and childbirth is of major concern, and new parents of both sexes need education and support.

One of the things that happen as a person ages is that the body processes begin to slow. Many individuals who have been in good health for almost all their lives begin to face new kinds of problems, including arthritis, hypertension, cardiovascular diseases, chronic obstructive lung disease, diabetes mellitus, and numerous others. Most such conditions do not lead to long-term hospitalization but pose special problems for community health and home health care nurses. Each age is an age of transition, but old age is marked not only by retirement and changes brought on by the aging process but also by inevitable loss of friends and loved ones, inability to care for oneself, and concern over a growing helplessness.

In each age-group the nurse is important not only as an information giver, but also as one who can also intervene when necessary. The ability to anticipate problems and to defuse crises in any one of the age-groups is the mark of an expert nurse, and no one is more qualified to intervene in various phases of the life cycle as the nurse who is involved at the time.

Nursing Through the Life Span

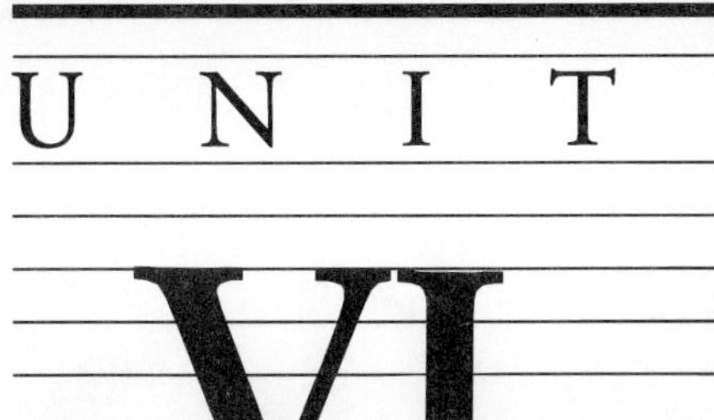

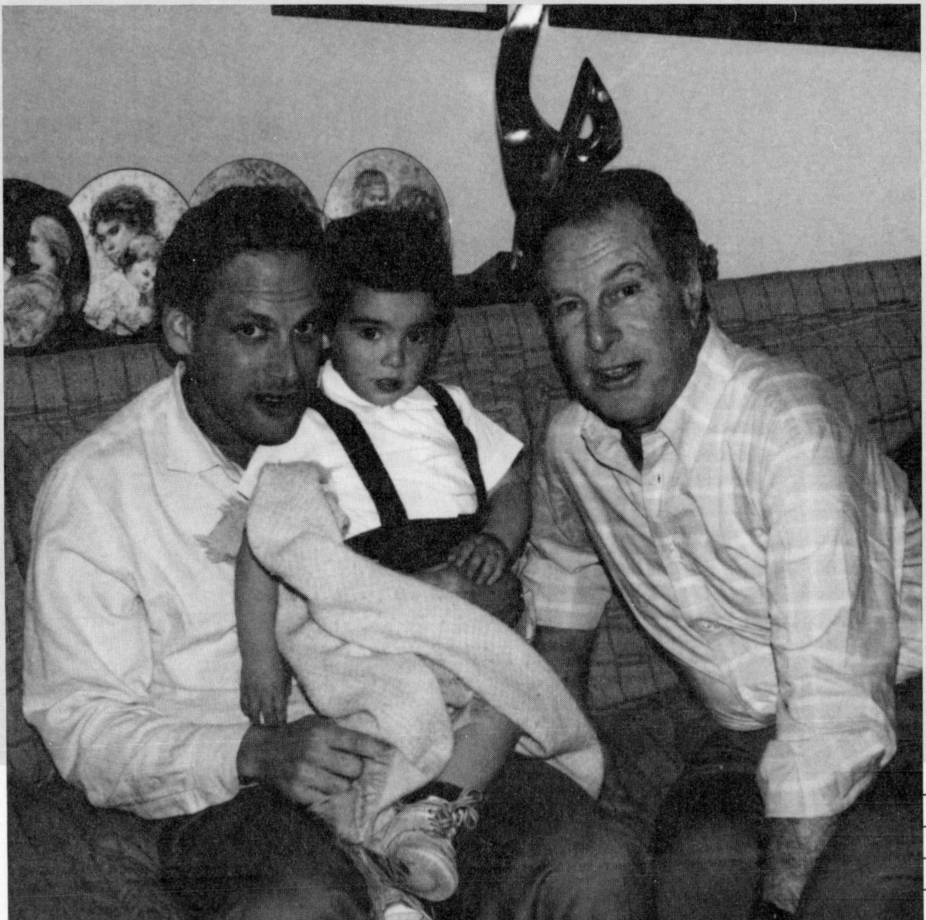

CHAPTER 15

Infants and Preschool Children

Constance D. Blair

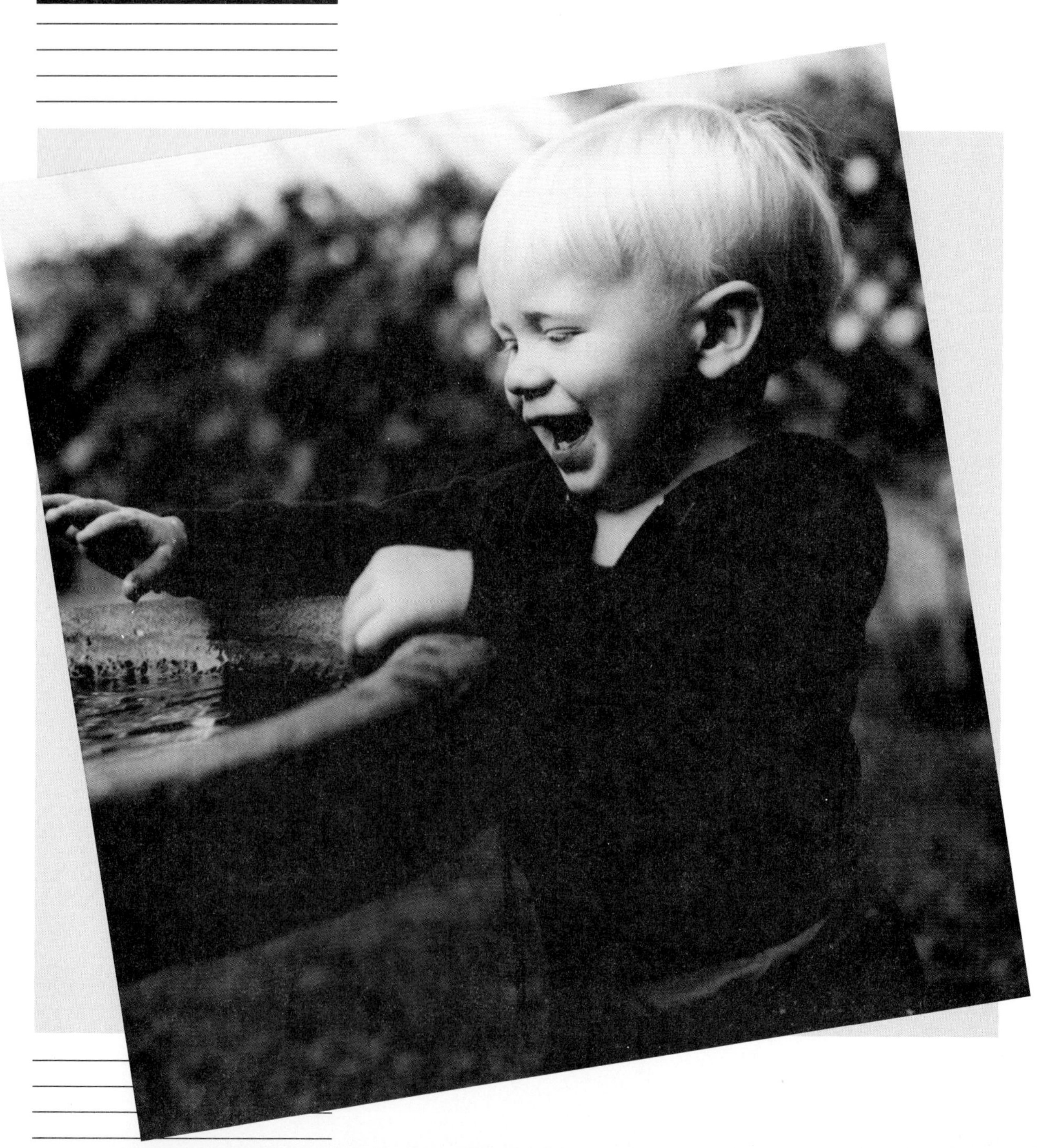

CHAPTER OUTLINE

Growth
- Premature and low–birth weight babies
- Measurement of growth

Development
- Assessing developmental progress
- Developmental screening

Health maintenance program
- Dental health
- Nutrition and nutritional assessment
- Vision and hearing screening
- Blood pressure screening
- Health education and anticipatory guidance

Common developmental and behavioral concerns
- Bowel habits of young children
- Toilet training

Common health problems
- Fever
- Upper respiratory infection
- Otitis media
- Gastroenteritis
- Skin rashes
- Diaper rash
- Yeast infections
- Eczema
- Impetigo
- Other rashes
- Sudden infant death syndrome

Immunizations

Summary

OBJECTIVES

After completing this chapter, the reader should be able to:

1. Discuss the growth and development of infants, toddlers, and preschool children.
2. Delineate general recommendations for child health maintenance and anticipatory guidance.
3. Identify common health problems in young children and make recommendations for management.
4. Outline specific recommendations for immunization of infants and children.

THIS chapter provides a basis for health promotion activities in the care of infants and young children. The chapter includes a discussion of the growth of infants, toddlers, and preschool children, as well as the various ways of assessing the developmental progress. Also included are recommendations for child health maintenance and anticipatory guidance. The chapter concludes with a discussion of common childhood health problems and current recommendations for immunization.

GROWTH

Early infancy is characterized by rapid changes in physical, physiologic, and behavioral systems. Change, not stability, is the hallmark of infancy. In the past, infants were thought to be relatively simple beings who were passive recipients of environmental stimuli. Research reveals that infants are far more complex than had earlier been thought. The newborn infant is not purely a product of genetic origin. Although genetic endowment is important, intrauterine nutrition, infection, and exposure to drugs, among other influences, can affect the development of the fetus. There is rapidly accumulating evidence that the newborn infant is already powerfully shaped even before delivery (Brazelton, 1984).

Birth weight of the newborn infant is determined by genetics, the mother's prepregnancy weight, and her weight gain during pregnancy. During the first week of life the infant commonly loses weight, which is usually regained by the tenth day. By 4 months of age most infants have doubled their birth weights, and by 12 months of age most infants have tripled their birth weights (Pipes, 1989). Racial differences have been noted in rates of growth. American black infants are smaller than American white infants at birth. However, American black infants grow more rapidly during their first two years of life. Asian-American children tend to be smaller than both black and white American children (Pipes, 1989).

Premature and Low–Birth Weight Babies

Weight curves are available for premature infants of varying gestational ages (GAs). The postnatal growth of premature infants resembles the growth pattern of fetuses of the same size rather than that of full-term infants of the same postnatal age (Howard, 1980). A distinction should be made between premature and low–birth weight babies. The infant's weight at birth is not necessarily a good indicator of the state of maturity of the infant. Classification of infants at birth by both weight and GA provides a more satisfactory method for predicting infant mortality (Whaley and Wong, 1987). By combining the weight of the infant and the GA, it is possible to determine whether an infant is small for gestational age (SGA), appropriate for gestational age (AGA), or large for gestational age (LGA). Fig. 15-1 shows the three classifications of infants by GA. The significance of these classifications is that low–birth weight and SGA babies have the highest mortality rates. AGA babies, even if preterm, are at lower risk of death than SGA babies, whereas LGA babies do better than either of the other two groups (Koops, Morgan, and Battaglia, 1982). To estimate the GA of the infant, scoring systems based on the neuromuscular and physical maturity of the infant are used.

Low birth weight as a factor in infant mortality in the United States continues to be a major public health problem. Although infant mortality rates have declined from 20 per 1000 live births in 1970 to 12.6 per 1000 in 1980 and 10.6 per 1000 in 1985 (American Public Health Association, 1985; National Center for Health Statistics, 1986), the United States still has a higher infant mortality rate than at least 15 other countries, and the U.S. rate is dropping more slowly than those of most of the 15 other nations. Officials from the U.S. Department of Health and Human Services have stated that

> the current slowdown could be due to the incapacity of ultra-modern intensive care units to push down mortality rates any further, or perhaps it may be due to other factors such as changes in the ages at which

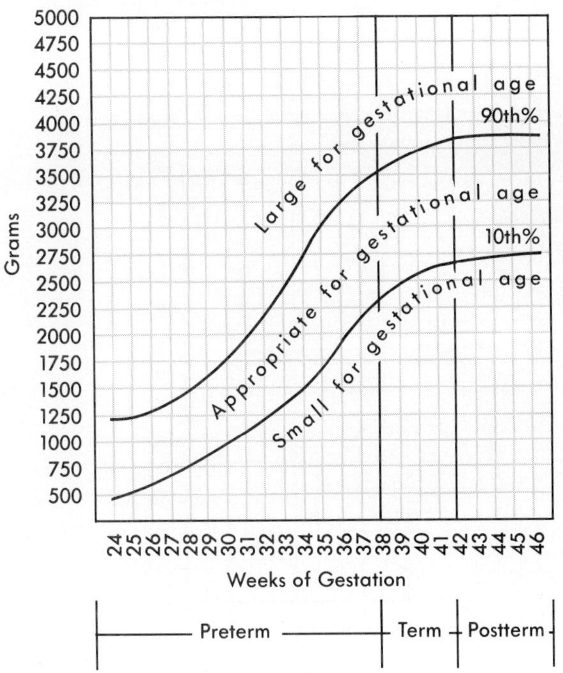

FIG. 15-1. Classification of infants by gestational age.

women are having children, or in the types of services they are getting (American Public Health Association, 1985).

Joel C. Kleinman, director of the division of analysis of the National Center for Health Statistics said that "low birth weight—the biggest factor associated with infants deaths—would drop by about 25% if women did not smoke" (American Public Health Association, 1985).

Measurement of Growth

Figs. 15-2 and 15-3 show examples of measurement grids that are used to plot an individual child's growth in height, weight, and head circumference. The grid reveals how consistently infants or children are maintaining their percentile relationships to children of the same age and sex. These growth charts (available from Ross Laboratories, Columbus, Ohio) have been formulated by research data compiled by the National Center for Health Statistics. The data were obtained by measuring a representative sample consisting of thousands of children throughout the United States over years of growth time.

For the charts to reflect the growth status of the child accurately, the child's measurements should be made in the same manner in which the reference data were secured. The weight values for the child younger than 36 months of age should be obtained with calibrated beam balance scales while the child is nude. Length values should be made with the child lying down. To use the charts specified for children between the ages of 2 and 18 years, measurements should be made with the child standing, in stocking feet and light clothing (gown or underwear as for an examination). Great care should be taken in the actual plotting of the measurement on the grid to ensure that the recording accurately reflects the true measurement (Hamill, 1979).

Interpretation of Growth Charts

Measurements that fall between the 25th and 75th percentiles are likely to represent normal growth. Measurements between the 10th and 25th and between 75th and 90th percentiles may or may not be normal, depending on the pattern of earlier and later measurements and on genetic and environmental factors affecting the child. Values above the 90th and below the 10th percentiles should be carefully checked for measurement and recording accuracy. Children whose measurements fall above the 95th and below the 5th percentiles deserve special attention and possible referral for further evaluation by a physician (Hamill, 1979). It must be emphasized, however, that there is no certainty as to what constitutes a dangerous degree of excess of less than normal weight for children (Gross and others, 1985). It should be noted that most children do not have a smooth growth curve as repeated measurements are made over time. Rather, there are normally

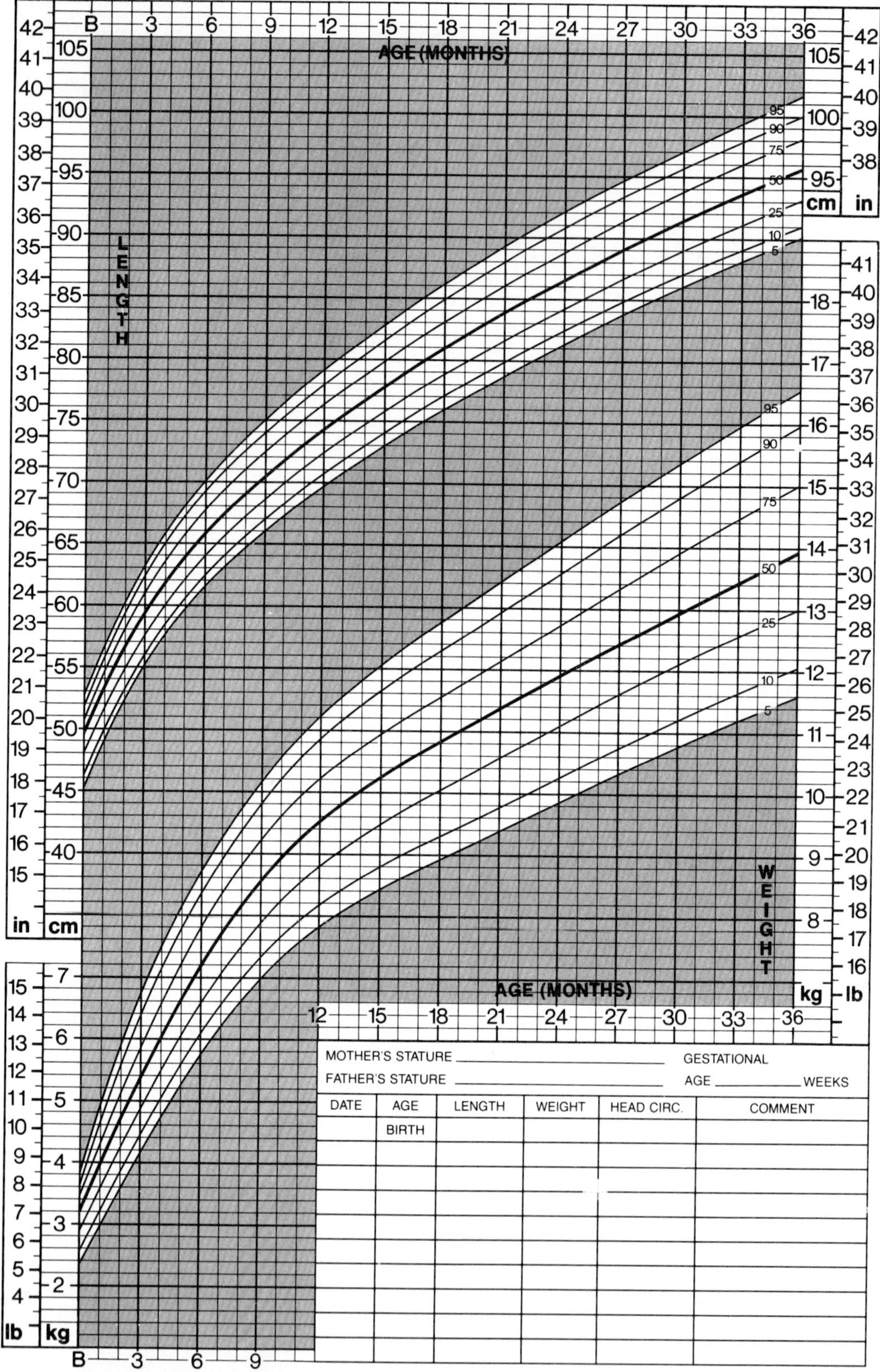

FIG. 15-2. Female infant growth chart. (Adapted from Hamill PVV, Drizd TA, Johnson CL, Reed RB, Roche AF, Moore WM: Physical growth: National Center for Health Statistics percentiles, Am J Clin Nutr 32:607, 1979. Data from the Fels Research Institute, Wright State University School of Medicine, Yellow Springs, Ohio. © 1982 Ross Laboratories.)

BOYS: BIRTH TO 36 MONTHS
PHYSICAL GROWTH
NCHS PERCENTILES*

NAME ____________________ RECORD # ____________

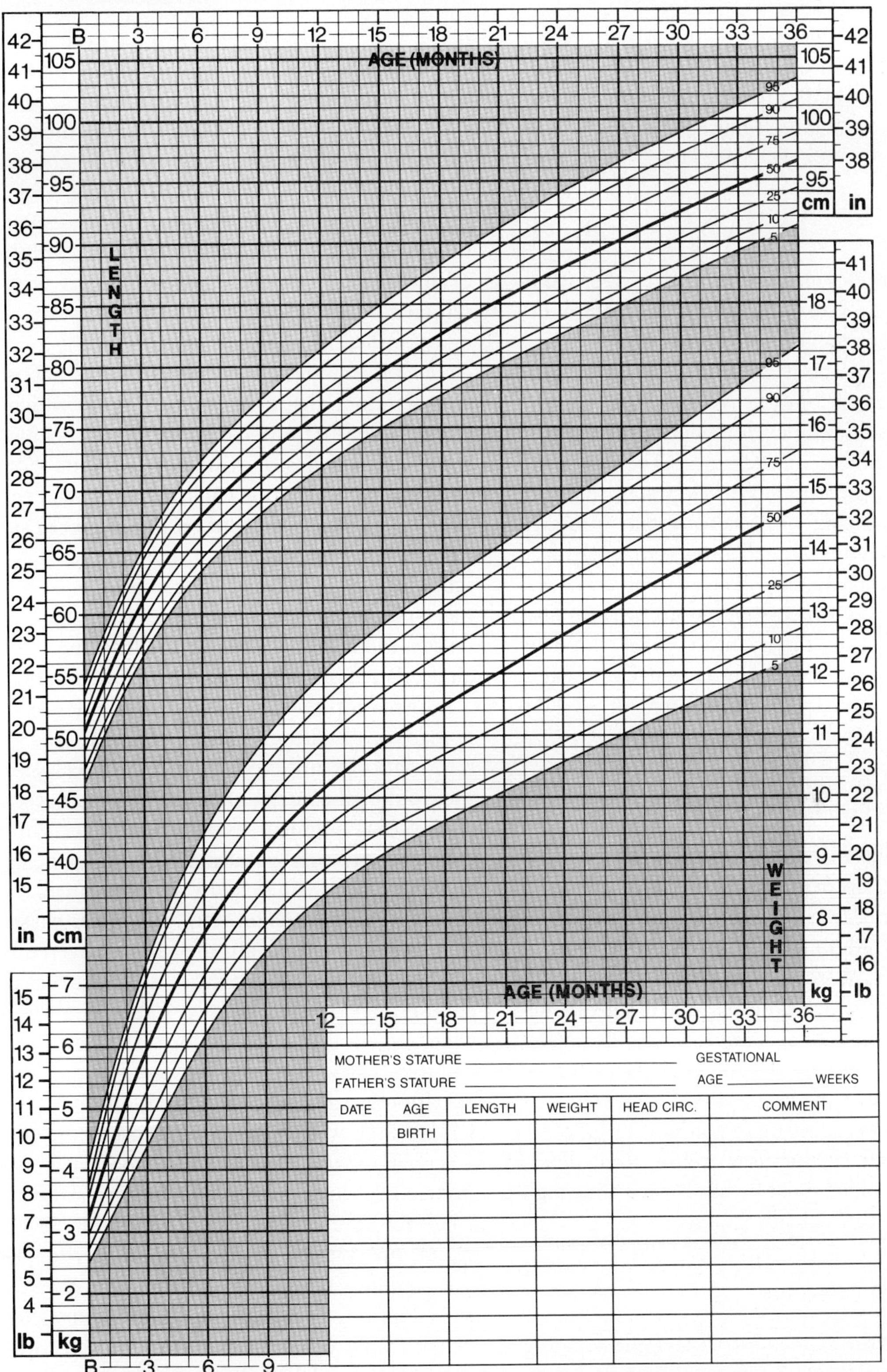

FIG. 15-3. Male infant growth chart. (Adapted from Hamill PVV, Drizd TA, Johnson CL, Reed RB, Roche AF, Moore WM: Physical growth: National Center for Health Statistics percentiles, Am J Clin Nutr 32:607, 1979. Data from the Fels Research Institute, Wright State Unversity School of Medicine, Yellow Springs, Ohio. © 1982 Ross Laboratories.)

periods of slowed and accelerated growth within a specific range. This gives an uneven appearance to an individual child's growth pattern as repeated measurements are plotted on the chart over time.

DEVELOPMENT

Physical development is defined as the acquisition of function associated with cell differentiation and maturation of individual organ systems. Every part of the body continues to mature and acquire increasing complexity. Simultaneous with physical growth and development is the psychosocial development of the child. There are numerous theories of human development that give a basis for nursing observations and interventions. Some examples of theories frequently used include Freudian theories, Piaget's cognitive theory, and Maslow's theory of hierarchy of human needs. Perhaps the theory most widely used by nurses for understanding human development is Erik Erikson's theory of social growth and development.

Assessing Developmental Progress

It is common for parents and grandparents to focus great concern on a child's developmental progress, seeing it as a direct result of their parenting ability. Although the sequence of stages in development is nearly uniform in all children, the precise ages at which children reach various developmental milestones vary considerably. Developmental screening of young children is based on comparison with the "normal" or "average" child as determined through study of large numbers of children. It therefore follows that developmental screening must be based on a thorough knowledge of normal (Illingworth, 1984).

Developmental Screening

Screening is the application of a simple accurate method for determining which children in a population are likely to need further evaluation or special services to develop optimally. Screening procedures should not be viewed as diagnostic; they simply divide a population into those who need diagnostic work and those who are not at risk for a condition (Foster and others, 1985).

Important in the developmental assessment of the child is a thorough health history and physical examination. The developmental history is an essential component within the health history of an infant or child. The developmental history includes information given by the child's parent or guardian to indicate the specific ages at which the infant or child acquired certain skills or behaviors, often called milestones of development. For an infant this information might include such things as the age at which the infant first began to smile, babble, sit, or crawl. For the toddler or preschooler the information includes ages at which the child began such things as walking, saying words, talking in sentences, and learning to dress alone. Often included as part of the health history is information about the child's activities of daily living, such as sleeping and eating patterns. This information, combined with direct observation of the child by the nurse, provides the data necessary to make a judgment as to whether the child is developing normally. Such a decision by the nurse is a crucial one, since many abnormalities, if discovered in early childhood, are much easier to correct or remedy than if they are discovered later in life. Parents also need the reassurance that their child is developing normally. Table 15-1 outlines developmental milestones for infants and young children. These should be assessed as part of the developmental history, although some may be observed directly during examination of the child.

Screening with a standardized tool, such as the Denver Developmental Screening Test (DDST), is a helpful adjunct in the assessment of developmental progress of an infant or child. The DDST is a common screening tool that was developed by William K. Frankenburg and his colleagues in Denver. The test is a device for the detection of developmental delays during infancy and the pre-

TABLE 15-1 Developmental Milestones from Birth to Age Six*

Age	Behavior
Birth to 2 months	Cries to express displeasure or needs Makes small throaty sounds Makes comfort sound during feeding Maintains eye contact with the mother Quiets in response to being held by mother Sleeps 16 to 20 hours per day
2 to 4 months	Smiles responsively Makes gurgling noises Comforted and quieted easily by mother Sleeps total of 15 to 16 hours per day Sleeps longer intervals at night Aware of separation from mother Lifts head Rolls from front to back
4 to 6 months	Smiles and makes babbling sounds Reaches out to touch and grasp Listens intently Shows recognition of familiar voices and sounds Interested in faces Enjoys being tossed lightly Sits with hands forward for support
6 to 9 months	Keen observer of movement, color, and sound Repeats syllables such as dada and mama Fascinated by and picks up small objects Learns to crawl Likes peek-a-boo and pat-a-cake
9 to 12 months	Crawls and climbs Pulls self to standing by holding on Walks holding on to furniture Insists on trying things on own Knows at least one word with meaning
12 to 14 months	Walks without support Pincer grasp complete Manipulates objects and turns knobs Insatiable desire to investigate surroundings
12 to 14 months	Knows two or three words with meaning
15 to 18 months	Climbs stairs up and down holding rail Removes clothing Feeds self, drinks from cup, and manages a spoon Jumps with both feet Points to three body parts on request
18 to 24 months	Runs and kicks a ball Uses jargon and phrases and names pictures Throws ball Puts on shoes, socks, and pants Likes to imitate and help with house chores Sleeps 10 to 15 hours per day, sleeps all night and takes naps Scribbles with pencil or crayon
2 to 3 years	Toilet trained Knows full name and sex Able to draw lines on paper with pencil Recognizes and names pictures of common objects Sleeps 10 to 12 hours at night with nap in day Expresses cold, hunger, and fatigue appropriately
3 to 4 years	Dresses and undresses fully with the exception of shoelaces Uses short sentences Able to balance on one foot Rides a tricycle Knows colors Turns to adults for support and help
4 to 6 years	Separates easily from mother Dresses self without supervision Able to hop Plays imaginative, interactive games with peers Draws objects with pencil and paper Regular sleep pattern established (10 to 12 hours at night and occasional daytime naps)

* The nurse should obtain the preceding developmental information from the parent or guardian if it is not possible to directly observe these behaviors displayed by the infant or child.

0-9 MONTHS (R-PDQ)

REVISED DENVER PRESCREENING DEVELOPMENTAL QUESTIONNAIRE

Child's Name ____________________

Person Completing R-PDQ: ____________________

Relation to Child: ____________________

For Office Use

Today's Date: ____ yr ____ mo ____ day

Child's Birthdate: ____ yr ____ mo ____ day

Subtract to get Child's Exact Age: ____ yr ____ mo ____ day

R-PDQ Age: (____ yr ____ mo ____ completed wks)

CONTINUE ANSWERING UNTIL 3 "NOs" ARE CIRCLED

Item	Answer	For Office Use
1. Equal Movements When your baby is lying on his/her back, can (s)he move each of his/her arms as easily as the other and each of the legs as easily as the other? Answer **No** if your child makes jerky or uncoordinated movements with one or both of his/her arms or legs.	Yes No	(0) FMA
2. Stomach Lifts Head When your baby is on his/her stomach on a flat surface, can (s)he lift his/her head off the surface?	Yes No	(0-3) GM
3. Regards Face When your baby is lying on his/her back, can (s)he look at you and watch your face?	Yes No	(1) PS
4. Follows To Midline When your child is on his/her back, can (s)he follow your movement by turning his/her head from one side to facing directly forward?	Yes No	(1-1) FMA
5. Responds To Bell Does your child respond with eye movements, change in breathing or other change in activity to a bell or rattle sounded outside his/her line of vision?	Yes No	(1-2) L
6. Vocalizes Not Crying Does your child make sounds other than crying, such as gurgling, cooing, or babbling?	Yes No	(1-3) L
7. Smiles Responsively When you smile and talk to your baby, does (s)he smile back at you?	Yes No	(1-3) PS
8. Follows Past Midline When your child is on his/her back, does (s)he follow your movement by turning his/her head from one side ***almost all the way to the other side?***	Yes No	(2-2) FMA
9. Stomach, Head Up 45° When your baby is on his/her stomach on a flat surface, can (s)he lift his/her head 45°?	Yes No	(2-2) GM
10. Stomach, Head Up 90° When your baby is on his/her stomach on a flat surface, can (s)he lift his/her head 90°?	Yes No	(3) GM
11. Laughs Does your baby laugh out loud without being tickled or touched?	Yes No	(3-1) L
12. Hands Together Does your baby play with his/her hands by touching them together?	Yes No	(3-3) FMA
13. Follows 180° When your child is on his/her back, does (s)he follow your movement from one side ***all the way*** to the other side?	Yes No	(4) FMA
14. Grasps Rattle ***It is important that you follow instructions carefully.*** Do ***not*** place the pencil in the palm of your child's hand. When you touch the pencil to the back or tips of your baby's fingers, does your baby grasp the pencil for a few seconds?	Yes No	(4) FMA

TRY THIS   NOT THIS

FIG. 15-4. Revised Denver Prescreening Developmental Questionnaire. (From Frankenburg W, MD, 1975, 1986. Used with permission.)

school years. It yields an overall developmental score with personal-social, fine motor–adaptive, language, and gross motor sectors. The DDST has undergone extensive reliability and validity testing involving more than 20,000 children. In addition, it has been adapted for use in screening more than 30 million children in more than 24 countries. The screening test's widespread popularity is due to its simplicity, pictorial representation, and extensive validation. Results of a DDST evaluation are classified as abnormal, borderline or questionable, untestable, or normal (Frankenburg, 1984).

The Revised Denver Prescreening Developmental Questionnaire (R-PDQ), which is completed by the parent or guardian, was developed more recently. The R-PDQ is used to identify children from birth to 6 years old who should be screened more thoroughly with the DDST. The second screening is important to prevent over-referral. Examples of the R-PDQ and DDST are shown in Figs. 15-4 and 15-5. (The R-PDQ questionnaire forms and standardized DDST manuals, kits, and scoring forms can be ordered from Denver Developmental Materials Inc., P.O. Box 20037, Denver, CO 80220-0037.) The instruction manuals for the Denver screening tests should be studied carefully and followed exactly in the administration and interpretation of the tests. There is always a danger of labeling a child falsely and unnecessarily alarming the parents simply because of a poorly administered or misinterpreted screening test. This can have detrimental effects on both the child and family.

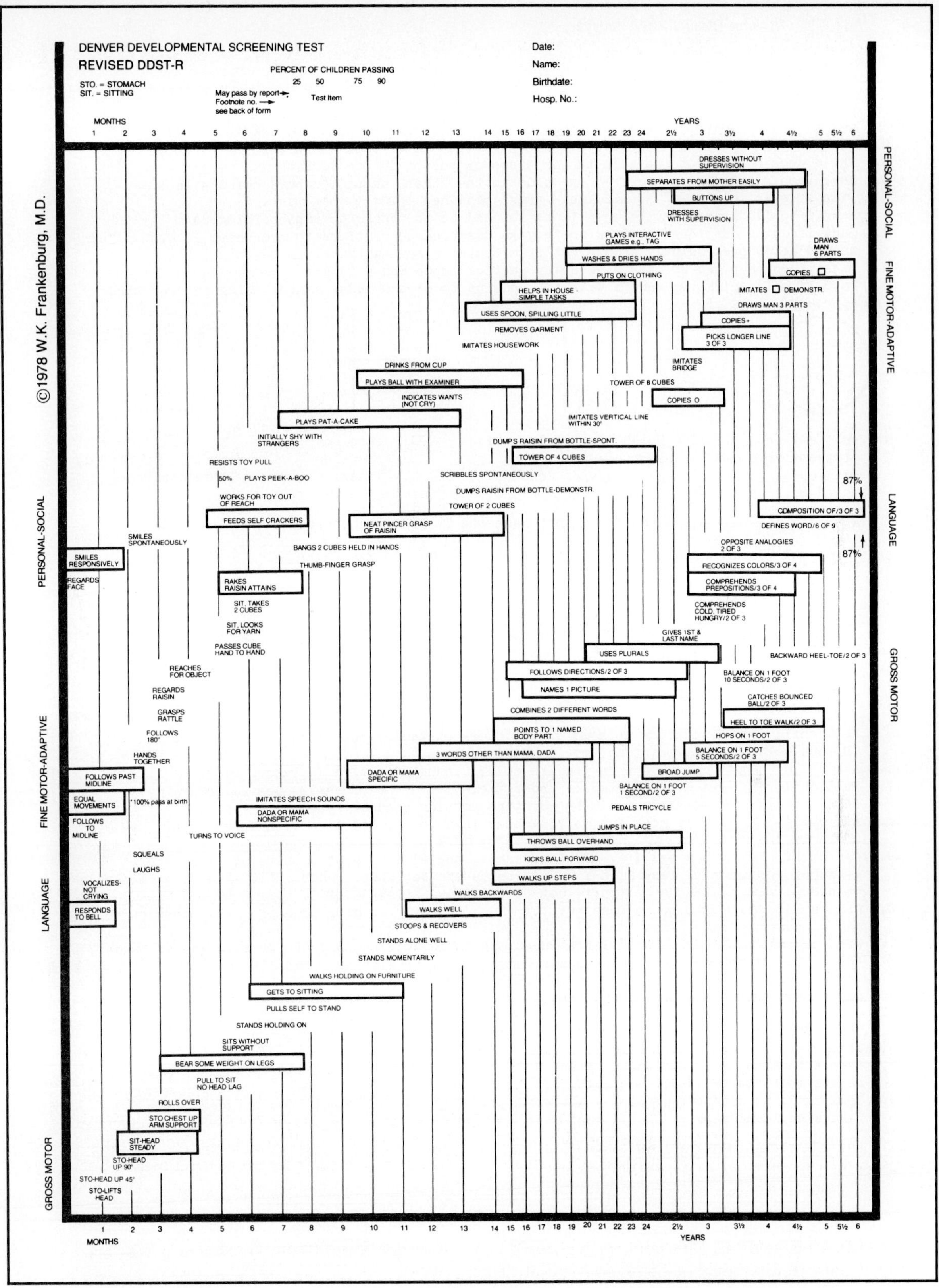

FIG. 15-5. Revised Denver Devlopmental Screening Test (DDST-R). **A,** This form, resembling a growth curve, places items at lowest age level starting at bottom left and progressing upward to right with increasing age. (From Frankenburg, WD, Sciarillo W, and Burgess, D: Newly abbreviated and revised Denver Developmental Screening Test, J Pediatr 99:995, 1981.)

Continued.

1. Try to get child to smile by smiling, talking or waving to him. Do not touch him.
2. When child is playing with toy, pull it away from him. Pass if he resists.
3. Child does not have to be able to tie shoes or button in the back.
4. Move yarn slowly in an arc from one side to the other, about 6" above child's face. Pass if eyes follow 90° to midline. (Past midline; 180°)
5. Pass if child grasps rattle when it is touched to the backs or tips of fingers.
6. Pass if child continues to look where yarn disappeared or tries to see where it went. Yarn should be dropped quickly from sight from tester's hand without arm movement.
7. Pass if child picks up raisin with any part of thumb and a finger.
8. Pass if child picks up raisin with the ends of thumb and index finger using an over hand approach.

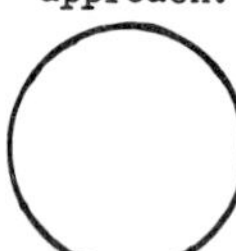

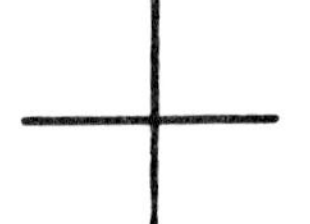

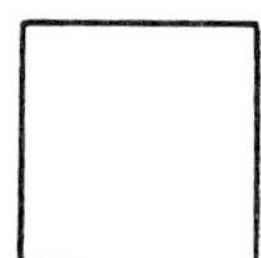

9. Pass any enclosed form. Fail continuous round motions.
10. Which line is longer? (Not bigger.) Turn paper upside down and repeat. (3/3 or 5/6)
11. Pass any crossing lines.
12. Have child copy first. If failed, demonstrate

When giving items 9, 11 and 12, do not name the forms. Do not demonstrate 9 and 11.

13. When scoring, each pair (2 arms, 2 legs, etc.) counts as one part.
14. Point to picture and have child name it. (No credit is given for sounds only.)

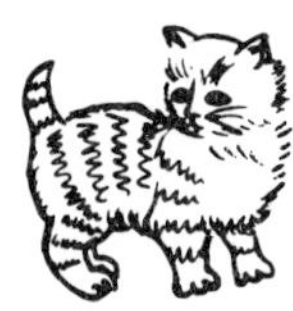

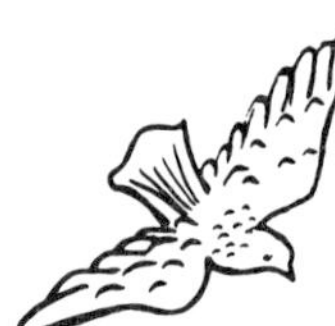

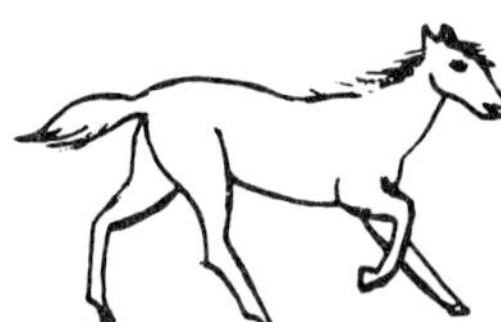

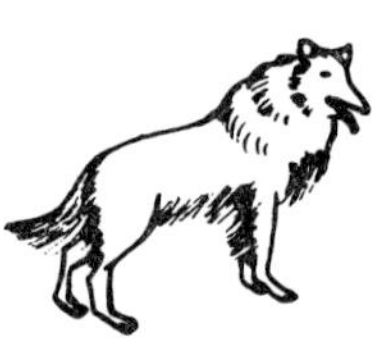

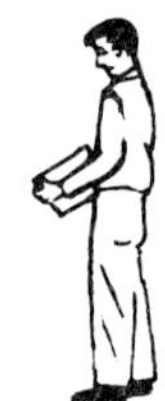

15. Tell child to: Give block to Mommie; put block on table; put block on floor. Pass 2 of 3. (Do not help child by pointing, moving head or eyes.)
16. Ask child: What do you do when you are cold? ..hungry? ..tired? Pass 2 of 3.
17. Tell child to: Put block <u>on</u> table; <u>under</u> table; <u>in front</u> of chair, <u>behind</u> chair. Pass 3 of 4. (Do not help child by pointing, moving head or eyes.)
18. Ask child: If fire is hot, ice is ?; Mother is a woman, Dad is a ?; a horse is big, a mouse is ?. Pass 2 of 3.
19. Ask child: What is a ball? ..lake? ..desk? ..house? ..banana? ..curtain? ..ceiling? ..hedge? ..pavement? Pass if defined in terms of use, shape, what it is made of or general category (such as banana is fruit, not just yellow). Pass 6 of 9.
20. Ask child: What is a spoon made of? ..a shoe made of? ..a door made of? (No other objects may be substituted.) Pass 3 of 3.
21. When placed on stomach, child lifts chest off table with support of forearms and/or hands.
22. When child is on back, grasp his hands and pull him to sitting. Pass if head does not hang back.
23. Child may use wall or rail only, not person. May not crawl.
24. Child must throw ball overhand 3 feet to within arm's reach of tester.
25. Child must perform standing broad jump over width of test sheet. (8-1/2 inches)
26. Tell child to walk forward, ⊂⊃⊂⊃⊂⊃⊂⊃→ heel within 1 inch of toe. Tester may demonstrate. Child must walk 4 consecutive steps, 2 out of 3 trials.
27. Bounce ball to child who should stand 3 feet away from tester. Child must catch ball with hands, not arms, 2 out of 3 trials.
28. Tell child to walk backward, ←⊂⊃⊂⊃⊂⊃⊂⊃ toe within 1 inch of heel. Tester may demonstrate. Child must walk 4 consecutive steps, 2 out of 3 trials.

<u>DATE AND BEHAVIORAL OBSERVATIONS</u> (how child feels at time of test, relation to tester, attention span, verbal behavior, self-confidence, etc,):

FIG. 15-5. cont'd B, Directions for numbered items on testing form. (From Frankenburg WK, and Dobbs JB, University of Colorado Medical Center, 1969.)

Therefore the nurse must use great care to administer and interpret screening tests in the manner the designers of the tests intended. Developmental screening tools are not diagnostic, cannot predict a child's future developmental capabilities, and should not be used to assign a child a developmental age. The findings of developmental screening are an estimate of a child's current abilities as compared with the average.

HEALTH MAINTENANCE PROGRAM

To enhance and promote the health of infants and young children, health professionals have recognized their role in supporting and assisting parents, the true providers of child health care. Health promotion does not consist of simply scheduling visits for children to receive immunizations. Rather, child health visits should include general assessment of the child's health, growth and developmental assessment, screening tests where appropriate, and teaching, counseling, support, and guidance for parents. Comprehensive child health care enhances the optimal physical, intellectual, emotional, and social growth of the child. Another goal is to develop self-confident parents through the provision of encouragement, reassurance, and other measures supportive of the parenting role (Chow, 1979). The developmental history and developmental assessment have already been discussed in detail. Discussion of dental assessment, nutritional assessment, vision, hearing, and blood pressure screening, as well as information for parents on nutrition and safety, is now presented.

Dental Health

The 20 deciduous teeth (temporary, or baby, teeth) begin to erupt at about 5 to 7 months of age. Tooth eruption continues until about 30 to 36 months. Toothbrushing with a soft baby brush should begin as soon as teeth appear. Toothpaste used can be any standard proprietary brand containing fluoride. Small children should visit the dentist, preferably with the parents, for regular checkups starting at 2 years of age. Deciduous teeth are just as important as permanent teeth. Early treatment, if necessary, is much easier and better than extraction. Waiting until pain is experienced may be too late for treatment (Gross and others, 1985).

Fluoride Supplements

Epidemiologic studies have shown an association between fluoride content of drinking water and reduction in dental caries. When the fluoride of drinking water is adjusted to a level of 1 part per million (ppm), the incidence of dental caries is reduced by about 60%. In areas where fluoride is not in the drinking water, supplements in the form of daily tablets or drops can be given. Combinations of fluoride and infant vitamin supplements are also available. It is important to check with the local water authority to determine the fluoride level already in drinking water. The Committee on Nutrition of the American Academy of Pediatrics recommends that supplemental fluoride dosages be adjusted to the fluoride content of the water supply. When fluoride concentrations of drinking water are more than 2 ppm, mottling (a brown staining of the teeth) can occur during tooth development. The incidence and severity of mottling increase as the fluoride content of the water increases.

Nutrition and Nutritional Assessment

The primary methods for assessing the nutritional status of a child are the measurement of physical growth and development and gathering other anthropometric data such as skinfold thickness and arm circumference. A useful adjunct in assessing nutritional status is the dietary history. The tools most often used for diet history in the clinical setting are the 24-hour recall and the three-day or seven-day food intake record. The interview is a key element in the assessment and is only as valid as the child's or parent's willingness to share information with the interviewer. Nevertheless, a diet history can identify children who may be at nutritional risk or discover patterns of intake that may indicate a particular nutrient is in short supply in the child's diet (Pipes, 1989).

Infant Nutrition

Breast milk or formula provides all necessary nutrients for an infant in the first six months of life. The breast of an adequately fed lactating mother or the nipple on a bottle of properly prepared formula gives a hungry infant both biochemical and psychosocial nurturance. When held in a semi-reclining position and offered the nipple, the infant sucks and receives the major portion of nourishment in the first 20 minutes of feeding. A flexible self-demand schedule is recommended. Newborn infants initially feed six to eight times a day at intervals of two to four hours and consume 2 to 3 ounces at a feeding. By 2 weeks of age most infants increase the amount of milk consumed at a feeding to 3 to 5 ounces and reduce the number of feedings to six per day. By 2 months of age most infants are fed five times a day.

Breast-Feeding

It is generally agreed that breast-feeding offers the best nutrition and psychosocial benefits to both mother and baby. Breast-fed babies have fewer infections, have lower incidence of allergies, and decreased incidence of dental caries. Advantages to the mother are promotion of involution of the uterus and decreased risk of postpartum hemorrhage. For most women, breast-feeding provides a satisfying emotional experience (Gross and others, 1985). Despite its benefits, breast-feeding of the newborn infant reached an all-time low of 18% in 1966. Renewed interest and support of breast-feeding has resulted in more than half of all infants being breast-fed at birth now. Nevertheless, after five to six months only as few as 25% may still be breast-feeding (Pipes, 1989). Although most women discontinue breast-feeding after several months, breast-feeding may be continued through 18 to 24 months of age.

Major determinants of whether a mother experiences success in breast-feeding include the support and education she receives from health professionals, as well as the support and encouragement she receives from her immediate family.

Mothers who choose to nurse their babies need support in understanding that, at least in the beginning, a good deal of trial and error and much patience are needed by both mother and baby to adjust to each other's needs and preferences. The following box outlines teaching points that can be offered by the nurse to support the mother in breast-feeding.

Bottle-Feeding

Infants who are not breast-fed may receive a cow's-milk formula. Milk-free formulas such as soy, meat base, or hydrolyzed casein formula are fed to infants who do not tolerate cow's milk (Pipes, 1989).

Parents who choose to bottle-feed may have to be helped not to feel guilty for choosing a "second-best" method of feeding. Even more common is the need to help parents who begin nursing and then switch to bottle-feeding to keep from feeling that they "failed." Both breast-fed and bottle-fed babies can grow up to happy, healthy children (Brown and Murphy, 1981).

Formula Preparation

Although studies have indicated that infants accept cold formula, most mothers warm milk to body temperature. Pipes (1989) offers the following information on formula preparation.

> Infant formulas are available in a variety of forms. Some come as liquid concentrates to be prepared for feeding by mixing equal amounts of the liquid with water. Ready-to-feed formulas that require no preparation are available in an assortment of sizes. Powdered formula that is prepared by mixing 1 level tbsp of powder in 2 oz of water is also available. Formula may also be prepared by mixing 13 oz of evaporated milk

with 2 tbsp of corn syrup and 18 oz of water. All of the formulas, when properly prepared, provide the nutrients necessary for the infant. Errors in dilution caused by lack of understanding of the proper method of preparation, improper measurements, or the belief of the parents that their child should have greater amounts of nutritious food can lead to problems. Anticipatory guidance of parents should include information on the variety of formulas available, the differences in methods of preparation of each product, and the dangers of overdiluted formula.*

Although sterilization of equipment for infant formulas is recommended, many parents do not follow this practice but prepare formulas by a clean technique. Several researchers have found no differences in incidence of illness or infection between infants fed formulas prepared by the clean technique and infants fed formulas prepared by the sterilization technique. If formulas are to be prepared by the clean technique, it is important that the person preparing the formula first wash the hands carefully. All equipment to be used in the preparation, including the cans that contain the milk, the bottles, and the nipples, must be thoroughly washed and rinsed. Once opened, cans of formula must be covered and refrigerated. After the formula is heated and the infant is fed, any remaining milk should be discarded. Warm milk is an excellent medium for bacterial growth (Pipes, 1989).

In the case of both breast-fed and formula-fed infants, air is swallowed by the infant during feeding, but less air is swallowed during breast-feeding. Holding the infant in an upright position and gently patting the back encourages expulsion of swallowed air and prevents distention and discomfort.

Adding Foods

Despite the fact that no nutritional advantage can be expected from the early introduction of semisolid foods, many mothers, on the advice of family, neighbors, and friends, introduce semi-

*Reproduced by permission of Pipes PL: Nutrition in infancy and childhood, ed 4, St Louis, 1989, CV Mosby Co.

INFORMATION FOR BREAST-FEEDING MOTHERS

Breast-feeding may be difficult the first few days. The baby is normally sleepy and may seem not to be interested in nursing, but this passes. Feeding behavior can be stimulated by stroking the infant's lips and the cheek on the side closer to the breast. The first few days the mother has colostrum, a yellowish liquid that precedes the breast milk. Human colostrum contains nutrients and is higher in protein and minerals than mature milk. Milk generally starts flowing the third or fourth day; mature milk is produced by about the tenth day.

Positioning the baby for breast-feeding is important. The nipple needs to be placed well back in the baby's mouth so that the baby's gums are able to press on the areola. If the baby's mouth is not far enough up on the nipple, the nipples can become traumatized and sore.

The baby should suckle each breast during a feeding. It may be as little as three minutes per breast at first and then gradually increased to 10 to 15 minutes per breast. The mother should start with the breast the baby finished with the last time to ensure that each breast gets emptied at every other feeding. A safety pin attached to a bra strap can be rotated each feeding and can serve as a reminder.

Mothers may worry about not having enough milk. The way to increase the milk is to allow the baby to feed longer and more often. The mother also needs a well-balanced diet and plenty of fluids. To ensure adequate fluid intake, the mother should drink enough liquid to supply 16 to 32 oz of milk per day for the infant.

Prematurity, cesarean section, and illness in mother or baby are not necessarily contraindications to breast-feeding.

Sore nipples and engorged breasts can be prevented by frequent feedings, proper positioning of the infant's mouth well up on the areola, air drying nipples, and placing warm moist heat (by shower or warm packs) on the breasts before a feeding.

Since the plastic nipple of a bottle is easier to manipulate than the human breast, the infant may learn to prefer the bottle if supplemental bottle feedings are offered. Supplemental bottle feedings should be kept to a minimum until after several weeks of well-established breast-feeding.

Breast milk can be expressed by hand or pump and frozen in a sterile container for several weeks, to be fed to the infant in the mother's absence.

Mothers should avoid drugs if possible, since most drugs are passed through the breast milk.

solid foods as early as 1 month of age. Because of concern about obesity and allergic reactions, health care professionals in the pediatric community recommend that foods not be introduced before 4 to 6 months of age. Even so, many parents are reported to continue to offer semisolid foods at an earlier age. If parents insist, cereal, fruits, or vegetables are all good for starters. No more than one new food should be introduced in a week, and no mixed foods should be given until the infant has had the ingredients separately first. Orange juice and egg whites should not be given before nine months of age, since they may produce allergies. Honey has been implicated as a source of spores of *Clostridium botulinum* during infancy. Foods should be given in small amounts by a spoon and should never be mixed in a bottle or given from a squeezer or syringe. Use of the spoon, despite the thrusting reflex of the infant's tongue, is advantageous for developing later feeding behaviors. What are sometimes called finger foods, or foods children can pick up and feed to themselves are also good. Foods that are small and round such as corn, popcorn kernals, and grapes, should not be given to the young children, since they might choke. Weaning from the bottle or breast to the use of a cup may be initiated at 8 to 12 months of age. There are no hard-and-fast rules for when to wean an infant, and much depends on the preference of the parents.

Vitamin Supplements

Vitamins are necessary for metabolic processes in the body. However, exact needs for vitamins are difficult to determine, and recommended daily allowances (RDAs) are continually revised. Most nutrition books contain tables that outline the RDAs for each vitamin and mineral for varying ages. Likewise, there have been conflicting recommendations on the use of vitamin supplements. From a review of current literature, the following represents a consensus of the most common recommendations:

1. A prophylactic intramuscular dose of vitamin K is usually given to infants at birth as a protection against hemorrhagic disease.
2. Breast-fed infants should receive vitamin supplements with iron.
3. Vitamins may be unnecessary for infants receiving commercially prepared formulas to which vitamins and iron are already added.

As an increasing variety of foods are added to the infant's diet, vitamin supplements may be discontinued. Some infants and children are at nutritional risk and should continue to receive vitamin supplementation. These include premature and low–birth weight babies, children who have suffered neglect or abuse, and children who have poor appetites or poor eating habits. All vitamin supplements, like any medication, should be made inaccessible to young children.

Feeding the Toddler and Preschooler

The infant who was normally considered a big eater may suddenly stop eating or become a small eater by 12 months of age. This happens because most babies grow enormously during the first year of life, usually tripling their birth weight, but their growth rate slows down considerably after 1 year of age. The natural consequence of the slowed growth is a decrease in appetite. Parents are often unaware of this phenomenon and may become concerned about the decrease in the child's appetite. Growth remains relatively slow during the years 1 to 6, and as a result children may become picky eaters, eating only one or two meals per day. The nurse should reassure parents that appetite reduction at this age is normal. To be sure that children get a balanced diet, a wide variety of foods should be made available to the child and the child should be permitted to choose among them. Given a choice of foods, most children choose a balanced diet for themselves. Snacks are fine provided they are nutritious. Cheese and fresh fruit make better snacks than cookies or potato chips.

Desserts should not be offered as a reward for eating. Offering sweets as a reward gives them unnecessary value, which later may lead to cravings for sweets and possible obesity. Desserts should be given no more emphasis than the rest of the meal. Limiting milk intake to 16 ounces in 24 hours for children in the preschool years may also help increase the appetite for other foods. One food should not be emphasized over another, for example, cooked vegetables, over raw vegetables or fresh fruits. The same nutrients may be gained from these alternatives. Toddlers and preschoolers should be allowed to choose their portions and feed themselves. If a child is not hungry at mealtime, little should be said. Skipping one meal does not lead to starvation (von Hippel, 1984).

Vision and Hearing Screening

Vision Screening

Vision screening should be part of any periodic physical examination and should be incorporated into all programs that undertake the total care of children. Observation of visual behavior is one of the most important procedures for detecting visual problems. This should be an ongoing process performed by all persons who are in contact with children, including parents, friends, relatives, teachers, aides, volunteers, and health care personnel. If an eye problem is suspected at any time, the child should have an eye examination immediately. No child is too small for an eye examination if a problem is suspected (Patterson, 1980).

As matter of routine, the eyes should be inspected during every physical examination from birth onward. Signs of eye disease include crossed eyes (esotropia), wall-eyes or eyes that turn out (exotropia), eyes that are not vertically aligned (hypertropia), red, swollen, or encrusted eyelids, watery eyes, discharges from eyes, haziness in the pupil, droopy lids (ptosis), and unequal size of pupils (anisocoria). Behaviors in the young child that may suggest visual problems include holding items unusually close to or far from eyes, frequent blinking, squinting or rubbing of the eyes, shutting or covering one eye, and head tilting (Patterson, 1980). Young infants should receive an ophthalmoscopic examination by a physician or nurse practitioner at birth. Thereafter the follow-up examinations should include elicitation of the red reflex and the Hirschberg corneal light reflex test. This test is performed by shining a penlight into the eyes. The reflection of the light should be in exactly the same position on each pupil. If there is even a slight difference, strabismus may be present. This test is particularly useful in children with pseudostrabismus, which occurs when an epicanthal fold makes the eyes appear crossed even when they are not. Infants should also be observed for ability to fix eyes on an object and ability to follow the object with the eyes.

For children older than age 6 months, the cover-uncover test should be performed at every examination to detect any muscle imbalance that can lead to amblyopia. Amblyopia is a condition of dullness or dimness of vision that may result from strabismus (abnormal position or deviation of one or both eyes), refractive differences of the eyes, nystagmus, or a congenital problem. Amblyopia is estimated to be responsible for more loss of vision during the first four years of life than all other eye diseases and eye injuries combined (Patterson, 1977).

The cover-uncover test is easy to perform and is useful for detecting strabismus. When the test is administered, the child is instructed to focus on an object at least 12 inches away from the eyes. The eyes should be held as still as possible. The examiner then holds a small card in such a way that it occludes the vision of one eye but does not touch the eye, since both eyes must remain open. The card is held in front of the eye for several seconds and then quickly removed. The covered eye is observed closely as the card is withdrawn. There should be no movement of the eye. A slight jerking movement of the previously covered eye indicates the presence of eye deviation that may be due to muscle weakness. The other eye should be tested in the same manner. The uncovered eye should also be observed as the cover is placed over the other eye. Any adjustment of the uncovered eye may also indicate muscle weakness. Any eye deviation as this test is performed is cause for referral to an ophthalmologist for further evaluation (Brown and Murphy, 1981). It is crucial that these tests be performed on all young children, since most visual problems are more effectively treated in young children and some problems, such as amblyopia, may become much more difficult or even impossible to treat as the child reaches school age. Therefore eye and vision screening should not wait until the child reaches kindergarten.

The visual acuity of the child should be assessed to detect refractive errors. This can be done by the use of screening charts for children as young as 2½ years of age. However, the younger the child is, the more preparation is needed to ensure the child's understanding and cooperation with the test. One experiment, conducted by Brown and Collar (1982), showed that by sending home a practice kit called the "Vision Matching Game" two weeks before the well child visit, the parents could successfully prepare the children for screening with the use of the HOTV vision chart (The letters contained on the chart are H, O, T, and V). The HOTV chart is used with a set of cards presented by the parent and matched with a set placed in front of the child. The child does not need to learn the names of the letters but simply needs to be able to match the shapes. The emphasis should be on making the experience a pleasant, nonpressured game (Brown and Collar, 1982). "Tumbling E" charts and picture charts are also used for assessing the visual acuity of young children. One problem encountered with the E charts is that the children sometimes have problems indicating the directions of the E. Likewise, the picture charts are sometimes a problem, since they assume prior experience with the item pictured and the ability to name the item. Special cards known as Allen cards may be used with the picture charts for matching of items so that the very young child is not required to name the item.

Referral criteria for vision screening may vary with different institutions, but some general guidelines indicating a need for further evaluation are as follows.

1. Visual acuity of 20/50 or poorer in one eye in 3-year-old and younger children.
2. Visual acuity of 20/40 or poorer in one eye in 4-year-old and older children.
3. All ages who have a two-line difference (on the chart) in acuity between each eye.

Hearing Screening

Early diagnosis of hearing defects is of great importance, since such problems may interfere with language development and learning. The health history should include asking the parent or guardian whether a hearing problem in the child is suspected. An otoscopic examination is also indicated with each physical examination of the child. For screening purposes, Table 15-2 describes methods that may be employed for hearing assessment of various age groups (Gross and others, 1985).

Audiometric screening is one method available for the detection of both conductive and sensorineural hearing losses. It is usually recommended for school-age children. Preschoolers are assumed to be too difficult to test, since they have trouble understanding the mechanics of the test. However, as with vision testing, Brown and Collar (1982) found that with minor modifications in instructions and administration and prior practice at home, children as young as 3 years of age could be successfully screened with audiometry. Any young child who does not cooperate with the

TABLE 15-2 Methods for Hearing Assessment at Various Ages

Age	Assessment method
Birth to 7 months	Do the parents think the child can hear normally? Is the young child startled by loud noises? Does the baby turn the head or eyes to the mother's voice?
7 to 12 months	Do the parents think the child hears normally? Use a rattle with a high pitched tone to see whether the child responds to the sound. Make sounds behind children as they sit on the mother's lap. The rattle should be held at ear level or below. The ability to locate sound above ear level does not develop until almost 2 years of age.
1 to 2 years	Do the parents think the child hears normally? Identify three toys and ask the child to point to or get each one. Is the child starting to talk? If the child is uncooperative, try earlier tests.
2 to 5 years	Do the parents think the child hears normally? See whether the child responds to a low voice spoken from 10 feet away. Is the child speaking in sentences? Ask the child to identify toys such as ball, doll, spoon, car, or block.

nurse should be referred to an audiologist for testing.

Impedance audiometry, also known as tympanometry, is being increasingly used in the testing of young children who are suspected of having ear problems. The test is conducted with a special probe that sends electronic waves through the ear canal. The waves bounce off the tympanic membrane and back to a sensing device within the probe. The direction and force with which waves bounce off the tympanic membrane are a function of the compliance of the membrane. In this manner the test indirectly determines eustachian tube function and presence of middle ear abnormality. The use of impedance testing for mass screening remains under debate, since it is expensive and requires specialized equipment and training. Further, since it is designed to assess only the status of the tympanic membrane, it is not an actual measure of hearing loss. However, advantages of impedance testing are that it can be used on children who are too young to cooperate with usual audiometric testing and it can pick up problems in asymptomatic children (Gross and others, 1985).

The use of acoustic reflex testing along with tympanometry can also help identify some hearing losses. In particular, acoustic reflexes are absent in all conductive hearing losses, such as those caused by otitis media and in severe to profound sensorineural hearing losses caused by damage to the inner ear or auditory nerve.

Blood Pressure Screening

Children 3 years of age and older should have an annual determination of blood pressure. In children younger than 3 years of age, blood pressure needs to be taken only when a child is hospitalized or when a specific indication is present. The use of a proper-sized cuff is important. An appropriate cuff usually covers about two thirds of a child's upper arm. The blood pressure measurement should then be compared with normative charts of children's blood pressures at the various ages. Generally speaking, a young child's blood pressure is much lower than that of an adult, but it differs with each age, and thus it is important to refer to the normative charts in the assessment. A blood pressure found to be above the 95th percentile for the child's age, either systolic or diastolic, is considered abnormal. Referral for further evaluation should be considered. The meaning and prognosis of high blood pressure in children is not fully understood, but it remains an important concern that is currently under study.

Health Education and Anticipatory Guidance

Perhaps the most important part of caring for young children is protecting them from harm (Fig. 15-6), as well as providing them with an environment that is supportive and nurturing. The information provided in Table 15-3 should be provided for parents at each well child visit. Safety is of paramount concern at all ages, since accidents are the leading cause of death in children.

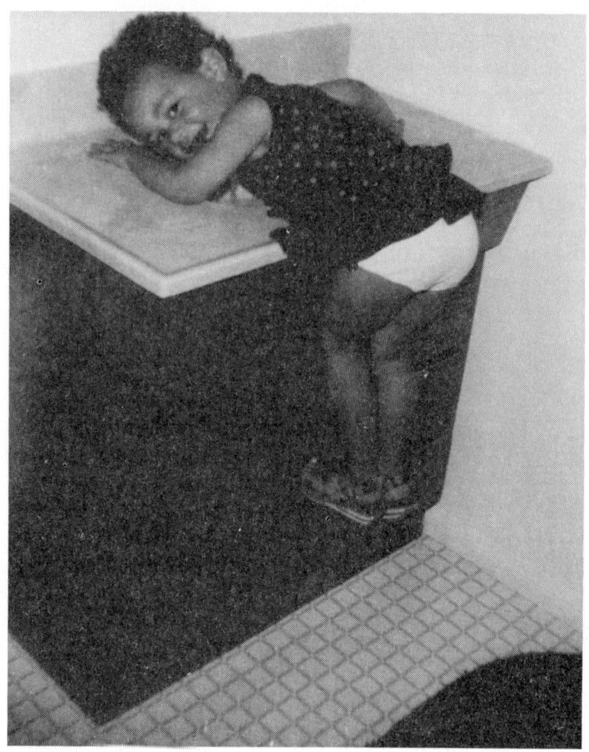

FIG. 15-6. Importance of anticipatory guidance.

TABLE 15-3 Education and Guidance for Parents of Young Children

Age	General	Safety
Birth to 2 months	Babies need warmth and security. Blankets should be wrapped tightly to provide body support. Babies like music such as lullabies sung by a parent or tapes and recordings. Gently rocking the baby provides comfort. A car ride or taking the baby outside provides a change of colors, sounds, and temperature.	An approved infant car seat should be used. Crib slats should be no more than 2 inches apart, and no loose plastic should be used as mattress cover. The baby should never be left alone for even one minute. The baby should sleep on the stomach so that the head can be turned from vomitus if necessary. Injuries at this age are somewhat unusual, and child abuse should be suspected if they occur.
2 to 4 months	Babies need a consistent schedule. Touching, rubbing and rocking are needed. Singing, smiling, laughing, and introduction of sounds such as running water, rattles, and household noises promote the learning of communication. Bright objects and moving objects help develop vision.	Keep crib away from window and curtain cords. Fire is a danger, so the baby should never be left in the house alone. Always use proper car seat. All objects smaller than 2 inches should be kept out of the baby's reach.

TABLE 15-3 Education and Guidance for Parents of Young Children—cont'd

Age	General	Safety
4 to 6 months	Babies are eager to explore surroundings and should be allowed to do so through touching, seeing, and hearing. Talking to the baby for language development at this age is important.	House should be babyproofed. New skills make constant surveillance necessary. Parents should know first aid for choking. Baby should never be left alone near water such as in a tub or wading pool. Continue use of car seat at all times.
8 to 14 months	Parents should be teaching the baby words and names. Babies like to name and point to body parts. Change of environment stimulates learning. Gross motor and fine motor skills such as walking, climbing, and removing clothes are being learned.	Accidents happen most frequently when the baby's usual routine changes (holidays, vacations, and illness in family), following stressful events for caretakers, and when caretakers are tired or ill. The baby needs increased mobility but must continue to be watched carefully. There needs to be a safe place such as a playpen to put the baby if the caretaker is out of sight, although the child should not be left there for extended periods. Emergency phone numbers should be nearby, and careful instructions for babysitter should be given.
18 to 24 months	Parents should play games such as hide and seek and "what is it?" with the child. Expectations should not be beyond the developmental capability of the child. Daily schedules should be regular and quiet. Overstimulation can reduce desire to learn.	Children need continued attention to prevention of accidents. The negativistic attitude of the toddler makes the toddler seem disobedient. Severe tone of voice should be saved only for emergencies. Parent should not trust that children's training will stop them from dangerous activity. Lack of behavior control and little memory can still lead to injury.
2 to 3 years	Children should be allowed to play with friends, but play should be supervised. Parent should accept masturbation as a normal occurence but should ask for guidance if concerned. Discipline may be imposed by limit setting and providing a consistent routine and safe environment. Unacceptable behavior should be corrected with as little attention as possible. Parent should set an exemplary standard and reward positive behaviors with praise.	Children still need constant watching as they explore surroundings. Environment should be safetyproof. Parent should insist that children remain buckled in car seat during travel.
3 to 5 years	Learning takes place by intuitive play. Children like to take on roles in imaginative games and learn activities easily from others. Sometimes children may be impulsive or quarrelsome. Parents should provide opportunitites for play with peers. Television watching should be selective and limited. Acceptable behavior may be promoted by providing a safe environment, a consistent daily schedule, and positive reinforcers such as hugs and praise. Beating fuels anger and violence.	Children begin to understand the consequences of actions, but continued teaching and supervision is needed. Magical thinking makes children think they can do the impossible. Emergency phone numbers should be posted and practiced. To prevent choking, children should not be allowed to run around while eating. Water safety should be emphasized.

COMMON DEVELOPMENTAL AND BEHAVIORAL CONCERNS

Bowel Habits of Young Children

For the first several months of life, an infant's bowel movements are frequent and soft. Breast-fed infants have bowel movements that usually have a loose, mustard-like consistency and color and vary a great deal in frequency. Some babies have one stool per feeding, whereas others have only one every few days. It is impossible for a breast-fed baby to become constipated. As the gastrointestinal tract matures, more fluid is absorbed from the stool allowing a firmer consistency and less frequency (by 4 to 6 months of age). From 8 to 14 months, babies who are not breast-fed may have a tendency to become constipated. This can be avoided by including large amounts of water, whole-grain cereals, and fruits in the diet. By 18 months of age most children have a regular pattern for their bowel movements, but it is still a little early for toilet training. By 2 to 3 years of age most children have regular, firm bowel movements, and they have learned bowel control. It is not necessary that a child have a daily bowel movement. It is entirely normal for some children to have a bowel movement only once every two or three days. Any use of laxatives or enemas in a young child should be avoided unless advised by a physician for an extreme condition.

Toilet Training

Toilet training is a big activity for parents during this stage of development. Some mothers begin the activity as their child approaches the first birthday. However, physiologically it is thought that children are probably not ready for toilet training until sometime between 32 and 44 months of age (Brown and Murphy, 1981). The best advice for parents is not to try toilet training too soon. Some 1-year-olds can indeed be taught to use the toilet, but the training is much quicker and easier if it is done later. Signals that indicate children may be ready for toilet training include a verbal signal by children when they need to go to the bathroom, dryness after a nap, ability to retain urine up to two or three hours, and attempts to pull down pants and actually use the toilet in an appropriate manner. However, just playing with the toilet and watching it flush does not indicate readiness for toilet training. Use of training pants, a small potty, modeling of older siblings, and use of praise are all helpful in toilet training. Punishment should not be used, since it may actually produce a mental block in the child and may prolong the process. Although some children may be bladder trained first and bowel trained later, Brazelton (1962) found that 80% of children attain bladder and bowel control at about the same time. The nurse should advise the parents not to aim at having their child be the first in the neighborhood to be toilet trained, but rather to aim for a child who is well adjusted to the process (von Hippel, 1984).

Enuresis

Enuresis is defined as repeated involuntary voiding of urine day or night after age 4 or 5 without an associated physical disorder (Gross and others, 1985). Before this age voiding accidents and bedwetting are common and there is no need for concern. Nurses should simply advise parents to have the child urinate before bedtime and perhaps to limit fluid intake in the evening. True enuresis may persist in as many as 15% of children even up to age 12 (Brown and Murphy, 1981). It occurs more often in boys and in those with a family history of enuresis. Management of a persistent problem is begun by taking a detailed history of the problem and of toilet training efforts. Laboratory tests and further medical evaluation may be indicated to rule out the possibility of infection or urologic abnormality. In most cases such abnormality is not detected. Management of enuresis is then directed at reducing the anxiety of the parents with the aim of fostering parental empathy so that excessive punishment or humiliation of the child is avoided. Behavioral modes of treatment include helping the child keep a chart with stars for dry nights and having the child routinely and matter-of-factly help change soiled bedding. Other regimens include enuresis alarms, drug treatment, and programs of urine retention training. Most of these regimens have only limited success. In these cases it is important to reassure the parent that the child will most likely outgrow the problem.

Encopresis

Encopresis is defined as involuntary movement of the bowels. Most children are bowel trained by 4 years of age but may have occasional accidents. As with accidental urination, this is not a cause for concern in young children. However, persistent soiling as the child gets older is definitely a problem. All children with this problem need a thorough history and physical examination including a rectal examination. The most common cause of soiling is constipation with overflow of diarrhea. These cases are generally managed with laxatives and enemas, followed by lubricants, stool softeners, high-fiber diet, adequate fluid intake, and bowel habit training. All such treatments should be carefully explained to the child and handled gently (Gross and others, 1985). Occasionally encopresis may be of psychogenic origin, in which case therapeutic counseling for the child and family may help. Rarer causes of encopresis include spinal cord lesions and anorectal stenosis (Chow, 1979).

COMMON HEALTH PROBLEMS

The immaturity of the infant and young child makes episodes of acute illness a common occurrence. The immune system of the infant and young child does not fully mature until later in childhood. Parents of young children are generally good at identifying illness in their child, but occasionally signs of illness can be missed or underestimated. It is important for the nurse to encourage parents to consult their health care professional whenever they suspect illness in their child. Likewise, it is important not to make light of or play down any visit initiated by the parent for concern about a child's illness even if the illness is mild. Children generally have a much narrower "margin of safety" in illness than do adults. In other words, what may appear to be a minor illness may suddenly become worse and, especially in the case of the neonate, can become a life-threatening problem in a short period. For this reason it is important to encourage parents to contact the physician or nurse practitioner for any concerns about their infant's or child's illness. Despite the fact that children can be susceptible to serious illness, by and large most childhood episodes of illness are minor and short-lived and the child recovers without complications. Following is a discussion of some of the common health problems in childhood and suggestions regarding their home management.

Fever

Fever is defined as body temperature in excess of 99.6° F rectally in an infant or child. It may be the first sign of illness onset. The temperature regulation mechanism of the infant and young child is immature and seems to be particularly sensitive to pyrogenic agents. Currently there is some thought that fever may be a physiologic response that actually helps the body fight infection. For this reason many pediatricians advise no treatment of fever unless the temperature exceeds 101° F rectally. Although a child's temperature is measured most commonly by the rectal route, there has been increasing popularity of measurement by the axillary route, especially for newborns. The rectal temperature reflects the body temperature at the core, whereas the axillary temperature represents a peripheral or surface body temperature. The axillary temperature is generally about 2° F less than the rectal. Most guidelines for treatment of fever in children refer to rectal, or core, temperature. If a mercury thermometer is used, it may take more than five minutes to obtain an accurate axillary measurement as opposed to two minutes for the rectal measurement. Most children younger than 4 years of age have difficulty keeping an oral thermometer in place, and thus this route is generally not useful for young children. In discussing a fever reported by the parent, it is important to ascertain the route by which the parent took the child's temperature.

Likewise it is important for the nurse to record the route by which the child's temperature is taken. Any fever in an infant younger than 8 weeks of age requires consultation with the pediatrician, especially if the fever is accompanied by feeding problems. For the child older than 8 weeks of age, who has only fever and no other major problems evident, the parent may treat the child at home first with antipyretic therapy. This includes treatment with acetaminophen (Tylenol, Tempra, or Liquiprin) according to the recommended dosage by age, keeping heavy blankets and excess clothing off the child to let body heat escape, and light sponging with lukewarm water (not to exceed 30 minutes of sponging in a two hour period). Sponging of the child is controversial among experts, since there is a belief that if the child becomes chilled during the process, shivering will result, which will actually raise the temperature. Therefore sponging should be done only with lukewarm water (not cold water or alcohol), and great care should be taken that the child does not become chilled in the process. Sponging may be a last resort if other methods fail to lower the temperature. Aspirin as a treatment for fever in young children is currently out of favor, since there have been reports of an association between aspirin treatment of viral illness and the subsequent development of Reye's syndrome, a syndrome of encephalopathy and fatty degeneration of the liver. Acetaminophen is currently the preferred drug. Any child who has a temperature higher than 104° F that does not respond to antipyretic measures or any child whose temperature continues to be elevated for three days should be seen by a pediatrician. Any child who has symptoms of vomiting, diarrhea, or lethargy accompanying the fever should also be evaluated promptly by the pediatrician.

Fever in an infant younger than 6 months of age is a special problem because signs of illness in this age group are nonspecific. Poor feeding, irritability, or lethargy with fever may be the only sign of sepsis or meningitis. For this reason, lumbar punctures are done frequently in infants. Babies younger than 6 weeks of age present an even more worrisome problem when they become febrile. Because of the immaturity of their immune system, they are readily invaded by both gram-negative and gram-positive organisms. Most physicians hospitalize infants younger than 6 weeks of age who have fever more than 100° F to evaluate them carefully for sepsis (Brown and Murphy, 1981).

Upper Respiratory Infection

The most common cause of illness in infancy and childhood is infection of the respiratory tract. Common symptoms are fever and nasal congestion. Occasionally there are accompanying cough, otitis, and even vomiting and diarrhea. Upper respiratory infections are most often of viral origin, for which no curative medicine is available. The parents can treat the symptoms through antipyretic measures (discussed previously) by providing plenty of fluids to maintain the child's hydration and placing a humidifier or vaporizer in the child's room to ensure that the child's nasal secretions remain liquified. If the child shows difficulty breathing, lethargy, persistent diarrhea or vomiting, or pulling at the ears, a referral to the physician or nurse practitioner is in order, since complications or serious illness are always a potential.

Otitis Media

Otitis media, or inflammation of the middle ear, is another frequent pediatric problem. Symptoms of otitis in infants and toddlers can be nonspecific. Any infant with symptoms of upper respiratory tract infection should be suspected of also having otitis, since the two commonly occur together. Common symptoms of otitis media include fever, irritability, pulling at the ears, and unusual waking at night with crying in apparent pain. Even diarrhea may be a presenting symptom. Young children who are bottle-fed and those who are in day-care centers are at high risk of otitis, although the majority of children have at least one episode of otitis by 2 years of age. Suspected otitis requires evaluation by the physician or nurse practitioner, and if it is confirmed by otoscopic examination, a course of antibiotics is most likely prescribed. Treatment of otitis in the young child is important, since if it is allowed to become chronic, it can lead to hearing problems with subsequent difficulties in speech development. On rare occasions, untreated otitis may lead to a more serious disease such as meningitis.

Gastroenteritis

Like upper respiratory infections and otitis, gastroenteritis is an illness that commonly occurs in infants and young children. Gastroenteritis is defined as inflammation of the gastrointestinal tract with the symptoms of vomiting, diarrhea, or both. Its most common cause is viral, although it may also be of bacterial origin or it may be the presenting complaint of a more serious underlying condition. Vomiting and diarrhea associated with viral gastroenteritis is short-lived and self-limited. The best treatment is to stop oral intake for about one hour and then to initiate fluid intake slowly, starting with clear liquids first, having the child take only 1 or 2 teaspoons every 20 minutes for the first hour. The intake can gradually be increased. Liquids such as Gatorade, flat 7-Up, and Jello water are good to use, since they help to replace important electrolytes that may have been lost. The major danger from gastroenteritis is the possibility of dehydration. Signs of dehydration include decreased tearing, dry mucous membranes, no urination in 6 hours, sunken fontanelle in infants, loss of skin turgor, and lethargy. Other danger signs associated with gastroenteritis are vomiting continuing for more than 12 hours, frequent vomiting (more than once every one to two hours), more than six watery bowel movements a day, or no improvement of diarrhea after 24 hours of a liquid diet. Any child exhibiting these signs and symptoms should have an evaluation by the physician or nurse practitioner (Brown and Murphy, 1981).

Skin Rashes

Skin rashes in babies and young children are common, since their skin is particularly sensitive. In many cases these rashes are harmless and quickly disappear and no treatment other than reassuring the parents is needed (Gross and others, 1985).

Diaper Rash

Diaper rash is a contact dermatitis that is usually caused by soiled or wet diapers being left unchanged for long periods. The rash is usually confined to the diaper area. Treatment is changing the diapers frequently, switching to cloth diapers from plastic disposable diapers, and not using plastic outer pants. The skin should be cleansed well after each diaper change to remove any urine from the skin, and the application of zinc oxide, Desitin, or A and D ointment before replacing the diaper may help. Leaving the diaper off for a time so that the skin is exposed to the air is also helpful.

Yeast Infections

Candidiasis, also known as yeast infection or Monilia, is the cause of a white patchy infection in the mouth, sometimes called thrush. Distinguishing thrush from milk curds in the mouth can be tricky. One way to make the distinction is to use a tongue blade to try to scape off one of the white patches. If it does not come off, it is probably thrush. The infection responds well to prescription antifungal agents such a nystatin. The diaper area can also become infected by yeast. It is distinguished by a red, glazed appearance of the skin and occurs commonly after the infant has had a course of antibiotic therapy. It is treated with antifungal cream.

Eczema

Eczema, also known as atopic dermatitis, is a common condition in which an itchy, papular rash develops in the child on the face or scalp, which may later involve the neck, wrists, and arms. It is thought to be allergic in origin, but the specific cause is not well understood. It tends to be chronic in nature, but the majority of children who have it outgrow it in time. Fortunately, it is usually mild and responds well to treatment with cortisone creams. Other control measures include keeping the skin soft and moist by adding bath oil to the bath water and avoiding overheating of the skin by not overdressing the child.

Impetigo

Impetigo is a bacterial skin infection characterized by vesicles that most commonly occur around the nose and mouth. The lesions break open and serum that turns to a honey crust oozes from them. The at-home treatment includes washing off the crusts with soap and water, applying hydrogrn peroxide followed by antibiotic ointment for a cleansing action, and leaving the lesions open to air. The lesions should be treated at least four times per day, but if there is no response or if the infection is severe, antibiotic treatment is indicated. The condition is contagious. Therefore children should have their own set of towels and should not be sent to preschool or day-care centers while the lesions are present.

Other Rashes

Other rashes may be the result of infectious diseases. Many viral illnesses have a prodrome of upper respiratory symptoms for several days before the appearance of a rash. Other infectious diseases of viral origin that cause maculopapular rashes are rubella, roseola, and exanthema subitum, or fifth disease. There is only one common vesicular pediatric exanthem—chickenpox. The word exanthem means rash associated with systemic disease (Brown and Murphy, 1981).

Sudden Infant Death Syndrome

Sudden infant death syndrome (SIDS) is defined as the sudden death of any infant or young child that is unexpected and in which a thorough postmortem examination fails to demonstrate an adequate cause for death. Although numerous theories have been proposed to explain SIDS, the cause remains unknown. Theories of causes relating to abnormalities or pathology of the respiratory tract are currently being studied, although the syndrome remains a mystery. Most SIDS infants die silently without struggle, and unobserved at home during the night while sleeping. Risk factors for SIDS include the following:

1. Low birth weight
2. Prematurity
3. Low socioeconomic group
4. Native American background
5. Winter months
6. Cigarette smoking in the mother
7. Maternal heroin addiction
8. Teenage mother
9. History of sudden infant death in antecedent sibling
10. Male sex

Babies who have frequent apneic spells are thought to be possibly at higher risk of SIDS. The use of home apneic monitors is discussed in Chapter 14.

SIDS occurs most often between the ages of 2 and 4 months. It is uncommon before 1 month and after 7 to 8 months of age (Chow, 1979). As

TABLE 15-4 Recommended Schedule of Active Immunization of Normal Infants and Children*

Recommended age	Immunization(s)	Comments
2 months	DTP and OPV	Can be initiated as early as 2 weeks of age in areas of high endemicity or during epidemics
4 months	DTP and OPV	Two-month interval desired for OPV to prevent interference from previous dose
6 months	DTP and OPV	OPV is optional, may be given in areas with increased risk of poliovirus exposure
15 months	Measles, mumps, and rubella (MMR)	MMR preferred to individual vaccines; tuberculin testing may be done
18 months	DTP and OPV	OPV may be given simultaneously with MMR at 15 months of age
18 months	HBPV	
4 to 6 years	DTP and OPV	At or before school entry
14 to 16 years	Td	Repeat every 10 years throughout life

Modified from American Academy of Pediatrics: Report of the committee on infectious diseases, Evanston, Ill, 1986, The Academy.

* For all products used, consult manufacturer's package insert for instructions for storage, handling, and administration. Biologicals prepared by different manufacturers may vary, and those of the same manufacturer may change occasionally. Therefore the nurse and the physician should be aware of the contents of the package insert.

DTP, diphtheria and tetanus toxoids with pertussis vaccine; *OPV,* oral poliovirus vaccine contains attenuated poliovirus types 1, 2, and 3; *MMR,* live measles, mumps, and rubella viruses in a combined vaccine; *HMPV, Haemophilus* b polysaccharide vaccine; *Td,* adult tetanus toxoid (full dose) and diphtheria toxoid (reduced dose) in combination.

a result of the devastating and unexpected death, acute grief reactions are intense for the parents. The nurse can do much to support the family throughout the grieving process. There are now numerous centers around the country that provide help and information on SIDS. To locate SIDS centers and materials, write or call National SIDS Clearinghouse, 3520 Prospect Street, NW, Suite 1, Washington, D.C., 20057, (202) 625-8410

IMMUNIZATIONS

Infectious diseases can be prevented by stimulating an active immunologic defense in preparation for meeting the challenge of future exposure to disease. In the United States, large-scale public health efforts with available vaccines have sharply curtailed diphtheria, measles, mumps, pertussis, poliomyelitis, rubella, and tetanus. Because these diseases persist in the United States, as well as in other countries, immunization procedures need to be continued. Routine immunization at the appropriate age is the best means of averting vaccine-preventable diseases. Preschool-age children currently have the highest age-specific incidence of measles, rubella, *Haemophilus influenzae,* and pertussis. Research on existing and new vaccines is continually being conducted with the result that immunization schedules are occasionally revised and new vaccines are added as they become available.

Active immunization consists of the administration of a modified or attenuated product of a microorganism. The goal is to mimic the natural infection by evoking an immunologic response that presents little or no risk to the recipient. The mechanics of immunization are critical to the success of immunization procedures. Recommendations for dose, route, technique of administration, and schedules must be followed for predictable effective immunization. Table 15-4 outlines the 1986 immunization recommendations of the Committee on Infectious Diseases of the American Academy of Pediatrics (1986). The parent or guardian of the child should be informed of the major benefits to be derived from vaccines in preventing disease and also the risks of those vaccines. The U.S. Centers for Disease Control has developed "Important Information" statements about the vaccines. These statements are used in public health clinics throughout the United States. There is emphasis now on making sure the information is understood and consent is given.

SUMMARY

Children are the future of any nation. Providing a good foundation for health care of children helps ensure the health of the entire population. Parents are the primary care providers of children, and the nurse can lend support and guidance to parents in their caring capacity. Periodic health screening examinations and the administration of immunizations to guard against infectious diseases not only promotes and maintains a child's health, but also assists parents.

QUESTIONS FOR DISCUSSION

1. Infants, toddlers, and preschool children have a number of health problems in common. List at least three such problems.
2. Infants, toddlers, and preschool children have some health problems that vary by developmental status in one of these three groups. List at least one problem that is unique to each of these developmental groups.
3. What is a health maintenance program, and what does it involve?
4. What kind of immunizations should be given to infants and preshool children, and what is the time frame for each of these immunizations?

REFERENCES

American Public Health Association: The nation's health 15:1, 1985.

Brazelton TB: A child-oriented approach to toilet training, Pediatrics 29:121, 1962.

Brazelton TB: Neonatal behavioral assessment scale, Philadelphia, 1984, JB Lippincott Co.

Brown MS and Collar M: Effects of prior preparation on the preschooler's vision and hearing screening, Matern Child Nurse J 7:323, 1982.

Brown MS and Murphy MA: Ambulatory pediatrics for nurses, ed 2, New York, 1981, McGraw-Hill Inc.

Chow MP: Handbook of pediatric primary care, New York, 1979, John Wiley & Sons Inc.

Foster C and others: Screening for developmental disabilities, 143:349, 1985.

Frankenburg WK; Developmental screening, Prim Care 11:535, 1984.

Gross E and others: The child health manual, Boston, 1985, Blackwell Scientific Publications, Inc.

Hamill PV and others: Physical growth: National Center for Health Statistics percentiles, 32:607, 1979.

Howard B: Growth and development. In Graef JW and Cone TE editors: Manual of pediatric therapeutics, ed 2, Boston, 1980, Little, Brown Co Inc.

Illingworth RS: Basic developmental screening: 0-4 years, Boston, 1984, Blackwell Scientific Publications, Inc.

Koops BL, Morgan LJ, and Battaglia FC; Neonatal mortality risk in relation to birth weight and gestational age: update, Pediatr 101:969, 1982.

National Center for Health Statistics: Monthly Vital Statistics Report, 35:1, 1986.

Patterson, JH: Vision screening techniques, Anchorage, Alaska, 1980, The Print Shop.

Patterson JH: Amblyopia, Anchorage, Alaska, 1977, The Print Shop.

Pipes PL: Nutrition in infancy and childhood, ed 4, St Louis, 1989, CV Mosby Co.

von Hippel M: More joy from parenting, Anchorage, Alaska, 1984, Stone Wall Press.

Whaley LF and Wong DL: Nursing care of infants and children, ed 3, St Louis, 1987, CV Mosby Co.

BIBLIOGRAPHY

Alexander MM and Brown MS: Pediatric physical diagnosis for nurses, New York, 1979, McGraw-Hill Inc.

American Academy of Pediatrics, Committee on Nutrition: Fluoride supplementation: revised dosage and schedule, Pediatrics 63:150, 1979.

American Academy of Pediatrics: Report of the committee on infectious diseases, ed 20, Elk Grove Village, Ill, 1986, The Academy.

Frankenburg WK and Coons CE; Home screening questionnaire: its valiidity in assessing home environment, Pediatr 108:624, 1986.

Graef JW and Cone TE, editors: Manual of pediatric therapeutics, ed 2, Boston, 1980, Little Brown & Co Inc.

Scipien and others: Comprehensive pediatric nursing, ed 2, New York, 1979, McGraw-Hill Inc.

CHAPTER

16

School-Age Child

Lucy Marion

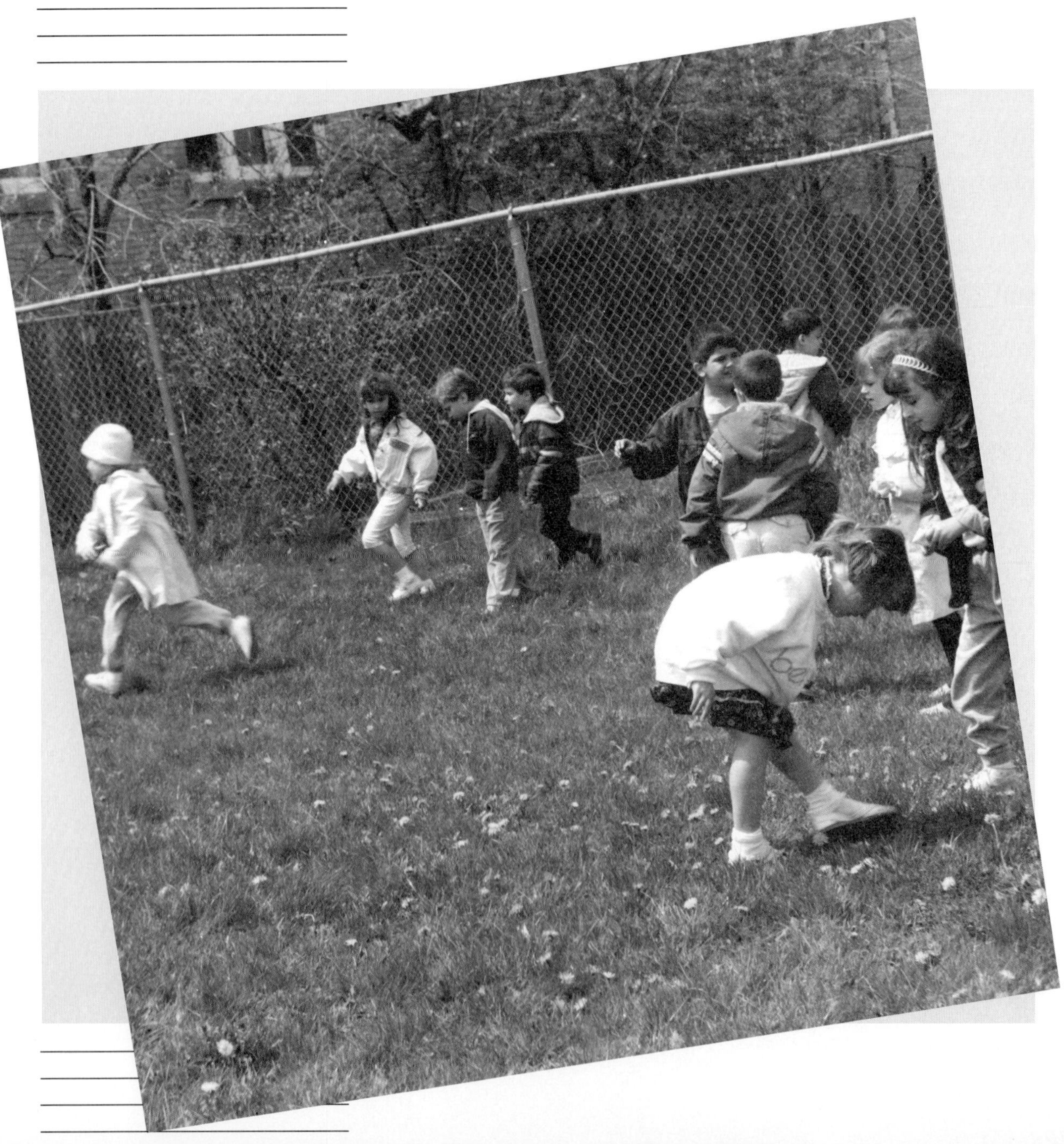

CHAPTER OUTLINE

School nursing

Other community nursing roles

Development

- Emotional development
- Cognitive development
- Physical development

Nutrition

Exercise

Health of school-age children

- Health care of the school-age child
- Child health visits
- Comprehensive school health programs

Common child health problems

- Common physical problems
- Common emotional problems
- Common cognitive problems

Special health problems

- Consequences of adolescent sexuality
- Substance abuse
- Acquired immunodeficiency syndrome
- Suicide

Summary

OBJECTIVES

After completing this chapter, the reader should be able to:

1. Discuss the emotional, cognitive, and physical aspects of the developmental process that take place during the school years.
2. Describe the role and functions of the school nurse and the school nurse practitioner.
3. Discuss the common physical health problems of school-age children including acute illnesses, chronic conditions, and problems related to the developmental process.
4. Understand the common emotional problems of children.
5. Discuss the topics that are particularly salient to the nurse who deals with adolescents, including the following:
   a. Sexuality
   b. Substance abuse
   c. AIDS
   d. Suicide

THE YEARS BETWEEN entry into kindergarten and graduation from high school are filled with numerous dramatic changes for every child. The student begins school life as a dependent being who often needs help with such simple daily tasks as tying shoestrings or opening milk cartons. When these years are over, the successful older adolescent is mature enough to start an independent life as a worker or advanced student. Each school category—primary, middle, and secondary—has associated sets of learning, behavior, and growth patterns and related potential and actual health problems. Because of the predictability of changes and health needs, the nurse has tremendous opportunity to improve the health of school-age children.

SCHOOL NURSING

School nursing is a specialty defined by the setting and age of the target population. The goal of school nursing is to develop and implement a school health program that prevents or corrects health problems interfering with learning. Another goal is to promote progressive self-care to achieve maximum wellness in each child. Clients of school nurses include individual children, their families, teachers, classes, groups of children with common problems, and the school as a whole. School nurses use the nursing process to guide activities to reach their goals.

Health promotion and disease prevention are the two components of *primary prevention*. The school nurse promotes health by teaching healthful practices to students, teachers, and community groups. The nurse is also an advocate for health promotion content within the total curriculum and selected school health practices such as exercise programs and well-balanced, appetizing lunches. Disease prevention, such as immunization and safety programing, is based on the risk factors of the children and resources of the community. An in-school, pregnancy prevention clinic for adolescents is essential for some areas, whereas community agencies meet this need for other school districts.

Secondary prevention encompasses early detection and treatment of problems to prevent progression of disease and to reverse illness indicators. Early detection of problems in schoolchildren is important because of the potential for loss of learning and other delayed development. Screening programs are based primarily on risk factors, screening tools, and the potential loss to the child. Cost effectiveness of every screening program must be determined repeatedly as new technologies emerge. Most early treatment is accomplished by referral to primary care providers in the community unless a school nurse has primary health care competencies and credentials such as a school nurse practitioner license.

Tertiary prevention is management of a health problem with irreversible damages to prevent further progression of the disease or to allow death with maximum comfort and dignity. School nurses assist in the management of diseases such as diabetes mellitus and leukemia and promote self-care at school. With the advent of Public Law 94-142 in 1975, children with severe physical, mental, and intellectual handicaps were brought into the schools. Tertiary prevention programs involving teams of nurses, teachers, and other school staff members were created to meet the urgent demand.

School nurses have a variety of educational backgrounds. Many have developed competencies of community health nursing without the benefit of a baccalaureate degree. Some have taken non–degree-granting programs to strengthen their knowledge and skill base. Nurses with baccalaureate degrees may have a nursing or an educational degree. Some school nurses have degrees in health education. Is the school nurse then primarily a generalist in health care or primarily a health educator? The role of school nurse is not

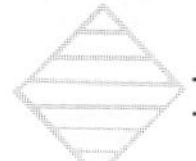

STANDARDS OF SCHOOL NURSING PRACTICE

STANDARD I. THEORY

The school nurse applies appropriate theory as basis for decision making in nursing practice.

STANDARD II. PROGRAM MANAGEMENT

The school nurse establishes and maintains a comprehensive school health program.

STANDARD III. NURSING PROCESS

The nursing process includes individualized health plans which are developed by the school nurse.

STANDARD IV. INTERDISCIPLINARY COLLABORATION

The school nurse collaborates with other professionals in assessing, planning, implementing, and evaluating programs and other school health activities.

STANDARD V. HEALTH EDUCATION

The nurse assists students, families, and groups to achieve optimal levels of wellness through health education.

STANDARD VI. PROFESSIONAL DEVELOPMENT

The school nurse participates in peer review and other means of evaluation to assure quality of nursing care provided for students. The nurse assumes responsibility for continuing education and professional development and contributes to the professional growth of others.

STANDARD VII. COMMUNITY HEALTH SYSTEMS

The school nurse participates with other key members of the community responsible for assessing, planning, implementing, and evaluating school health services and community services that include the broad continuum of promotion of primary, secondary, and tertiary prevention.

STANDARD VIII. RESEARCH

The school nurse contributes to nursing and school health through innovations in theory and practice and participation in research.

uniformly defined by credentials in many areas. The 1983 American Nurses' Association publication, *Standards of School Nursing Practice,* should help nurses and nonnurses understand the role (see box).

OTHER COMMUNITY NURSING ROLES

School-age children see nurses in a variety of community health settings, usually clinics and private offices (Table 16-1). A *child health nurse* is a professional nurse who is responsible for health appraisal, health maintenance, problem identification, referral, and follow-up of essentially well children. A *specialist* in child health nursing is a child health nurse with a master's degree who has advanced competencies in health appraisal and problem management of children. The specialist has an increased knowledge and skill base for clinical practice and additional preparation in public health sciences and program planning. This nurse may have nurse practitioner skills. A *pediatric nurse practitioner* is an advanced nurse who provides primary health care to children of all ages. A *school nurse practitioner* is a nurse practitioner who provides primary health care to children within the school setting.

TABLE 16-1 Nursing Roles for School-Age Children

Title	Education	Settings	Major functions
School nurse	Basic nursing	School Home	Health education Screenings Prevention through immunization and other preventive measures (fluoride rinses) First aid Problem management Teacher consultant
School nurse practitioner	Basic nursing Advanced, formal didactic and clinical preparation	School Home Clinics	School nurse functions Diagnosis and treatment of common illnesses Management of chronic illnesses
Specialist in nursing: school health	Master's degree in school health nursing	All settings with school-age children	School nurse functions Nursing management of complex health problems Program development and evaluation Research consultation and administration in school health Use of school resources to promote health for entire community
Specialist and nurse practitioner in school health	Master's degree in school health nursing Care management preparation		Combination of school nurse practitioner and specialist roles

DEVELOPMENT

Development generally refers to functional or nonorganic changes (contrasted with growth, which is organic). In children it relates to orderly physiologic, psychologic, and environmental processes occurring in stages and at varying rates. The pattern of development is usually consistent, but there are many exceptions, and careful assessment is required for individuals.

The child is not simply an entity of separate, interacting, or even unified parts and functions. The child is a whole whose development is a single progression toward maturity. Students of human development assign stage phenomena to categories. Nurses who work with children know that attending to only one facet of development does not usually result in designed change of the whole person. Nurses know and use developmental data to understand the child, to plan care holistically, and to evaluate outcomes.

A family role is to assist its children in their development. The family promotes independence through educational and experiential opportunities while setting limits for safety of the children and reasonable comfort for the family. Society has not adjusted to the needs of today's families, which are no longer the stereotypical Daddy, Mommy, Johnnie, and Janie. Many families experience the stress of divorce, single parenting, and post-marital strife, with a host of related problems. After-school activities for younger children of working parents are inadequate and for adolescents are almost nonexistent. Jobs for adolescents are rarely available until they are almost finished with high school.

Rearing children to lead satisfying, productive adult lives is a highly stressful process in today's society for most families, regardless of strengths and resources. As the oldest child goes through developmental stages, so does the family. Part of gaining independence is questioning family values. This process can be painful to the developing person and to the developing family as well. The child or adolescent rebels against family expectations, and the family rebels against the child's behavior. Outpourings of stormy emotions including disapproval, dislike, fear, and doubt are frequent. The healthy family survives this stage partially by adapting limits to increasing needs for independence and by maintaining a sense of humor. Negative outcomes may occur as the children and the families struggle with developmental tasks. Less resourceful families need assistance from a variety of health professionals, family, and friends. Chaotic families may need to relinquish their children to a more stable and enriching environment, but few opportunities exist in the average community for a stable environment for children from these families.

Emotional Development

One approach to conceptualizing emotional development of school-age children is to use the stages described by Erik Erikson (1963). His summarizing terms describe both positive and negative resolutions of emotional developmental tasks.

The child entering school as a 5-year-old kindergartner may not have yet developed a sense of *initiative.* Well kindergartners are still happy to explore new situations, be aggressive in competitive situations, be productive without comparing their products with others', and do for the sake of doing. The child usually enjoys making models, playing games, and using movement for play without feelings of superiority or inferiority. The unfortunate child whose initiative is impeded by adults who foster *fear* and *guilt* frequently develops a sense of being a person who is bad and feels bad about this self-image.

The child in primary grades has the task of developing a sense of *industry.* No longer are lopsided cakes, crooked letters, or strike-outs in baseball acceptable. The 6- to 12-year-old not only wants to produce, but also has standards to meet. Standards initially are set by expectations of families and teachers, and the feedback concerning success is usually prompt. Later, children internalize these standards for their own. They also set expectations by comparing themselves with their peers and striving to meet at least the average of the group. When their products are consistently at or above the norm, a positive sense of industry develops. If not, a negative sense of *inferiority* can develop. Adults such as parents and teachers can diminish or reverse this process with praise and encouragement, open acceptance of the child experiencing failure, and advocacy for the child experiencing peer ridicule.

Adolescence is a time of conflict for most individuals and their families in the United States. If teenagers achieve success in trust, autonomy, initiative, and industry, they can attend to the task of developing a sense of *identity.* Developing identity requires observation of adults in their various work and interactional roles and acting out different and sometimes opposing roles. The teenager may pursue a job with vigor and then quit because it interferes with dating. Teenagers may smoke for a while but stop because it does not fit an image of themselves as an athlete or intellectual. Adolescents' difficulty in emotional development may be acted out in roles to the extreme, resulting in problems such as perfectionism, anxiety, depression, anorexia nervosa, recklessness, addictions, and promiscuity. Most causes of adolescent morbidity and mortality are related to extremes in behavior characteristic of this stage of development.

Young schoolchildren generally accept the values and views of their parents, teachers, and other adults in their lives. Prepubescents have learned that the family point of view is not necessarily the only one and often choose peer group preferences over all others. To achieve a clearly separate identity of self and no longer of someone's child, the adolescent goes through active rebellion with rejection of parental values. This rejection is often modified or even reversed by the end of this stage. The young adult, with a stronger sense of self, is ready to pursue life's goals of satisfying work and lasting relationships. Unsuccessful resolution of adolescent developmental tasks may result in *role diffusion* with a lack of direction and difficulty in developing independence.

Cognitive Development

As described by Jean Piaget, cognition develops in a progressive fashion (Piaget and Inhelder, 1969). Young children's cognitive stage of development, *preoperations,* is predominated by egocentrism, intuition, and fantasy. They do not have refined intellectual skills that allow them to reason logically in problem solving and understanding. By kindergarten age, however, children use insight and symbols, continue the formation of concepts (time, space, numbers, class, and causality), and begin to cope with more than one thing at a time. Memory and attention spans are adequate for structural learning experiences. The kindergarten environment and curriculum are designed to capitalize on a child's ability to increase logical reasoning.

Most of the school-age period coincides with Piaget's stage of *concrete operations.* The child experiences marked progress in concept formation, logical thinking, and therefore decreasing egocentrism. These changes occur over time, but at about 7 years of age, the average child approaches work and problem solving with a higher level of cognition. Thinking during school age is concrete and present oriented, but new intellectual competencies increase understanding of relationships and others' points of view. The school-age child can now acquire much more knowledge and logical problem solving and develop social skills required for effective group functioning.

The next stage of intellectual development, Piaget's stage of *formal operations,* begins around 11 years of age in many, but not all, children. Ability and experience determine the probability that an individual will progress to a higher level of cognitive functioning. Many adults remain at the stage of concrete operations and lead normal, productive lives. People who acquire formal operations are more abstract than concrete. They can see clearly from many points of view and can scrutinize their own biases more objectively. Rather than being bound to trial and error, these adolescents are capable of creating and testing different hypotheses to reach conclusions. This is a time of great intellectual growth leading to serious questioning of previously accepted, comfortable values. Debates over political, ethical, and religious issues are characteristic of bright adolescents at home and school. Intellectual ability leads to inner turmoil during the period of awakening and adds to the stress of the age. The older adolescent develops a relatively stable, personal view of reality with the recognition that others exist.

Moral development is dependent on intellectual ability, exposure to morality concepts, and sociocultural influences. Young, school-age children are still egocentric, so they justify their behavior by some rationalization. For young children the badness of wrongdoing is related to the quantity of the misdeeds, not intention. For example, a young child may think that breaking several glasses accidentally is worse than deliberately destroying one glass. If this justification fails, children may protect themselves by lying or cheating. The approach seems logical to them, but they learn with time that others do not view them positively when they lie or cheat. Their consciences control their behavior fairly well by 8 years of age. Older children progress considerably in their understanding of right and wrong, but their understanding is based on the concrete reactions of others to them. The intellectually advanced child is beginning to use formal logic and reasoning about moral and spiritual concerns. During adolescence serious questioning of established moral codes is common among children with abstract capabilities. They study themselves—their ideas, beliefs, and behaviors. Children look at consequences of behavior—their own, their country's, and those of historical events—and the way behavior affects the individual, the earth, and the universe. Children decide which part of society's moral code is applicable to them and their relationships to such things as people, religion, and politics. Adults who stay at a concrete level continue to see right and wrong in terms of societal responses and not in universal terms of consequences to others.

Physical Development

The child's body changes dramatically in size, proportion, and physiologic functioning during the 13 school years. Changes occur in periods of acceleration, plateaus, and deceleration, which are predictable according to the child's past patterns, age, sex, race, nutritional and health status, and family characteristics. Kindergartners have all their deciduous teeth and struggle to maintain control of bladder sphincters, whereas the older adolescent has a mature reproductive system and has reached full adult height and body proportions.

Size

Early school-age growth is relatively steady with gains of about 5 cm (2.4 inches) in height and 3 kg (6.6 lb.) per year until the prepubertal spurt. The average child is near 135 cm (56.25 inches) and 32 to 41 kg (70.5 to 90.3 lb.) when the rapid growth begins.

The pubertal growth stage in girls usually begins at 11 years of age and lasts approximately two years. Annual gains in height are about 9 cm (3.75 inches) and about 5 kg (11 lb.) in weight during the peak of the growth stage. Around age 13 years, boys begin their growth spurt, which lasts approximately two years, and gain about 11 centimeters (4.58 inches) in height and 6 kg (13.2 lb.) annually during peak periods. Completion of pubertal physical changes takes 1.5 to 3 years in girls and 1.8 to 4.7 years in boys. The earlier the onset of puberty is, the earlier the completion will be; that is, the boy who becomes taller than his peers at 11 years of age will complete his growth in a shorter time. Late puberty is associated with a longer growth time. Skeletal growth stops with the closure of the epiphyseal plates in the long bones. The shorter growth period in girls is attributed to increased estrogen levels occurring in the menstrual cycle (Figs. 16-1 to 16-4).

Body Proportions

The school-age child does not experience significant proportional changes until the pubertal stage. Until such time, average children appear to grow more up than out. Their arms and legs grow faster than their trunks and their heads grow little, giving them more adultlike proportions.

Pubescence is characterized by more growth of hands, feet, arms, and legs. Many children experience an increase in adipose tissue and look chubby before getting taller. Skeletal growth in males and females involves increases in leg length, hip width, chest breadth, shoulder width, length of trunk, and anterior-posterior diameter of the chest. Hormonal changes in boys bring about greater increases in shoulder breadth, leg length, and arm length, especially the forearm. Development of the facial skeleton, especially the mandible and the maxilla, results in a more angular, mature-looking face in just a few months. Female hormonal changes increase the width of the hips and overall size of the pelvis.

Changes in muscle tissue mass occur in boys and girls at different rates, amounts, and distri-

Text continued on p. 384.

GIRLS: 2 TO 18 YEARS
PHYSICAL GROWTH
NCHS PERCENTILES*

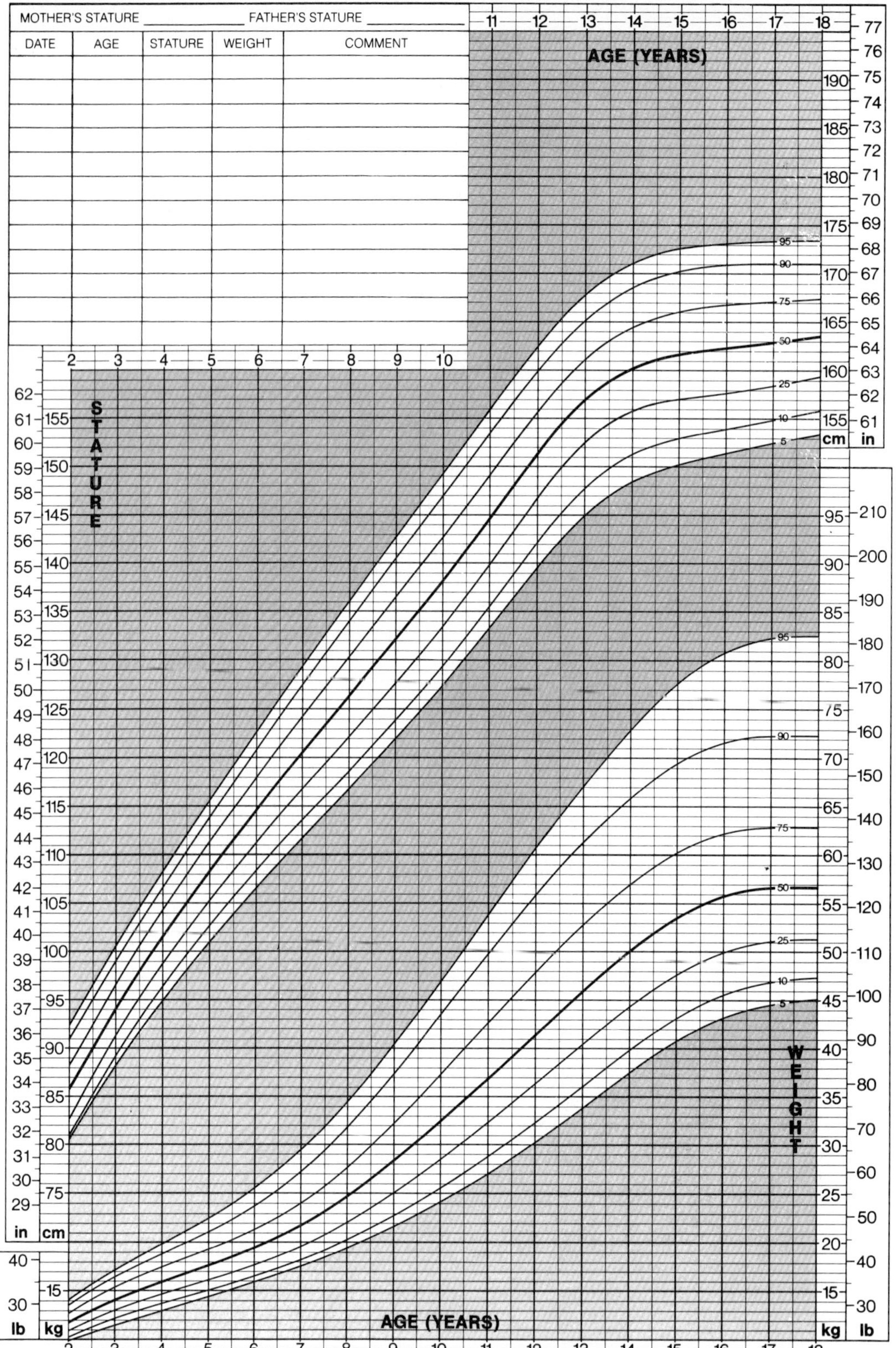

FIG. 16-1. Girls 2 to 18 years, physical growth NCHS profiles. (Adapted from Hamill PVV, Drizd TA, Johnson CL, Reed RB, Roche AF, and Moore WM: Physical growth: National Center for Health Statistics percentiles, Am J Clin Nutr 32:607, 1979. Data from the National Center for Health Statistics [NCHS], Hyattsville, Md. © 1982 Ross Laboratories.)

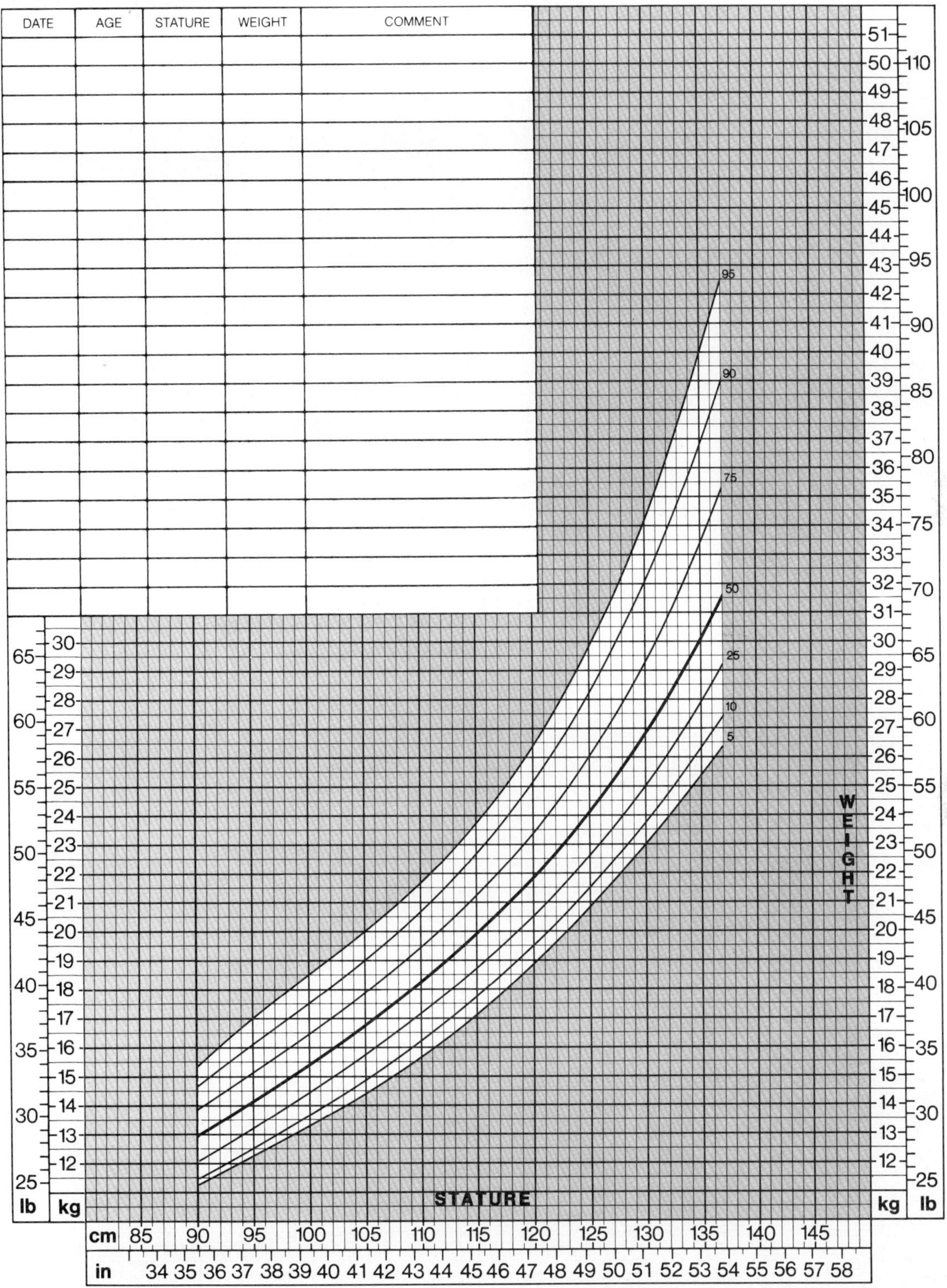

FIG. 16-2. Girls: Prepubescent physical growth NCHS percentiles. (Adapted from Hamill PVV, Drizd TA, Johnson CL, Reed RB, Roche AF, and Moore WM: Physical growth: National Center for Health Statistics percentiles, Am J Clin Nutr 32:607, 1979. Data from the National Center for Health Statistics [NCHS], Hyattsville, Md. © 1982 Ross Laboratories.)

BOYS: 2 TO 18 YEARS
PHYSICAL GROWTH
NCHS PERCENTILES*

NAME ______________________ RECORD # ______________

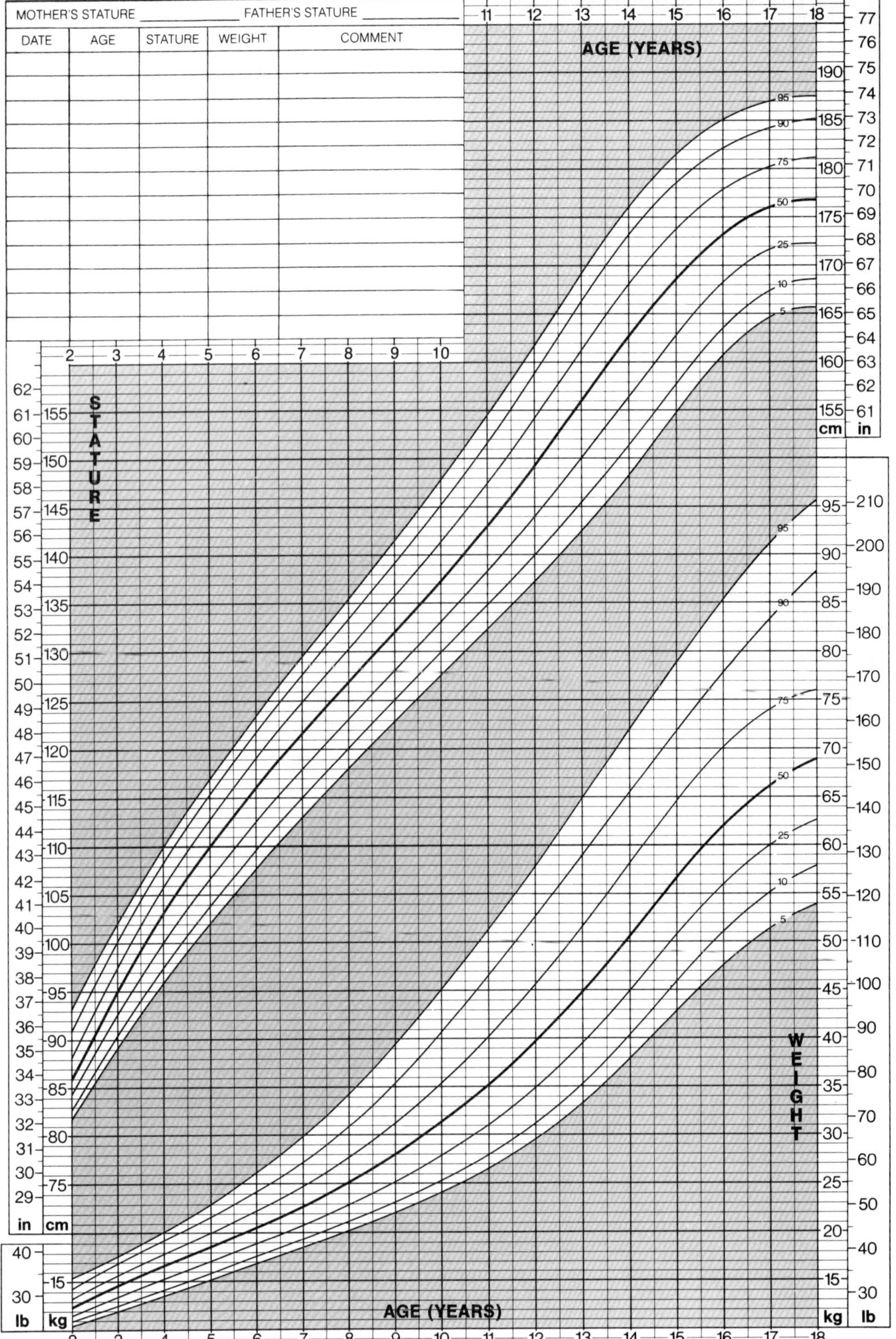

FIG. 16-3. Boys 2 to 18 years NCHS percentiles. (Adapted from Hamill PVV, Drizd TA, Johnson CL, Reed RB, Roche AF, and Moore WM: Physical growth: National Center for Health Statistics percentiles, Am J Clin Nutr 32:607, © 1979. Data from the National Center for Health Statistics [NCHS] Hyattsville, Md. © 1982 Ross Laboratories.)

BOYS: PREPUBESCENT PHYSICAL GROWTH NCHS PERCENTILES*

NAME ____________ RECORD # ____________

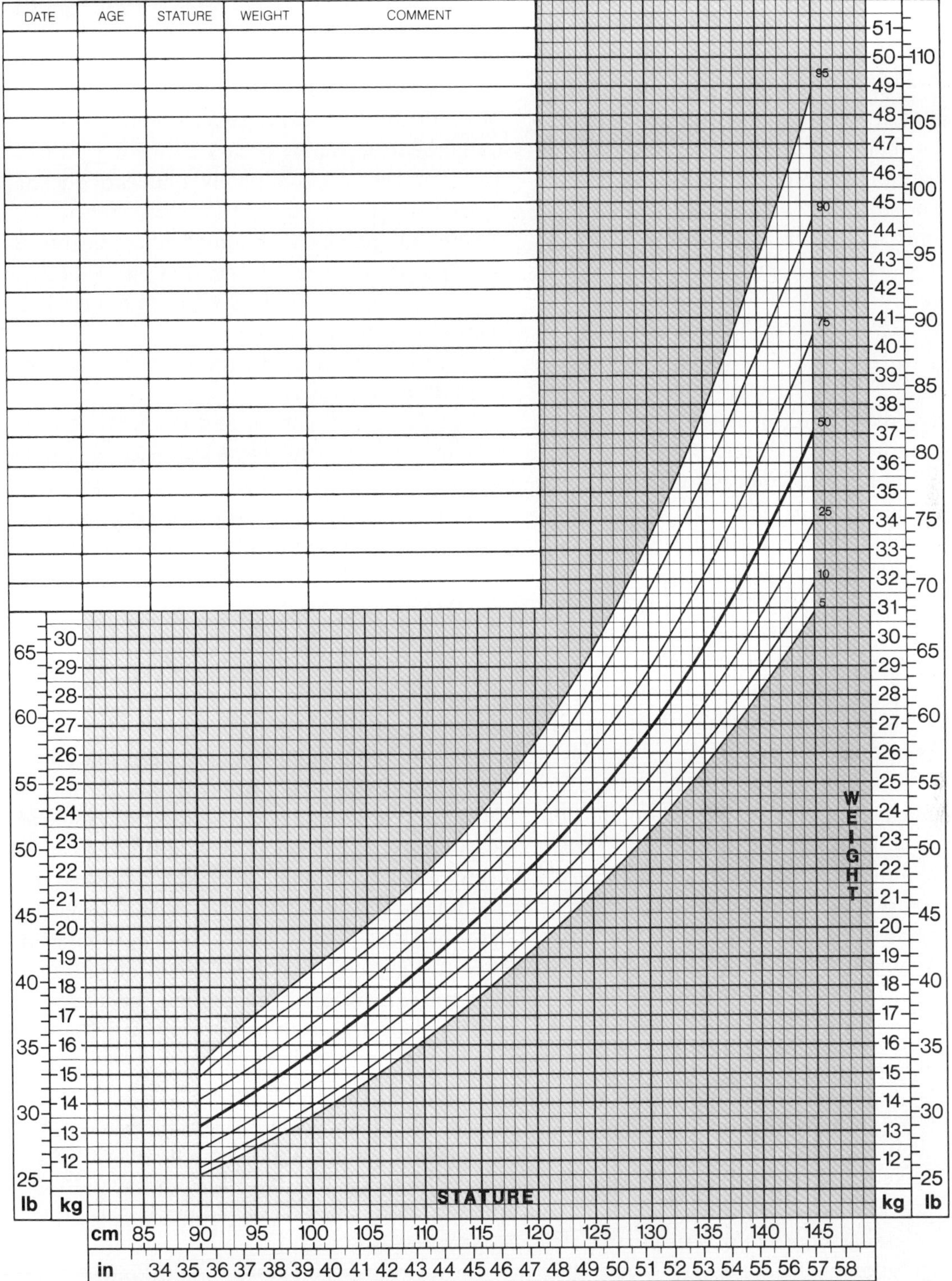

FIG. 16-4. Boys: Prepubescent physical growth NCHS percentiles. (Adapted from Hamill PVV, Drizd TA, Johnson CL, Reed RB, Roche AF, and Moore WM: Physical growth: National Center for Health Statistics percentiles, Am J Clin Nutr 32:607, 1979. Data from the National Center for Health Statistics [NCHS], Hyattsville, Md. © 1982 Ross Laboratories.)

bution. Girls have reached their peak in number of muscle cells by the time of menarche, but boys continue to produce more muscle cells for 18 months after reaching maximum height. Boys also have a greater distribution of muscle tissue in the shoulder and back. Adipose tissue (the bane of the adolescent girl's existence in today's world) is increased and distributed in the breasts, lower abdomen, hips, and thighs of girls. Boys have less adipose tissue but higher proportions are found in the trunk.

Physiologic Changes

Just as growth and proportions change during the child's journey through school, so does the body's functioning. Each body system matures at varying rates and reaches adult stage at different ages during childhood and adolescence.

Reproductive system changes profoundly affect appearance, feelings, and behavior of every person. This process is primarily a result of hormonal changes influenced by the central nervous system. Physical changes in both sexes follow an orderly pattern. The first indication of puberty in boys is the enlargement of the testes followed by gradual lengthening of the penis and textural changes in the scrotum. There usually is a small amount of long, fair pubic hair at this point. As the penis and testes continue to enlarge, spermatogenesis begins. These primary changes usually occur after the first year of testicular growth. Nocturnal emissions may begin at this phase. Many boys experience tender, swollen breast tissue that subsides after a few months to three years. During the second year, the genitals further enlarge and pubic hair darkens and curls. Voice changes and axillary and facial hair appear approximately two years after pubic hair. Completion of these physical changes can take from approximately two to five years.

The breasts and genitals are organs greatly affected by hormones in girls at puberty. About the same time the growth spurt begins, breasts become slightly elevated, enlarged, and tender. This is followed almost immediately by fine, sparse hair on the genitals. Pubic hair increases and darkens and breasts continue to enlarge for one and one half to three years. Menarche, the first menstrual period, usually occurs between 12 and 14 years of age, approximately one and one half years after first breast development. At menarche, nipples and pubic hair assume adult appearances. The first menses may normally occur as early as 9 years of age or as late as 17 years of age. Early menses may be irregular and sparse as a result of immature functioning of the hormones and the central nervous system.

The changes in genital and secondary characteristics are not in the same sequence or rate for all boys and girls. It is important to remember that the information is based on averages of many individuals and does not represent the average person. Girls especially may show deviation from the average but still be quite normal.

Other body systems mature in less radical fashion. Cardiovascular system changes include a slowing of heart rate to 60 to 65 beats per minute and a rise in blood pressure to 120/60 mm Hg, both average for healthy young adults. Blood volume and blood components increase in general during adolescence. The respiratory system becomes more efficient as the rate of respirations decreases and the vital capacity increases. The immune system is essentially mature at 8 years of age when such organs as tonsils stop growing and later atrophy. The urinary system is able to function efficiently during infancy but remains more vulnerable to infection in girls primarily because of the short urethra and proximity to the anus. The integumentary system often is problematic, with increases in skin thickness, sebaceous secretions, sweat, odors, and body hair caused by pubertal hormonal changes. The senses are fully mature during early years, but some changes in sensitivity may occur.

The neuromuscular system of the kindergartner is adequate for gross motor activity such as running, climbing, jumping, and swinging. Fine motor capability includes drawing a relatively straight line, painting with a large brush, and using a fork. Young school-age children are motivated to improve motor skills. They are better able to play a variety of skill games, since they become less egocentric at this age and can cooperate as team members. Opportunity and support are also important for gross motor development in some children, especially with the enormous amount of passive entertainment available to children today. Fine motor coordination improves remarkably during school age. Each side of the brain matures and specializes further in such areas as speech and drawing. The average child shows a clear preference for use of the right or left hand during early school age. Fine motor coordination improves rapidly during the first and second grades, so the second grader can learn cursive writing. The adolescent simply refines motor skills of early school years and develops more complicated ones. During peak growth periods, clumsiness may be a problem that is self-limited to the average adolescent.

Nutrition

Children in primary grades have a slow growth rate, prepubescents acquire a reserve for growth, and pubescents have a major growth spurt. Adolescents grow according to gender and when the growth spurt started. Growth rates, sex, size, energy usages through activity, and basal metabolism determine individual nutritional requirements. The range varies widely. Rarely does a U.S. schoolchild have a health problem caused by insufficient intake of nutrients. Usually sufficient calorie intake increases other essential nutrients enough to prevent disease. The most significant nutritional problem of children in school is obesity. Nutritional patterns established in childhood, however, usually continue and may create risks to health throughout adulthood.

Life-styles of schoolchildren are not always conducive to good nutrition. Children have more money, more access to convenience stores or fast-food products, and more control over when they eat than in past years when families sat down daily to cooked meals. Television, sports, various lessons, and other activities compete with the family function of dining. Schools have attempted to satisfy current eating preferences of students by offering à la carte selections such as french fries, hot dogs, pizza, and salads, as well as balanced meals. Some nutrition-conscious or weight-conscious individuals select foods wisely. Others make poor choices such as fries and soft drinks for lunch. Snacks after school and on weekends are consumed regularly. Parents have the opportunity to improve overall nutrition of the age group by having dairy products, fruits, and vegetables available as snacks and avoiding salty, fatty, or greasy foods.

Peer groups play a special part in food selection throughout the school years. The rewards of being part of the group during the social event of dining are great enough to tempt the staunchest nutrition advocate to eat pizza or fast foods regularly. Television and other forms of media help create fads with children through commercials for sweetened cereals and other potentially harmful foods. Almost all extracurricular activities, such as sports and dances, have some association with foods that have predominantly no nutritional value.

Food is equated with love in many families, and therefore some babies are overfed, preschoolers are bribed to eat, and children are forced to clean their plates. By school age, struggles for control over eating habits exist with some parents and children around mealtimes. It is no wonder that some individuals eat and actually enjoy new food at a friend's home or on a group outing when they refuse it at home. Some children associate hunger with anxiety in anticipation of conflict. They do not learn to control their own eating patterns and may acquire eating disorders reflective of family dysfunction.

Promotion of healthful nutrition in school-age

children includes increasing their knowledge, assisting them in decision making about food and providing essential nutrients through school and other community resources when necessary. Helping the family avoid power struggles over food intake and dining practices improves many situations. Use of selected media, for example, a television documentary on sugar's effect on the body, may get the attention of children and adults better than traditional teaching methods. The school nurse has the additional task of promoting nutrition within the school system. This may require consulting with dietitians and administrators for provision of nutritional foods in the cafeteria and snack machines such as low-fat milk, fresh fruit, and sugarless drinks and elimination of popular but low-nutrient foods such as sticky sweets and fried potatoes. School nurses also provide individual and group guidance for obese persons and refer those with severe eating disorders such as anorexia nervosa to specialists.

Exercise

The young school-age child still enjoys body movement for the sake of moving. Most run, skip, jump, and climb with limited interference from rules, scores, or stress. By age 8, the child has acquired enough gross motor, cognitive, and emotional ability to begin participation in organized sports. Since children can compare themselves with peers, the potential for developing a sense of industry or of inferiority in relation to physical activity exists. The former tradition of neighborhood games has almost disappeared with the competition of television, after-school day care, and organized sports. Schools in many communities are so large that only superior athletes are eligible to play on teams. Physical education may be limited to selected grades and then may be limited in time and actual activity for students. Community centers provide youth opportunities ranging from a few activities to outstanding programs for all ages.

Many children do not have transportation to participate in organized sports because of working parents, costs, and geographic consideration. A circular problem exists for girls in that there may be few programs for them, and recreation planners say few programs exist because few girls are interested.

In view of the restraining forces in many current environments, the community health nurse who wishes to promote healthful exercise in children faces multiple challenges. Clearly exercise leads to such positive outcomes as cardiovascular fitness, sense of well-being, weight control, and social interactions. In addition to traditional nursing roles of guidance of children and families by providing knowledge and encouragement, the nurse is an advocate for exercise in schools and communities. The nurse consults with physical and health educators and administrators to assess the level of physical activity provided in the school and to plan for increases when indicated. The nurse also supports programs for special populations such as children with physical or emotional handicaps. Community involvement at political and policymaking levels are required to encourage programing for children without afternoon transportation, for girls, and for others without adequate opportunities.

Children who have regular exercise and participate in organized sports have additional health needs. Calories in the form of carbohydrates and fluid requirements increase, but other nutritional requirements remain essentially the same in active and quiescent children. Strenuous, prolonged exercise may lead to mild potassium and sodium depletion, but a diet with any food variety meeting caloric needs usually replenishes losses. Planning for appropriate activity reduces accidents and injuries. The small child may need to avoid contact sports. The child with asthma may need to plan medication or to avoid outdoor sports during peak pollen times. The prepubescent boy should postpone weight lifting until muscles are developed sufficiently through androgen influences.

The child health nurse collaborates with a variety of professionals in managing the special needs of children who are active in sports.

HEALTH OF SCHOOL-AGE CHILDREN

Children in schools of the United States are remarkably well. Most enter schools with little danger of exposure to the infectious diseases responsible for morbidity and mortality of past years. Congenital anomalies resulting in death during earlier years are usually corrected or controlled by school age. Illnesses that do occur are usually treated promptly, and there are fewer complications. Risks to children's well-being have changed from disease and disability to stresses of life-style such as obesity and adolescent pregnancy. Accidents, the most common cause of death and a major cause of mordibity in children, can be attributed in part to life-style and to related developmental and family characteristics. In view of the trend toward increased preventable programs and decreased disease, primary prevention of child health problems is of the utmost importance to the community health nurse. That children are seldom hospitalized increases the responsibility of community health nurses in secondary and tertiary prevention (see box).

Health Care of the School-Age Child

Promotion and maintenance of health in school-age children require a system of periodic health evaluations, prompt treatment of abnormal findings, education concerning risk reduction, and support of efforts to change health behaviors. In the United States the system is often fragmented in terms of delivery settings and types of services and providers. The child may go to a public health clinic for well child visits, to a hospital clinic for acute illness, to another setting for management of a chronic problem, and to the school health room for life-style problems. Traditional retrospective fee-for-service payment is illness oriented and rarely covers immunizations or well child visits to primary care providers. The more recent prospective payment systems usually, but not always, cover and encourage these prevention efforts. Prevention-of-illness measures, such as immunizations, have drastically changed the health of children. Prevention of accidents and life-style consequences within a loose framework of providers and payment mechanisms are major challenges of today's nursing.

Child Health Visits

Child health assessments include an age-specific health history, physical examination, screening tests, case finding procedures specific to risk factors, prompt intervention for positive findings, and counseling, education, and support for positive changes. Much disagreement exists over when and where the examinations should occur, who should provide the services, and what components should be included. The school-age child who has a history of regular examinations and immunization during preschool, has no complaint or risk factor, and has school screenings for height, weight, hearing, vision, scoliosis, and blood pressure probably does not need a physical examination or any further objective health testing until pubescence.

The most important service of these visits is probably the education and encouragement toward good health practices, prevention of accidents, and control of life-style stresses. A major focus of the educational component is anticipatory guidance to prepare child and family for expected changes of the next developmental stage and strategies for positive outcomes. Adolescents also have few physical problems, but the increase in morbidity and mortality rates for life-style and developmental problems suggests a need for regular assessment and intervention throughout this period. The health visit that includes only illness-directed history, physical examination, and

RISKS TO CHILDREN'S HEALTH HAVE CHANGED

Children in the United States are remarkably healthy. Medical, social, and economic progress have all contributed to a substantial decline in risks to children's health. These gains have been made largely through a highly successful assault on the infectious diseases that formerly were the leading causes of childhood illness, disability, and death.

Paralleling and supporting medical progress since 1900 were improvements in the environment—sanitation, housing, drinking water—improvements in nutrition and product safety, and for most American families, markedly increased real incomes. Simultaneously, higher family incomes, the advent of various federal and state child health programs, and an increase in physicians and other health services have improved children's access to care.

Despite the positive impact on health of these important trends, there remain several rationales for school districts to become involved in expanded health services programs. The Robert Wood Johnson Foundation's program concentrated on only the first of these:

- The improvements in health and access to medical care that are enjoyed by most American children are not yet enjoyed by all. Those from families who are minority, poor, uneducated, or living in remote rural areas or urban ghettos—these children lag behind the rest for many measures of health. These are also the children most likely not to have a regular source of care (see Fig. 16-5 on opposite page).
- New, more subtle, and perhaps more intractable, child and adolescent health problems have emerged—deficits in physical capacity, learning ability, or emotional development. Many of these problems could be prevented and many more of them remedied. Despite great concern about behavioral and developmental problems, many parents are reluctant to discuss such matters with pediatricians. The schools, rather than the health care sector, find themselves the social agencies that must cope with these problems.
- At least 4.3 million American public school children are enrolled in special education programs serving mentally retarded or emotionally disturbed children, children with vision, hearing, orthopedic, or multiple handicaps, and children with chronic illnesses and specific learning disabilities. A 1975 federal law (P.L. 94-142) requires that states make available a "free appropriate public education" to all handicapped children ages 3 to 21, regardless of the severity of their disabilities or their families' ability to pay for services. At the local level, schools must offer individualized instruction and related supporting services—including health services.
- Risky behavior is a hallmark of adolescence, but it exacts a heavy toll—70% of all deaths among adolescents 12 to 17 are from injuries and violence—and all of these deaths are at least theoretically preventable. Because of high U.S. rates of fatal auto injuries and violence, death rates for American teenagers are half again those of their contemporaries in other industrialized nations (Trunkey, 1983).
- Nearly one-quarter of teenage girls have sexual relations before age 15. Yet, teenagers usually delay a year after first having intercourse before seeking contraceptive services (Zelnik and Shah, 1983; Zelnik, Koenig, and Kim, 1984).
- Teenage pregnancies are increasing, with 1.1 million in 1981. That year, nearly 10,000 babies were born to girls 14 and younger. One study has predicted that "If patterns do not change, four in ten young women will get pregnant at least once while still in their teens" (Teenage Pregnancy, 1981).
- Fewer high school seniors report themselves as "frequent users" of marijuana, tobacco, or alcohol than a few years ago, but drug use among U.S. youth is still "the highest in the Western industrialized world;" almost one adolescent in five has an acute drinking-related problem, including driving while intoxicated; and one high school senior in eight smokes at least a half-pack of cigarettes daily. These habits have life-long adverse consequences for health.

Social and economic changes affect not only child health, but also child health care. Several of these trends also might influence school districts' interest in embarking on an expanded school health services program.

Working mothers find it difficult to obtain health care for their children during the day. In 1983, 59 percent of children ages 6 to 17 had mothers in the work force, up from 42 percent just a decade earlier.

Nearly 13 million U.S. children—one child in five—live with their mother only. In these families, it is not just the lack of a father, but the lack of a father's income that creates barriers to health care. In 1983, the median family income in two-parent families with children was $27,286; in one-parent families, it was $11,789. This income level is only slightly over the 1983 poverty threshold for a family of four, $10,178. Nearly half of all black families are headed by women, and, at any one time, nearly half of black children are living in poverty.

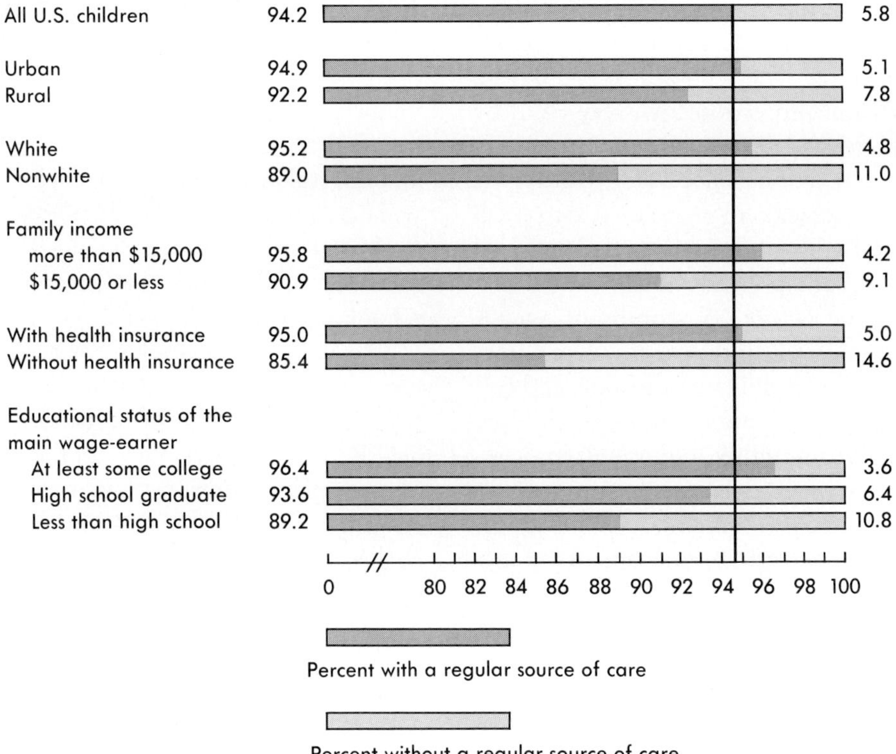

FIG. 16-5. Characteristics of children younger than 17 years of age with and without a regular source of care.

screening tests falls far short of the needs of young people.

Screening

Screening for health problems in schoolchildren is a priority school nurse function. The child with an undetected vision or hearing handicap or undetected scoliosis may require costly and painful treatment or have permanent disability. Screening programs are designed to focus on prevalent or serious problems that would benefit from early detection and have diagnostic and treatment mechanisms. Screening tests are selected according to their accuracy, simplicity, cost, safety, and client acceptability. Once the program is established, the school nurse decides if, when, and how to use volunteers to perform first screening tests. The nurse also trains volunteers, rescreens any children identified by volunteers, refers children to community resources as necessary, and follows progress of treatment. Use of volunteers is a necessity in schools where there are only itinerant nurses, but screening by school nurses increases the chance of finding targeted problems and problems in general.

Immunization

Protection from many childhood infectious diseases is provided in the United States through a loose network of health care agencies, private offices, and schools that administer immunizations. The system of administration and documentation is dependent on parents' willingness to return to provider sites as scheduled and keep records of every immunization. The school health program works toward full protection for every child by kindergarten entry and to maintain immunity through reimmunization as necessary. During the mid-1980s an outbreak of measles occurred in adolescents and young adults who had received the live measles, mumps, and rubella viruses in a combined vaccine before 15 months of age. A massive immunization initiative involving government and private providers in schools and colleges followed. School nurses tracked children with questionable immunity, reimmunized or referred as necessary, and documented coverage on the school health record. Immunization programs are time consuming and tedious but more successful under the direction of school nurses.

Dental Health

Promotion of the dental health of school-age children includes good nutrition, brushing twice daily, flossing once daily, use of fluoride in water, rinses, and toothpastes, and regular dental checks with application of sealants to vulnerable areas. By far the most cost-effective public health method of preventing tooth decay in children is communal water fluoridation, but the best combination of prevention measures and specific ages has not yet been determined (APHA, 1986). Orthodontics is a growing specialty that requires special attention to dental hygiene. Braces were at one time an embarrassment to pubescents but are more a status symbol in today's society. Use of the appropriate provider of dental care is a growing controversy among hygienists, generalists, and specialists of dentistry. With the decrease in caries of young people, generalists are extending their practice to orthodontics and other fields.

Comprehensive School Health Programs

Some schools provide an innovative mode of care delivery (Robert Wood Johnson Foundation, 1985). Primary health care needs are met in the school setting by a school nurse or a school nurse practitioner with medical preceptors in the community. In addition to staffing the health room for such things as minor complaints, screenings, and referral to community agencies for public assistance, nurses also deliver primary care. Common acute illnesses are diagnosed, treated, and followed, and health assessments required for school activities are performed at the school (Table 16-2). Some adolescent health clinics also provide human sexuality counseling and contraception. Although most students have personal health care providers, they use the clinics because of convenience, low cost, and acceptability to the student body in general. Comprehensive school health clinics are rare in the United States because of limiting payment mechanisms, laws restricting nurse practitioner practice, community values against direct care to children, and turf-guarding by other professionals. The most recent major constraint to providing health care in the schools is the exorbitant cost of liability insurance. This issue compounds the controversy over whether the educational institutions or the health care institutions will provide health services.

COMMON CHILD HEALTH PROBLEMS

There are many ways to approach health problems of school-age children. Mortality and morbidity rates are important aspects of such study. Because the reasons for death and illness are not always the same, both sets of problems require specific programing for identification and treatment. Another approach is to separate acute and chronic problems, for example, upper respiratory infection from asthma. Expected developmental problems, whether physical, emotional, or cognitive, may be targeted for mass intervention programs, such as one for accident prevention, or integration into all other programs. All categorization of health problems requires arbitrary placement of some problems that do not clearly

TABLE 16-2 Distribution of Children's Problems by Diagnostic Category and Source of Identification, School Health Services Program, 1980-1982

Type of problem	Primary care	Physical examination	Screening	Total
Respiratory	6012	264	0	6276
Musculoskeletal	3196	251	1	3448
Trauma	2987	31	0	3018
Dermatologic	2596	353	13	2962
Vision	417	205	2211	2833
Hearing	1698	205	623	2526
Medications	2438	8	0	2446
Miscellaneous	2187	234	2	2423
Dental	1349	592	2	1943
Gastrointestinal	1571	58	0	1629
Otitis media	1342	84	0	1426
Eye	1066	163	0	1229
Genitourinary	804	201	0	1005
Speech, learning, and behavior	624	245	0	869
Scoliosis	142	90	607	839
Tonsillitis	609	29	0	638
Headache	571	16	0	587
Blood pressure and cardiovascular	317	92	158	567
Height and weight checks	3	0	426	429
Heart murmur	164	221	0	385
Obesity or underweight	155	199	0	354
Anemia	77	105	0	182
Neurologic	119	53	0	172
Allergy	128	6	0	134
Neoplasm	87	28	1	116
Total	30,659	3,733	4,044	38,436

Modified from Meeker RJ and others: An evaluation-driven school health initiative, unpublished manuscript, 1984.

fit a category. Occasionally problems are so detrimental that they require an individual grouping. All problems share some characteristics, especially since children are whole and separation of mind, body, and environment is impossible.

Common Physical Problems

The school-age child has physical health problems that, for this chapter, are categorized into common developmental problems, acute illnesses, and chronic conditions.

Common Developmental Problems

Structural and functional changes throughout childhood result in risks to the child's health and self-esteem. The problem may or may not be severe physically, as with progressive scoliosis, but the human reaction may be most troublesome to the child. However, the vast majority of children have changes such as growth and change in body proportions, beginning of menses and ejaculation, and skin imperfections. The problems may be handled with basic nursing services for child and family or may require medical intervention. Table 16-3 gives an overview of developmental physical problems. Please note that all have a psychosocial component that may also require nursing intervention.

Acute Problems

Acute health problems generally are considered to be illness or injury of short duration and in need of medical attention or restricted activity. Type and incidence of acute problems in schoolchildren may be determined by reports of diagnoses from physicians' offices and clinics, presenting complaints in school settings (Table 16-2), and reasons given for school absenteeism. Acute problems in general have declined with improvements in the standards of living and better disease prevention programs. Acute problems are fewer during school years than earier years as the immune system matures and the body responds to infectious exposures more effectively. Once the school-age child develops an acute illness, there is a longer recovery period than for younger children. One area of increase in infectious disease during school years is sexually transmitted disease. In addition, accidents continue to cause significant rates of illness and disability throughout these years. Nurses in schools and other child health settings are challenged to manage the care of children with acute problems, to prevent the spread of the problems to other children, and to plan and implement primary prevention programs.

Most acute health problems are self-limited, so teaching self-care skills is an important nursing role. Even young schoolchildren can learn to manage their own colds and prevent spread of the infection. They can also learn the basics of first aid, temperature measurement, and the values and dangers of over-the-counter medication. By the end of high school, adolescents should be ready to assume full responsibility for self-care, including how to recognize the need for professional health care.

Respiratory Conditions

Respiratory conditions account for the majority of acute illnesses is school-age children. The common cold is the most frequently occurring respiratory problem, causing absenteeism from school by most children each year. Unless complications such as otitis media and bronchitis occur, upper respiratory infections are self-limited and professional care is not necessary. Self-care measures include determining the presence of fever, using appropriate antipyretic measures, increasing fluid intake and rest, and preventing spread of microorganisms to others. The school nurse may need to send the child home, depending on school policy, the child's discomfort, and indicators of complications. The school nurse practitioner may diagnose and treat the complications according to nurse and physician protocols and parental permission.

Pharyngitis

Pharyngitis is a common upper respiratory problem of school-age children. The most frequent type of pharyngitis is viral, but the less frequent streptococcal pharyngitis is more serious in that it is usually more painful, results in a higher fever, and has the potential complications of rheumatic fever and acute glomerulonephritis. There is no way to rule out streptococcal pharyngitis without sophisticated laboratory procedures, but screening tests are increasingly sensitive, specific, inexpensive, and quick. Some school nurses screen for streptococcal infections and provide penicillin (or alternative medications for those allergic to penicillin) according to protocol. The

TABLE 16-3 Common Developmental Physical Problems

System	Change	Risk of problem	Potential human responses	Nursing interventions
Skeletal	Increase in length and diameter	Height above or below norms	Body image disturbance	Explain growth potentials Support Refer adolescents whose height is above the 95th percentile or below the 5th percentile for medical intervention
		Scoliosis	Pain Progression of curvature	Medical referral
Reproductive	Breast growth	Males—gynecomastia	Body image disturbance	Explain time limitation Refer for surgical consideration if severe
		Females—hyperplasia or hypoplasia	Body image disturbance	Support—stress positive attributes Discuss surgical alterations for later periods in life
	Menarche with hormonal fluctuations	Amenorrhea Irregular bleeding Excessive bleeding	Disturbance in internal body image Fear of pathology Anemia	Discuss normal feelings and fears Explain normal physiology Medical referral to rule out pathology Support
		Unstable moods	Erratic behavior Depression Elation	Support Avoid overreaction Explain physiologic basis Recommend regular exercise, sufficient sleep, and avoidance of excessive sweets
	Increase in size of genitals	Hypoplastic penis	Body image disturbance	Discuss penile functioning
	Production of semen or vaginal secretion	Appearance of unexplained body fluids	Fear Anxiety Powerlessness	Teach origin of emission and secretion of body fluids in males and females
Integumentary	Increase in production of sebum by sebaceous glands	Acne	Inflammation Painful lesions Body image disturbance	Teach cleansing techniques Over-the-counter preparations, healthful nutrition, and exercise patterns Refer for medical intervention Support
			Body image disturbance	Teach hair removal techniques
		Folliculitis	Painful lesion of axilla and groin	Teach cleansing techniques Refer for medical intervention Support
	Stimulation of epocrine gland	Body odor	Social isolation	Teach cleansing techniques and use of antiperspirants and deodorants

child with streptococcal pharyngitis is generally considered contagious until 24 hours after initiation of antibiotic therapy. Viral pharyngitis requires self-care of fever and sore throat, since no antibiotic affects the course of the disease. Studies indicating that some pharyngitis is caused by bacteria other than the streptococcus will probably lead to further diagnosis and treatment protocols and improve the management of this problem.

Varicella

Varicella (chickenpox) is a common viral childhood disease that has no immunization to date. This highly contagious exanthematous disease can spread rapidly in a school setting. Children with varicella are isolated at school and sent home as soon as possible. They can return to school when all lesions are crusted over. Varicella is usually a self-limited disease, and care is directed toward alleviation of itching with antihistamines and topical preparations and prevention of secondary bacterial infections of the skin.

Parasitic Infections

Parasitic infections including *pediculosis* (lice) and *scabies* are conditions requiring careful classroom and home observation for spread of the parasite, immediate treatment, and preventive measures. Outbreaks of these and other parasitic infections, although rarely life threatening, can result in significant numbers of days lost from school and require that much time and effort be expended by school and health personnel.

Injury

Injury to school-age children is the leading cause of death and a major cause of acute illness. Common injuries include fractures, sprains, strains, lacerations, and contusions. Risky behaviors increase with age in schoolchildren, and peer pressure is a frequent cause (Lewis and Lewis, 1984). The adolescent becomes even more daring, somewhat because of the need to deny mortality and also because of sensation-seeking tendencies. Prevention of injury is based on getting the attention of society as a whole, changing attitudes toward safety precautions, limiting child and adolescent exposures to danger, and establishing safe habits such as wearing seat belts in automobiles. The community health nurse requires regular continuing education to maintain current first aid and cardiopulmonary resuscitation skills and should review and revise first aid protocols for school, clinic, and home settings. Such issues as management of bee stings in allergic children should be established and on file before an incident occurs.

Digestive System Disorders

Digestive system disorders, including various upper and lower gastrointestinal tract disorders, are acute conditions resulting in days lost from school. These are almost always self-limited with self-care directed toward fluid and electrolyte maintenance until recovery. Handwashing is a preventive measure to be taught to all schoolchildren, and bathrooms should have ample supplies of soap and warm water.

Chronic Health Problems

Children in school infrequently have chronic physical health problems, since they have had little exposure to life-style and environmental stressors. Chronic problems are usually caused by congenital anomalies, allergic conditions, injury, or neoplasms. Public Law 94-142 (1975) mandated that all children have the right to a free education appropriate to their abilities. Suddenly public school teachers found children with major physical handicaps in their classrooms. Nurses began to provide services to these children in health rooms and to teach teachers how to manage needs of children with special conditions such as colostomies and numerous orthopedic devices. The question of where children with significant problems should be educated is still debated. Currently they generally attend classes with "normal" children as much as possible and attend special classes as necessary. Homebound teachers may be provided during periods of exacerbation. Providing a safe, accepting, comfortable learning experience for children with chronic illness or disability is a major challenge to the school system.

Congenital Anomalies

Congenital anomalies are predominantly orthopedic, hearing, and visual impairments. A team approach is required to meet these children's needs. The nursing role is holistic, including comprehensive health assessment of the child, the classroom environment, the home, and the family, management of medications and treatments, referral to community health agencies, teaching of self-care, and advocacy for the child in general.

Allergic Conditions

Allergic conditions, especially asthma, are chronic disorders with periods of acute illness. Children with allergic conditions may be well controlled for much of the year with medication and activity and environmental restrictions but miss several days or weeks during peak pollen seasons or other illnesses that exacerbate asthma. To maintain adequate learning experiences, the school nurse may be responsible for administering multiple medications in a timely manner to maintain blood levels without interrupting classes or making the child feel uncomfortable in front of classmates. For example, sensitive nurses may plan administration of nebulized medication in their offices and not in the classroom. The nurse also may assess the child and determine the need for immediate medical attention or provide a quiet spot for medication to relieve wheezing. Coordination of care between home and school certainly requires collaboration with the family, primary care provider, and teachers and may require collaboration with other members of the child health and education team.

Injury

Injury may result in prolonged recovery and permanent orthopedic, visual, or other disability. Homebound instruction and perhaps home health nursing are required, followed by adjustment of the school environment and self-care instruction of the child to provide for mobility, pain control, and treatments. Children learn to manipulate casts, crutches, braces, and wheelchairs with the help of teachers and classmates. The goal of care is to facilitate rehabilitation whenever possible and to prevent any complications. As with all long-term health problems, a team approach is helpful in assisting the child in achieving optimal health.

Malignant Neoplasms

Malignant neoplasms at one time resulted in fairly rapid deaths of victims. Today children survive long periods, and many are cured of their diseases. Treatment, however, is traumatic, causing pain, nausea and vomiting, weight loss, hair loss, and a host of emotional stresses including fear of death. Classmates, teachers, and all others involved with children with malignancies experience mixed emotions. Affected children may receive messages of concern, love, caring, grief, pity, rejection, ridicule, curiosity, fear, and overprotection. Children with malignant neoplasms need acceptance from their peers, expectations of work according to their abilities, limits on their behaviors according to the class standard, and discomfort control and support from teachers and nurses. The teacher or nurse may collaborate with the parents and decide how to involve classmates. One class designed an official class cap that all the children wore during the ill child's alopecic period. When a child dies, the class needs permission to grieve openly. Several children will inevitably experience some behavioral and emotional changes, especially an increase or recurrence of death anxiety.

Common Emotional Problems

Emotional problems during school years are often developmental or situational and usually self-limited if there is an adequately functioning family. Some emotional disorders are familial, with genetic and environmental causes, and may range from minor to severe, requiring a variety of professional and support services from the school and community. The school nurse may be first to note a problem by assessing the number and type of complaints an individual child has or may consult with a teacher who has concerns about a child. Depending on school staffing of mental health professionals, the nurse may have the delicate task of informing and gaining trust of the parents, assessing the home environment and family dynamics, coordinating referral services, and reporting all cases of suspected abuse or neglect to authorities. Nurses should assess the emotional status of the child client and the family's competence, and intervene according to need. Anticipatory guidance for the child and family can increase skill in handling a problem or decrease the risk of developing complications.

Death Anxiety

Sometime during elementary school, the child begins to comprehend death as an irreversible event with all the separation connotations. This may be hastened by illness or death of a family member, including a pet, or be delayed by almost no exposure to death, but the phenomenon is actually a result of increased cognitive skills. Some children experience this awareness with relative ease and discuss their feelings with parents and others. Some children react with alarm and experience anxiety with behavioral components such as delaying separation from parents at bedtime and schooltime, crying for no apparent reason, and performing poorly in school. The astute observer of child health recognizes this normal developmental event. Anticipatory guidance prepares parent and child for the need for open discussions about death, family beliefs about life after death, and the expectation that the child will develop some acceptance of the finality of death.

School Phobia

Fear of school occurs in varying degrees in children, but "school phobia" is a term generally reserved for persistent, severe fears. School phobias are related to situational events at home, such as the illness of a parent, and at school, such as a harsh teacher, and to dysfunctional separation anxiety between parent and child. If the problematic situation can be identified, a rational problem-solving approach with emotional support for the child usually suffices. For example, the child with a baby sibling may need increased individual attention from parents. The child with an unduly harsh teacher may require assistance to establish a comfortable working relationship or a class change. The family experiencing separation difficulties may need counseling or psychotherapy. The school nurse frequently identifies school phobia by noting repeated functional complaints such as stomachaches and headaches. These complaints increase at the beginning of school, after holidays, and during test time. The primary care provider usually is the professional who rules out organic disease. Regardless of the cause or planned interventions, the child must go back to school. Only by attending school can children learn that they can, indeed, manage anxiety.

Depression

In the past, our society has denied the existence of most mental disorders in young people. Child and adolescent depression often are not recognized or not considered an important finding. In actuality, many children and adolescents experience depression, which disturbs eating and sleeping habits, creates hopelessness, interferes with parental and peer relationships, and decreases interest in achievements such as school grades. Reasons for depression include death in the family, divorce, and any of multiple losses the children experience as they give up childhood ways and familiar tendencies. Some schools and community mental health centers have groups for depressed children. Maintaining routine activities minimizes insecurities during depressed periods. Exercise, especially in groups, enhances the sense of well-being. Increasingly, antidepressant medications are prescribed for children and adolescents with prolonged depression, in addition to traditional counseling and support of the child and family. Most depression improves with time, but prolonged, severe depression may require intensive efforts on the part of the health team (see Suicide). Anticipatory guidance of families experiencing loss can lessen or shorten some of the negative effects on the child.

Eating Disorders

Compulsive behaviors, low self-esteem, and distorted body image are common to most disorders that include misuse of food to solve life's problems. *Anorexia nervosa* is extreme undernutrition with at least 25% loss of original body weight. *Bulimia* is characterized by an abnormal increase in episodes of hunger that leads to eating large amounts of food and may be followed by induced vomiting, ingestion of laxatives, or both. *Obesity* is weight in excess of 20% of optimal body weight and is by far the most common eating disorder. Through screenings, abnormal height to weight ratios cue the nurse to assess further. Classmates may tell the nurse or teacher their concerns. During physical examinations, the primary care provider may discover additional abnormalities including excessive or inadequate skin folds, abnormal laboratory studies, striae of the abdomen, thighs, and breasts, and maybe such extreme findings as rectal bleeding. Suspicion of an eating disorder requires a complete history with diet recall, menstrual history, family history, and changes in emotional and activity status and ability to manage expectations of society. The adolescent with an eating disorder may be adept in hiding abnormal behaviors or may be relieved to be found out and describe patterns of food abuse and perhaps abuse of other substances including laxatives, diuretics, and mind-altering drugs. The child with a severe eating disorder requires lifesaving hospitalization and intensive care including individual and group education and community health psychotherapy and family therapy. Nurses identify and refer the child, and later may provide portions of the treatment plan such as monitoring and support. Eating disorders such as anorexia nervosa and bulimia increase with the adolescent's drive to meet society's, expectations of the perfect body.

Common Cognitive Problems

Schoolchildren may have problems with cognition that impair their learning. Children who fall short of a classroom standard for achievement may have functional problems including headaches, stomach pains, short attention spans, and hyperactivity. Specialists in educational assessment and school psychology have numerous tools and techniques for identifying and minimizing learning problems and refer students to appropriate professionals.

Specific Learning Disabilities

There are several blocks to learning that are clearly identifiable phenomena. The disability may be a developmental delay, a result of brain injury, or a genetic defect. Teaching strategies for children with specific disorders have been developed. One example of a specific learning disability is dyslexia, inability to read or interpret written letters, but ability to understand the spoken word. Letters have little or no meaning to these children, and they must develop an alternative way to give meaning to letters. They can learn with the assistance of audiotapes and other forms of learning aids, since their intelligence is usually average or above average. They also learn to recognize certain symbols and signs, enabling them to participate in activities such as driving.

Minimal Brain Dysfunction

Minimal brain dysfunction (MBD) is a nonspecific term in that it includes a variety of physical, psychosocial, cognitive, and behavioral disorders that interfere with a child's ability to learn in the average classroom setting. MBD is usually attributed to minimal injury to the brain and results in such problems as distractibility, short attention span, clumsiness, hyperactivity, and immature behaviors. Careful structuring of the learning environment to exclude unnecessary stimuli usually improves learning. This disorder is usually frustrating to parents and teachers because it is hard to define and definitely difficult to manage. Some children improve with medication, and most achieve more self-control with time.

Mental Retardation

Children who have frank intellectual deficits are mentally retarded (MR). Most children are *educably mentally retarded* (EMR), with an IQ of 50 to 70. Children with IQs of 30 to 50 are classified as trainable mentally retarded (TMR), and those with profound retardation require custodial care and have severely limited intellect. Schools have programs to meet the learning needs of these children. One category of children who frequently are unrecognized, and therefore unattended, are slow learners, or "no-man's-land" children. Because their IQs are not quite normal (70 to 90 IQs), they too often fall behind classmates and need remediation. Children such as these are often at greater risk for other health problems that the school nurse identifies and manages with the assistance of the school team of professionals.

Mixed Learning Disorders

Unfortunately, children may have a combination of learning disorders, compounding the struggle of child, teachers, and family. MBD may be associated with slow learning classifications. Children then may have impaired intellect plus an inability to sit still in their seats for more than brief periods. These children need careful planning, patience, and persistence to meet educational goals.

Giftedness

The child who is gifted in relation to peers has a special set of concerns. If gifted children do not receive educational challenges appropriate for their abilities, they may have negative reactions. Some gifted children learn to do their work quickly, glossing over the assignments but still achieving at a higher level than their peers. They develop poor study habits and must relearn how to study when and if they are challenged later. Others simply give up with boredom and become the classic underachievers. Many gifted school-age children achieve at high levels in many walks of life and are well-adjusted, happy people.

These gifted children do need special attention. They may need some counseling to help them understand themselves and why they experience stress in the face of such ability. Teaching them about health requires different techniques in that they often are already knowledgeable and expect fast-paced, interesting presentations to keep their attention.

SPECIAL HEALTH PROBLEMS

Some health problems are so devastating to the child, and society as a whole, that they need special consideration by the student of community health nursing. Three of the four problems selected for discussion occur generally in adolescence, but causative and associated factors include life-style patterns set by society and family traits that begin influencing the child early in life.

Consequences of Adolescent Sexuality

Adolescent sexuality is usually problematic to the child, the family, and every facet of society. Even the well-adjusted, healthy child must incorporate new feelings, body image, and body functions into the self-image, as well as deal with changing interpersonal relationships. Several surveys indicate that a majority of Americans favor sex education in public schools, but a vocal minority are in strong opposition. Controversy about the value versus the dangers of sex education continues, often preventing implementation of effective educational programs and contraceptive services. The literature does reveal conflicting findings, but data from the 1981 National Survey of Children show that 15- and 16-year-olds who have been exposed to sex education are less likely to be sexually experienced (Furstenberg, 1986). Sex education programs include the standard anatomy, physiology, and contraception content, and, increasingly, wise decision making about sex, how and when to choose abstinence, and ways to handle peer pressure.

The adolescent who chooses to be sexually active may have one or more of the following problematic consequences:

1. Pregnancy (rate of about 1 million adolescent pregnancies per year in the United States)
2. Sexually transmitted disease (rate of 2.5 million adolescent cases per year) (Tolsma, 1988)
3. Lowered self-esteem
4. Family alienation

Each of these consequences has a set of related preventive measures and treatments that are often managed and delivered by a nurse. The school nurse and the nurse practitioner (family, family planning, and school nurses) are nurses who deal with adolescent sexuality on a daily basis. However, the United States falls far short of adequately managing the consequences and rates even worse in preventing the consequences and moving toward healthful sexual practices. Our adolescents do not have the clear message to use contraception with every act of intercourse. The erroneous message is, "Do not have intercourse, and do not plan for intercourse," or, "If you find you must have intercourse, either do not get pregnant and contract diseases or get pregnant and show the world that you can produce something special and valued." This is a simplistic view of mixed messages given to adolescents. Unfortunately, mixed messages and lack of adequate sex education, support for abstinence, and family planning services have resulted in high rates of unplanned adolescent pregnancies, infant mortality, sexually transmitted diseases, abortion, and a host of negative educational and socioeconomic factors affecting particularly the young mother and her child. The nation is finally addressing the problem, but there is not yet an effective system to deal with adolescent sexuality and its problems.

The school nurse role includes teaching human sexuality in the classroom, providing individual counseling and sexuality information, referral for family planning services or management of pregnancy, and supporting school reentry after pregnancy. The school nurse is also part of the program planning team that deals not only with the student population as a whole, but also with the community at large. The nurse is often the professional most knowledgeable about the value of sex education and actual adolescent sexual practices in the face of a vocal minority insisting that abstinence is the only solution. The nurse also serves as consultant to parents and parent groups. Delivery of services related to adolescent sexuality requires a clear understanding of laws, ethics of confidentiality, community and family values, developmental and reproductive physiology, signs and symptoms of pregnancy and sexually transmitted disease, and much more. This role is critical to schoolchildren and should be greatly expanded throughout the U.S. school system.

Substance Abuse

Adolescent substance abuse is a major public health problem. Numerous studies have been done to identify types of abused substances, causes and predictors of abuse, periods of vulnerability, patterns of initiation and progression, and decline of drug use. Trends of use have been researched in relation to world events (wars and international trafficking), fads (rise in popularity of new substances), other life-style trends, and geographics. As the picture of substance abuse becomes clearer, diagnoses and prognoses have become more accurate and treatment plans are more effective.

Identified risk factors for substance abuse are many. Certainly gender is a factor, since males use drugs more often and more heavily than females. A longitudinal study of adolescents in a Los Angeles high school revealed the following risk factors in increasing order (Newcomb, Maddahian, and Bentler, 1986):

1. Poor self-esteem
2. Psychologic distress
3. Poor academic achievement
4. Low religiosity
5. Poor relationship with parents
6. Sensation seeking
7. Early alcohol use
8. Adult drug use
9. Deviance (low law abidance)
10. Peer drug use

A cohort study of former New York State adolescents indicated that initiation of cigarettes, alcohol, and marijuana is completed, for the most part, by 20 years of age. Alcohol and marijuana use begins to decline at 20 to 21 years of age. This contrasts sharply with cigarettes, which exhibit highest use through the end of the study period—25 years of age (Kandel and Logan, 1984). Sequences of progression found in the same group were from one class of legal drug (alcohol or cigarettes), to marijuana, then to use of other illicit drugs. Alcohol, cigarettes, and marijuana were found to precede use of prescribed psychoactive drugs. The most striking difference between males and females is that cigarettes can precede marijuana in the absence of alcohol use among young women, whereas alcohol, even with the absence of cigarettes, consistently precedes marijuana use among men (Yamaguchi and Kandel, 1984). Adolescents may or may not progress to the end of the cycle before the decline of young adulthood.

Alcohol use is a problem in primary and middle school children, as well as adolescents because of its availability. Up to 90% of high school seniors have tried alcohol, and 40% to 45% drink regularly. Approximately 10% use marijuana daily. Cigarette, alcohol, and marijuana use is decreasing somewhat, but the use of cocaine has increased dramatically in older adolescents and young adults.

Obviously, treatment of substance abuse requires identification of those who are at risk for abuse, who are abusers, and who are addicted. Knowing the sequence is helpful for planning prevention programs involving youths, parents, teachers, and any others working with adolescents. Further studies are necessary to determine successful prevention programs. One risk-reduction program resulted in increased knowledge, but an erosion of attitudes toward smoking occurred (Dignan and others, 1985). Referral to community treatment centers, including residential care and follow-up care in the school, is frequently necessary. Peer assistance groups of recovering abusers are a highly effective method of treatment. Nurses perform a variety of roles on the heath team in dealing with substance abuse. The nurse must see substance abuse as a problem requiring objectivity in evaluation and referral and must avoid inadvertently enabling the adolescent to continue this destructive behavior.

Acquired Immunodeficiency Syndrome

Acquired immunodeficiency syndrome (AIDS) and its earlier stages have caused the U.S. school system phenomenal stress. Each level of prevention is critical to the well-being of children with and without the AIDS virus.

The following are three major sources of the disease in the school-age population:

1. Contaminated blood products or perinatal transmission
2. Infected sexual contacts
3. Illicit drug usage

Although school-age victims compose a small portion (approximately 2%) of the total AIDS virus–infected population (Tolsma, 1988), the number of school-age children who contract the virus but whose infections are undetected for an average of five years until young adulthood is estimated to be significant. Again the health care system is faced with a growing need to prevent exposure to the virus with promotion of abstinence or safe sex practices and avoidance of illicit drugs. Studies to date indicate that many risk factors exist, and that the adolescent, as usual, does not recognize the risk to the self and does not usually act to prevent the possible consequences.

The children with transfused or transmitted viruses require secondary and tertiary prevention for themselves. There are no known cases of transmission from these children to other children in aggregate conditions such as day care or schools. The issues surrounding whether to allow AIDS virus–infected children to attend school with other children have created marked controversy among decision makers, including parents, teachers, school administrators, school boards, health care providers, and others. Fear is based on the unknown, and regardless of the reports from the Centers for Disease Control, some still do not believe that attendance at school when an AIDS virus–infected child is not having symptoms such as diarrhea is safe (CDC, 1988). The fear is that the reports are wrong and that all of the facts are not in.

The nursing role in AIDS prevention and treatment is as diverse as it is with the other complex, issue-laden problems in schoolchildren. Risk reduction in the face of adolescent behavioral patterns is a formidable task for teams of professionals. Knowledge of the disease and methods of prevention is the basis of all risk-reduction programs, but much more is required. Certainly providing social support and teaching peers to abstain from sex or practice safe sex is worth the effort. Increasing a sense that one can control sexual urges to protect health is also a promising endeavor. Community awareness and support of a risk reduction program in conjunction with everything else is a must. Blood and body secretion precautions are used appropriately to protect the nurse and others.

Human responses to problems are the targets of nursing care. Individual children and those involved with their daily lives in the school may have responses requiring intervention. Establishing protocols for when to send a child home, when to offer care at school, and when the child is safe to attend school with other children may be a function of the nurse in conjunction with the school health team. Primary care nurses outside of the school may also be involved in this process. When the child is ill, the home heath nurse is often the primary care provider of health care. The unit of service includes the parents, who are faced with their child's impending death and are in great need of all the support the nurse in every setting can give.

Suicide

Suicide is listed as the third leading cause of death in adolescents but probably would be listed as the second leading cause if all suicides could be determined not to be accidents. This major health problem occurs more frequently in males who have a history of previous attempts, depression, distant interpersonal relationships, and a family history of suicide. The suicide or suicide attempt is often preceded by a recent loss, giving away of prized possessions, marked change of eating and sleeping patterns, and extreme moods. A precipitating event such as a failing grade or fight with a friend or family member may occur.

Nurses in the community often see some signs of suicidal behaviors and must decide when and how to act. School nurses may consult with teachers, psychologists, and family members, as well as the child, to assess emotional status. Nurses in primary care settings may find assessment more difficult, since the client may be distant. Once the nurse decides that the potential for suicide exists, the adolescent should be told of the nurse's concern. The youth needs to understand why confidentiality cannot be maintained in life-threatening situations. Immediate treatment includes notifying parents, providing a safe environment with observation for no less than 48 hours at home or in a hospital, and arranging for care management by a qualified psychotherapist. Continuing care of family, therapy, and support groups may prevent further suicide attempts. The client needs skills in managing crises of all types and in obtaining help when emotions are no longer manageable. The nurse may be responsible for coordinating care on return to clinic or school. A trusting, enduring, and encouraging relationship is important to this role.

SUMMARY

No single chapter can cover all issues and health needs faced by community health nurses working with school-age children. The field of study and practice is rich with opportunity to manage all phases of health care for individuals, groups, and whole populations, to work as a member of a team dedicated to the welfare of children, and to interact with the community at large to protect its future generations. Although the types and causes of health problems have changed, the school-age population continues to have numerous needs requiring quality nursing care.

QUESTIONS FOR DISCUSSION

1. Outline the physical, moral, and emotional developmental patterns of the school-age child.
2. What kind of health education should school-age children receive?
3. List and illustrate three of the common health problems of the school-age child. What should the role of the nurse be in dealing with these?
4. What are some special health problems of the school-age child? How can the nurse help the child deal with these?

REFERENCES

American Public Health Association: Review of national preventive dentistry demonstration program, Am J Public Health 76:434, 1986.

Centers for Disease Control: Guidelines for effective school health education to prevent the spread of AIDS, J Sch Health 58:142, 1988.

Dignan MB and others: Evaluation of North Carolina risk reduction program for smoking and alcohol, J Sch Health 85:103, 1985.

Erikson EH: Childhood and society, New York, 1963, WW Norton & Co Inc.

Furstenberg FF, Kristin AM, and Peterson JL: Sex education and sexual experience among adolescents, 75:1331, 1986.

Kandel DB and Logan JA: Patterns of drug use from adolescence to young adulthood. I. Periods of risk for initiation, continued use, and discontinuation, Am J Public Health 74:660, 1984.

Lewis CE and Lewis MA: Peer pressure and risk-taking behaviors in children, Am J Public Health 74:580, 1984.

Newcomb MD, Maddahian E, and Bentler DM: Risk factors for drug use among adolescents: concurrent and longitudinal analysis, Am J Public Health 76:525, 1986.

Piaget J and Inhelder B: New York, 1969, Basic Books Inc, Publishers.

Robert Wood Johnson Foundation: Special reports, Princeton, NJ, 1985, Roper & Ward Johnson Foundation.

Teenage pregnancy: The problem that hasn't gone away, New York, 1981, The Alan Guttmacher Institute.

Tolsma D: Activities of the Centers for Disease Control in AIDS education, 58:133, 1988.

Trunkey DD: Trauma, Sci Am 249:28, 1983.

Yamaguchi K and Kandel DB: Patterns of drug use from adolescence to young adulthood. II. Sequences of progression, Am J Public Health 74:668, 1984.

Yamaguchi K and Kandel DB: Patterns of drug use from adolescence to young adulthood. III. Predictors of progression, Am J Public Health 74:673, 1984.

Zelnik M and Shah FK: First intercourse among young Americans, Family Plann Perspect 15:64, 1983.

Zelnik M, Koenig MA, and Kim YJ: Sources of prescription contraceptives and subsequent pregnancy among young women, Family Plann Perspect 16:6, 1984.

BIBLIOGRAPHY

Bergman AB: Use of education in preventing injuries, Pediatr Clin North Am 29:331, 1982.

Berwick DM: Scoliosis screening: a pause in the chase, Am J Public Health 75:1373, 1985.

Boynton RW, Dunn ES, and Stephens GR: Manual of ambulatory pediatrics, Boston, 1983, Little, Brown & Co.

Epstein MH and Cullinan D: Depression in children, J Sch Health 55:10, 1986.

Felice ME and Friedman SB: Behavioral considerations in the health care of adolescents, Pediatr Clin North Am 29:399, 1982.

Igoe JB: Changing patterns in school health and nursing, Nurs Outlook 28:486, 1980.

Igoe JB: Professionally speaking—what is school nursing? A plea for more standardized roles, MCN 5:307, 1980.

Johnson TR, Moore WM, and Jeffries JE, editors: Children are different: developmental physiology, Columbus, Ohio, 1986, Ross Laboratories.

Lewis CE, Siegel JM, and Lewis MA: Feeling bad: exploring sources of distress among preadolescent children, Am J Public Health 74:117, 1984.

Long KA: Are children too young for mental disorders? Am J Nurs 85:1254, 1985.

Maceyko SL and Nagelberg DB: The assessment of bulimia in high school students, J Schl Health 55:135, 1985.

Morais T, Bernier M, and Turcette F: Age-and-sex specific prevalence of scoliosis and the value of school screening programs, Am J Public Health 75:1377, 1985.

Newacheck PW, Budetti PO, and McManus P: Trends in childhood disability, Am J Public Health 74:232, 1984.

O'Malley PM, Backman JG, and Johnston LD: Period, age, and cohort effects on substance use among American youth, 1976-82, AJPH 74:602, 1984.

Pipes PL: Nutrition in infancy and childhood, ed 4, St Louis, 1989, CV Mosby Co.

Robbins LN: The natural history of adolescent drug use, AJPH 74:656, 1984.

Schwab EK and Conners CK: Nutrient-behavior research with children: methods, considerations, and evaluation, J Am Diet Assoc 86:319, 1986.

Steiger NJ and Lipson JG: Self care nursing: theory and practice, Bowie, Md, 1985, Brady.

Valanis BB: Patterns of morbidity and mortality in childhood and adolescence. In Valanis BB, editor: Epidemiology in nursing and health care, Norwalk, Conn, 1986, Appleton & Lange.

Wachter EH, Phillips J, and Holaday B: Nursing care of children, Philadelphia, 1985, JB Lippincott Co.

White DH: A study of current school nurse practice activities, J Schl Health 55:52, 1985.

Woods NF: Human sexuality, ed 3, St Louis, 1984, CV Mosby Co.

CHAPTER

17

Young and Middle Adulthood: The Working Years

Mary Ann Parsons
Gwen Felton

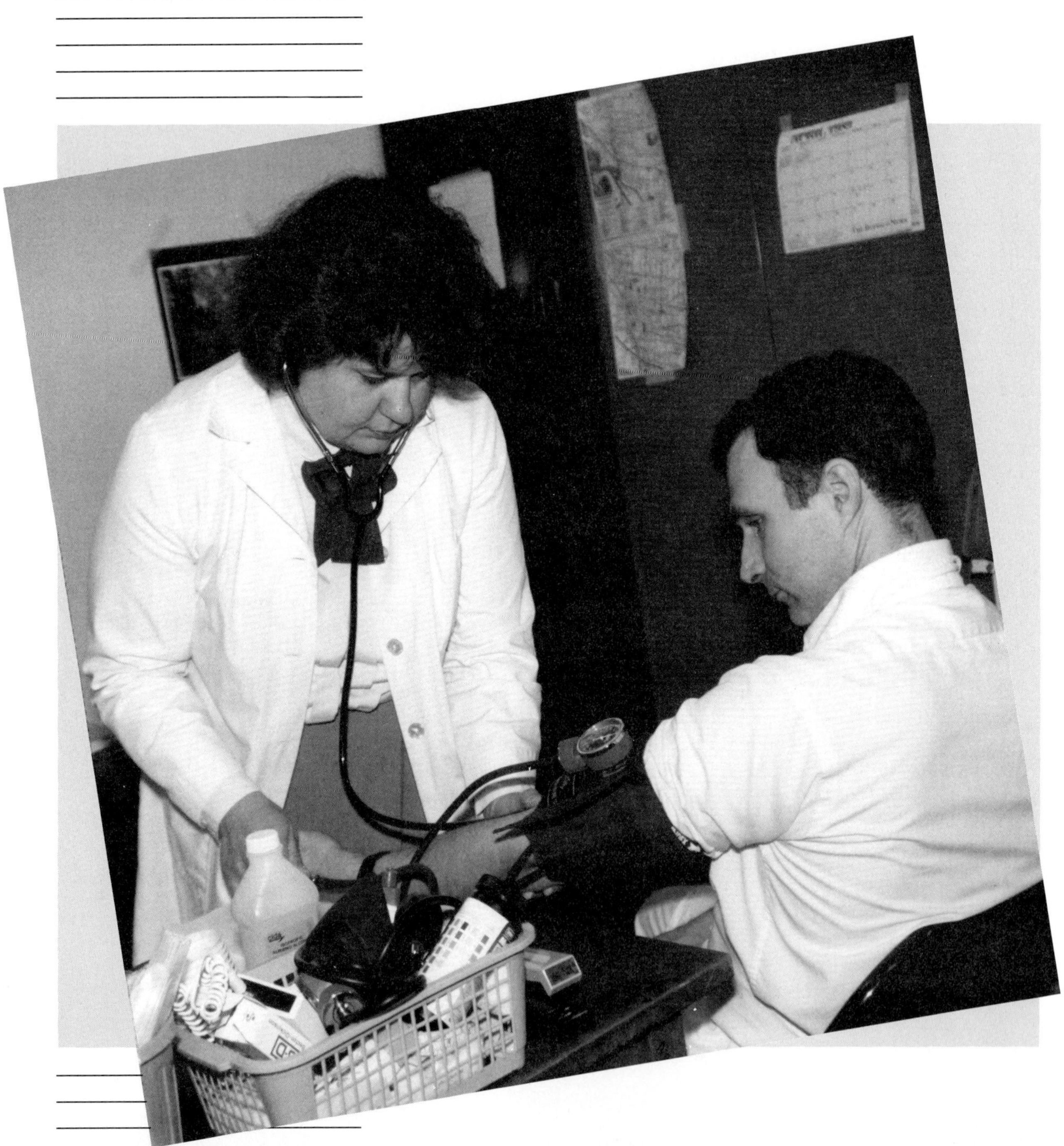

CHAPTER OUTLINE

Assessment of the health and environment of the working population
- Individual within the context of family and community
- Cognitive and psychologic development of young and middle-aged adults
- Health considerations of young and middle-aged adults
- Work environment in the United States

Legislation affecting the work environment
- Occupational Safety and Health Act of 1970
- Toxic Substance Control Act of 1976
- Worker's compensation
- Rehabilitation Act of 1973

Workplace hazards and associated health problems
- Chemical toxins
- Carcinogens
- Ionizing radiation
- Infectious agents
- Physical trauma, safety hazards, and homicide
- Noise-induced hearing loss
- Psychologic and social stresses

Social and ethical considerations in the workplace
- Women in the work force
- Sexual harassment
- Pregnant workers
- Female-intensive occupations
- Men and women who work as homemakers
- Minorities in the work force
- Workers with nonoccupational health problems

Role of community health nurse in occupational health
- Role of occupational health nurse

Nursing interventions in the workplace
- Stress management
- Nutritional programs
- Exercise programs
- Substance dependency programs

Summary

OBJECTIVES

After completing this chapter, the reader should be able to:

1. Identify the cognitive and psychosocial development and health considerations of young and middle-aged adults.
2. Discuss the environment of the worker populations in relation to the impact of federal legislation.
3. Describe the social and ethical considerations of women and minorities in the work force.
4. Define the emerging nurse's role in occupational settings.
5. Evaluate the health services available for workers in occupational settings.

THIS CHAPTER FOCUSES on young and middle adulthood, which are divided into the following age-groups:

1. Young adulthood (18 to 24 years)
2. Young middle adulthood (25 to 39 years)
3. Older middle adulthood (40 to 59 years).

Since these years are usually the healthiest time of one's life, emphasis is placed on the changing life-styles and health needs of these groups. Only problems significantly influenced by life-style are discussed. Recent attention to this phase of adult development has been stimulated by a population that is becoming increasingly older in the United States. The adult years have taken on a new meaning as middle-aged adults in the United States have sought to maintain the physical appearance and vibrancy of their youth (Breslow and Somers, 1977).

Recognizing that chronologic age and developmental tasks vary for individuals, an artificial division of age provides a framework within which health goals can be established based on health promotion and maintenance needs, away from the more traditional illness orientation. For each age-group, health goals and health care services are discussed with an emphasis on the community health nurse as a provider and coordinator of services.

ASSESSMENT OF THE HEALTH AND ENVIRONMENT OF THE WORKING POPULATION

A nursing assessment of the health of the working community is systematic and continuous. It includes the past, present, and future health and safety of individual workers, their families, and their communities. The community health nurse assesses the adult workplace in terms of human-environmental interrelationships so that the health of the community can be promoted and protected.

Individual Within the Context of Family and Community

The individual cannot be understood outside the context of family and community. The family and community are the two major determinants of development throughout the life span. There are several ways to define family. The more traditional definition is based on ties between individuals who are biologically or legally related by such things as blood, marriage, and adoption. However, the community health nurse must recognize the diversity of the number and type of structures that conceptualize the family in our modern society. Experimental family forms include open marriage, communes, cohabitating couples, group marriages, and homosexual unions. There are no "right," "wrong," "proper," or "improper" family structures. Families must be accepted and understood for what they are. Just as community health nurses must understand the uniqueness of individuals, they must understand the uniqueness of each particular family. Society places conflicting demands on people, and thus a range of family forms can coexist. Nurses must accept differing family forms and recognize that "ideal" forms are dependent on the specific needs of individuals (Friedman, 1981). The major functions of the family, regardless of its makeup, are the physical care of dependent members, the socialization of its members, the creation of a sense of belonging, and the provision of love and affection (Freibert, 1979). As the family is an important determinant in the development of the individual, so too is the community. The community provides the structure within which the values and beliefs instilled by the family can be tested and allows individuals to meet their needs and realize their goals. One must have membership in many communities for growth and achievement to occur.

Although nurses must be aware of the profound impact of the family and community in the development of the individual, they must always be cognizant of the uniqueness and complexity of the individual. Individuals are part of the past, connected to the present, and always changing as they strive to meet future goals.

Cognitive and Psychosocial Development of Young and Middle-aged Adults

In the process of maturing, adults acquire knowledge and develop skills and behaviors that improve the abilities developed in adolescence. Development of intellectual maturity also influences the selection of behaviors and attitudes that affect health and well-being. Continued learning is found throughout adulthood in areas such as reasoning, vocabulary, and spatial perception. Decreases may be seen, however, in recall time, reaction time, and cognitive flexibility as one ages (Kudzma and Quinn, 1986).

Innate ability and cognitive development obviously influence one's learning. However, achievement motivation contributes to successful learning far more than innate ability and cognitive ability alone (Freiberg, 1979). Nurses need to capitalize on the achievement motivation factor to enhance attainment of the client's health goals, especially for those clients 30 years of age and older. Older individuals tend to perform at higher levels than their younger counterparts because of the achievement motivation factor.

Health Considerations for Young and Middle-aged Adults

Concern for one's health varies according to age. Those in their twenties seem to have the least concern about health. The major threats to health in this age-group include violent death resulting from motor vehicle accidents (36 deaths per 100,000 population), suicides (20 deaths per 100,000 population), and homicides (11.8 deaths per 100,000), alcohol and drug abuse, and unwanted pregnancies (U.S. Department of Health and Human Services, 1985). After 35 years of age the sense of immortality has faded. The recognition of limitations caused by increasing physical and mental stresses, economic concerns, occupational choices, and, in particular, a diminishing sense of well-being is present. The physical well-being of this age-group, like young adults in their twenties, is threatened primarily by life-style factors such as alcohol, smoking, and stress. Many chronic diseases, such as chronic bronchitis and hypertension, have their onset in the thirties but because of lag time tend not to become serious threats until later adulthood.

Around 40 years of age the midlife transition begins and serves to bridge young middle and older middle adulthood. This midlife crisis is a developmental crisis one can compare only to the crisis experienced in the teenage years. As in all transitions, the individual must come to terms with the past and prepare for the future. This period requires that one reappraise the past so that the past and future can coexist in the present, adjust the meaning life had in the thirties and begin the development of a renewed satisfaction and acceptance of life in the forties, and become more individuated, that is, turn inward to the self with an emphasis on the process of living rather than the attainment of specific goals.

The community health nurse needs to be particularly sensitive to the struggles of those in their midlife transition. Many adults are not aware of the developmental tasks they are experiencing. They only know that there are unrest, frustration, and often anger with which they must deal. These internal changes may be conscious and openly expressed or covert and subtly expressed. Some may react to these internal feelings by making dramatic life-style changes. Regardless of the nature of the changes that occur during this midlife transition, the meaning an individual gives to life in the forties is profoundly different from the meaning given in the thirties (Levinson and others, 1978).

TABLE 17-1 Value Orientation Shift During Adult Life

Value orientations	Adult phases: Young adulthood	Core of the middle years	The new middle years	Late adulthood
"The great American dream"			"Live and let live"	
Human nature	Good		Neutral or mixture of good and evil	
Man-nature-supernature	Mastery over		Harmony with	
Time	Future		Present	
Activity	Doing		Being-in-becoming	
Relational	Individualism		Collaterality	

From Stevenson J: Issues and crises during middlescence, New York, 1977, Appleton & Lange.

During the forties one may have excellent health or may experience increasing disability because of illness. The leading threats to health in the forties are cancer, heart disease, accidents, cirrhosis, cardiovascular diseases, and suicide (U.S. Department of Commerce, Bureau of the Census, 1985). The individual's life-style and predisposition to disease influence the incidence of these life-threatening conditions.

Usually, by 50 years of age most adults have come to terms with their emotions, feelings, and relationships. Value reorientation occurs as the older adult focuses on what has been learned in the thirties and forties and moves toward living in the present. Older adults tend to have an appreciation of feelings of joy, sorrow, tenderness, affection, faith, and trust. Fewer adults report reactions of intense anger, jealousy, hatred, resentment, or self-pity (Dean, 1962). These feelings do occur but are reserved for significant happenings. The findings of a study of 524 women and men in seven age-graded groups help researchers understand the value orientation shift of those between 50 and 60 years of age and those in younger age-groups. For example, respondents between 50 and 59 years of age placed minimal importance on the item: "I don't make enough money to do what I want." Younger respondents placed great importance on the item. Although younger respondents rated themselves as more important than their spouses, older respondents rated their spouses as more important than themselves (Gould, 1975). Changes in value orientation occur gradually over time. The shift in value orientation during adult life can be viewed in Table 17-1.

Heart disease, cancer, cardiovascular disease, accidents, and cirrhosis are the major threats to those 50 to 59 years of age (U.S. Department of Commerce, Bureau of the Census, 1985). The middle-aged adult also has a greater incidence of diseases known to be associated with genetics, for example, diabetes, hypertension, and Huntington's chorea. A major health problem of women and men in the middle years is obesity, which is associated with a sedentary life-style (Overfield, 1980).

Work Environment in the United States

In the United States it is expected that an individual will begin some type of work after the age of 18 years. This expectation may be delayed by a preparation period for work or initiated earlier for those who do not complete high school. Although this discussion of occupational health

TABLE 17-2 Employed Civilians by Industry and Occupation, 1982 to 1983 (in millions rounded to tenths)

Industry	Total employed	Managerial and professional specialty	Technical, sales, and administrative support	Service occupations	Precision production, craft, and repair	Operators, fabricators, and laborers	Farming, forestry, and fishing
Agriculture	3.4	0.1	0.1	0.0	0.1	0.1	3.1
Mining	1.0	0.2	0.2	0.0	0.4	0.2	0.0
Construction	5.8	0.7	0.8	0.0	3.1	1.2	0.0
Manufacturing	20.3	3.1	4.3	0.4	3.5	8.8	0.1
Transportation and public utilities	6.6	1.2	2.6	0.2	1.3	2.2	0.0
Wholesale and retail trade	20.8	3.4	9.2	3.9	1.5	2.6	0.0
Finance, insurance, and real estate	6.3	1.4	4.4	0.3	0.1	0.1	0.1
Services	30.3	11.8	7.5	7.4	1.6	1.3	0.4
Public administration	5.2	1.5	1.6	1.2	0.3	0.2	0.1

From US Dept of Labor, Division of Labor Statistics: Handbook of labor statistics, Bulletin 2217, 1985.
*Because of rounding, components may not add to the totals.

focuses on men and women who are gainfully employed in settings outside the home, some attention is given to those engaged in cottage industries and homemaking. The role of the community health nurse includes the assessment of health problems related to work in the home. However, the role of the community health nurse engaged in occupational health is limited to the care of aggregates in the workplace.

The transition from school to work is a stressful period for everyone. Work requires more self-discipline, since there is a loss of autonomy and one's output is measured by standards of productivity. The rewards of work are twofold—monetary compensation and the sense of achievement and self-worth. For many people the world of work is merely time spent in labor at backbreaking or mindless chores, whereas others can be creative and receive satisfaction from their work.

One quarter of the 101 million Americans in the work force have professional, managerial, or supervisory employment, with some degree of control or autonomy over their work (U.S. Department of Labor, Bureau of Statistics, 1985). Most workers take jobs that are available and do whatever they need to do to keep them. That work is an economic necessity tends to obscure the fact that work in itself is important to people. Work is important because of the social interaction at the workplace, the desire to be needed, and the desire to contribute to the common good.

American workers, members of an "at-risk" group, spend almost one fourth of their time at work. Despite improved working conditions, the high degree of automation, and computerization, hazards have not been eradicated in the workplace. Many workers are exposed to dust, chemicals, noise, and dangerous machinery. Table 17-2 categorizes the almost 101 million workers in the United States by industry and occupation. Women constitute more than 43% of the work force in the United States, and most workers are

TABLE 17-3 Number of Occupational Injuries and Illnesses by Industry (in thousands)

Industry: Private sector	Injuries	Illnesses
Total	4751.0	105.6
Agriculture, forestry, and fishing	83.3	3.7
Mining	109.2	1.4
Construction	473.5	5.4
Manufacturing	1754.4	59.3
Transportation and public utilities	398.1	5.8
Wholesale and retail	1146.2	10.2
Finance, insurance, and real estate	93.7	1.5
Services	692.4	18.4

Modified from US Department of Labor, Division of Labor Statistics: Occupational injuries and illnesses in US by industry, 1982, Bulletin 2196, Washington, DC, 1982, US Government Printing Office.

employed by small businesses that do not provide occupational health services.

Work-Related Injuries and Illnesses

A reported 48 million work-related injuries and almost 106,000 new work-related illnesses occur each year. Labor statistics indicate a decrease in the number of occupational diseases and injuries reported each year. Table 17-3 categorizes reported injuries and illnesses by industry division and category of illness. These statistics, although helpful, do not represent the true magnitude of work-related health problems. Many health problems go unidentified as work related. Those problems more easily identified, such as skin diseases (see Table 17-4), are reported more frequently.

Factors that contribute to the lack of identifi-

TABLE 17-4 Number of Occupational Illnesses by Industry Division and Category of Illness, 1982 (in thousands)

		Number of illnesses by category						
Industry division	Total illnesses	Skin diseases or disorders	Dust diseases of the lungs	Respiratory conditions caused by toxic agents	Poisoning	Disorders caused by physical agents	Disorders associated with repeated trauma	All other occupational illnesses
	105.6	41.9	2.0	8.8	3.4	8.3	22.6	18.6
Agriculture, forestry, and fishing†	3.7	2.5	‡	.1	.2	.2	.1	.5
Mining	1.4	.4	.3	.1	.1	.2	.1	.2
Construction	5.4	2.2	.1	.6	.3	.8	.3	1.0
Manufacturing	59.2	22.5	1.2	4.7	1.4	4.6	20.0	4.8
Transportation and public utilities	5.8	2.2	.1	.7	.3	.7	.7	1.0
Wholesale and retail trade	10.2	4.0	.1	.7	.4	.6	.6	3.6
Wholesale trade	3.5	1.4	.1	.2	.3	.2	.4	1.0
Retail trade	6.7	2.6	‡	.5	.2	.4	.2	2.6
Finance, insurance, and real estate	1.5	.5	‡	.1	.1	.1	.1	.6
Services	18.4	7.6	.1	1.6	.5	1.1	.6	6.8

*Because of rounding, components may not add to the totals.
†Excludes farms with fewer than 11 employees.
‡Fewer than 50 cases.

cation of work-related health problems can be categorized as related to the employee, the employer, and the health care professional. Often employees may not recognize a health problem as being work related or may not report a problem for fear of losing their jobs. Some employees choose not to recognize new problems because to do so implies a self-responsibility to do something about the problem. The employer may not report new work-related problems because work reporting requirements are not strict. The occupational health professional may fail to identify work-related problems because of the long period between exposure and onset of symptoms. It is often difficult to differentiate between occupational and nonoccupational hazards to which workers have been exposed.

Occupational health nurses must be diligent in obtaining an occupational health history and know when to suspect a work-related problem so that they can ask the appropriate questions to determine whether the problem is work related. The most distinguishing characteristic of occupational diseases is that they are, in principle, preventable.

LEGISLATION AFFECTING THE WORK ENVIRONMENT

Occupational Safety and Health Act of 1970

The federal government assumed an active role in the creation and enforcement of standards for a safe and healthy workplace through the enactment of the Federal Coalminer Safety and Health Act of 1969 and the Occupational Safety and Health Act (OSHAct) of 1970. OSHAct established the Occupational Safety and Health Administration (OSHA) within the Department of Labor. OSHA's major responsibilities include encouraging employers and employees to reduce hazards in the workplace, implementing safety and health programs, developing and enforcing mandatory occupational safety and health standards, requiring employers to maintain records related to work injuries and illnesses, and collecting and analyzing health and safety data. The OSHAct was also responsible for the creation of the National Institute for Occupational Safety and Health (NIOSH). NIOSH is located in the Department of Health and Human Services and is a component of the Centers for Disease Control of the U.S. Public Health Service. NIOSH's primary responsibility is to investigate health and safety hazards in workplaces when requested to do so. Other responsibilities include conducting research and implementation of demonstration projects, developing of occupational standards for toxic materials, and publishing of an annual list of known toxic substances. NIOSH is not empowered to issue citations to violating employers. However, it can issue warnings to employees and employers and report its findings to OSHA, which has the power to enforce the federal standards.

The passage of OSHAct created great controversy, since many feared federal regulations would be costly and possibly ineffective. Even though the programs are costly, the benefits in reduced injuries, illnesses, and mortality have been significant and justify the cost.

Toxic Substance Control Act of 1976

A more recent piece of legislation was the enactment of the Toxic Substance Control Act of 1976 for the purpose of regulating commerce and protecting the environment and individual health through the control of specific chemicals. The Environmental Protection Agency (EPA), responsible for administering the act, has authority to regulate and take action concerning new chemicals that present an unreasonable risk to health or the environment. Although the economic impact of the Toxic Substance Control Act has not been determined, the need to prevent tragedies from uncontrolled toxic substances is unquestioned.

Worker's Compensation

Worker's compensation is a legal system designed to set reimbursement guidelines for persons disabled from injuries and illness arising from the workplace. This law holds the employer responsible for some of the costs incurred from lost wages and health care and rehabilitation expenses. Worker's compensation is a no-fault system and does not require the worker to prove that the injury was caused by employer negligence. The following three conditions must be met for a worker to qualify for benefits in the United States:

1. An injury or illness must be present.
2. The injury or illness must have occurred on the job or as a result of employment.
3. The injury or illness must incur health cost, rehabilitation costs, lost wages, or disfigurement.

Sometimes cases occur in which it is difficult to determine the relationship of the injury or illness to employment. In these situations employees may institute legal proceedings against the employer. These cases are the exception and not the rule. In most situations the employee files a claim for benefits with the employer. The claim is accepted and paid for by the employer either directly or through the worker's compensation insurance carrier. One of the flaws in the system is the determination of when the worker is ready to return to work. Although the amount of reimbursement under worker's compensation is limited by law, the system has benefited the worker but not without abuse.

Rehabilitation Act of 1973

The Rehabilitation Act of 1973 provided that handicapped persons not be discriminated against in any program or activity receiving federal financial assistance. In 1977 a new regulation provided guidelines to implement the nondiscriminatory practices.

WORKPLACE HAZARDS AND ASSOCIATED HEALTH PROBLEMS

Specific hazards found in the workplace that result in illness or injury include the following:

1. Chemical toxins
2. Carcinogens
3. Ionizing radiation
4. Infectious agents
5. Physical trauma, safety hazards, and homicide
6. Noise and hearing impairments
7. Psychologic and social stressors

All workers are at risk for illness or injury resulting from one or more of these hazards. For many years hazards were monitored for short-range effects. More recently, it has been recognized that serious, life-threatening conditions can result from prolonged exposure to hazards in the workplace. Recognizing hazards and attenuating their effects on the worker can reduce the number of health problems resulting from occupational injuries and illnesses.

Chemical Toxins

Toxins encountered in the workplace are classified as dusts, fumes, mists, vapors, gases, liquids, and solids. Toxins are substances that are harmful to biologic systems, depending on the dosage received by the worker. Workers are exposed to many new chemical substances. It has been estimated that more than 1000 new chemical products are introduced into industry each month (Ray, 1985). Most of these products have not had the rigorous laboratory testing necessary to fully determine their toxic effects. Damage to the individual may be temporary, permanent, or passed on to the next generation. To determine the toxic effects of chemicals, the absorption, distribution, metabolism, and excretion patterns need to be analyzed.

Chemicals are absorbed by the respiratory system, skin, and gastrointestinal tract. Some chemicals may be absorbed through the mucous membranes and open lesions. Airborne particles are absorbed through the respiratory tract and have a pathologic effect on the lungs. Gases, vapors, and mists, also absorbed through the respiratory tract, pass through the lungs into the bloodstream for a systemic effect. Absorption through the skin occurs through epidermal cells, hair follicles, and sebaceous glands. Factors such as body site, wetness, vascularization, and the properties of the chemical itself influence absorption. Cutaneous exposure may have a local effect, systemic effect, or no effect at all. Gastrointestinal absorption occurs in workers who are mouth breathers or gum and tobacco chewers or workers whose hands are in contact with their mouths while they are in the work area. For this reason, workers should be discouraged from eating, drinking, or smoking on the job. The gastrointestinal tract itself has several functions, such as excretion of gastric and pancreatic juices, that reduce the toxicity of chemical substances. However, substances retained in the body, such as mercury and lead, are the most dangerous.

Some toxins have only a local effect as mentioned above, whereas others enter the bloodstream and are transported to other parts of the body. The toxins may be stored or may exert an immediate toxic effect on the body. The distribution of a particular toxin is determined by its ability to cross various membrane barriers and its affinity for particular body sites. The most important barriers of the body are the blood-brain barrier and the placenta. The blood-brain barrier hinders the passage of toxins to the brain, and the placenta blocks the transport of some toxins to the fetus. These two barriers are unable to block all substances. Therefore for the worker to be protected, the properties of the chemical substance must be known.

When a substance has an affinity for a particular site and accumulates, it can result in a toxic effect. This effect may occur at the storage site or more likely, at a different site. For example, lead is stored in the bone but exerts a toxic effect on soft tissue. Toxins may be released systemically years after the exposure.

The body can convert foreign chemicals through the process of metabolism. This process usually reduces the toxicity of foreign chemicals, but sometimes it can increase their toxicity. For example, methanol acts through its metabolite formaldehyde and forms acid to cause optic nerve damage and blindness.

The chemical changes that occur in the body must be understood, and literature regarding metabolic processes must be interpreted carefully. These processes differ among humans and animals, so results of animal research may not always apply to humans unless an animal species with a pathway similar to that of humans is used. General health, age, nutrition, sex, and genetic factors are human factors that influence response to toxins.

The major route of excretion is the kidneys, and the liver is the second major organ of excretion. The kidneys handle toxins essentially the same way they handle other substances. The liver secretes toxins with the bile into the gastrointestinal tract. The bile is then excreted with the feces unless it is reabsorbed. The gastrointestinal tract can excrete substances directly if they are not absorbed. The lungs can excrete volatile gases and vapors through passive diffusion. However, fat-soluble gases tend to linger in adipose tissue and take more time to be excreted by the lungs. The lungs excrete vapors absorbed through the skin or ingestion. For example, gasoline absorbed through the skin can result in bronchial irritation when the vapor is exhaled from the lungs. It must be remembered that toxins can also be excreted in breast milk and may pose a risk to the nursing infant. Additionally, it is possible for toxins to be excreted in sweat, hair, and saliva (Frumkin, 1983).

Carcinogens

Cancer is a growing concern because of the increased number of chemicals identified as carcinogenic. To compound this problem it is estimated that thousands of products in common use have not been tested to determine their teratogenicity, carcinogenicity, or both (Hill and Kleinberger, 1984).

The morbidity and mortality associated with work-related cancers are often unrecognized. Clinical observations of an unusually high number of cases of a specific malignancy in a cluster of workers exposed to a common hazard may lead to the identification of links between carcinogens found in the workplace and the resulting malignancy. Epidemiologic studies are the most valid approach to determining carcinogenicity. Many factors, such as repeated exposure to carcinogens over time and nonoccupational risk factors, such as smoking, tend to interact in such a way as to result in a malignancy. The period of time between exposure and a diagnosis of cancer may be years, leading health professionals to overlook the relationship between occupational exposure and disease. Often when the relationship is suspected, it is difficult to document because of insufficient record keeping. This situation is particularly true for workers who were employed before the enactment of laws that require monitoring of employee exposure to known carcinogens.

Cancer is the second leading cause of death in the United States. Approximately 700,000 new cases of cancer (excluding skin cancer and in situ cancer of the uterine cervix) are diagnosed each year. It is estimated that 60% to 90% of all cancers are caused or influenced by environmental factors such as diet, smoking, exposure to hazards in the workplace, and consumer products (Frumkin and Levy, 1983). Although specific occupational carcinogens have been identified (Table 17-5), many unknown carcinogens remain in the workplace. The identification of work-related cancer requires a thorough, detailed occupational history of all exposures to hazardous chemicals, including contacts with workers who have contaminated clothing.

The principle of dose-response must be considered in that the greater the intensity of exposure, the more likely a malignancy will occur. The extent and duration of exposure to a carcinogen must be assessed in the occupational history. Consideration must be given to other factors that may interact with the occupational hazard and increase the risk of cancer. For example, a worker who is exposed to asbestos hazards has a chance of developing cancer that is five times greater than that of the general population. If the worker smokes, the risk is increased tenfold (Frumkin and Levy, 1983). Since there may be a 20- to 30-year span between onset of exposure and diagnosis, the health professional must include a detailed history of all previous jobs to determine work-related cancer.

Ionizing Radiation

Ionizing radiation is the type of radiation that is most likely to cause biologic damage. The units commonly used for the measurement of radiation are the curie, roentgen, and rem. The rem (roentgen-equivalent-man) is the most useful unit and measures the biologic effect of radiation on a person. The subunit of a rem is the millirem—1 rem equals 1000 millirems. Maximum permissible amount of annual organ dose is available through the Nuclear Regulatory Commission. The maximum permissible annual dose for the whole body is 5 rems. Acceptable exposures for specific organs vary. For example, the lung dose is lower than the thyroid dose. In addition, the maximum acceptable dose is different for those who are at lower risk for exposure, such as nursing students, clients, and family members as opposed to radiologists. In the United States 7 million workers may be at risk for exposure to ionizing radiation. Several occupational groups are at particular risk for work-related exposure. These include nurses, radiologists, x-ray technicians, nuclear plant employees,

TABLE 17-5 Principal Sites of Occupational Cancer

Site of cancer	Carcinogens	Occupations
Lung	Arsenic; asbestos; chromium; coal products; dusts; iron oxide; mustard gas; nickel; petroleum; ionizing radiation; bis-chloromethyl ether (BCME)	Vintners; miners; asbestos workers; textile workers; insulation workers; automobile brake and clutch mechanics; tanners; smelters; glass and pottery workers; electrolysis workers; radium dial painters; exposed medical personnel; chemical workers; coal tar and pitch workers; iron foundry workers
Pleura and peritoneum	Asbestos	Asbestos workers; textile workers; insulation workers; automobile brake and clutch mechanics; construction workers; shipyard workers
Nasal cavity sinuses	Chromium; isopropyl oils; nickel; wood and leather dusts	Glass, pottery, and linoleum workers; nickel smelters, mixers, and roasters; electrolysis workers; wood, leather, and shoe workers
Bladder	Coal products; aromatic amines; leather dusts	Asphalt, coal tar, and pitch workers; gas stokers; still cleaners; dyestuffs users; rubber workers; paint manufacturers; leather and shoe workers; textile dyers
Skin	Arsenic; sunlight; coal soot, coal tar, and other products of coal combustion; petroleum and petroleum products	Insecticide makers and sprayers; oil refiners; vintners; smelters, farmers; gashouse workers; asphalt, coal tar, and pitch workers; cokeoven workers; miners; workers in contact with lubricating, cooling, or fuel oils
Liver	Arsenic; vinyl chloride	Tanners, smelters, vineyard workers; plastic workers
Bone marrow	Benzene; ionizing radiation	Benzene, explosives, and rubber cement workers; distillers; dye users; painters; exposed medical personnel

Modified from Levy BS and Wegman DH, editors: Occupational Health, Boston, 1983, Little, Brown & Co.

and some military personnel. These workers are exposed to small, recurring doses over a long period. Any increase in radiation exposure has the potential for injury or damage to the worker. Not every case of radiation exposure results in cancer, leukemia, or genetic defects (Gillette, 1972). Disease induction is influenced by many factors. These include type of radiation, age, sex, genetic background, nutritional status, and exposure to cocarcinogens. Although ionizing radiation is a known carcinogen in animals and humans, health professionals find it difficult to identify a worker's disease as radiation-induced because of the time between onset of exposure and diagnosis. It may take 3 to 10 years for leukemia to develop and 15 to 40 years for carcinoma to occur. The known risks of ionizing radiation and the number of workers exposed makes it imperative that radiation exposure be carefully monitored and potential for exposure be minimized.

Infectious Agents

The primary group at risk for occupational infections are health care employees. The hazards of hospital-acquired (nosocomial) infectious diseases are well documented. The major infections are hepatitis A, hepatitis B, non-A, non-B hepatitis, tuberculosis, rubella, cytomegalovirus, and laboratory-associated infections such as typhoid fever, brucellosis, coccidioidomycosis, Q fever, and psittacosis.

Infectious diseases in non–health care workers are those diseases of animals that are transmitted to humans (zoonoses). The major occupational groups at risk are farmers, veterinarians, butchers, and slaughterhouse workers. These infections are viral, bacterial, rickettsial, chlamydial, parasitic, and fungal.

Work-related bacterial diseases are uncommon but should be considered when a worker has a skin lesion and lymphadenopathy and supporting work history of exposure to animal sources. Bacterial diseases include anthrax, brucellosis, leptospirosis, plague, salmonellosis, and tularemia. Common animal sources are cattle, sheep, horses, dogs, cats, rabbits, poultry, and mice. The best protection includes immunizations and the use of protective clothing and gloves.

Occupational viral infections do occur, but they account for few of the infectious diseases diagnosed in workers. The most common viral diseases are rabies, cat scratch fever, and encephalitis. These diseases are caused by animal, mosquito, and tick bites. Vaccination of domestic animals provides protection against rabies. Anyone bitten by a nonimmunized animal is a candidate for postexposure immunization. Workers who handle nondomestic animals or who come in contact with them should wear protective clothing. Cat scratch fever does not usually result in the sequelae of other viral diseases, since it can be easily treated. Agriculture and forestry workers and especially entomologists are at particular risk for encephalitis. Clothing and insect repellants provide some protection for those at risk.

Other infectious diseases, particularly Rocky Mountain spotted fever and Lyme disease carried by ticks, pose a threat to foresters and farmers. Protection against tick bites is needed. Psittacosis is a *Chlamydia* disease and usually results in pneumonia. Those working with birds are at greatest risk for *C. psittaci.* Occupational fungal diseases acquired from inhaling spore-containing dust include histoplasmosis and coccidioidomycosis. Histoplasmosis is endemic to the states of Tennessee and Kentucky, and there is a high incidence in the Ohio and Mississippi valleys. Workers at particular risk are those who work with the soil such as bulldozer operators and farmers. The risk may be reduced by spraying contaminated soil with 5% formalin solution. Coccidioidomycosis is also found in the soil and occurs most frequently in the Southwest. There is no known protection from this naturally acquired disease (Gantz, 1983).

Physical Trauma

Reported work-related accidents injure 4.7 million workers each year (U.S. Department of Labor, Bureau of Statistics, 1985). It is estimated that as many as 20 million accidents occur, although a much lower number is reported. The needs for emergency care will vary to some degree in all settings. The work setting and the age range of the workers determine which accidents are of primary concern. Programs such as cardiopulmonary resuscitation (CPR) and emergency first aid procedures are integral to the safety of all work sites. The highest incidence of accidents occurs in manufacturing and wholesale retail.

Accidents and Safety Hazards

Whereas the cause of an occupational injury is clear when the injury is immediately preceded by an accident, not all occupational injuries occur in this manner. A worker who lifts 20 pounds routinely at work and notices a herniated disc while at home most likely has an occupational injury (Ray, 1985). This is called cumulative trauma and results from repeated minor insults to a particular part of the body.

Occupational injuries are preventable. The type of accidents and injuries depend on the kind of activities on the job. The American National Standards Institute (ANSI) classifies work accidents as follows:

1. Struck by
2. Overexertion
3. Falls from elevation
4. Falls from some level
5. Caught in, under, and between
6. Motor vehicles
7. Other causes of physical trauma.

Education in accident prevention, safety measures, and the enforcement of safety regulations can help reduce the number of occupational accidents. Attempts to decrease accidents and injuries by rewarding workers for days without accidents have increased worker awareness. The focus on the worker as the causative agent rather than on factors inherent in the work situation may result in unsafe conditions that contribute to accidents. Recent evidence suggests that unsafe conditions are primarily responsible for accidents. Prevention of occupational trauma is best accomplished through engineering designs such as covering of moving parts of machines and grounding of electric wires. A second protective measure designed to preserve the health of the worker is training and supervision of employees in the use of personal protective equipment. Controls must be placed on the amount of exposure. This can be accomplished by the worker rotating to various work sites to reduce risks. The personal protective equipment issued is dependent on the type of job hazard. These include use of safety glasses for metal grinding operations, masks for cotton fiber exposure, and ear plugs for loud noises. More dangerous jobs may require use of respirators, radiation suits, and face shields. Workers may not always value protective gear. They need to be educated about the need for personal protection. Administrators need to have policies and procedures to deal with employees who do not adhere to safety standards.

Ergonomics (human factors engineering) is an applied science concerned with the design of work equipment and work tasks that are compatible with human physical and psychologic characteristics. Ergonomic methods may be applied to most occupational safety hazards. The application of ergonomics at the work site can reduce accidents and increase productivity.

Homicide

Each year an estimated 1600 workers die by homicide on the job (Dietz and Baker, 1987). Individuals such as policemen, security officers, taxi drivers, operators of eating and drinking establishments, and service station and convenience store employees have the highest mortality. The National Institute of Occupational Safety and Health (NIOSH) reported that shootings accounted for 4.5% of all at-work deaths in 1980-1981 (Centers for Disease Control, 1984). Discrepancies exist in the reporting of work-related homicides, so the actual number of annual homicides occurring during work-related activities is unknown. Occupational homicide and injury caused by assaults is gaining attention as a community health concern (Kraus, 1987).

Noise-Induced Hearing Loss

Approximately 15 million workers are exposed to hazardous noises in the workplace. Approximately 6 million of these workers suffer hearing loss (Jaffe, Bell, and Irwin, 1983).

The intensity, or loudness, of sound is measured in decibels (dB). The threshold of normal hearing is 0-3 dB HL (hearing level). The noise level in a quiet home is approximately 30 dB HL, and the level of average conversational speech is approximately 50 dB HL. A jet plane produces 117 dB

HL, and textile machinery produces 106 dB HL. The threshold of pain for most individuals is 100 dB HL.

A worker can be exposed to an average noise level of 80 dB HL for eight hours in a 24-hour period without sustaining damage more significant than the population in general. If the 80 dB HL level is exceeded, hearing loss is likely to occur. According to OSHA regulations, higher noise levels are allowed for only limited periods, with the amount of time cut in half for each 5 dB increase in noise level. A worker may be exposed to 85 dB HL of noise for eight hours in a 24-hour period but to 90 dB HL for only four hours under these regulations. At 110 dB HL, only 15 minutes of exposure is allowed in a 24-hour period.

Hearing loss caused by noise exposure generally affects the higher frequencies first, with the greatest damage occurring at 4000 Hz. Most sounds contained in human speech are in the range of 500 to 2000 Hz. Since these frequencies are not affected at first, the person may not notice any difficulties with everyday communication until substantial damage has occurred.

The first symptoms of hearing loss are frequently tinnitus (ringing or buzzing in the ear) and a blocked or full sensation in the ear. Because the hearing loss progresses gradually, someone other than the worker is often the first to notice that there is a problem.

To determine the extent of hearing loss, audiometric testing is conducted. An audiometer is used to measure the threshold (least audible sound) of the person's hearing at frequencies from 250 to 8000 Hz. Testing is carried out in a noise-free environment, preferably in a soundproof booth.

Once hearing loss is determined, it is the health professional's responsibility to recommend whether the worker should be removed from the work situation. Persistent changes in audiogram results of workers should alert the occupational health nurse to assess noise levels and to control excess noise exposure. Managers have the responsibility to maintain a work environment that protects the worker from those noise hazards that are within their control. Some engineering techniques for reducing noise include room absorption, barriers, mufflers, and machine enclosures. It is also the responsibility of the employer to provide personal protection devices such as ear plugs, ear muffs, helmets, or all three. The worker is responsible for consistently using the devices that prevent hearing loss. Staffing patterns that move workers from one site to another reduce the workers' exposure to excess noise. Although this method introduces more workers to excess noise levels, it shortens the individual worker's total exposure and reduces the incidence of hearing loss (Jaffe, Bell, and Irwin, 1983).

A hearing conservation program should be a priority in those industries where noise is a hazard. Preplacement baseline audiograms with annual audiograms for comparison for each employee should be required. The program should educate employers and employees regarding the nature of hearing loss. Worker participation is necessary for any hearing conservation program to be successful. Workers should be informed that hearing loss is irreversible and that prevention is the best method to reduce hearing loss.

Even low-level noise can result in psychologic and physiologic stress that can be damaging. Physiologic changes include an increase in blood cholesterol level and blood pressure, ulcers, digestive upsets, and an increase in perspiration. Psychologic changes can range from irritability to personality disorders. The body attempts to adapt to this low-level noise and in most cases body functions return to normal when there is a change in environment.

Psychologic and Social Stressors

Stress is a major hazard in the workplace. Work-related stress has an impact on interpersonal relationships, job satisfaction, and productivity. It can also negatively affect nonoccupational health problems such as diabetes mellitus.

Individual characteristics, the job, and working conditions including work load and organizational structure contribute to work-related stress.

Personality traits and predispositions affect how one handles work stress. Type A behavior characterized by competitiveness, aggressiveness, impatience, restlessness, and striving for achievement puts one at risk for stress-induced problems. The ability to adapt, cope, and use defense mechanisms has an impact on how one responds to stress. How workers manage the demands of the job in relation to their own personalities requires understanding of their previous responses to stress and willingness to modify their own behaviors.

Job stress falls into three categories—frustration, excessive stimulation, or lack of stimulation. Frustration is the impediment of progress toward a desired goal. If stress is a result of a lack of congruence between a worker's needs, skills, and abilities and the job demands, an occupational change that reduces the stress should be considered. Or the worker may analyze goals and if the specific goal can be met outside the job through other activities, the worker may be able to reduce frustration and be satisfied with the current job.

Other stress-producing factors in a job may be shift work and physical and clinical hazards in the work environment. Shift work is a significant stressor. Workers whose shifts rotate once a week have their social life disrupted and experience a disruption in time-oriented patterns such as sleeping and eating. Jobs that are boring may result in stress. Many workers cannot adapt to the monotony of the job. Jobs that produce excessive stimulation resulting in prolonged sensory overload are just as likely to produce stress in the worker. Additionally, the acquisition of new skills may create rather than reduce stress if the job requirements remain the same.

If working conditions are stressful, there is a spillover effect into other areas of functioning. The impact of a stressful job is cumulative and poses a serious threat to the worker's health. If the workload is fast ‸aced and physically demanding with long hours and high discrepancy between job demands and job rewards, the worker may experience depression and anxiety. Ideally, the job should be mentally challenging, provide appropriate rewards, have safe working conditions, allow for personal growth, and provide a support system that deals with work-related problems. The organizational structure of the workplace impacts on job satisfaction and absenteeism and has been linked to the mental health status of workers. Large organizations with a traditional bureaucratic structure have the highest levels of absenteeism and job dissatisfaction. Those in decision-making positions are less likely to experience job dissatisfaction than those in staff positions. It is important for the employer to be aware of the effect of organizational structure on employee satisfaction and productivity (Kasl and Cobb, 1983).

SOCIAL AND ETHICAL CONSIDERATIONS IN THE WORKPLACE

Women in the Work Force

The type of work available to men and women traditionally was dictated by culture and not by physical and sexual differences. As technology reduced the physical strength needed for many jobs, social factors began to account for work assignments. Today most work can be handled equally well by men or women. The emerging view is that women are no better or less capable of parenting than men, just as men are no better or less capable than women of handling jobs traditionally limited to men. However, more than one half of the working women in the United States are still in female-intensive occupations (Brunt and Hricko, 1983; Rytina and Bianchi, 1984). The representation of women in heavy industrial jobs and the building industry is small but increasing. This small number may be a result of early legislation that was designed to protect women from environmental hazards in the workplace. Women were limited in the number of hours they could work and the amount of weight they could be required to lift. These laws that were designed to protect women were later used as justification for not hiring them. Current laws require that hiring practices be based on an individual's ability to perform a given job without regard to sex.

Although women have played a significant role in the work force since World War II, only recently have the numbers of working women reached such a level as to mandate that the needs of women in the workplace be addressed. Women now constitute about one half the nation's work force. Economic necessity is one of the major reasons for a consistent increase in the number of working women. Although there was a tendency in the past for women to leave the work force for marriage and childbearing, the current trend is for women to remain in the work force throughout their adult life. In 1984, the percentage of women in the work force by marital status was 25% single, 59% married, and 16% widowed or divorced (U.S. Department of Commerce, Bureau of the Census, 1985). Currently, women who work full time earn 60 to 65 cents for every dollar earned by men. This gap has persisted at approximately the same level over several decades (Shack-Marquez, 1984).

Many working women, even in two-parent families, continue to be responsible for both child care and housework. Despite the women's movement and other social forces, men have not shared equally in family maintenance functions. With women earning income, power bases tend to shift in the family causing family conflict. In addition to this conflict, being tired, often feeling the social pressure to stay at home with small children, negotiating child care arrangements, and experiencing guilt for any misconduct of their children contribute to the stress of the working woman.

There are also many sources of stress on the job. The jobs into which most women are placed can best be described as low paying, demanding, monotonous, lacking in autonomy, and inherently stress producing. Male-dominated occupations pose particular risks for female workers. Safety equipment, usually designed for men, exposes women to hazards caused by poorly fitted safety equipment. Women workers often encounter hostility from their male coworkers who assign them difficult tasks that the women are not prepared to perform. When men set women coworkers up for failure, additional stress is produced for the women.

Sexual Harassment

An analysis of hazards of working women reveals that the single most widespread occupational hazard is sexual harassment (Horgan and Reeder, 1986). The term sexual harassment is described as "any repeated or unwanted verbal or physical sexual advance or sexually explicit derogatory statement" (U.S. Dept of Labor, Women's Bureau, 1980). Although sexual harassment is difficult to define in behavioral terms, it exists. A situation in which a female employee is explicity told that her job will be threatened unless she submits to sexual demands occurs less often than subtle forms such as suggestive language or unnecessary body contact. Rape does occur but often goes unreported because of fear of job loss, embarrassment, or self-imposed guilt. Many women in the work force often do not know how to handle unwanted sexual advances that contribute to job stress. Some states have granted worker's compensation benefits to employees for stress-related health problems attributed to sexual harassment. The Federal Equal Employment Opportunity Commission (EEOC) handles sexual harassment complaints like other complaints of job discrimination. Although recourse is open to women, sexual harassment is commonplace and accepted by many as a norm. This erroneous perception is a barrier in preventing this occupational hazard.

Pregnant Workers

With young women of childbearing age comprising a major portion of the work force, the protection needs of this at-risk population must be addressed. The Federal Civil Rights Act of 1964 was amended in 1978 to protect women from job discrimination on the basis of pregnancy, childbirth, or related health conditions. The Pregnancy Discrimination Act prevents women from being dismissed or denied work because of pregnancy or abortion. This right to work must be considered along with the worker's health, job hazards, and the worker's ability to perform during pregnancy. The majority of jobs can be performed by healthy pregnant women. Although job performance may not be decreased, the pregnant women may be more susceptible to infectious agents and chemical toxins. In the United States 30% of spontaneous abortions (miscarriages) were found to have chromosomal alterations that can be caused by toxic chemicals (Fogel and Woods, 1981). Fetal development may be altered by chemicals, radiation, and biologic agents. The first trimester is the period of greatest vulnerability for teratogenic insult.

There is a recognized lack of data on reproductive hazards for women in the workplace. Thousands of women who work in high-technology industries are working with chemicals that have not been tested for their effect on reproduction. The goals of current legislation and health care professionals are not to close industries but to find ways to protect all workers exposed to harmful agents.

The postpartum period continues to put the infant at risk of chemicals ingested or inhaled through breast-feeding. Heavy metals such as lead, cadmium, and mercury, many pesticides, polybrominated biphenyls (PBBs), and polychlorinated biphenyls (PCBs) have been identified in the breast milk of women occupationally exposed to these toxic substances. Currently, evidence of harm to infants is insufficient to support control of exposure of nursing mothers to these substances. However, women should be informed that breast milk can be contaminated and toxic levels can be determined.

All women should have a rubella titer assessment before their first pregnancy to determine their immunity. If the titer is determined to be insufficient, the woman is a candidate for rubella immunization. Women at particular risk are those who work with small children, such as teachers, day-care workers, and pediatric nurses.

Female-Intensive Occupations

Despite the increase in the number of women in nontraditional jobs and occupations, 57% of women work in 25 occupational categories, 15 of which were classified as female intensive in 1980. The percentage of women employed in these occupations and the changes in employment over the last decade are shown in Table 17-6. The major change occurred in the managerial category.

By 1980 management was the largest occupation for men and the sixth largest for women. The number of women in these positions increased by 27% during the 1970s. Occupational segregation in employment had declined by 1980 because of the increase of men and women in sex-neutral occupations. The number of men in female-intensive occupations has not changed substantially since 1970. The number of women in male-intensive occupations has increased in the area of management and in a few professional occupations such a law, medicine, and engineering. However, the increase in the overall number of women in male-intensive occupations has been minimal and has not had an impact on labor statistics.

Hazards Affecting Workers in Traditional Female-Intensive Occupations

In the United States female-intensive occupations have been considered hazard free, but this assumption is without validity, since little re-

TABLE 17-6 Percentage of Females Employed in Certain Occupations and the 1970 to 1980 Change in that Percentage in the 25 Occupations with the Largest Number of Women in 1980

Detailed 1980 occupational title	Number of women	Women's proportion in 1980	Women's proportion in 1970	1970 to 1980 change in female percentage
Secretaries	3,949,973	98.8	97.8	1.0
Typists	716,449	96.8	94.8	2.0
Practical nurses	420,412	96.6	96.1	0.5
Registered nurses	1,232,544	95.9	97.3	−1.4
Receptionists	525,290	95.8	95.3	0.5
Sewing machine operators	860,848	94.1	94.9	−0.8
Child care workers	570,794	93.2	92.5	0.7
Bank tellers	464,139	91.1	86.9	4.2
Bookkeepers	1,700,843	89.7	80.9	8.8
Food servers	1,325,928	88.0	90.8	−2.8
Nursing aides	1,209,757	87.8	87.0	0.8
Hairdressers	490,785	87.8	90.0	−2.2
Cashiers	1,565,502	83.5	84.2	−0.7
Office clerks	1,425,083	82.1	75.3	6.8
Maids and housemen	510,277	75.8	94.3	−18.5
Teachers, elementary school	1,749,547	75.4	83.9	−8.5
Salesworkers	1,234,929	72.7	70.4	2.3
Handpackagers	415,925	66.8	67.0	−0.2
Cooks	771,878	57.2	67.2	−10.0
Teachers, secondary school	486,603	56.5	49.6	6.9
Assemblers	841,158	49.5	45.7	3.8
Machine operators	471,011	33.5	30.2	3.3
Supervisors, sales	445,492	28.2	17.0	11.2
Managers, n.e.c.	1,407,898	26.9	15.3	11.6
Janitors and cleaners	498,623	23.4	13.1	10.3

From Rytina NF and Bianchi SM: Occupation reclassification and change in distribution by gender, Monthly Labor Review 104:16, 1984.

search has been done on these occupational groups. Studies done in other countries indicate that hazards are present in female-intensive occupations in both industrial and nonindustrial settings.

Ozone is a respiratory and mucous membrane irritant that can cause headache, chest pain, respiratory distress, and pulmonary edema. It has also been identified as a mutagen. Ozone is a byproduct of many copy machines. If a copy machine is not properly maintained, ozone emission can reach levels that exceed safety standards. Emission levels of ozone must be monitored regularly, and workers must be educated about signs and symptoms of ozone exposure. Flight attendants are at particular risk during long-distance flights at high altitudes, since this can result in high concentrations of ozone in the airplane cabin.

Methanol, a common duplicating machine chemical, is known to cause eye irritations, headache, dizziness, insomnia, and visual problems. Personnel in schools that use "spirit" duplicators are at high risk for hazardous exposure. Air concentrations of methanol need to be monitored for safe levels, which are set by OSHA. High levels of methanol often go undetected because schools are generally considered safe. A NIOSH study of one school district found that 60% of the teacher aides had symptoms of methanol toxicity (National Institute for Occupational Safety and Health, 1980).

Halogenated hydrocarbons are chemicals found in many products used by those in laundry and dry-cleaning, clerical, cosmetical, and housekeeping occupations. The hazards of short-term exposure include liver toxicity, headache, fatigue, narcosis, and mucous membrane irritation. Long-term exposure can result in liver necrosis and cancers of the lung, liver, and skin (Fogel and Woods, 1981). The groups of workers in contact with halogenated hydrocarbons, in particular, cosmetologists and housekeepers, are not monitored for the ill effects of these substances.

Other carcinogens, such as benzene, benzidine-based dyes, and asbestos, are known to cause leukemia, bladder cancer, and lung cancer. Benzene and benzidine-based dyes are used in the textile industry. Asbestos, a common construction material used between 1958 and 1973, is present in the ventilation systems of many office buildings.

Teratogens are present in anesthetic gases, thereby exposing operating room personnel, nurse anesthetists, and anesthesiologists to a health hazard that is believed to increase the risk of spontaneous abortion, congenital abnormalities in offspring, and liver and renal disease (Brodsky, 1983). The single most correctable source of pollution is careless anesthesia techniques. The best method of control is installing a scavenger system and improving techniques of administration (Wright, 1979). Dental and medical assistants, veterinary personnel, and laboratory workers are also exposed to teratogens in their work settings.

Radiation exposure of hospital personnel and clients has received increased attention but primarily in relationship to exposure during pregnancy. Research efforts need to be directed toward the incidence of breast, thyroid, and other types of cancer in women exposed to radiation. Although it is difficult to prescribe specific radiation protection measures, programs for radiation protection need to focus on methods to minimize the exposure of women. This can be done by providing clear explanations of the physical and biologic principles of radiation, shielding the worker from radiation, reducing exposure time, maintaining distance from the source, performing regular assessments of workers' adherence to safety standards and their knowledge of sources of radiation, and maintaining safe equipment (Kahn and others, 1983).

Health care workers, particularly nurses, used hexachlorophene (pHiso-Hex) extensively during the 1960s and 1970s until studies reported the dangers associated with this chemical. Halling (1979) reported a significant increase in congenital abnormalities of infants born to nurses exposed to hexachlorophene. Other studies (Check, 1978; Hill and Kleinberger, 1984) found measureable blood levels of hexachlorophene in cord blood of mothers using this chemical and in persons who washed frequently with hexachlorophene.

Skin disorders are prevalent in many female-intensive occupations. The high-risk industries, which require the use of disinfectants, drugs, and cleaners, include hospitals, hotels, restaurants, and hairstyling shops. Exposure to these substances may cause contact dermatitis, which accounts for 90% of all skin disorders. Signs and symptoms include redness, swelling, crusting, and scaling, or skin thickening with excoriation (Arndt, 1983).

Microbial hazards are common problems faced by individuals who work with sick persons and in clinical laboratories. Hepatitis B is the most frequent work-related infectious disease with 200,000 new cases estimated each year (Centers for Disease Control, 1982). Blood and blood by-products are the major sources of the infection, although the virus is found in saliva, semen, and feces. The incidence of hepatitis B has increased for those who work in kidney dialysis units, oncology units, operating rooms, dental offices, and wash areas for supplies and equipment. Although hospitals have infection-control protocols, they do not always have procedures for handling and disposing of potentially infectious materials. An effective vaccine is available and recommended for workers in high-risk preexposure situations and for postexposure following breaks in skin or mucosa.

Tuberculosis, the second most common infectious disease, is prevalent in health care workers. A total of 26,846 new cases was reported to the Centers for Disease Control in 1983. A low index of suspicion of the disease has resulted in reduced detection efforts. Personnel who are exposed to clients with undiagnosed tuberculosis have six times the increase in the rate of positive tuberculin skin tests when compared with nonexposed personnel. Annual skin test screenings are recommended for at-risk groups who have not previously converted. Isoniazid (IHN) may be administered according to the Centers for Disease Control recommendations. Bacillus Calmette Guérin (BCG) vaccination is not recommended for hospital personnel unless there is an unusually high number of persons who have skin test conversions.

Acquired immunodeficiency syndrome (AIDS) caused by the HTL-VIII virus is a growing national health problem. AIDS is rapidly becoming a major concern of health care workers. Researchers have documented seven cases involving health care workers becoming infected with the human immunodeficiency virus (HIV) after accidental exposure to contaminated blood (The American Nurse, 1987). The Centers for Disease Control has issued guidelines to prevent transmission of AIDS in the workplace. The guidelines recommend the use of protective clothing including gloves, gowns, masks, and eye coverings (depending on the circumstance) when there is risk of exposure to blood or other body fluids. The issue of mandatory testing of all health care workers and clients is being debated. Currently, voluntary HIV testing is being promoted.

Women in the work force are at particular risk for job-related injuries in nonindustrial settings. One of the primary contributing causes of injury is improper footwear. Back injuries are another major health problem for workers in female-intensive occupations. Studies have shown that lifting, slips, trips, and falls are the primary causes of back injury. Such injuries are costly because of time away from the job and health care cost. One survey of hospital workers indicated that 40% of the nurses who left nursing did so because of back pain (Brunt and Hricko, 1983). The best predictor of individuals at risk for back injury is the general condition of the employee (Frymore, 1984). Spinal x-ray films have not proved an effective predictor (Ustby, 1981).

Although research has not demonstrated that education in proper lifting techniques reduced the incidence of back injuries, instructions in lifting technique are recommended (Yu and others, 1984). Prework exercise programs have been reported to reduce the incidence of back injuries.

Women and Men Who Work As Homemakers

A large population of women (40%) are not protected by any occupational regulations—at particular risk are the 29.4 million women who work in the home (U.S. Department of Labor,

Bureau of Statistics, 1985. The number of men who work in the home is increasing, and they are subject to the same risks as women. The lack of attention given to this population by health care professionals including community health nurses may be attributed to the value attached to housework. The value that society places on this occupation influences the self-esteem of those who choose this work. Although there are hazards in the home such as physical stress, accidents, and high noise levels, household chemical hazards pose the greatest threat to women and men who work as homemakers. Petroleum products, carbon monoxide, pesticides, and drugs, including aspirin, barbituates, and tranquilizers, account for 30% to 36% of the accidents and 40% of the fatalities in the home (Oakley, 1974; Laws, 1979).

Physical hazards are more easily prevented. It is the social hazards that are the most difficult to overcome. Dissatisfaction with housework is reported by 70% of full-time homemakers. Monotony was identified as the greatest cause of dissatisfaction, and autonomy was the most valued characteristic of this occupation (Oakley, 1974; Laws, 1979). Homemakers report a mean work week of 77 hours, spending as much time in housework as their grandmothers did. This time spent in housework supports the adage that work expands to fill the available time. Homemakers engaged in housework often express a lack of power in family decision making because they do not make a financial contribution to the family budget.

The homemaker's world often revolves around children if they are present in the home. Homemakers often experience social isolation and tend to neglect their own psychosocial needs. Along with the responsibility of children, homemakers often care for infirm clients and relatives. In this role as caregiver, the homemaker's need for support and time management must be included in the community health nurse's plan of care for the family.

Minorities in the Workforce

The minority worker is at risk for occupational diseases. When clusters of workers can be identified to be at greater risk than the general population of workers, the needs of the subpopulation must be addressed in the occupational setting.

Minority workers include blacks, Asians, Hispanics, and Native Americans. Although blacks constitute 10% of the work force and are the majority of minority workers, Hispanic workers constitute 5% of the American work force and their number is rapidly increasing (U.S. Department of Labor, Bureau of Statistics, 1985).

People who immigrate to the United States have traditionally worked in the least desirable jobs. These subgroups tended to be replaced in these jobs by the following wave of immigrants. The current patterns of employment suggest that minority groups (blacks, Asians, Hispanics, and Native Americans) have experienced discrimination in hiring practices and have not been as successful as many earlier European immigrants. Consequently, these minority groups are still in the least desirable jobs.

Nonwhite workers are concentrated in manufacturing and service industries, which have the highest rates of occupational illnesses (see Table 17-1). Because of these employment patterns, black workers have a 37% greater risk of occupational injury or illness and have a 24% greater risk of death from an illness or injury (Kotelchuck, 1978).

The data and resulting statistical findings show the concentration of minority workers in particular jobs, but research efforts have not been directed toward studying the influence of race on occupational disease patterns. Although research linking job hazards among minority workers with work-related diseases is minimal, sufficient evidence exists to suggest that the general health status of minorities may place them at greater risk for occupational injury and disease than the general population. Research data that are available are limited to the health status of the black worker.

Blacks have higher morbidity and mortality than whites for most major diseases. Blacks have higher incidences of lung, colo-rectal, prostate, and esophageal cancers. Blacks, particularly black women, are more likely to have diabetes than whites. It has been estimated that diabetes develops in blacks 20% more often than in whites. Age-adjusted death rates for blacks are five times that of whites for tuberculosis. Hypertension is found in 27% of blacks and only 15% of whites. More specifically, there is an increased incidence of hypertensive heart disease and higher mortality. The average life expectancy for blacks is about seven years less than that for whites (Jarvis, 1981). Given that there is a difference in the general health status of blacks, epidemiologic studies are needed to examine the relationship between health problems and occupation.

Workers with Nonoccupational Health Problems

Although the working years are usually the healthiest time of life, nonoccupational health problems that impinge on the worker's health and productivity are present in a significant number of American workers. For the individual with a documented medical problem who seeks employment, the health professional should consider the job requirements and recommend placement that is within the person's mental and physical capabilities, compatible with the existing health problem, and not hazardous to other workers. Individuals who have medical problems but who are otherwise healthy may have an unrealistic perception of their ability to perform in a particular job. For example, a healthy man who lost vision in one eye as a child threatened legal action when told he was not eligible for a position as a correctional officer. The nurse had to help the young man understand that the position had stringent visual requirements to protect the worker from harm and to ensure that the worker could perform the job.

A worker with a nonoccupational–related illness is protected by antidiscrimination laws, collective bargaining agreements (if unionized), and privacy considerations. The rights of the employer are limited to information pertinent to the employee's return-to-work status, job performance, and effect of illness on coworkers. Health professionals have an ethical and legal responsibility not to disclose information regarding an employee's illness. The health professional does have the obligation to provide the employer information regarding the employee's ability to return to work.

Discussion of the following three nonoccupational medical problems covers some of the major issues the occupational health nurse (OHN) must be aware of to promote the health of the individual while maintaining productivity.

Epilepsy can be controlled by medication, and workers with epilepsy are capable of doing most jobs. Workers should not be placed in job situations where their safety or that of coworkers is jeopardized. The OHN should request that workers with seizure disorders be seen periodically for assessment and medication review. Also, the employee's immediate supervisor must be taught how to respond if a seizure occurs. With the worker's permission the nurse should contact the worker's private provider to coordinate job activities and management regimens. Changes in work hours such as shift rotation and overtime may place individuals with seizure disorders at particular risk. The contribution of the worker with special health needs usually far outweighs the concessions made by management.

Substance use among employees is one of the major health problems affecting the workplace. More than 80% of 141 businesses surveyed reported problems with employee substance abuse (Schreier, 1983). Substance abuse cost the American economy $25.8 billion in absenteeism, lost productivity, medical and treatment costs, and crime-related expenses (Lodge, 1983). Work characteristics of the abuser include "late 3 times more often, requires time off 2.2 times more often, has 2.5 times as many absences of eight days or more, uses 3 times the normal level of sick benefits, is 5 times more likely to file a workman's compensation claim, and is involved in accidents 3.6 times more often than other employees" (Lodge, 1983). It is estimated that in any company approximately 10% of the employees have alcohol-related problems. It is estimated that 30% of the alcoholics in the work force are women (U.S. Department of Health and Human Services, 1980). The exact relationship of workplace stress and substance abuse is not known, but the work environment can contribute to this preexisting problem. The time pressures created by work requirements are related to substance use and frequency of use. Other factors in the work environment associated with alcohol and drug abuse levels include lack of feedback regarding performance, additional work, role stress, and the institutional work environment.

Diabetes mellitus is a chronic disease that affects 2% of the American population with 5% to 10% being insulin dependent. More than 55% of diabetics are female. Since 80% of the cases begin in adulthood when individuals are already in the work force, changes in work assignments may be necessary. Insulin-dependent diabetics have more hypoglycemic reactions and may pose more of an employment risk. The health professional needs to evaluate the employee's level of control. Acceptable control includes infrequent insulin reactions and hyperglycemic episodes, supervision by a private health care provider, and infrequent absenteeism caused by the disease.

Diabetics in general should avoid changes in work patterns that could interfere with the employee's ability to control blood sugar levels and eating and sleeping patterns. The employment situation needs to be flexible enough to allow the employee to perform self-care activities.

Insulin-dependent diabetics do have some federal job restrictions such as driving heavy vehicles, operating cranes, or driving passenger-transporting vehicles in interstate commerce. Many states have similar restrictions.

ROLE OF THE COMMUNITY HEALTH NURSE IN OCCUPATIONAL HEALTH

Most workers are employed in work settings with fewer than 500 employees and do not have the benefits of safety and health professionals on the job. It is estimated that 75% of workers do not have access to the services of an OHN. This lack of on-site health services mandates a role for the community health nurse in the workplace (Brown, 1986).

Nurses who work in private and public community health agencies can significantly affect the well-being of the community by promoting and protecting the health of workers in the home and small industries and businesses. The community health nurse has the preparation and skills necessary to function as a consultant to workers, their families, and their employers. The identification of work-related problems through the systematic collection, analysis, and dissemination of data on workers in the community serves to effect change in the workplace. Surveillance can result in improved health of the worker and the community. The nurse's extensive knowledge of community resources and the referral process may facilitate the recovery and return to work of the individual who has sustained a work-related illness or injury.

The community health nurse must initiate health promotion and screening programs for at-risk populations in marginal-profit (small business) operations. For example, screenings for hypertension, cervical cancer, and hearing loss at the worksite are more effective than screenings conducted at a community agency site. Although time away from the job must be negotiated with the employer, the benefit of a healthy worker population is cost effective. Community health nurses must broaden their concept of community to include the workplace. The concept of the workplace as community serves to promote the health of workers and increases the effectiveness of the community health nurse.

Role of The Occupational Health Nurse

Practice in the workplace differs from practice in health care delivery agencies in the following three ways (Ray, 1985):

1. The worker's health is secondary to the product or service goals of the industry or business. The worker's health is valued in relation to the worker's productivity.
2. Health care services to workers are a direct cost to the employer. These costs include the nurse and other providers who deliver on-site services and the worker's time away from the job to obtain services. An increase in health services including screenings, wellness programs, and surveillance activities results in an increase in cost to the employer.
3. OHNs must justify their positions and services to employers. Since businesses operate to make profit, health professionals must demonstrate how their activities contribute to a decrease in the number of work-related illnesses and injuries, absenteeism, worker turnover, and workman's compensation costs.

The OHN is responsible for protecting and promoting the health of a group of workers. Nurses who are employed by an industry or business and whose primary responsibility is protecting and promoting the health of the workers in that particular industry or business are, by setting, labeled OHNs. The community health perspective is the foundation of occupational health nursing. This foundation is reflected in the independent provider role and interdependent collaborator role of the OHN. More than 50% of the OHNs who responded to a national survey indicated they were the primary provider of services at the worksite. Although 48% reported on-site physician backup, the physician was usually a part-time employee (Cox, 1985). In the workplace the OHN consults with other health professionals, but often the nurse has primary responsibility for maintaining the on-site health program.

The OHN's responsibilities include direct care, administration, and collaboration. The major activities of the OHN are listed in the following box. These activities are directed toward the individual worker, groups of workers, management, and the company.

The average OHN spends 49% of the time providing services such as counseling, assessing health problems, referring, and screening (Cox, 1985) to individual workers at all levels. Workers who are at risk for particular health problems or safety hazards are important clients for the OHN. Specific health programs are developed and targeted toward at-risk groups. The OHN communicates with management to protect the worker from hazards in the workplace and interprets the health needs of the workers. The company as employer and client of the OHN must be made aware of the benefits of health programs and services for the company and the individual worker.

The level to which the OHN assumes these responsibilities is dependent on the educational preparation of the nurse. As the role of the OHN expands to meet the complex health needs in the workplace, the baccalaureate degree is the minimal level of preparation for the occupational generalist. There is a documented need for specialists prepared at the graduate level in occupational health nursing. The OHN practitioner with a master's degree has an important role in health promotion and illness and injury prevention in the workplace. The diversity and complexity of the workplace requires a well-prepared OHN to interact with the physician, industrial hygienist, safety engineer, toxicologist, and management personnel. The occupational field is in a stage of growth and development. Well-prepared nurses have an opportunity to claim an important role in the field of occupational health.

RESPONSIBILITIES OF THE OCCUPATIONAL HEALTH NURSE

DIRECT NURSING CARE SERVICES

1. Provide direct care for work-related injuries, illnesses, and diseases.
2. Monitor nonoccupational health problems that impinge on workers' productivity.
3. Conduct health assessments, including preplacement and periodic screenings, and return-to-work health evaluations.
4. Provide first aid and emergency service.
5. Provide health education and counseling services.
6. Conduct workplace "rounds" to identify actual and potential health problems.

ADMINISTRATION

1. Formulate and coordinate health promotion and surveillance programs.
2. Evaluate the effectiveness of health and surveillance programs.
3. Ensure compliance with state and federal regulations.
4. Maintain employee health records.
5. Interpret health and medical information to management.
6. Monitor occupational health and safety programs.

COLLABORATION

1. Participate in management decisions that affect the health and safety of workers.
2. Coordinate community resources to meet worker and management needs.
3. Participate with other health professionals in research efforts to determine at-risk workers.
4. Develop evaluation plans in conjunction with safety and health professionals and labor representatives.

Data from Ossler C: Distributive nursing practice in occupational health and safety. In Hall D and Weaver B, editors: Distributive nursing practice: a systems approach to community health, Philadelphia, 1985, JB Lippincott Co; Ray L: Community health nursing at the worksite. In Archer S and Fleshman R, editors: Community health nursing, Monterey, Calif, 1985, Wadsworth Inc.

NURSING INTERVENTIONS IN THE WORKPLACE

Occupational health programs in the workplace are developed to promote the health of the entire workplace community including the worker's family. Worksite health programs can be viewed as having four generations. First-generation programs are initiated for reasons unrelated to health. Policies such as "no smoking" are imposed for safety and productivity. Second-generation programs focus on specific risks and selected interventions for a particular population. The recipients of these programs are generally upper management. In the first and second generations, programs' health benefits are secondary outcomes.

Third-generation health programs target the entire workplace community and offer a more comprehensive approach for reducing a variety of risk factors. Fourth-generation programs include a wellness strategy that is reflected in all activities, policies, and decisions that affect the health of the workers, their families, and the community. All four generations of health programs exist in American business and industry (O'Donnell and Ainsworth, 1984). The widespread enthusiasm for the fourth-generation programs has been tempered by questions such as, "Should business and industry assume the high cost of health care for workers?" and "Is the consumer willing to pay higher prices for products and services to cover health care costs?"

The decision of whether to provide health promotion programs is not easy to make. As decreasing productivity and rising costs add to the dilemma regarding the benefits of workplace health programs, business and industry must weigh the advantages and disadvantages. The costs and time away from the job, hiring personnel or contracting for the training, and convincing management of the worth of health programs are definite disadvantages. There is, however, a growing awareness on the part of corporations of the need to combat low productivity, absenteeism, and high turnover rates. In the end no one profits from neglecting efforts to establish workplace health programs. In reducing risks and overcoming limitations both the individual worker and the business profit.

Stress Management

It is estimated that one in four persons has severe emotional stress (President's Committee on Mental Health, 1978). More than $30 billion are lost annually in industrial productivity because of stress-related problems. In 1980 more than 50% of the worker's compensation cases in California were for stress-related disorders (O'Donnell and Ainsworth, 1984). It appears that these figures alone support the need for stress management programs in the workplace.

Approaches to helping workers manage stressful situations include habitation, change avoidance, time blocking, time management, environmental modification, and counterconditioning.

Often unrecognized as a stress reducer, habits or routines decrease the amount of physical and psychologic energy needed to perform tasks where other behavioral options are unavailable. Habituation serves as a stabilizing force. Positive routines and habits of workers should be supported during high-stress periods. The OHN can help the worker establish new routines when work tasks or work assignments change.

Change avoidance is indicated for workers who are experiencing stress caused by significant life changes. A worker should be advised not to make any unnecessary changes during a particularly stressful time. Multiple change is synergistic in that several small changes occurring simultaneously can cause significant stress. The worker should understand that any change is stress producing. Therefore unavoidable change can be handled more effectively when planned change is postponed.

Time blocking is a stress-management method that allocates specific time to focus on a stressor and develop strategies for coping. For instance, a worker experiencing on-the-job trauma to the shoulder must set aside time to learn exercises for rehabilitation and time to perform them. The use of time-blocking technique can reduce anxiety and frustration.

Without mastery over time, stress management techniques cannot be effective. Time management requires that one identify and prioritize goals. Once priorities are set, one can determine how to allocate time. Overcommitment and unrealistic expectations of oneself are two major sources of stress that require time management. Learning to say "no" and knowing what one can realistically accomplish are important factors in achieving control over one's time. Two basic concepts of time management are scheduling and delegation. Scheduling allows an increase in control over daily activities. It also allows division of tasks into smaller units and reduces the feeling of overload. When a task is broken down into smaller units, it is easier to accomplish. Delegation of secondary responsibilities when appropriate can save the time needed to accomplish the primary goal.

Environmental modification is an important means of controlling job-related stress. Workers must identify experiences and personalities that are stress producing and reduce their exposure to them. Some individuals are stress carriers and should be avoided if possible. Contact with stress-producing individuals requires assertive behavior. Assertiveness allows workers to share their perceptions and feelings with others in a way that enhances personal or group productivity. It is not always possible for the physical environment to be changed. The worker may choose to change companies or seek another position within the same company. The immediate interpersonal environment of the worker can be modified to reduce environmental stress.

Another stress-management technique, counterconditioning, seeks to control physiologic responses to stress. The goal of counterconditioning is to reduce stress with muscle relaxation and increased parasympathetic functioning. The three interventions most frequently used to accomplish counterconditioning are relaxation techniques, biofeedback, and imagery (Pender, 1987). Each of these interventions requires training on the part of the OHN and worker and is beyond the scope of this chapter.

TABLE 17-7 Potential Economic Benefits from Improved Nutrition and Dietary Habits

Health problem	Potential benefits
Obesity	80% reduction of incidence and potential problems caused by obesity. Reduction of costs of medical care and quick weight loss methods.
Heart and vascular problems	25% reduction of incidence of heart and vascular problems (reducing the $50 billion annual cost)
Diabetes and carbohydrate disorders	50% of cases prevented or improved (reducing the $10 billion annual cost)
Digestive problems	15% fewer digestive problems (reducing the $10 billion annual cost)
Alcoholism	33% savings of costs from absenteeism, lowered productivity, and accidents (costs estimated at $100 billion annually)
Cancer	25% reduction of incidence, deaths, and related costs
Dental	50% reduction of incidence, severity, and expenditures

Modified from O'Donnell MP and Ainsworth TH: Health promotion in the workplace, New York, 1984, John Wiley & Sons Inc; US Senate Select Committee on Nutrition and Human Needs: Benefits of human research, Appendix A, Nutrition and Health II, Washington, DC, 1976, US Government Printing Office. An individual benefit is improved work efficiency with a 5% increase in on-the-job productivity (with improved diet alone, not considering health problems) and a 25% reduction of working days lost.

Nutritional Programs

The American diet is rapidly changing. People are consuming more saturated fats, cholesterol, refined and processed sugar, salt, and alcohol. In the United States 30% of meals are eaten out, and preprocessed and packaged foods make up 60% of the American diet. Many convenience foods are high in fat and low in fiber. The fast-food industry's share of the food dollar is more than 50% (Koniz-Booher and Koniz, 1986) and demonstrates an irreversible social change. The nutritional implications of this trend warrant investigation.

Additional study is also needed to understand the nutritional needs of those between 20 and 50 years of age. Attention should be paid to dietary patterns, maintenance of ideal body weight, meeting the vitamin and mineral recommended daily allowance (RDA), and compliance with known dietary recommendations.

Strong evidence suggests that positive dietary modification can reduce several of the major risk factors associated with cardiovasclar disease. Well-designed primary prevention efforts have reduced mortality and demonstrated that nutritional counseling is effective in maintaining long-term adherence to changes in life-styles (O'Donnell and Ainsworth, 1984). Evidence is mounting that nutrition is the single most basic factor in maintaining health and averting disease. The U.S. Senate Select Committee on Nutrition and Human Needs estimated the potential economic benefits from improved nutrition and dietary habits; these figures are found in Table 17-7.

Nutritional intervention programs can be categorized into the following three approaches (O'Donnell and Ainsworth, 1984):

1. Nutritional awareness
2. Behavior change
3. A health food program

Nutritional awareness programs enhance the workers' understanding of the benefits of good dietary habits. These programs emphasize the benefits of good nutrition in reducing health risks. Such programs incorporate self-help materials, various types of group presentations, and opportunities to apply principles of nutrition to one's own dietary habits. Programs need to be developed on sound teaching and learning principles and on the concepts of adult learning. Nutritional awareness programs often focus on the relationship of eating habits to health, nutrition as a way of reducing risks, altering eating habits, food economy and marketing, nutrition through the life cycle, and the harmful effects of fad diets.

Behavioral change programs may be introduced into the workplace for the purpose of preventing or treating nutrition-related health problems. Dietary modification is within the worker's control but is one of the most difficult changes to effect because of the multicausal nature of eating behaviors. The occupational health nurse must understand that the determinants of eating behaviors are biologic, psychologic, sociocultural, and environmental.

The techniques used in behavior change programs include self-monitoring, operant conditioning, and stimulus control. Self-monitoring is basic to any behavioral management program. This process is a powerful technique for change, since it increases self-awareness, forces the identification of eating problems, and requires individuals to monitor their own progress.

Operant conditioning and in particular positive reinforcement of desirable eating patterns has the best outcome. Contingency contracting, another operant conditioning technique, identifies the parameters of behavior to be engaged in and the conditions and rewards to be obtained when the contract is fulfilled. Personal commitment through contracting is a useful technique for promoting dietary change.

Stimulus control is the modification of the environment to decrease the cues that precipitate negative eating behaviors and increase cues that promote positive eating behaviors. For instance, eating may be due to the availability of food and not actual hunger. The worker needs to develop awareness of the particular cues that trigger eating behavior and control these cues. Self-discipline is the cornerstone of stimulus control (Pender, 1987).

The healthy foods program is the most cost-effective nutritional intervention in the workplace. Theoretically, the OHN can influence one third of the nutritional intake of workers. The availability of nutritious foods is an indication of the value the business or company places on the worker's general health status, as well as the worker's nutritional status. Incentives such as discounts and speciality advertisements can be used to influence the worker's food selections. Replacing junk foods with nutritious snacks can also alter the worker's eating behavior. The OHN's participation in decisions regarding food service can improve the quality and selection of foods available to workers.

Exercise Programs

Perhaps the single most important factor affecting health other than dietary patterns is the type and amount of exercise performed by the worker. The average American worker has for many years neglected the need for exercise. The National Center for Health Statistics 1975 study reported that 49% of Americans exercised weekly. Although 49% of adults claim to exercise, their level of fitness remains unknown.

Haskell (1980) estimated that fewer than 30% of the people who exercise get an effective workout. The health conditions related to poor fitness are costly. Cardiovascular disease alone is estimated to cost $2.5 billion per year in direct health care cost and $11.2 billion in lost earnings (Hartunian, Smart, and Thompson, 1980). Since 1965, health care costs have soared from $39 billion to $322 billion (O'Donnel and Ainsworth, 1984). Absenteeism is a major expense associated with poor fitness. Heart attacks account for 132 million lost workdays per year.

Studies continue to document the benefits of physical fitness (Bjurstrom and Alexiou, 1978; Paffenbarger and others, 1986). The decline in fatal coronary artery disease is attributed to positive health habits including exercise. Since the employer assumes 50% of health care expenditures, promoting the health of workers through fitness programs will continue to gain attention.

The major types of exercise programs are aerobic, muscle development, and flexibility. Aerobic exercises are rhythmic activities that stimulate the heart and lungs to take up and deliver oxygen to the body tissue. For an exercise to be considered aerobic, the frequency, intensity, and time criteria must be met. The recommended frequency of exercise ranges from three to six times per week. The intensity is the maximum heart rate (target heart rate) needed for an exercise to be considered aerobic (see box). The maximum rate is a sustained heart rate at 70% to 80% above the resting heart rate for 20 to 30 minutes.

Exercises that develop muscles are important in preventing injury and in the rehabilitation of workers who have experienced an injury. The major types of muscle development exercises include calisthenics, weight training, and a few sports such as skiing and mountain climbing. Cooper (1981) stated that calisthenics not only builds muscle strength but increases agility and coordination. Flexibility is an important dimension of fitness. It is defined as the ability of joints and muscles to move through their full range of motion. A decrease in flexibility indicates inactivity. Stretching to increase flexibility is important in preventing injury during exercise. Stretching should be performed before and after sustained exercise.

The goal of an exercise program is to provide an effective efficient method of fitness, protect against injury and overexertion, and maintain interest and continued participation. The exercise program must be based on the worker's fitness status, the goals and interest of the worker, and the resources available to perform the exercise. An exercise program must be individualized to ensure adherence to the program (O'Donnell and Ainsworth, 1984).

AEROBIC EXERCISE: HOW TO CALCULATE YOUR TARGET HEART RATE

ACTIVITY CATEGORY

Sedentary to Moderate = 60% to 70%

Active to Very Active = 71% to 80%

TARGET RATE FORMULA

220 − age = Maximum Heart Rate (MHR)
MHR − Resting Heart Rate (RHR) = Heart Rate Reserve (HRR)
HRR × Low Range Activity + RHR = Minimum Target Rate
HRR × High Range Activity + RHR = Maximum Target Rate
Cardiovascular Fitness = Minimum to Maximum Target Rate

Substance Dependency Programs

Increased exposure and use of substances such as tobacco, alcohol, stimulants, and depressants can lead to addictive behavior that causes problems at work and home. Addiction is a syndrome with definable and recognizable behaviors. There are common elements in addiction regardless of the addictive substance. The characteristics of addictive substance dependency are increased usage, distress when regular use is interrupted, the recognition that more of a drug relieves the stress that results from abstinence, an intense craving for the substance, and the inability to remain substance free. Intervention programs must be based on an understanding of the nature of the relationship between the substance and the user.

Tobacco Dependency

Tobacco use is the nation's primary health problem and the most preventable cause of premature morbidity and mortality in the United States. Lung cancer is a leading cause of death in the United States, and cigarette smoking is a factor in 90% of the cases. One third of the coronary artery disease deaths are attributed to smoking, with 70% of the deaths caused by emphysema and bronchitis related to smoking. It is estimated that 53 million people, or 35% of the population, smoke. Of the 65% who identified themselves as non-smokers, one third were former smokers. Of every 10 smokers, nine express a desire to quit. Of the smokers who initiate cessation programs, one third are reported to relapse after one week. Of those who quit smoking, 25% remained cigarette free for six months (Gallup, 1981).

It is estimated that health care cost for an adult smoker is $164 per year more than for a nonsmoker over a lifetime. Insurance expenses are a direct cost to business and industry, and absenteeism and reduced productivity are indirect costs. Individuals who smoke at least one pack of cigarettes a day have a 50% higher rate of hospitalization than nonsmokers. The illness-related cost of smoking in the United States is $11 billion annually (Kristein, 1977 and 1980).

The intervention strategies available for cigarette smoking cessation range from individual self-help methods to organized group programs. Both commercial concerns and nonprofit organizations offer information and programs.

Pharmacologic aids have been developed to relieve the symptoms of nicotine withdrawal. Controlled studies have found these to be no better than placebos. Behavior modification strategies include self-monitoring, contingency contracting, and adversive conditioning techniques. These techniques have been somewhat successful in maintaining abstinence, with up to 36% of the participants remaining cigarette free up to 18 months.

The success rate is increased with programs using a combination of techniques. Eclectic programs offer some hope for smokers. Hypnosis and group educational techniques have essentially the same success rates as the modification programs. For all the programs, the relapse rate is high with only 25% remaining cigarette free for a year.

For those industries that permit workers to smoke, designated areas must be provided that protect nonsmokers from passive cigarette smoke. The nurse should monitor the workplace for excessive concentrations of smoke and improve ventilation where indicated.

A growing concern is the use of smokeless tobacco. This health problem has only begun to be recognized for its potential damage to users. Tobacco is addictive regardless of form and is a known carcinogen. It is safe to assume that the risks associated with smoking tobacco are as great for smokeless tobacco.

Alcohol and Drug Dependency

The cost of alcoholism and related disorders was $11.9 billion in 1976, with $20.6 billion lost in earnings. A report to Congress from the National Institute of Alcohol Abuse and Alcoholism estimated that 11% of the adult population are alcoholics. Homeless persons constitute 3% of alcoholics, 50% of alcoholics have attended college, 25% hold white collar jobs, and 45% are in managerial positions. Alcoholism is the third leading cause of death in the United States (Rakel, 1984). Occupational risk for alcoholism includes availability of alcohol during work hours, strong social pressure in occupations such as sales, and jobs characterized by social isolation or minimal supervision.

Drug abuse and dependency are common in today's society. Marijuana, heroin, and cocaine have spread to the suburbs and farms. The problem permeates all socioeconomic groups and occupations. The employer's perception of the extent of drug use in the workplace is often inaccurate. A survey of executives and employees from 20 companies found that 5% of management did not perceive drug use to be a problem, whereas 35% perceived it as a minor problem. However, 79% of the employees reported using drugs. The drugs workers most frequently cited were marijuana, amphetamines, barbiturates, and cocaine. The most prevalent drug used on the job was marijuana (Trice, 1980).

Employee assistance programs (EAPs) are designed to reduce alcohol-and drug-related problems and reduce the employer's costs that result from dysfunctional work behavior. Existing data from EAPs have demonstrated that participants referred through work-based programs tend to recover rapidly and that businesses and industries that have established programs have realized an equal return on their investment.

Four trends affecting management's response to employee dependency are a growing awareness that dependency problems are treatable, an increasing desire by employers to find humane and cost-effective ways of assisting dysfunctional employees, local, state, and federal funding to stimulate community support for employee assistance programs, and an increase in legal decisions and state and federal statutes that require employers to provide programs to handle dependency problems in employees.

SUMMARY

The young and middle-aged years are usually the healthiest and most productive time of one's life. The well-being of these age-groups is threatened primarily by life-style factors such as alcohol consumption, smoking, and stress. Since this age-group spends almost one fourth of the time at work, hazards in the work environment place workers at risk. Labor statistics indicate a decrease in the number of occupational diseases and injuries reported each year, yet many problems go unidentified as work related.

The role of the community health nurse in occupational health is essential, since approximately 75% of workers do not have access to the services of an OHN. Community health nurses must broaden their concept of community to include the workplace. The community health nurse has the preparation and skills necessary to affect the well-being of the community significantly by promoting and protecting the health of workers. The OHN who is employed by an industry or business has the primary responsibility to protect and promote the health of workers in a particular industry or business. The major activities of the OHN include direct nursing care services, administrative duties, collaboration with management, workers, and other health professionals, and the development of evaluation plans to ensure a safe work environment. A growing awareness of the need to promote health at the worksite has resulted in programs in stress management, nutrition, exercise, and substance dependency including tobacco, alcohol, and drugs.

QUESTIONS FOR DISCUSSION

1. Which law do you consider the key federal legislation to protect workers?
2. What are the occupational hazards related to nursing?
3. What are the major nonoccupational health problems of young and middle aged adults?
4. How does the work of an occupational health nurse differ from that of other community-based nursing roles?

REFERENCES

Arndt K: Skin disorders. In Levy B and Wegman D, editors: Occupational health, Boston, 1983, Little, Brown & Co Inc.

Bjurstrom L and Alexiou N: A program of heart disease intervention for public employees, J Occup Med 20:521, 1978.

Breslow L and Somers A: The lifetime health-monitoring program, N Engl J Med 296:601, 1977.

Brodsky J: Exposure to anesthetic gases: a controversy, AORN J 38:132, 1983.

Brown ML: The quality of the work environment. In Spradley B, editor: Readings in community health nursing, Boston, 1986, Little, Brown & Co Inc.

Brunt M and Hricko A: Problems faced by women workers. In Levy B and Wegman D, editors: Occupational health, Boston, 1983, Little, Brown & Co Inc.

Centers for Disease Control: Leading work related diseases and injury in the US, MMWR 33:213, 1984.

Centers for Disease Control: Inactivated hepatitis B virus vaccine, MMWR 24:318, 1982.

Check W: New study shows hexachlorophene is a teratogenic in humans, JAMA 240:513, 1978.

Cooper K: The new aerobics, New York, 1981, Bantam Books.

Cox A: Profile of the occupational health nurse, Occup Health Nurs 33:591, 1985.

Dean L: Aging and the decline of affect, J Gerontol 17:441, 1962.

Dietz P and Baker S: Murder at work, Am J Public Health 77:1273, 1987.

Fogel C and Woods N: Women in the workplace. In Fogel C and Woods N, editors: Health care of women, a nursing perspective, St Louis, 1981, CV Mosby Co.

Freiberg K: Human development: a life-span approach, North Scituate, Mass, 1979, Duxbury Press.

Friedman M: Family nursing theory and assessment, New York, 1981, Appleton & Lange.

Frumkin H: Toxins and their effects. In Levy B and Wegman D, editors, Occupational health, Boston, 1983, Little, Brown & Co Inc.

Frumkin H and Levy B: Carcinogens. In Levy B and Wegman D, editors: Occupational health, Boston, 1983, Little, Brown & Co Inc.

Frymore J: Helping your patients avoid low back pain, J Musculoskeletal Med 1:65, 1984.

Gallup G: Poll shows drop in U.S. smokers, The San Francisco Chronicle, p 4, August 31, 1981.

Gantz N: Infectious agents. In Levy B and Wegman D, editors: Occupational health, Boston, 1983, Little, Brown & Co Inc.

Gillette R: Radiation standards: the last word or at least a definitive one, Science 178:966, 1972.

Gould R: Adult life stages: growth toward self-tolerance, Psychology Today, 8:74, 1975.

Halling H: Suspected link between exposure to hexachlorophene and malformed infants, Ann NY Acad Sci 320:426, 1979.

Hartunian N, Smart C, and Thompson M: The incidence of economic cost of cancer, motor vehicles, coronary heart disease and stroke: a comparative analysis, Am J Public Health 70:1257, 1980.

Haskell W: The physical activity component of health promotion in occupational settings, Public Health Rep 95:109, 1980.

Hill L and Kleinberger F: Effects of drugs and chemicals on the fetus and newborn. II. Mayo Clin Proc 59:755, 1984.

Horgan D and Reeder G: Sexual harassment, AAOHN Journal 34:83, 1986.

Jaffe B, Bell D, and Irwin K: Workplace noise and hearing impairment. In Levy B and Wegman D, editors: Occupational health, Boston, 1983, Little, Brown & Co Inc.

Jarvis L: Community health nursing: keeping the public health, Philadelphia, 1981, FA Davis Co.

Kahn K and others: Ionizing radiation. In Levy B and Wegman D, editors: Occupational health, Boston, 1983, Little, Brown & Co Inc.

Kasl S and Cobb S: Psychological and social stresses in the workplace. In Levy B and Wegman D, editors: Occupational health, Boston, 1983, Little, Brown & Co Inc.

Koniz-Booher P and Koniz M: Nutrition and lifestyle. In Edelman C and Mandle C, editors: Health promotion throughout the lifespan, St Louis, 1986, CV Mosby Co.

Kotelchuck D: Occupational injuries and illnesses among black workers, Health PAC Bulletin 11:33, 1985.

Kraus J: Homicide while at work: persons, industries and occupations at high risk, Am J Public Health 77:1285, 1987.

Kristein M: Economic issues in prevention, Prev Med 6:252, 1977.

Kristein M: How much can business expect to earn from smoking cessation. Paper presented at the National Interagency Council on Smoking, Chicago, January 9, 1980.

Kudzma E and Quinn J: Young adulthood. In Edelman C and Mandle C, editors: Health promotion throughout the lifespan, St Louis, 1986, CV Mosby.

Law JL: The second X sex role and social role, New York, 1979, Elsevier Science Publishing Co Inc.

Levinson D and others: The seasons of a man's life, New York, 1978, Ballantine Books.

Lodge J: Taking drugs on the job, Time, p 52, 1983.

National Institute for Occupational Safety and Health: Methyl alcohol toxicity in teacher aides using spirit duplicators, MMWR 29:437, 1980.

Oakley A: The sociology of housework, New York, 1974, Pantheon Books.

O'Donnell M and Ainsworth T: Health promotion in the workplace, New York, 1984, John Wiley & Sons Inc.

Ossler C: Distributive nursing practice in occupational health and safety. In Hall D and Weaver B, editors: Distributive nursing practice: a systems approach to community health, Philadelphia, 1985, JB Lippincott Co.

Overfield T: Obesity: prevention is easier than cure, Nurse Pract 5:25, 1980.

Paffenbarger R Jr and others: Physical activity, all cause mortality, and longevity of college alumni, N Engl J Med 314:605, 1986.

Pender N: Health promotion in nursing practice, Norwalk, Conn, 1987, Appleton & Lange.

President's Commission on Mental Health: Report of the President's commission on mental health, Washington, DC, 1978, US Superintendent of Documents.

Rakel R: Textbook of family practice, Philadelphia, 1984, WB Saunders Co.

Ray L: Community health nursing at the worksite. In Archer S and Fleshman R, editors: Community health nursing, Monterey, Calif, 1985, Wadsworth Inc.

Schreier J: A survey of drug abuse in organizations, Personnel J 6:478, 1983.

Shack-Marquez: Earnings differences between men and women: an introductory note, Monthly Labor Review 107:15, 1984.

Trice H: Drugs, drug abuse and the workplace. In Dupont RL and Basen MM, editors: Control of alcohol and drug abuse in industry: A literature review, Rockville Md, 1980, National Institute of Drug Abuse.

US Department of Commerce, Bureau of the Census: Statistical abstracts of the United States, ed 105, Washington, DC, 1985, US Government Printing Office.

US Department of Health and Human Services: Health: United States, 1980 with prevention profile, Hyattsville, Md, 1980, National Center for Health Statistics.

US Department of Health and Human Services: Health: United States, DHHS Pub. No PHS 85-1232, Washington, DC, 1985, US Government Printing Office.

US Department of Labor, Bureau of Statistics: Handbook of labor statistics, Bulletin 2217, Washington, DC, 1985, US Government Printing Office.

US Department of Labor, Women's Bureau: Facts on women workers, Washington, DC, 1985, US Government Printing Office.

Ustby R: Pre-employment back x-rays—an unnecessary practice: try another approach, Occup Health Nurs 29:20, 1981.

Wright S: Operating room pollution—or is it contamination? AANA 47:313, 1979.

BIBLIOGRAPHY

Centers for Disease Control: Annual summary 1983: reported morbidity, mortality in the US, MMWR 54:54, 1983.

Rytina N and Bianchi S: Occupational reclassification and changes in distribution by gender, Monthly Labor Review 104:11, 1984.

Selby TL: Nurses care for prisoners with AIDS, Am Nurse 20:1, 1987.

Yu T and others: Low-back pain in industry: an old problem revisited, J Occup Med 26:517, 1984.

CHAPTER

18

Women's Health Care in the Reproductive Years

Sherrie Bernat
Linda Snell
Lisa Monagle

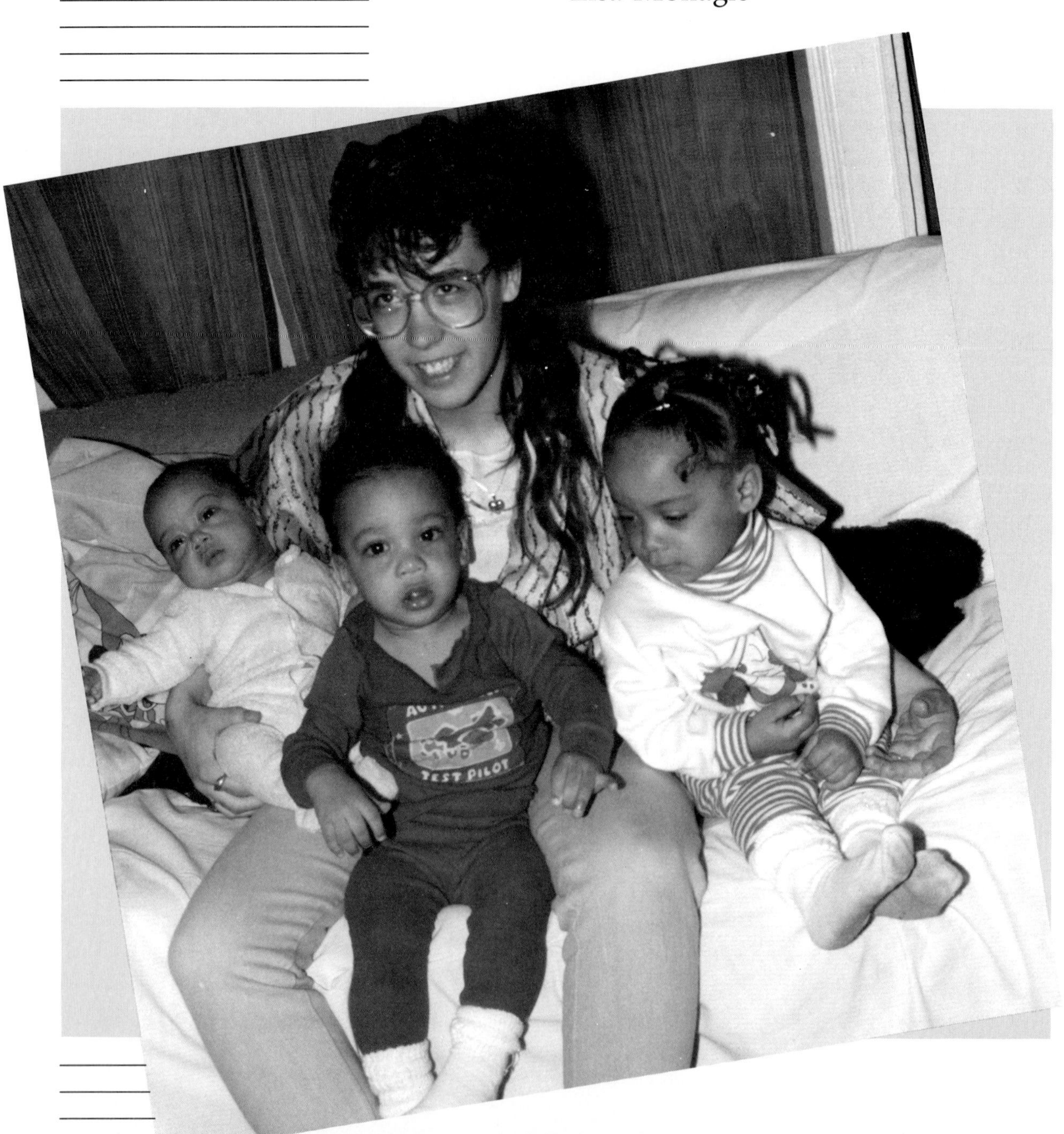

CHAPTER OUTLINE

Prenatal care
- Diagnosis of pregnancy
- Initiation of prenatal care
- Health education of the prenatal client
- Common discomforts of pregnancy
- Postpartum care

High-risk pregnancy
- Diabetes
- Pregnancy-induced hypertension
- Low birth weight
- Teenage pregnancy
- Role of the community health nurse in high-risk pregnancy

Contraception

Abortion
- Historical perspective
- Impact of abortion practices on health outcome
- Surgical methods of abortion

Trends in birthing practices
- Historical perspective
- Current birth settings and health care providers

Summary

OBJECTIVES

After completing this chapter, the reader should be able to:

1. Identify goals of prenatal care on an individual, community, and worldwide level.
2. Offer guidance, support, and information to the normal pregnant client regarding routine prenatal care, health education, pregnancy discomforts, and the postpartum period.
3. Identify the role of the community health nurse in high-risk pregnancy, including knowledge of risk factors for poor pregnancy outcomes and knowledge of common high-risk pregnancy complications such as diabetes, pregnancy-induced hypertension, and intrauterine growth retardation.
4. Discuss the individual and community implications of teenage pregnancy and provide specific counseling to the pregnant adolescent regarding diet and life-style.
5. Discuss with clients the different contraceptive method options, taking into consideration the woman's unique situation.
6. Identify trends in abortion practices, explain various surgical procedures used, and identify those at low and high risk for abortion complications.
7. Identify contemporary trends in birthing practices and discuss with childbearing clients the increased choices available to them.

THE COMMUNITY HEALTH NURSE'S GOAL is the coordination of health care activities with the needs, goals, and resources of the whole community. In the area of prenatal care and the health care of women in their reproductive years, national health priorities have been to provide improved care to the medically underserved population, train and use nurse clinicians, promote research, and develop effective methods of educating the general public about preventive health care. In addition to community health nurses' interest and role in activities addressing national health priorities and wellness promotion, they also observe health patterns and programs functional at the community or societal level. Accordingly, this chapter addresses the community health nurse's role in prenatal care, pregnancy complications and risk factors associated with poor maternal and fetal pregnancy outcomes, how to offer contraceptive guidance, and historical and current societal trends in women's health care, including abortion practices and birthing alternatives in the United States.

PRENATAL CARE

There are numerous educational, physical, and emotional needs of pregnant women and their families that can be considered universal. These prenatal concerns can be successfully addressed individually or in community and group settings. A major prenatal care guideline developed by the committee on maternal health care and family planning of the American Public Health Association states that "prenatal care services should be available, accessible, and acceptable to all pregnant women, and should respect individual differences" (Barnes, 1978).

The community health nurse needs to understand the goals of prenatal care on an individual, community, and worldwide level. The World Health Organization (WHO) defines maternity care as follows (Barnes, 1978):

> The object of maternity care is to ensure that every expectant and nursing mother maintains good health, learns the art of child care, has a normal delivery, and bears healthy children. Maternity care in the narrower sense consists of the care of the pregnant woman, her safe delivery, her post-natal care and examination, the care of her newly-born infant, and the maintenance of lactation. In the wider sense it begins much earlier with measures aimed to promote the health and well-being of the young people who are potential parents, and to help them to develop the right approach to family life and to the place of the family in the community. It should also include guidance in parent craft and in problems associated with infertility and family planning.

Community health nurses who know the needs of women on all levels can become catalysts in providing comprehensive prenatal, postpartum, and interconceptional nursing care. These forward-looking nurses have the satisfaction of knowing that their efforts have helped present and future generations achieve the highest level of wellness possible.

Diagnosis of Pregnancy

Before the prenatal care plan can be formulated and implemented, it is essential to obtain an accurate diagnosis of pregnancy, since most women come to their health care provider's office or clinic with only suspicions that they are pregnant. The most common subjective (or presumptive) signs of pregnancy are an absence of menstruation, breast tenderness, enlargement, or both, changes in skin pigmentation, nausea and vomiting, fatigue, frequent urination, and increased vaginal discharge. Although each of these symptoms could be caused by something other than pregnancy, taken together they represent a classic set of pregnancy symptoms.

Objective (or probable) signs of pregnancy include positive serum tests, urine pregnancy tests, or both, uterine and abdominal enlargement, and palpation of a fetal outline. The presence of fetal heart sounds, fetal movement, and sonographic evidence of a fetus are considered positive signs of pregnancy. Any woman experiencing presumptive, probable, or positive signs of pregnancy should receive immediate medical attention so that a definitive diagnosis can be made and prenatal care begun.

Initiation of Prenatal Care

The first step in developing a comprehensive prenatal plan of care is to take a detailed health history. The health history provides important facts that can help date the pregnancy, screen for high-risk factors, and identify educational needs specific to the individual woman. For example, a smoker needs to be informed of the risks to her fetus and provided with help by the appropriate resources so that she can stop smoking. A woman who previously gave birth to a baby with a birth defect or has a family history of birth defects should be referred immediately for genetic counseling and given extra emotional support.

The second step in client assessment is a thorough physical examination. Vital signs need to be recorded. The thyroid, heart, lungs, breasts, abdomen, pelvis, and extremities need to be thoroughly examined to determine the woman's current health status and to provide a baseline in case problems in a body system develop later. The pelvic examination can diagnose any vulvar, vaginal, or cervical abnormalities. The size of the uterus is assessed and compared with the anticipated size based on the last menstrual period. The pelvic diameters are measured to determine whether the size of the pelvis is adequate for vaginal delivery. If the pregnancy is advanced 12 weeks or more, the uterus is palpable abdominally. Fundal height can then be measured to indirectly determine fetal size and fetal growth. In addition, at 12 weeks fetal heart sounds can be heard with a fetal Doppler scanner. If the pregnancy has progressed 20 weeks or more, the health care provider assesses the position and presentation of the fetus.

Nägele's rule is the most commonly used method to determine the estimated date of confinement (EDC), which is the approximate date of delivery based on the first day of the last menstrual period (LMP). To find the EDC using Nägele's rule, subtract three months from the date of the LMP, and add seven days. A pregnancy date wheel (see Figure 18-1) is an invaluable aid in determining the EDC and the approximate gestational age of each woman throughout her pregnancy. By placing the line labeled FIRST DAY OF LAST PERIOD on the proper date, the EDC and weeks of gestation are immediately available.

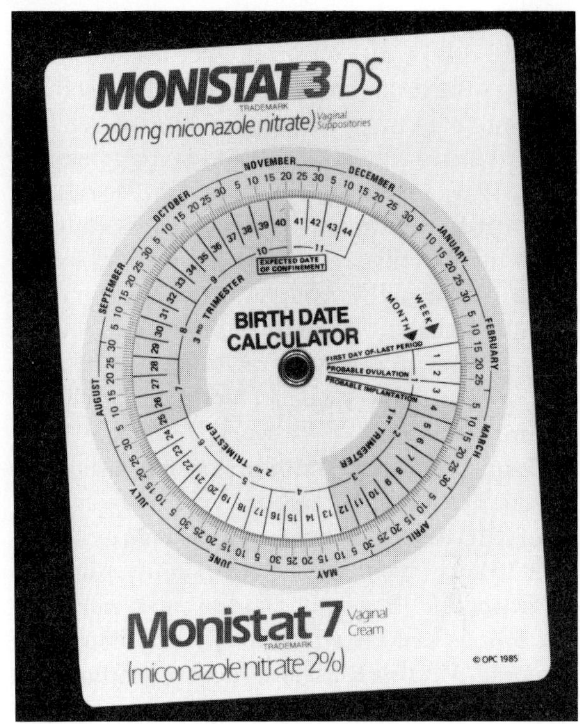

FIG. 18-1. Birth date calculator. Courtesy Ortho Pharmaceutical Corp.

Although Nägele's rule and the pregnancy wheel are helpful aids in dating a pregnancy, they must be used in conjunction with objective physical findings. Women should start prenatal care in the first trimester of pregnancy to obtain the best gestational age estimations. If uterine size is inconsistent with the woman's dates, an ultrasound examination is warranted to determine gestational age of the fetus more accurately and to rule out such conditions as multiple gestation, fetal anomaly, and intrauterine growth retardation. If menstrual periods are often irregular or if the LMP was abnormal, using the LMP for dating the pregnancy is more likely to be inaccurate than when the periods are regular. Ultrasound examinations done for determination of gestational age are more reliable when done in the first 20 weeks of pregnancy. Ideally two or three examinations are performed to provide a more accurate clinical picture.

Certain laboratory tests are essential in the evaluation. The following box describes a typical protocol of tests perfomed throughout a normal pregnancy. A complete blood cell count is done to check for the presence of anemia and infection. The mother's blood type is obtained to determine potential ABO or Rh blood incompatibility with the fetus. If the woman is Rh negative, a Coombs' test is done initially and several times throughout pregnancy to determine whether she is developing antibodies against the baby's blood type. The mother is also screened for syphilis, gonorrhea, and chlamydia. Black women should be tested for sickle cell trait. A rubella titer should be drawn. If the results indicate that the woman is not immune to rubella, she is cautioned to be especially careful to avoid exposure to children with German measles in her first trimester of pregnancy and is encouraged to receive a rubella vaccination immediately after delivery. A Papanicolaou (Pap) smear is performed to rule out cervical cancer. A urinalysis is performed to screen for kidney disease and urinary tract infections. Glucose tests are ideally ordered at a specified point in the pregnancy, with the 50 g glucose screen being most useful in identifying gestational diabetes between 24 and 30 weeks' gestation. Finally, nonstress tests are commonly performed from 40 weeks' gestation until the baby is delivered to further evaluate the adequacy of the placental functioning. Although this is a typical protocol of laboratory tests during pregnancy, women with specific problems should have additional tests ordered at intervals appropriate for their needs.

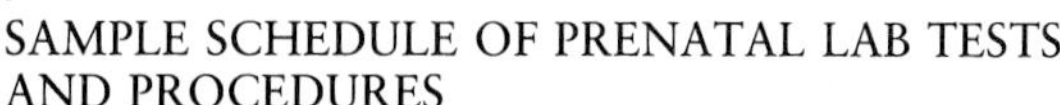

SAMPLE SCHEDULE OF PRENATAL LAB TESTS AND PROCEDURES

At the first prenatal visit a detailed health history should be taken and initial laboratory examinations should be done, including a complete blood cell count, blood typing, rubella, syphilis, and gonorrhea cultures, a Papanicolaou (Pap) smear, urinalysis, a urine culture and sensitivity, and sickle-cell screening for black women.

At 16 weeks an ultrasonographic examination should be done, and serum α-fetoprotein levels should be checked if desired (screening test for neural tube defects in the fetus.)

At 24 to 30 weeks 50 g glucose should be administered to the client to screen for gestational diabetes.

At 26 weeks screening for Rh antibodies should be repeated in Rh-negative mothers.

At 28 weeks Rh_o (d) immune globulin (RhoGAM) should be administered intramuscularly to Rh negative mothers, and a complete blood cell count should be done on all mothers.

At 36 weeks antibody screening should be repeated for Rh negative mothers, gonorrhea and chlamydia cultures should be examined, and weekly pelvic examinations should begin and continue until delivery.

At 38 weeks serum estriol and human placental lactogen levels should begin being checked weekly until delivery.

At 40 weeks a nonstress test should begin being administered weekly until delivery.

For the first 32 weeks of pregnancy, a pregnant woman is customarily checked at four-week intervals. From 32 to 36 weeks gestation she is usually evaluated at two-week intervals. After 36 weeks gestation a pregnant woman needs to be seen weekly until delivery. At each visit her weight, blood pressure, and fundal height are recorded. Figure 18-2 shows the approximate fundal height throughout the 40 weeks of pregnancy. A urine sample is checked at each appointment for the presence of sugar and protein. Spilling of glucose could indicate the presence of gestational

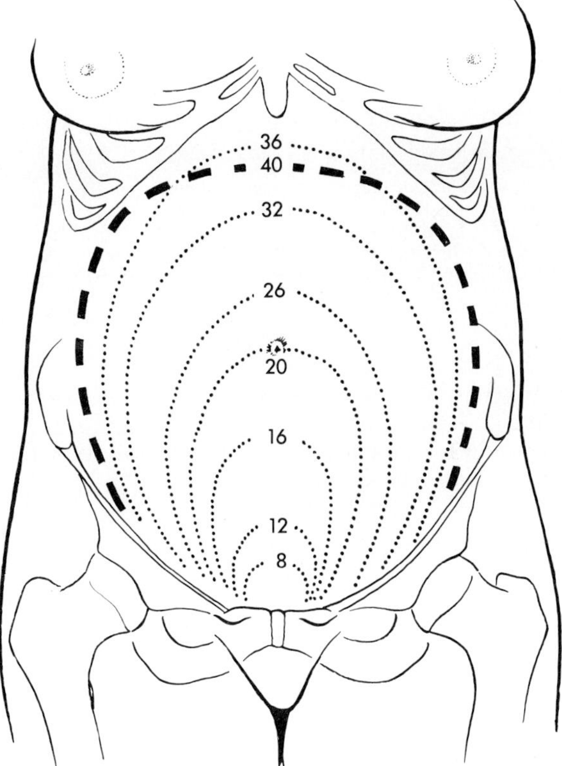

FIG. 18-2. Uterine placement weeks 8 to 40.

diabetes, whereas protein in the urine could be a sign of developing preeclampsia. Fetal heart rate, pattern of fetal movement, fetal position, and presentation are assessed. In the last four weeks of pregnancy a vaginal examination is performed weekly to determine the softening, dilatation, and effacement of the cervix, along with the descent of the baby's head into the maternal pelvis. Danger signs during pregnancy include a cessation or decrease in fetal movement, vaginal bleeding, headaches, edema, visual disturbances, epigastric pain, leg pain, fever or chills, fluid leaking from the vagina, abdominal pain, sudden increase in blood pressure, sudden increase in weight, and abnormal or absent fetal heart sounds (normal range is 120 to 160 beats per minute heard after 12 weeks). Any pregnant woman who experiences one or more of these symptoms must be immediately evaluated to determine whether a problem is developing so that the appropriate treatment regimen can be started.

Health Education of the Prenatal Client

Women are especially motivated to make positive changes in their behavior during pregnancy. Knowledgeable community health nurses are often in a position to help prenatal clients identify changes in life-style that would be positive. A therapeutic relationship between the nurse and the pregnant woman encourages the woman's efforts to provide the best possible prenatal environment for the growing fetus.

The community health nurse may encounter pregnant women suffering from malnutrition, anemia, pica, extreme fatigue, depression, lack of social support, and drug or alcohol abuse. Although these problems can occur in all social strata, they are primarily observed among poor women and, as a group of problems, represent a special challenge to the community health nurse. As part of the health education planning for each pregnant woman, the previously outlined problems should be investigated and either ruled out or incorporated into the overall mutually agreed on plan for improving the client's overall health.

First, the pregnant woman's diet is discussed. A nutritious diet is essential to maternal and fetal well-being. Prenatal vitamins with iron are particularly essential, since even an exemplary diet would fail to meet the increased iron demands during pregnancy. To accurately evaluate the diet of a pregnant woman, it is helpful to have her do a 24-hour diet recall at the first prenatal visit and periodically throughout her pregnancy. This enables the nurse to reinforce the proper food choices and make suggestions to increase any nutrients that are deficient. Dietary habits are sometimes difficult to assess because of cross-cultural miscommunication, personal biases, and the time-consuming nature of the diet history for the client

TABLE 18-1 Nutritional Requirements During Pregnancy

Nutrient	RDA	Best sources
Calories	2400	Meat, fish, poultry, fats, fruits, grains, legumes, and nuts
Protein	74 to 100 g	Meat, fish, poultry, eggs, milk, milk products, legumes, and grains
Calcium	1200 mg	Milk (all forms), yogurt, cheese, leafy green vegetables, clams, oysters, and almonds
Iron*	18 mg	Liver, meats, fish, poultry, whole grain and enriched cereals and breads, legumes cooked in an iron pan, leafy green vegetables, dried prunes and apricots, and raisins
Folic acid*	800 μg	Liver, yeast, leafy green vegetables, legumes, whole grains, fruits, and assorted vegetables
Pyridoxine (B)	2.5 mg	Wheat germ, meat, liver, whole grains, peanuts, soybeans, and corn

Modified from Worthington-Roberts B, Vermeersch J, and Williams S: Nutrition in pregnancy and lactation, St Louis, 1985, CV Mosby Co.

* It is recommended that pregnant women supplement their diets with iron, 30 to 60 mg per day and folic acid, 400 to 800 μg per day.

and the nurse. The nurse must avoid being judgmental. Open-ended questions that let the client provide information instead of questions with only yes or no answers give the nurse a better background with which to work. The 24-hour recall is a relatively simple and accurate method that can provide a peephole view into the pregnant client's dietary life. The client takes an average day that she considers normal for her and lists everything she ate or drank from rising to retiring. The diet of a pregnant woman should include a variety of foods from the basic four food groups. See Table 18-1 for the recommended dietary allowances for pregnant women.

If the nurse has developed a good rapport with the client, the client is more likely to be honest than to present an ideal, yet false, picture of her situation. The client's economic situation, proximity to shopping, kitchen facilities, amount of physical activity, job description, and stress and social pressures, as well as numbers and ages of other people with whom she lives also affect her eating habits. Perhaps the client is the last to sit down to a meal and she eats only after everyone else has been served and has eaten. Sometimes this cultural habit can be broken by making the family aware that while this woman is pregnant she must have adequate quantities and types of food that help her stay healthy and have a healthy baby. She may live alone or with her other children and may not be motivated to fix nutritious meals for herself. Instead she may fix simple meals that children enjoy but that are often high in carbohydrates and fats and low in protein and vitamins she and her children require. Preparing nutritious meals can be especially difficult if her partner's emotional and financial support are available only intermittently.

The nurse may suggest easily prepared meals such as macaroni and cheese, chili con carne with rice, and hearty soups that use less expensive cuts of meat or dried beans as a source of protein. The children may enjoy these meals as well. The client can be reminded that her complete nutrition need not come from only three meals a day. This may give her a different perspective on her eating habits, and she may use nutritious snacks between meals to supplement her diet. Peanut butter on whole wheat crackers is a nutritiously portable high-protein snack that will help her fulfill daily requirements. If the woman has iron deficiency anemia, foods high in iron can be discussed and the nurse can suggest how those foods can be easily increased given the family's usual dietary habits.

All pregnant women should be asked whether they experience any unusual food cravings during their pregnancy. Unusual cravings include food and nonfood items such as flour, starch, refrigerator frost, and red clay. Although women may be embarrassed to discuss these cravings a nonjudgmental approach on the part of the community health nurse is helpful in dealing with these problems, which are highly associated with anemia and malnutrition.

The overweight client needs particular care and guidance in food selection. She may not be aware of how much she actually eats or may feel the need to hide actual quantities of food she eats. The nurse must be forthright and nonjudgmental without denying the client her privacy in encouraging less fatty, high-calorie foods and more nutritious, low-calorie foods to substitute for those the client normally eats, such as 2% milk instead of whole milk or an apple instead of a piece of cake. She may also need help arranging her food budget so that she can afford the more expensive, leaner cuts of meat and poultry.

Pregnant women who lack economic resources should be referred to the Women, Infants, and Children (WIC) program. WIC is a supplemental food program run by the U.S. Department of Agriculture for the benefit of pregnant women, nursing mothers, infants, and children. Research has demonstrated that women participating in this program give birth to babies with significantly higher birth weights (Metcoff and others, 1985). Families in economic need should also be referred to the food stamp program. It is essential for the community health nurse to be familiar with local sources of help such as food banks so that clients can be advised appropriately to receive the help they need.

Weight gain is an important indicator of a pregnant woman's nutritional status. The pattern of weight gain is also significant. A gain of 2 to 4 pounds during the first trimester is optimum. After the first three months a gain of ¾ to 1 pound per week is reasonable. Ideal weight gain is partly dependent on prepregnancy weight. Although a gain of 25 pounds is a suitable goal for women of ideal weight, underweight women should gain more. They would aim for a weight at term equal to 120% of their ideal weight. Overweight women should not go on a reduction diet during pregnancy. However, they can safely gain less weight than thinner women. A gain of approximately 16 pounds is believed to be most appropriate for obese women (Rosso, 1985). When weight gain is either delayed or excessive, further nutritional counseling is required.

Pregnancy is the optimal time to discuss client preferences regarding infant feeding. Information regarding the superiority of breast milk over formula, as well as the advantages and disadvantages of breast- and bottle-feeding, should be provided. Once the feeding method is chosen, the community health nurse can be instrumental in providing support and instruction for the method of choice. Written materials are valuable for reference. Mothers choosing to breast-feed often find referrals to groups such as LaLeche Leauge helpful in providing emotional support and practical information about breast-feeding. Family members or friends who have successfully nursed infants are also invaluable resources for the new breast-feeding mother.

It is essential to instruct each pregnant woman regarding the use of alcohol, tobacco, and drugs during pregnancy. It is widely recognized that alcohol adversely affects the fetus. Babies born to alcoholic mothers may be born with fetal alcohol syndrome, a syndrome accompanied by physical defects and mental disabilities including mental retardation. Since it is not known what amount of alcohol is safe, abstaining from alcohol during pregnancy is recommended. Clients identified as alcohol or drug abusers should be strongly encouraged to join treatment programs. Ideally, the community health nurse is aware of such community resources and can reinforce the client with information and support during the nurse's regularly scheduled contact with the client.

Numerous studies have been conducted regarding the adverse effects of smoking on the fetus (Allen and Ries, 1985; Davidson, 1981; Diebel, 1980). Smokers give birth to low–birth weight babies and have a higher incidence of miscarriages and stillbirths than do nonsmokers. Ill effects persist after birth with increased rates of sudden infant death syndrome and respiratory disease in children born to smoking families. A major goal of nursing care of a pregnant woman who smokes is to provide emotional support for the client attempting to cut down or quit smoking. Referrals should be made to the American Cancer Society or other appropriate local agencies that provide smoking cessation information and programs.

Most drugs cross the placenta and have an effect on the developing fetus. During the first trimester the fetus is particularly susceptible to damage from drug exposure. Women must be counseled to avoid drug use (including many over-the-counter drugs) during pregnancy.

Expectant parents often have concerns regarding sexual activity. In a normal pregnancy, intercourse is considered safe throughout gestation. Couples should refrain from intercourse if there is any vaginal bleeding, leaking of amniotic fluid, pain, or signs of labor. Women who have had a history of repeated miscarriages or premature labor are sometimes advised to avoid sexual activity for part or all of their pregnancy.

Other frequent areas of concern to pregnant women include exercise, hygiene, travel, and working during pregnancy. Moderate exercise should be encouraged throughout pregnancy. Walking and swimming are especially suitable. Exercise should not be pursued to the point of pain or severe shortness of breath. Sports requiring a good sense of balance such as skiing, horseback riding, and skating should be avoided as the pregnancy progresses because the woman's center of gravity shifts and she is more prone to falls.

It is permissible for pregnant women to take a tub bath unless the membranes are leaking. The main concern is that she does not fall in the tub and can lift herself out of the bathtub in the last weeks of pregnancy. Douching should be avoided. There is no available treatment for the prevention of stretch marks. Keeping the skin supple with cocoa butter or other moisturizers is a comfort measure. Women can be reassured that stretch marks fade in the months after delivery.

Travel is generally unrestricted during a normal pregnancy. Several helpful guidelines include frequent stops for changes in position to prevent venous stasis, avoiding remote areas where medical care would be unavailable, and staying within an hour of the health care provider during the last month of pregnancy in case labor should begin.

The decision to continue working during pregnancy needs to be considered carefully by a woman and her health care provider. Generally a woman experiencing an uncomplicated pregnancy can continue working until delivery. The exposure of the woman to chemicals, heavy lifting, or any number of other possible hazards may necessitate a leave from work or a transfer to another position within the employment setting. The community health nurse can offer emotional support to the pregnant woman undergoing employment changes caused by her pregnancy while referring her to appropriate agencies to determine the benefits to which she is entitled.

Fatigue, depression, lack of social support, and lack of information about pregnancy and delivery might be observed among some of the pregnant women with whom the community health nurse has contact. Childbirth education classes can be helpful to all women but often are not readily available to those who are socioeconomically deprived. These classes can be especially useful as a source of social support and information. These classes can provide information about pregnancy, labor, delivery, the postpartum period, infant care, and hospital procedures and may decrease anxiety. A group setting is particularly useful for women to learn from one another about neighborhood resources and infant care and for generally supporting one another in their pregnancy complaints and concerns. During the pregnancy the most effective education is in peer group sessions when experienced mothers can share with others. Attendance of the father is of value in sharing open discussion, answering his questions, and decreasing his anxiety. Most hospitals have childbirth classes free to their clients or for a small fee that can be waived as the case warrants. Other educational programs such as smoking cessation, weight reduction, improved nutrition, and stress alleviation are also available in most areas.

Common Discomforts of Pregnancy

Unfortunately, pregnancy is often a time of multiple discomforts. Although these discomforts are generally not serious, they can tax the coping ability of the woman and disrupt her life-style. With knowledgeable health counseling, most women can help minimize their symptoms to tolerable levels. Stressing the temporary nature of most of the discomforts is often helpful.

Nausea with or without vomiting is probably the most common discomfort of pregnancy. It affects as many as 80% of all pregnant women. Despite its common title of morning sickness, it can occur at any time of day. Usually nausea and vomiting taper off after the first trimester. Eating small, frequent meals often helps relieve symptoms. Women should be advised to avoid fried, greasy, and spicy foods. Eating dry crackers or toast before rising from bed helps some women. Persistent vomiting resulting in weight loss of 10 pounds or more, dehydration, or both need to be evaluated further by the woman's health care provider.

Headaches are common in the first trimester of pregnancy. Although headaches in the last trimester can be a sign of pregnancy-induced hypertension, headaches early in pregnancy are generally not considered ominous. Acetaminophen often provides adequate pain relief. Persistent, severe headaches during pregnancy should be evaluated by a neurologist.

Most pregnant women notice increased urinary frequency, especially during the first trimester when the growing uterus puts pressure on the bladder. As the uterus rises out of the pelvis in the second trimester, frequency often abates somewhat. Urinary frequency increases again during the last trimester as the fetal head descends into the pelvis and presses against the bladder. Although urinary frequency is physiologic in most cases, each woman must be assessed for symptoms of urinary tract infection such as pain and burning while voiding. Many women also notice increased vaginal discharge during pregnancy. Although this symptom is also physiologic, any foul odor, itching, or irritation is cause for further assessment. Vaginal yeast infections are especially common in pregnancy.

The increased levels of estrogen and progesterone play a part in many discomforts of pregnancy. High progesterone levels tend to relax smooth muscle, thus promoting constipation and varicose veins. As the uterus increases in size and weight, the increased pressure further accentuates these problems. Often the use of support hose and frequent resting with the legs elevated can relieve varicose veins. Increased activity, fluids, and fiber-rich foods can help alleviate constipation. It is important to prevent constipation, since it is the most frequent cause of hemorrhoids, another common discomfort of pregnancy.

Backaches can occur as the growing uterus places increasing amounts of strain on the lower back. Women need to be instructed in proper posture and body mechanics to avoid back injury. Wearing low-heeled support shoes and regular gentle abdominal-toning exercises can also help minimize back symptoms.

The expanding uterus also puts pressure on the diaphragm, causing shortness of breath. This discomfort generally decreases somewhat during the last few weeks of pregnancy as the baby moves farther down into the mother's pelvis.

Pressure on the stomach promotes gastric reflux leading to heartburn. Pregnant women should avoid greasy, spicy foods and heavy meals. Small, frequent meals are usually better tolerated. Eating just before bedtime is another frequent cause of gastric reflux. Antacids can be used as a last resort in the smallest effective dose. Baking soda and other antacids high in sodium should be avoided.

The uterine ligaments often spasm under the stress of supporting the increased uterine weight, causing a moderate to severe "catching" sensation. These spasms (referred to as "ligament pain") seem to increase in severity with each successive pregnancy. Women should be reassured that the pain does not affect the fetus in any way, nor does it contribute to maternal morbidity. Although there is no specific treatment of these spasms, the avoidance of heavy lifting and sudden position changes often minimizes the painful episodes.

Leg cramps are another common discomfort of pregnancy. Massage and gentle stretching of the muscle are often effective in relieving the cramp. Calcium supplementation has also been found helpful in preventing leg cramps.

During the last two months of pregnancy the uterus begins mild, irregular contractions in preparation for labor. These Braxton Hicks contractions are generally not painful, and most pregnant women just need reassurance that their pregnancy is progressing normally.

Postpartum Care

Many women in preparing for the birth of their baby do not think beyond the pregnancy or birth because of a variety of factors. Perhaps the pregnancy was unplanned. Perhaps the mother is financially unable to prepare for the infant. Perhaps she is denying the reality of the childbirth and subsequent parenting role thrust on her. Teenagers in particular have difficulty planning for the future or relating their present activities to future consequences. The nurse can help the mother plan ahead for the postpartum period.

The mother's physical needs in the postpartum period need to be considered. The nurse can explain about lochia, which lasts for several weeks and gets progressively lighter, and tell the new mother that she will need sanitary supplies for this. The nurse can explain about the excessive thirst and perspiration the mother will experience, since this is one mechanism her body has of getting rid of extra fluid she has retained during her pregnancy. If the mother's breasts become sore, suggested comfort measures may include cold cloths and tight bras if she is bottle feeding, or warm soaks and more frequent nursings if she is breast-feeding. Many women are not prepared for the extreme fatigue that accompanies the immediate postpartum period. The new mother needs help at home if possible. She needs someone to assume the household chores and tasks while she sleeps and takes care of her new baby and her own physical needs. The nurse can help her decide who that person should be, a family member, a friend, a neighbor, or the baby's father. The new mother needs someone to "mother" her if at all possible, at least for the first postpartum week. She also needs to eat nutritious meals, especially if she is nursing. The best diet is to continue her pregnancy diet with vitamin and iron supplements for several months so that she can regain her strength and nourish her baby properly. The mother may need help acquiring equipment for the baby, such as a crib, diapers, blankets, and baby clothes. If laundry facilities are not readily available, the mother will need a supply of disposable diapers for emergencies or for everyday use.

It is important for the new mother to develop an attachment to her baby. As the nurse assesses her postpartum situation in the home, she must observe the mother interacting with her child and encourage a loving attitude. The mother should be encouraged to hold her new baby as often as she wants and as the baby needs to be held. Babies need to feel the mother close to them and to have their needs met readily so that they will become acquainted with the mother and begin to trust her. The nurse should encourage and praise the mother in her efforts to stroke her baby and talk or sing to her baby. The quicker the mother develops a feeling of closeness to her baby, the better her attempts at mothering will be. Adjusting to a new infant is difficult under the most ideal circumstances, but when the mother starts to love her baby the job becomes easier. Occasionally the mother develops postpartum blues with symptoms of crying, sadness, anorexia, and sleeplessness. If this appears to interfere with the mother's handling of and caring for the baby or lasts more than two weeks, the mother must be referred to her medical caregiver for attention. She may just be exhausted and need more help at home or, more rarely, may be developing postpartum depression, which requires medical attention.

It is important for the mother to interact with other mothers and babies. Mothers learn a great deal from one another about community resources, baby sitters, and childrearing practices. If she does not have friends in her neighborhood or a social circle in which she can meet other new mothers, there are parent support groups to which a mother or both parents may belong. Depending on the community, a partial list of these agencies would include the following:

1. International Childbirth Education Association
2. American Society for Psychoprophylaxis in Obstetrics/Lamaze Parent Group
3. LaLeche League
4. Parents Anonymous
5. Mothers of Twins
6. Church or temple women's groups

HIGH-RISK PREGNANCY

In 1977 the U.S. Public Health Service established a goal of only nine infant deaths per 1000 live births by the year 1990. Infant mortality and maternal mortality have been declining steadily for many years, but the 1990 goal currently seems unattainable as the speed of decline has slowed to an imperceptible pace in the past few years.

Maternal mortality, defined as the number of deaths for any cause during the pregnancy cycle per 100,000 live births, has declined to 7.9 deaths per 100,000 live births from 29.1 in 1966 and 83.3 in 1950 (Romney and others, 1981). In 1982 the decline included a drop in maternity deaths from abortion as more states legalized abortion and techniques became safer. Persisting causes of maternal mortality, however, are hypertensive disorders (21%), infection (18%), hemorrhage (14%), and other chronic diseases such as cardiac disease and diabetes mellitus (46%) (U.S. National Center for Health Statistics, 1982).

Infant mortality, defined as the number of deaths at less than 1 year of age per 1000 live births, is falling, but the decline is limited by the prematurity rate, which has remained constant since 1950. The decline is mostly attributable to a reduction in neonatal mortality, which is the number of deaths before 28 days of life per 1000 live births. Leading causes of neonatal and infant mortality are congenital anomalies, respiratory distress syndrome, and problems related to preterm labor and low birth weight (LBW). Infant mortality varies also across racial groups. Infant mortality rates in 1984 for blacks were 18.4 deaths per 1000 live births and for whites were 9.4 deaths per 1000 live births (Topics, 1987). This obvious disparity in pregnancy outcome among racial groups is mediated by factors such as socioeconomic status, maternal education, health insurance coverage, and access to prenatal infant health care. A variety of ways exist to improve maternal and infant outcomes, including good prenatal care, nutrition, and care of high-risk pregnant women such as those with diabetes, pregnancy-induced hypertension, and suspected intrauterine growth retardation. Barriers to implementing these factors include the high cost of health care, the expense of developing new programs, and problems in motivating clients to accept and participate in the care provided.

Diabetes

Before the discovery of insulin in 1921, diabetic mothers and their infants often died during pregnancy, in labor, or during the postpartum period. In pregnant women with diabetes, maternal mortality was 30% and fetal mortality was 65% (Hellman and Pritchard, 1971). Today mortality of infants born to diabetic mothers is 10% to 20% and maternal mortality is less than 1%. This encouraging statistic is partly due to the fact that more is known about diabetes and how pregnancy and diabetes are related. The important step in securing good health in pregnant women is to control their blood sugar. As the mean blood sugar approaches normal, infant mortality rates decline.

Diabetes is diagnosed on the basis of client symptoms and laboratory tests showing elevated glucose levels in urine and blood. Diabetes is divided into types depending on the age of onset, the length of time the person has had it, and the severity of sequelae accompanying the diabetes as shown in Table 18-2. The common signs of diabetes are polyuria (frequent urination), polydipsia (excessive thirst), weight loss, and excessive hunger.

During a normal pregnancy the nondiabetic woman experiences changes in her metabolism caused by the insulin antagonism of the placental hormones and altered insulin use. The diabetic woman also experiences these changes and most likely must alter her insulin, exercises, and diet to keep a normal balance.

Diabetes that develops during pregnancy is called gestational diabetes. Gestational diabetes develops in approximately 2% to 3% of all pregnant women. Women at risk for gestational diabetes include the following (Public health, 1986):

1. Women who are at least 25 years of age
2. Obese women, especially those older than 25 years of age
3. Women who have a family history of diabetes or gestational diabetes
4. Women who previously had large infants, infants with congenital anomalies, or stillborn babies

Diabetes is a cause of a large number of adverse pregnancy outcomes. The longer a woman has been a diabetic, the more she and her infant are at risk, especially if she has had poor control of her disease over the years. Problems for which women are at risk related to diabetes in pregnancy can be severe. They are more prone to hypertension in pregnancy, especially if they are diabetic before pregnancy. Diabetic women have stillbirths 1% to 4% of the time, and 5% of babies born live to diabetic mothers have congenital anomalies. A greater percentage of babies are overweight with increased body length and fat, increased spleen and liver size, respiratory problems, or hypoglycemia in the first few days of life. These women are at increased risk for delivering prematurely or having problems with a vaginal delivery such as shoulder dystocia or other birth trauma because of the large size of the infant.

The goals of management of the pregnant diabetic woman are universal goals that include a healthy mother, a normal fetus who will grow and develop normally, and prevention of future problems in the mother and child. The role of the nurse is to ensure appropriate care for women diagnosed as diabetics (either established or gestational); to ensure postpartum follow-up and continuing care of women with established diabetes; to maintain good blood glucose control before pregnancy and throughout subsequent pregnancies; and to ensure postpartum follow-up of women with gestational diabetes to detect previously undiagnosed established diabetes.

Early diagnosis of pregnancy in the diabetic woman and early diagnosis of diabetes in pregnancy are important so that blood sugars can be controlled, diet can be adjusted, and complications can be prevented. Once gestational diabetes is diagnosed, the preventive health care related to this diagnosis can be implemented. Ultrasound is performed routinely throughout pregnancy to

TABLE 18-2 Conditions with Glucose Intolerance

Category	Characteristics
Diabetes mellitus	
Type I: insulin-dependent diabetes mellitus (IDDM)	Dependent on exogenous insulin to maintain life Ketosis-prone Usually occurs before age 40 but can occur at any age
Type II: non–insulin-dependent diabetes mellitus (NIDDM)	Not usually dependent on exogenous insulin to maintain life; under stress exogenous insulin may be needed transiently to prevent excessive catabolism Obesity common trait Ketosis-resistant Usually occurs after age 40 but can occur at a younger age Strong inheritance tendency Insulin receptor or postreceptor defects present
Secondary diabetes mellitus	Includes a variety of diseases that result in glucose intolerance severe enough to meet the diagnostic criteria of diabetes mellitus Associated with pancreatic insufficiency, endocrinopathies, and drug reactions
Gestational diabetes mellitus (GDM)	Glucose intolerance developing during pregnancy Associated with increased perinatal risk and fetal mortality Hormonal interplay and insulin resistance partly responsible Requires reclassification after pregnancy
Impaired glucose tolerance (IGT)	Usually asymptomatic Impaired glucose tolerance but not diabetes mellitus Associated with endocrinopathies, hepatic disease, drug reactions, stress, certain genetic disorders, and malignancy Increased susceptibility to atherosclerosis and neuropathic diseases May decompensate to overt diabetes at 4% to 5% per year

Modified from Kaye D and Rose LF, editors: Fundamentals of internal medicine, St. Louis, 1983, CV Mosby Co.

identify exact gestational age, growth patterns, gross malformations, or polyhydramnios (more than 2000 ml of amniotic fluid present in the uterus), which are common in diabetic pregnancies. The pregnant diabetic should be given nonstress tests (NSTs), contraction stress tests (CSTs), or both once or twice a week later in the pregnancy, depending on the individual mother, to determine fetal health.

The CST evaluates respiratory reserve of the uterine-placental-fetal function and transporting capacity of the placenta. With contractions it is normal to have a decreased blood flow to the placenta. Normal fetuses tolerate this well as they do in labor. If there is insufficient placental reserve, the test shows the fetal heart rate decelerating as the contraction ends. The NST includes using a fetal monitor to observe the baseline variability of the fetal heart rate (FHR) noting accelerations of the FHR with fetal movement. Accelerations imply an intact fetal central nervous system and autonomic nervous system with no intrauterine hypoxia. Loss of variability is significant, and follow-up would be a CST. CSTs are done weekly starting at 32 to 34 weeks depending on the individual mother. If the CST is positive, that is, if decelerations are observed, an amniocentesis might be done to check lung maturity, especially if the infant will be delivered before 37 weeks. In any case the baby may need to be delivered by cesarean section at the time of a positive CST. Timing and management of the delivery are crucial so that the infant is mature enough to be viable outside the uterus but not too postmature to risk deterioration of the placenta to the detriment of the fetus.

In the postpartum period the gestational diabetic may expect to revert to her prepregnancy nondiabetic state 90% of the time. The insulin-dependent diabetic needs less insulin postpartum for several days after the delivery, which can be confusing to the woman. She should understand that, if insulin is not required or a lower dose is used postpartally, this is not a permanent arrangement. Her insulin needs will return to her prepregnancy requirements in a few days.

Cooperation and agreeability of the pregnant woman and her family are of utmost importance for compliance. Her understanding of why certain things are required of her will help ensure compliance. The nurse may educate and counsel the client regarding changes in her health habits and may refer the client to other resources for educational materials or professional information on diabetes. Some agencies that help are listed in the box.

There are chapters of these organizations in larger cities and resources can be mailed to the client or the community health nurse for their use.

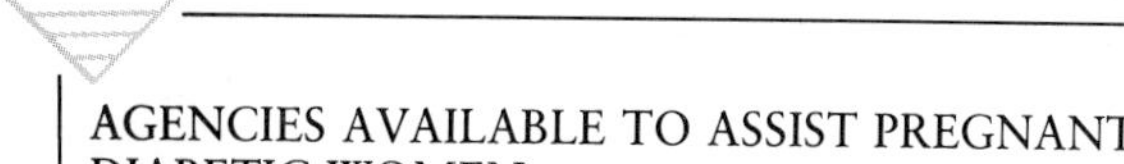

AGENCIES AVAILABLE TO ASSIST PREGNANT DIABETIC WOMEN

American Association of Diabetic Educators
American College of Obstetricians and Gynecologists
American Diabetic Association
Division of Diabetes Control, Center for Prevention Services
Communicable Disease Center
National Diabetes Information Clearing House
March of Dimes

Pregnancy-Induced Hypertension

Another complication of pregnancy is hypertension that develops during pregnancy. Young women, especially teenagers, black women, primiparas, those with a family history of preeclampsia, and those carrying multiple fetuses are at risk for pregnancy-induced hypertension (PIH).

PIH is a leading cause of maternal mortality in the United States. It occurs in 5% to 7% of pregnant women (Olds, London, and Ladeweig, 1984). It usually occurs in the third trimester of pregnancy after the twenty fourth week but can occur earlier, especially if the woman had hypertension that went undetected until pregnancy occurred. If untreated, PIH can progress to eclampsia, seizures, coma, and kidney failure. PIH may be detrimental to the fetus as well. If the mother has PIH, the circulation to her large organs, as well as the placenta, may be impaired. This can prevent the fetus from growing properly. PIH is associated with growth retardation, low birth weight, and preterm labor.

Women at risk for PIH need to be aware of the signs and symptoms related to it such as severe headaches, blurred vision, and swelling in the face, hands, or legs. These symptoms may indicate that PIH has already been present for some time and that the woman needs to be hospitalized for treatment.

The pregnant woman with PIH needs frequent prenatal visits. Her urine should be tested to detect proteinuria. Protein in the urine may indicate fluid imbalance, constriction of blood flow to kidneys with decreased renal plasma flow, and decreased glomerular filtration. Her reflexes should be checked to make sure she is not hyperreflexive. This is another indicator of a change in fluid balance causing increased intracellular sodium, decreased intracellular potassium, and muscle and nerve irritability. This and lower extremity edema can be early signs of PIH even before the blood pressure rises. A sustained blood pressure of 140/90 mm Hg or a rise in systolic pressure of 30 mm Hg, a diastolic rise of 15 mm Hg above her usual levels, or both are an indication of PIH. These levels must be observed on two separate occasions at least six hours apart.

Fetal evaluation of the client with PIH should be more aggressive at 30 weeks. Besides appointments for fetal heart tone and fundal height measures, the client may be scheduled for weekly or biweekly NSTs and CSTs; ultrasonographic examination to check for fetal growth retardation should be done as needed. The biophysical profile, a discussion of which follows, may also be used to assess fetal well-being. This profile is helpful in recognizing fetal asphyxia in utero and preventing poor outcomes. Women with high-risk pregnancies are at particular risk for increased perinatal mortality. With information received from the biophysical profile and other obstetric and maternal data, a proper management plan and delivery time may be formulated with a more positive fetal outcome (Manning and others, 1985).

Biophysical Profile Testing

A biophysical profile consists of an NST with the addition of four observations made by real-time ultrasound. A biophysical profile test includes the following:

1. Reactive NST—observations by real time of normal biophysical profile
2. Fetal breathing movements (one or more episodes of 30 seconds or more in 30 minutes)
3. Fetal movements (three or more discrete body or limb movements in 30 minutes)
4. Fetal tone (one or more episodes of extension with return to flexion)
5. Quantitation of amniotic fluid volume (one or more pockets of 1 cm or more in two perpendicular planes)

With this method a score of 2 (normal) or 0 (abnormal) is assigned to each observation. A score of 8 or 10 is normal; a score of 6 is considered questionable; and a score of 4 or less is abnormal.

The nurse can help the client understand the meaning of these tests and the importance of them in her individual case. The nurse will reinforce with the client how to assess fetal movement, which is another indicator of fetal well-being. One technique that can be used to explain to the mother how to count movements follows. On rising or at 9 A.M. she should begin to mentally count fetal movements, noting the time of the tenth movement. She will normally complete the count in several hours. If she has not felt the tenth movement by 6 P.M., if there is no movement all day, or if it takes longer each day to count the tenth movement, she should contact her prenatal care provider. Often the characteristics of the fetal movements are different for each baby. Some move 10 times in 30 minutes. Some move 10 times in eight hours. It is especially ominous if vigorous frequent movements suddenly stop. Counting fetal movements is an easy, noninvasive way to involve the client in her care and to help reassure her that the baby is doing well. The nature and frequency of the movements may change during the pregnancy. These movements can be described as kicks, swooshes, swishes, flips, and hiccups (Cohen, 1985).

Strong movements increase in frequency until about 37 weeks and then decrease until term. Weak movements that start occurring at 20 weeks decrease in frequency until 36 weeks and then increase until term. That strong movements decrease near term and weak ones increase does not

TABLE 18-3 Common Fetal Movements

Time (weeks)	Movement
7 to 10	Twitching and flutters
10 to 12	Independent limb movements
16	Combined limb, head, and torso movements
20 to 24	Respiratory effort
18 to 29	Increased movement and grander large movements
29 to 38	Peak movement can be seen
38 to 40	Decreased movement until delivery

signal fetal distress (Cohen, 1985). Table 18-3 gives an indication of the progression of fetal movements throughout the pregnancy as seen on sonogram by Birnholz, Stevens, and Faria (1978).

The previous chart can help nurses explain to the client what she is feeling and reassure her that what she feels is normal or clue her to an abnormality that needs medical attention. For example, some babies are active only in the early evening hours according to the mother, so having her count fetal movements from 9 AM to 6 PM when there are few would worry the mother needlessly. Some assurance that the fetus will have a unique rate and rhythm of movement should be made, but if the pattern changes dramatically, the mother should call her medical caregiver.

Finally, in the postpartum period the mother who had high blood pressure during her pregnancy may continue to have an elevated blood pressure. She may need close medical supervision, and a special diet or medication may be required. The client needs encouragement to follow the required regimen and reassurance that she can lead a normal life despite her medical problem.

Low Birth Weight

In the United States the incidence of low–birth weight infants (infants weighing less than 2500 g at birth) is becoming an increasingly important factor in the cause of infant deaths and has been identified as a principal risk factor in poor perinatal outcome. There is a broad-based public health and educational program being implemented to improve infant mortality by decreasing the numbers of low–birth weight infants. Low–birth weight infants still account for two thirds of the neonatal deaths in the United States (Behrman, 1985). Surviving low–birth weight babies are at greater risk than infants of normal birth weight for neurologic sequelae, congenital anomalies, and lower respiratory tract problems. Low birth weight results from preterm delivery and intrauterine growth retardation; often a combination of both is seen.

The cause of prematurity remains unknown and speculative. The mechanisms for maintaining and directing normal labor remain unknown as well. There are conditions associated with premature labor such as abruptio placentae, PIH, premature rupture of membranes, multiple pregnancy, and urinary tract infection. Some cases of preterm labor cannot be associated with any factor.

Causes of intrauterine growth retardation are usually related to circulation and function of the placenta, congenital problems of the fetus, or health and nutrition of the pregnant mother (Hobel, 1984). The most frequent problems associated with intrauterine growth retardation are hypertension, diabetes, and maternal cardiovascular problems that interfere directly or indirectly with oxygen and nutrition to the fetus. Risk factors associated with low–birth weight infants are listed in the following box. Many of these factors can be identified before pregnancy occurs with possible interventions at that time.

Age is a particularly important factor in the incidence of low–birth weight infants. Teenagers are at greater risk for this complication, particularly black mothers who are more likely to be teenagers than are other ethnic groups (Topics, 1987). Black women have a relative risk of giving

PRINCIPAL RISK FACTORS FOR LOW–BIRTH WEIGHT INFANT

DEMOGRAPHIC RISKS

Age (younger than 17 years of age or older than 34 years of age)

Low level of education

Low socioeconomic status

Race (black)

Unmarried

MEDICAL RISKS PREDATING PREGNANCY

Diseases such as diabetes and chronic hypertension

Genitourinary anomalies or surgery

Low weight for height

Maternal genetic factors such as low maternal weight at own birth

Nonimmune status for infections such as rubella

Parity (zero or more than four)

Poor obstetric history, including previous low–birth weight infant and multiple spontaneous abortions

MEDICAL RISK IN CURRENT PREGNANCY

Anemia or abnormal hemoglobin

Fetal anomalies

First-trimester or second-trimester bleeding

Hyperemesis

Hypertension, preeclampsia, or toxemia

Hypotension

Incompetent cervix

Isoimmunization

Multiple pregnancy

Oligohydramnios or polyhydramnios

Placental problems such as placenta previa or abruptio placentae

Poor weight gain

Selected infections such as symptomatic bacteriuria, rubella, and cytomegalovirus

Short interpregnancy interval

Spontaneous premature rupture of membranes

BEHAVIORAL AND ENVIRONMENTAL RISKS

Alcohol and other substance abuse

Diethylstilbestrol exposure and other toxic exposures, including occupational hazards

High altitude

Poor nutritional status

Smoking

EVOLVING CONCEPTS OF RISK

Cervical changes detected before onset of labor

Events triggering uterine contractions

Inadequate plasma volume expansion

Progesterone deficiency

Selected infections such as mycoplasmal or chlamydial disease

Physical and psychosocial stress

Uterine irritability

HEALTH CARE RISKS

Absent or inadequate prenatal care

Iatrogenic prematurity

birth to a low–birth weight infant that is more than double that of white women (Institute of Medicine, 1985). This is because Blacks are more likely to be of lower socioeconomic status and to have less education, less prenatal care, and more PIH, which all contribute to low–birth weight (MMWR, 1987). Infections such as rubella and urinary tract infections are related to low–birth weight and preterm labor. Relationships of intrauterine growth retardation and low–birth weight to infections caused by such organisms as *Mycoplasma* and *Chlamydia* are being studied.

Nutrition has a positive influence on birth weight but is negatively intertwined with socioeconomic status and age. Risks of having a low–birth weight baby increase if there is poor nutritional status of the mother before pregnancy, or inadequate food consumption, poor maternal weight gain, or drug abuse including alcohol and smoking during pregnancy.

Reducing the incidence of low–birth weight is a major public health concern. The nurse who knows the risk factors may have an impact on this by influencing the people with whom she comes in contact. She may counsel her clients who are teenagers and women of childbearing age to reduce their risks before they become pregnant. To this end, Behrman (1985) suggests that general health education in community schools be expanded to include the following:

1. Factors placing a woman and her fetus at risk, including low–birth weight
2. The importance of reducing risks before conception
3. The importance of early pregnancy diagnosis, early continuous care, and knowing locations for obtaining such services
4. The importance of immunizations for young women and the relationship of maternal infection to fetal risk
5. The value of altering health habits such as smoking and alcohol consumption
6. The vulnerability of the fetus to environmental and behavioral changes during the early weeks of pregnancy
7. The value of family planning services to prevent pregnancy in high-risk women or teenagers until they are ready, willing, and able in all aspects of their lives to bear children

Early prenatal care for the high-risk woman is essential to detect and manage behavioral risks such as smoking, nutritional inadequacies, and alcohol and substance abuse, to date pregnancy precisely, to prevent iatrogenic prematurity, and to detect intrauterine growth retardation or premature labor. Good early prenatal care of which the nurse is a part is less expensive socially and economically than care for a woman whose PIH or diabetes is uncontrolled or for a baby who is compromised. Costs of quality prenatal care are one tenth the cost of hospitalization for low–birth weight infants. Potential saving of public assistance funds in one year if the low–birth weight rate was reduced to 10% is $12,439,470. If the low–birth weight rate dropped to 9% by 1990, which is the goal of the surgeon general, the saving would more than double. Reductions of low–birth weight from 11.5% to 10% to 9%, the goal of the surgeon general, represent an ultimate 22% reduction on low–birth weight rates. This is a realistic goal that could be easily attained through quality prenatal programs directed toward high-risk women.

The community health nurse can supplement and augment the pregnant woman's ordinary prenatal care with much-needed counseling that will improve her pregnancy outcome. The nurse could do nutrition assessments and counseling, being careful to take into account the woman's ethnic and socioeconomic background. A psychosocial assessment may also be done for several purposes. It may reveal addictive behaviors of the client or of family members who affect the client. It can disclose how the client and family feel about the pregnancy; how prepared they are psychologically and financially for the baby; and what their plans are for the care of the infant if both parents work. If both parents are working and one will retire for the purpose of full-time child care, how will they cope? What support systems does the pregnant woman have—friends, family, neighbors, or the baby's father? If the woman needs public assistance or financial help for food or transportation to the prenatal clinic or child care, this need can be identified and proper referrals can be made.

The community health nurse is an integral part of this health team providing good prenatal care. She is an important liaison between the client and the prenatal care provider. The nurse may take referrals from a clinic or private source such as a family friend or neighbor. The nurse is in a position to assess the needs of the woman and her family in the home environment and make her own referrals as needed—to the nutritionist for dietary problems or the social worker for economic, financial, housing, or family support problems. If the community health nurse discovers wife or child abuse, there are child protection agencies and women's shelters where a woman may be taken. Clients may be directed to support groups provided by community agencies. Many women are socially isolated from family, friends, or other support persons. Parenting under these circumstances is extremely difficult, and the mother needs all the support available to her. Finally, the nurse may use other community agencies to secure maternity clothes, coats, shoes, baby clothes and equipment, bottles, a crib, formula, and diapers.

Teenage Pregnancy

The United States has the seventh highest teenage pregnancy rate in developed countries (Neinstein and Stewart, 1984). An upward trend in teenage pregnancy became evident in the 1950s. In the 1980s the rate has slowed but teenage pregnancy still represents a major health problem. Every year 1.1 million teenagers between the ages of 15 and 19 years become pregnant. Of these pregnancies, about half result in delivery. Why do so many teenagers become pregnant? Teenagers can be effective users of contraceptives, but many use them sporadically if at all. For many unmarried teenagers, the current trend is to continue the pregnancy and raise the infant, which presents a serious challenge to health professionals and in particular the community health nurse who is involved in the planning and provision of health care to pregnant teenagers and their families (Logan, 1986).

Adolescent pregnancy prevention is a goal of all health care providers, parents, and most adolescents. Most teenage pregnancies are unintentional. The decision to become sexually active is consciously or more often unconsciously made without regard to consequences. Nonmarital sexual activity has begun earlier than in years past, with 25% of 15-year-olds and 69% of 19-year-olds having had nonmarital sexual intercourse (Alan Guttmacher Institute, 1981). Teenage pregnancies result in live births 48% of the time and in abortion 38% of the time. The remaining 14% end in miscarriage or stillbirth (Dryfoos, 1982).

Adolescent pregnancy is a serious health problem because teenagers are at a higher risk than adult women for PIH, poor nutrition, complications during labor and delivery, premature delivery, maternal mortality, poor parenting skills, and having infants at higher risk of infant mortality and morbidity, including morbidity associated with low–birth weight such as mental retardation and neural abnormalities (Menkin, 1985). The pregnancy puts the teenager at an educational, psychologic, social, and economic risk for many years. These risks are great when the woman is younger than 18 years of age and even greater if she is younger than 16 years of age. Adolescence is a time of transition. Physical changes during adolescence, which are under hormonal control, include skeletal growth, increased muscle mass, and sexual development (Leppert, 1984). Pregnancy is also a time of great physiologic change, including changes in uterine muscle mass, breast size, and metabolism. When the physiologic changes of pregnancy are superimposed on the changes of adolescence, the demands are heavy and the fetus and mother may suffer.

Prevention is a key factor that can reduce almost all risks in a pregnant teenager. Primary prevention is the best strategy to employ. This involves developing programs to help prevent adolescent pregnancy, including helping young people learn decision making and how to make responsible choices regarding their life-styles and life goals and knowing resources in the community for supervised after-school social, athletic, and scholarly activities. The nurse can provide sex and family education to male and female teenagers and teach family planning to groups of teenagers at risk for pregnancy with information concerning their sexuality and decision making. Groups for parents of teenagers may be conducted in schools and community centers. The parents need to be actively involved in their children's lives and education, since they are directly affected if the teenagers' activities result in pregnancy. Most parents welcome direction and education regarding communication with their teenagers to help them grow into mature, responsible adults. Male and female adolescents should be targeted for outreach. Boys are often as misinformed as girls about sexuality and contraception and need to understand the important role they play in the prevention of pregnancy.

Once the teenager becomes pregnant and chooses to continue with the pregnancy, minimizing the risks to her health is the focus for the care of the client. The teenager needs to know what options are available to her in the community. Any mature decision-making skills that the teenager has learned as well as communicating openly with the teenager's parents if at all possible, are useful at this stage. Quality nurse-adolescent interaction is shown to be an important aspect of good contraceptive and prenatal compliance (Nathanson and Becker, 1984; Tyrer and Duarte, 1984).

Early and quality prenatal care is especially important for the teenager because of increased risks during the pregnancy for herself and the infant. This may be the teenager's first pelvic examination, and there is a good deal of needless anxiety surrounding this event. Ideally she will have a support person attending the visits with her such as her mother or sister. The community health nurse can encourage the teenager to arrange this. The nurse can introduce the teenager to fetal growth and development. This enhances the understanding of the importance of good nutrition and other preventive measures.

Good nutrition can be a particularly difficult habit for the pregnant teenager to develop. Fad and fast foods are often staples of her diet. These foods have low nutritive value and high salt, additive, and sugar content. Usually teenagers do not cook for themselves, but rather parents cook meals for them. This can be a positive aspect if the mothers of the teenagers are aware of or can be taught good nutritional habits. Family and friends should be enlisted to help the nurse and nutritionist encourage the teenager to eat well. Good nutrition is essential during pregnancy and especially during teenage pregnancy when both fetus and mother are growing. Table 18-2 (p. 451) has outlined recommended daily requirements of essential nutrients and their food sources to aid the community health nurse in her dietary counseling.

The job of the community health nurse is not finished with the delivery of the teenager's baby. Further prevention strategies are aimed at helping the teenager develop good parenting skills and adjust to the role of parent while balancing her own developmental tasks of growing into a mature, autonomous adult. The teenager needs sex education and contraceptive information for both herself and the baby's father, if he is present, to prevent further pregnancies. She needs help to see her responsibility as a parent while still maintaining some peer contact and, it is hoped, adjusting to family life and child care so that she can finish school. The community health nurse may work with the new mother by being with her, giving her suggestions, and praising her efforts so that she learns to handle the baby easily and gains confidence in her skills as a new mother.

The nurse encourages the teenager to take the child to a well-baby clinic for regular checkups, physical examinations, and immunizations. The new mother may need help obtaining child care during school hours, financial support from public assistance for herself and the new baby, or transportation to the child-care or well-baby clinic. The community health nurse refers the teenager as needed and acts as an advocate for her and her family in getting them through the system to proper agencies. It is hoped that this keeps the adolescent, her family, and her new baby as happy and healthy as possible.

Role of the Community Health Nurse in High-Risk Pregnancy

The role of the community health nurse in a high-risk pregnancy is important. The nurse must attend to certain aspects of the home care. Because of the close prenatal supervision required for the pregnant diabetic, the community health nurse encourages the mother to keep every appointment. The frequent visits can be stressful to the family if transportation is a problem, if child care is difficult to obtain, or if a woman works or attends school. If she is unemployed, she may be under economic pressure to skip appointments because of cost.

The diabetic mother may come home from her clinic appointment with instructions for home urine or blood glucose testing that may need clarification. The nurse should become familiar with the equipment used so that she can guide the mother in their correct use and meaning. If special equipment such as an insulin pump or an autolet for blood glucose testing is necessary, financial support may be needed. The pregnant woman may be newly insulin dependent and will need instruction in correct injection technique and changing sites every day. The nurse, having gained the confidence and trust of the pregnant woman, can stress the importance of continued prenatal visits and explain procedures that she might be experiencing. The woman's family must understand the importance of following outlined procedures so that they can support her in such needs as correct dietary intake, good hygiene, proper rest and exercise, and keeping clinic appointments. She may need help in scheduling her time so that she gets the rest she needs while caring for other small children. The pregnant diabetic may need suggestions as to whom she could call for help; her mother, a neighbor, or a schoolgirl after school to take the children for a walk or, if the neighborhood is unsafe, play with them quietly in another room while the mother naps for an hour are all possible sources of help.

The pregnant diabetic needs nutrition counseling that will help her maintain normal blood glucose levels early in her pregnancy. This reduces the risk of infant and maternal mortality. The nutrition plan suggests a diet that contains 35 to 38 cal/kg of ideal body weight (2200 to 2400 cal/day) and is appropriately balanced with carbohydrates, fats, and proteins. Clients divide their calories among three meals and several snacks.

Pregnant women with PIH also need nutritious diets that are well balanced from the four food groups with extra protein (90 mg total per day). Protein is important for the hypertensive client because there is a fluid imbalance and obligatory protein is lost from the urine. It must be replaced for proper fetal growth. The extra protein may be difficult for her to secure because of expense or inability to shop frequently. The nurse helps these women plan menus that are inexpensive but high in protein. Ethnic heritage must be considered in selecting foods that are palatable for her.

Other preventive management items on the PIH client's list are bed rest and lying in the left lateral recumbent position for two hours every day. This increases circulation to the major organs, including the uterus, kidneys, and liver, as well as the placenta, which are often compromised during a pregnancy complicated with hypertension. This also helps decrease the edema in the extremities. The amount of time a pregnant woman is required to spend resting depends on the severity of her disease. The nurse can help the client understand the importance of this regimen to herself and her baby. She may need help arranging her schedule and gathering her support network to allow time every day for this important aspect of her prenatal activity.

The woman with a possible low–birth weight infant also needs help planning nutritious meals and adjusting her activity and rest according to her individual needs. Often the woman needs encouragement to gain weight; a minimum weight gain of 16 pounds is associated with healthier babies and decreased infant mortality. Teenagers have a particular problem with this because they try to keep the thin body contour that society encourages. They do not realize that this compromises their infant. This can also be a result of their denying the pregnancy, and this possibility needs to be explored with the client as well. Stressors in the woman's life such as economic difficulties, family problems, or even boredom can affect the woman's eating pattern. The community health nurse who has developed a good rapport may be able to explore these factors with the client and think of solutions that might help her feel better about the pregnancy and therefore take better care of herself.

CONTRACEPTION

The choice of a contraceptive method is an extremely personal decision. Ideally both sexual partners are involved in the prevention of an unwanted pregnancy. The community health nurse can play an important role in the choosing of a contraceptive method by providing factual information about the available contraceptives and helping couples explore their own needs and preferences.

One of the most important issues in regard to contraception is the reliability of each method in preventing pregnancy. Clients must realize that no contraceptive method is 100% effective. Sterilization and oral contraceptives are considered the most effective methods of preventing pregnancy. See Table 18-4 for the estimated effectiveness rates of various contraceptives. Couples should be informed that careful and consistent use of the chosen method is essential in the prevention of pregnancy. For instance, the effectiveness of barrier methods significantly increases if they are used with every act of intercourse.

The frequency of intercourse is an important consideration in choosing a contraceptive method. A woman having infrequent intercourse might want to avoid oral contraceptives, which need to be taken daily and would expose her to possible side effects. Women engaging in frequent intercourse might prefer the convenience of oral contraceptives. Partner preference is also crucial in this decision. If either the woman or her partner finds a particular method objectionable, it is likely that it will be used inconsistently if at all.

TABLE 18-4 A Guide to Contraceptive Methods

Method	Estimated effectiveness* %
Birth control pills	98
Intrauterine device (IUD)	95
Diaphragm with spermicide	81
Vaginal spermicides	82
Vaginal sponge	80-90
Condom	90
Natural family planning (rhythm)	76
Sterilization	>99

Actions	Risks	Noncontraceptive benefits	Convenience	Availability
Combinations of estrogen and progesterone, which suppress ovulation	Increase with age and smoking and include blood clots, hypertension, gall bladder disease, liver tumors and nausea	Menstruation is lighter and less painful Protects against ovarian and endometrial cancer Protects against ovarian cysts and pelvic inflammatory disease	Must be taken daily Does not interfere with spontaneity	Prescription only
Changes uterine lining so that implantation is prevented	Cramps, increased bleeding, pelvic inflammatory disease, and uterine perforation	None	Continuous protection until removal	Must be inserted by the health care provider
Diaphragm blocks the cervical entrance, spermicide stops sperm movement	Allergic reaction (rare), bladder infections, and toxic shock syndrome	Possibly protective against some sexually transmitted diseases	Must be inserted just before intercourse	Diaphragm must be fitted by the health care provider Spermicide available OTC
Blocks cervical entrance and stops sperm movement	Allergic reactions (rare)	Possibly protective against some sexually transmitted diseases	Must be inserted just before intercourse	OTC
Acts as a barrier at the cervix, continuous release of spermicide to stop sperm movement	Allergic reaction (rare) Toxic shock syndrome	Possibly protective against some sexually transmitted diseases	May be inserted up to 24 hours before intercourse	OTC
Collects semen, which prevents sperm from entering the cervix	Irritation, allergic ractions (rare)	Good protection against sexually transmitted diseases	Must be applied just before intercourse	OTC
Partners learn to recognize the woman's fertile days and avoid intercourse at those times	None	None	Daily evaluations of woman's fertility, periods of abstinence	Instructions from the health care provider
Fallopian tubes are surgically burned or cut so that sperm cannot reach the egg	Surgical risks	None	No further steps needed after surgery	Surgical procedure

*Estimated effectiveness was derived from Schirm A and others: Contraceptive failure in the United States: the impact of social, economic and demographic factors, Family Planning Perspectives, 14:68, 1982. Careful and consistent use of each method can give better results than reported rates in actual use for average users.

Prevention of sexually transmitted diseases should be a factor in the selection of a contraceptive. Women with more than one sexual partner are at increased risk for sexually transmitted diseases. Although condoms cannot be considered completely effective in the prevention of sexually transmitted diseases, they are currently the most effective prevention available. The other barrier methods may also offer some protection (Table 18-4).

Another contraceptive issue is cost and accessibility. Clients need to consider whether they can afford a contraceptive method and whether they can receive the medical care needed for several of the methods. The community health nurse's knowledge of community resources can be invaluable in referring clients to low-cost family planning clinics when necessary.

Medical problems can be a determining factor in the choice of a contraceptive. Women with a medical history of hypertension, blood clots, strokes, and heart attacks cannot take oral contraceptives. Smoking is another possible contraindication to oral contraceptive use. The IUD would be contraindicated in women with a history of pelvic inflammatory disease. A careful personal health history is essential in determining which contraceptive would be safe for each individual woman.

Every client has a right to informed consent before starting a new method of contraception. Informed consent includes being told the benefits, risks, and alternatives to the method. The client is given an opportunity to ask questions about the method and given an explanation of its use and the option of not starting or not using the contraceptive at any time. The client must not be coerced into any contraceptive choice, and the informed consent procedure must be documented.

The health of the family and therefore the community will improve when all pregnancies are wanted and planned. Unwanted pregnancies are a threat to a woman's mental, physical, economic, and social health. To prevent these unwanted pregnancies, it is essential that all women have access to high-quality contraceptive counseling.

ABORTION

In the past two decades the issue of abortion has moved from a private dilemma to the center stage of public concern (Luker, 1984). Although herbs, roots, and medications have been used throughout history in a variety of ways to induce labor and terminate pregnancy, abortion as a public debate is a recent one. Despite the complex emotional, social, and political issues surrounding the abortion controversy, abortions are being performed at a rate of 42.5 per 100 live births (1985 statistics) (U.S. Bureau of the Census, 1989). Therefore, because induced abortion constitutes a significant portion of women's health care and because of the influence values and attitudes have on the delivery of health care to women, there is a need for the community health nurse to examine the topic and provide accurate, factual information to the client considering different pregnancy options. Accordingly, this section on women's health care provides a brief historical review of abortion, a summary of the current legal status of abortion, a description of the varying methods of abortion, and the community health nurse's role in providing information and minimizing abortion-related complications. Luker (1984) concludes that the moral status of the embryo has always been ambiguous and that, given the lack of agreement among theologians, philosophers, physiologists, and physicians on basic issues surrounding the definition of life, the abortion moral debate is not about facts but how to weigh, measure, and assess facts. Although the community health nurse recognizes that the two opposing sides share no common premises and little common language, it is important to adopt an information-giving role that is supportive of the client in whatever her pregnancy-related decision may be.

Historical Perspective

As previously stated, induced abortion is one of the oldest methods of fertility control. The morality of abortion over time, however, has varied according to period and culture, and even within the same religious doctrine, views on abortion have varied significantly (Fogel and Woods, 1981). In the Roman Empire, a number of Roman authors noted the high frequency of abortion, and a list of prescriptions for drugs that would accomplish abortion was compiled by the natural historian Pliny. In 1100 the Catholic church debated the morality of abortion, condemning abortion but holding that abortion of the "unformed" embryo was not homicide. At that time the formation of an embryo was considered to occur at 40 days for a male embryo and at 80 days for a female embryo. In effect this ruling, which remained intact until the 19th century, did not treat first-trimester abortions, or abortions occurring during the first 13 weeks of pregnancy, as murder. It was not until later in the nineteenth century in America that the morality of first-trimester abortions came into question. Luker (1984) notes that at this time physicians played a major role in the changing moral and legal views of abortion at any time in the pregnancy. In 1859 the American Medical Association (AMA) passed a resolution condemning abortion and urging state legislatures to outlaw it. In 1864 the AMA awarded a prize to the authors of the "best anti-abortion book written for the lay public" (Luker, 1984). By 1880 almost every state had a law restricting abortion to situations where the mother's life was threatened (Fogel and Woods, 1981).

From the 1880s until the early 1970s, abortion went underground, occasionally with disastrous results. On January 22, 1973, however, the U.S. Supreme Court announced its decision regarding two cases related to abortion, Roe v. Wade and Doe v. Bolton. A summary of the decisions is as follows:

1. In the first trimester an abortion decision and its performance must be left to the judgment of the pregnant woman and her physician.
2. In the second trimester the state, in promoting its interest in the health of the pregnant woman, may choose to regulate the abortion decision in ways that are reasonably related to her health.
3. For the state of pregnancy subsequent to viability, the state, in promoting its interest in the potentiality of human life, may, if it chooses, regulate and even proscribe abortion where it is necessary, according to appropriate medical judgment for the preservation of the life or health of the pregnant woman (Hatcher, 1988).

The U.S. Supreme Court decision regarding Roe v. Wade and Doe v. Bolton struck down any state laws preventing a woman from choosing to terminate her pregnancy before viability. The Supreme Court left the parameters of induced abortion even after a pregnancy reached viability to the states for interpretation. If the woman's health, which is a broad term, or life were in danger, abortion at any gestational age would be justified.

Since 1973 many states and the federal government have slowly but surely limited this decision. In 1977 the Supreme Court ruled that states are not required under joint federal-state medical assistance programs (Medicaid) to pay for abortions that are "not medically necessary." The Hyde amendment implemented this by transferring the federal share of the Medicaid payment for most abortions to the states. Most of the larger states in which 83% of Medicaid abortions were performed continued to pay for these services from state funds (Tietze, 1983). By 1981, however, New York, the District of Columbia, and a few other areas were the only places Medicaid funding for abortion was available (Tietze, 1983).

Since the Reagan era began in 1981 with its concomitant tide of conservatism, the abortion issue had become a legal battle. Every year the Supreme Court is petitioned to hear a case that might overturn the Roe v. Wade decision of 1973. In 1989, the court heard Webster v. Reproductive Health Services and upheld a Missouri law prohibiting the use of public funds or facilities for abortions. Although Roe v. Wade was not overturned, states can now limit abortion rights severely. Additional cases are scheduled to be heard by the Supreme Court in 1990, and the availability of legalized abortion could be further limited.

Impact of Abortion Practices on Health Outcome

Only since the liberalization of abortion laws has induced abortion become readily accessible for scientific study. Two major points have emerged thus far from the examination of abortion-related statistics. First, the increase in legal abortions has had a positive impact on the nation's infant and maternal health care statistics. The rise in the number of legal abortions was the single most important factor in reducing neonatal mortality between 1973 and 1977 (Miller, 1985). Further, the widespread availability of legal abortion is associated with declining maternal mortality and morbidity related to abortions. Second, it has been suggested that long-term detrimental effects of legal abortion on subsequent reproduction exist. Scattered reports in the obstetric literature suggest that women who have had two or more abortions are less likely to carry a subsequent pregnancy to term. Because these studies are preliminary, more research is needed to examine the long-term effects of abortion. This need is felt strongly among health care providers responsible for the welfare of women seeking induced abortions. Data that are available on the short-term safety of selected surgical methods of abortion follow.

Surgical Methods of Abortion

Surgical methods of inducing abortion are currently the most widely employed procedures for pregnancy termination in the United States. There are three methods of inducing abortion that are commonly used in pregnancies up to 16 weeks after the beginning of the last menstrual period. The nurse, using this information, can briefly describe the procedures to interested clients.

Vacuum Curettage

Perhaps the most widely used method of abortion is vacuum curettage. It is a simple, effective technique that involves a complete emptying of the uterus by suction after a small cervical dilation is made. The use of local anesthesia during vacuum curettage rather than general anesthesia is especially important in reducing complications related to the procedure. Vacuum curettage is a method that can be used up to 16 weeks' gestation and can take place in a private office setting on an outpatient basis.

Dilation and Curettage

In dilation and curettage (D and C) a metal curette is used instead of a vacuum curettage. The walls of the uterus are scraped, resulting in pregnancy loss. Disadvantages of this method include increased blood loss, increased pain, more cervical dilation, and less complete uterine evacuation.

Dilation and Evacuation

Dilation and evacuation (D and E) incorporates aspects of the more traditional D and C and the more widely used vacuum curettage. This procedure is primarily used in the 13- to 16-week gestation period, although it has been used as an abortion method up to 20 weeks' gestation. General anesthesia is commonly required, as well as an intravenous flow of oxytocin to encourage uterine contractions. Because of the use of general anesthesia and the relatively late date of the abortion, the D and E is associated with more complications than the other two methods.

Menstrual Extraction

Menstrual extraction is the withdrawal of menstrual fluid and products of conception up to 50 days after the last menstrual period (Corson, 1985). Menstrual extraction is often performed without positive diagnosis of pregnancy. Until 1979, urine pregnancy tests could not detect a pregnancy of less than 6 weeks gestation, so women who wanted to prevent or abort pregnancy could use this method. Newer pregnancy tests can diagnose pregnancy earlier and may decrease further use of menstrual extraction.

Medical Methods of Abortion

Medical methods of induced abortion are currently being used for second-trimester terminations. These methods include prostaglandin $F_{2\alpha}$ and prostaglandin E_2 hypertonic saline and hypertonic urea. The prostaglandins are used to induce contractions by acting on the uterine muscle to make it contract and dilate the cervix. Prostaglandin $F_{2\alpha}$ is injected into the amniotic fluid. Prostaglandin E_2 is a vaginal suppository. Side effects of these agents include gastrointestinal symptoms, thermoregulatory changes, and possible delivery of a live fetus.

Hypertonic saline is also injected into the amniotic fluid causing fetal death, which, coupled with the increased amount of fluid expanding the uterus, causes contractions and expulsion of the products of conception. Hypertonic urea injected into the amniotic sac also causes fetal death. It is usually used in combination with one of the prostaglandins to facilitate contractions.

These medical methods of induced abortion are administered to a woman in a hospital setting. There is a slightly higher incidence of maternal morbidity and mortality associated with these methods, since the maternal morbidity and mortality increase proportionately with gestational age regardless of outcome (MMWR, 1988).

A future medical method of abortion is administration of the drug RU486, which is in clinical use in Europe but has not been approved by the Food and Drug Administration in the United States. RU486 is an oral progesterone antagonist that may be used as an early abortion agent and midcycle contraceptive (Nieman, 1987). When administered within 10 days of the missed menstrual period, it produces a complete abortion in 85% of women by disrupting hormonal support of the endometrium. If taken in the midluteal phase before the menstrual period, it induces menses in 72 hours with no risk of pregnancy. RU486 as a method of abortion could have a tremendous impact on women's access to induced abortion if Roe v. Wade is ever overturned.

As part of counseling clients considering an abortion, it is important for the nurse to be aware of those at lower risk and conversely those at higher risk for complications. Hatcher (1986) offers the following list identifying situations associated with lower risk for abortion-related complications:

1. The pregnancy is early.
2. The client is healthy.
3. The clinician is well trained and experienced with abortion techniques.
4. The uterus is not acutely anteverted or retroverted.
5. The client understands the warning signs for potential postabortal problems.
6. Prompt follow-up care is available on a 24-hour basis.
7. Careful examination of the aspirated or curetted tissue is undertaken to rule out the possibility of a molar or ectopic pregnancy.
8. Rh immune globulin is given to an Rh-negative woman.
9. The client does not have gonorrhea or chlamydia.
10. The client is not ambivalent about having the abortion performed (or can cope with the feelings if she is ambivalent).
11. The abortion is carefully and fully completed, (that is, the uterus is emptied.)
12. Local anesthesia is used.
13. Laminaria to dilate the cervix is used.

In summary, abortion as a solution to unwanted pregnancy is as old as recorded time. The morality of abortion has varied through the centuries, but not until recently has the abortion debate been the topic of major public controversy. Despite the legal status of abortion and numbers of abortions currently being performed in the United States, the moral controversy remains as heated as ever. The community health nurse, in recognizing the historical lack of agreement regarding abortion facts, may play an important role in women's health care by giving information and ideally supporting the client's decision for or against abortion.

TRENDS IN BIRTHING PRACTICES

Historical Perspective

The change from the home to the hospital as the common place of birth and the change from the midwife to the physician as the usual maternity health care provider in the United States has been recent, occurring only in the last 50 years.

In 1900 less than 5% of all babies born were delivered in a hospital (Institute of Medicine Report, 1982). Not until 1940 was the percentage of babies born in the hospital greater than the percentage of babies born outside the hospital. From 1940 to 1970 a dramatic decline in the proportion of babies delivered outside the hospital was observed—from 44% in 1940 to 0.6% in 1970 (National Center for Health Statistics, 1984). Since 1970, however, there has been a slight rise in the proportion of deliveries performed outside the hospital setting, although the proportion as of 1979 had not risen above 1%.

Likewise, a dramatic decline in the use of midwives as maternity health care providers and an increase and a dominance of physicians in the field of obstetrics occurred. For centuries, obstetrics, defined by many dictionaries as the practice of the art of midwifery, was the sole providence of the midwife. As a result of a number of social and political events occurring since the turn of the century, by the early 1970s 97% of all births were attended by physicians (Institute of Medicine, 1982). Some of the many sociopolitical reasons for the reversal in health care providers follow. First, the obstetric branch of the medical profession had grown in influence, and they took a stance that strongly opposed midwives on grounds that midwives' practice inhibited the growth and advancement of obstetrics as a recognized medical specialty, and that the midwives lacked standardized training. Second, a public health campaign against disease, malnutrition, dirt, and uncleanliness was growing, and because midwives were largely associated with lower socioeconomic classes, the work of the midwife was seen as substandard and unclean. Third, a major concern among health caregivers about high infant mortality rates developed in the 1920s, and again because of the nurse-midwife's involvement in the care of pregnant women from lower socioeconomic classes, the midwife was seen by the establishment as being associated in part with poor pregnancy outcomes.

The move toward hospital birth occurred quickly, but because of the lack of standardized obstetric training among the physicians themselves, their high use of sometimes harmful obstetric instruments and interventionist approaches, and the continued lack of access by the poor to medical care, maternal and infant mortality remained high. Public health officials suggested that implementing a standardized training program for nurse midwives might fill the gap in access to medical care and contribute to the care of the obstetric client with an uncomplicated pregnancy. This suggestion was not supported by the medical profession until after the Frontier Nursing Service nurse-midwives demonstrated excellent outcomes and the Maternity Center Association, a training program for nurse midwives, was opened in the 1930s. From the 1930s to 1970 the growth of nurse-midwifery in the United States has been slow but steady.

Current Birth Settings and Health Care Providers

Since the 1970s interest has developed in psychologic factors surrounding the birth experience. The changing social contexts in which contemporary childbirth interests are expressed include the women's movement, consumerism, the desire for more natural deliveries, and the concern about rising health care costs. The effect of this new consumer interest has been a reexamination of obstetric practices and the increased involvement of nurse-midwives, lay midwives, family practice physicians, and other health care practitioners in the care of the childbearing family.

The proportion of nonhospital births of babies has increased slowly since the low point in 1970. Concomitant with the recent rise in nonhospital deliveries is the growing number of hospital births attended by certified nurse-midwives (a registered nurse who has obtained additional education in the care and delivery of essentially healthy and normal mothers) and an increase in the estimated number of births attended by lay midwives. Although national information on the number of midwife deliveries in hospitals has been available only since 1975, the number of such births has risen from 19,686 (0.6% of all births) in 1975 to 44,496 (1.3%) in 1979 (Institute of Medicine, 1984).

Currently, the range of birth settings available to the pregnant client includes traditional hospital maternity units, conventional hospital perinatal units, hospital birthing rooms, hospital-based birth centers, freestanding birth centers, and home delivery (Institute of Medicine Report, 1982). Although the majority of births still occur in traditional hospital maternity units, perinatal units, or hospital birthing rooms, the number of birth center births and home deliveries has increased slowly and steadily. Births at home are now estimated to be about 1% of the total number of births per year. The number of freestanding birth centers grew from three in 1975 to about 130 in 1982 (Institute of Medicine Report, 1982). Washington, North Carolina, Texas, California, and Oregon are states with the highest number of nonhospital births.

Currently, controversy surrounds out-of-hospital deliveries, primarily planned-birth-center and home-delivery births. Birth centers and home deliveries constitute an alternative health movement that has developed to promote practices associated with individual choice in the activity of the laboring woman, a homelike atmosphere for the birth and family participation, and control in the birth process in contrast to conventional obstetrics, which tends to emphasize procedures to deal with group risks such as infection, monitoring fetal and neonatal well-being, and a hospital atmosphere with nearness to equipment and use of technology. The primary controversy surrounding the use of birth centers and home delivery surround safety issues. Although each group of health care providers hold strong opinions on the safety of hospital, birthing center, and home births, it is apparent that the literature is insufficient for conclusive determination. Data collection is ongoing to compare the outcomes of home and birthing center births with hospital deliveries for women with similar risk factors. At present, however, opinions range from the hospital as the only safe place for all deliveries to hospital practices being harmful to those having normal childbirth. As the data become available, the community health nurse will be able to evaluate them and use them in counseling of clients regarding childbirth options. Until then a recognition of the availability of choices both in obstetric health care providers and in the place of birth will be helpful to the community health nurse in discussing childbirth options and philosophies with childbearing clients.

SUMMARY

Health teaching to support good pregnancy outcomes should start long before a pregnancy occurs because young women should be immunized against rubella and other infectious diseases, their life-styles should be oriented towards good health, and they should understand the problems that can occur with a pregnancy during adolescence before pregnancy occurs.

An early diagnosis of pregnancy is important for all clients so that they can be warned to avoid alcohol, smoking, and teratogenic drugs. It is even more important to diagnose pregnancy early if the client has diabetes or hypertension. Clients with these problems are considered to be at high risk, so early and continued monitoring and treatment by both nurses and other members of the health care team is essential.

The choice of a contraceptive or even the decision not to contracept is a personal decision, but the nurse can play an important role in the decision by providing accurate, up-to-date information. Abortion is an even more personal decision, but the nurse can again provide accurate and thoughtful information.

QUESTIONS FOR DISCUSSION

1. List four of the common discomforts of pregnancy and explain their physiologic origins.
2. Using Nagel's rule calculate the expected date of confinement (EDC) for a woman whose last menstrual period (LMP) started January 5 of the current year.
3. Plan a community-focused project aimed at coping with the problem of the high incidence of low–birth weight infants.
4. Who should be responsible for teaching young persons about contraceptives? What is the role of the nurse in this area?

REFERENCES

Allen C and Ries C: Smoking, alcohol, and dietary practices during pregnancy: comparison before and after prenatal education, J Am Diet Assoc 85:605, 1985.

Barnes F, editor: Ambulatory maternal health care and family planning services: policies, principles, practices, Crawfordsville, Ind, 1978, RR Donnelly & Sons.

Behrman R: Preventing low birth weight: a pediatric perspective, J Pediatr 107:842, 1985.

Birnholz JC, Stephens JC, and Faria M: Fetal movement patterns: a possible means of defining neurological development milestones in utero, Am J Roentgenology 130:537, 1978.

Cohen AW: Movement as a yardstick for fetal well-being, Contemp Obstet Gynecol 26:61, 1985.

Davidson S: Smoking and alcohol consumption: advice given by health professionals, J Obstet Gynecol Neonatal Nurs 10:256, 1981.

Diebel P: Effects of cigarette smoking on maternal nutrition and the fetus, J Obstet Gynecol Neonatal Nurs 9:333, 1980.

Doe v Bolton citation. Supreme Court of the United States. Doe et al v Bolton and Attorney General of Georgia et al. Supreme Court of the United States, Opinion No 70-40, January 22, 1973.

Dryfoos J: The epidemiology of adolescent pregnancy: incidence, outcomes and interventions. In Stuart I and Wells C, editors: Pregnancy and adolescence: needs, problems and management, New York, 1982, Van Nostrand Reinholt Co Inc.

Fogel CI and Woods NF: Health care of women, a nursing perspective, St Louis, 1981, CV Mosby Co.

Hatcher R and others: Contraceptive technology 1986-1987, ed 14, New York, 1988, Irvington Publishers.

Hellman L and Pritchard J: Williams obstetrics, ed 14, New York, 1971, Appleton & Lange.

Hobel CJ: Prevention of preterm delivery. In Beard RW and Nathanials DW, editors: Fetal physiology and medicine, New York, 1984, Marcel Dekker Inc.

Institute of Medicine, Division of Health Sciences Policy and National Research Council Commission on Life Sciences: Research issues in the assessment of birth settings: report of a study by the committee on assessing alternative birth settings, Washington, DC, 1982, National Academy Press.

Institute of Medicine: Committee to Study the Prevention of Low Birth Weight: Preventing low birth weight, Washington, DC, 1985, National Academy Press.

Leppert P: The effects of pregnancy on adolescent growth and development. In Golub S, editor: Health care of the female adolescent, New York, 1984, Haworth Press.

Logan B: Adolescent pregnancy. In Logan B and Dawkins C, editors: Family centered nursing in the community, Menlo Park, Calif, 1986, Addison-Wesley Publishing Co Inc.

Luker K: Abortion and the politics of motherhood, Berkeley, 1984, University of California Press.

Manning F and others: Fetal assessment based on fetal biophysical profile scoring: experience in 12,620 referred high risk pregnancies, Am J Obstet Gynecol 151:343, 1985.

Menkin J: Teenage childbearing: its medical aspects and implications for the U.S. population. In Wescoff C and Park R Jr, editors: Demographic and social aspects of population growth, Washington, DC, 1975, US Government Printing Office.

Metcoff J and others: Effects of food supplementation (WIC) during pregnancy on birth weight, Am J Clin Nutr 41:933, 1985.

Miller CA: Infant mortality in the US, Sci Am 253:31, 1985.

Nathanson C and Becker M: The influence of client provider relationships on teenage women's subsequent use of contraception, Am J Public Health 75:33, 1984.

National Center for Health Statistics: Midwife and out-of-hospital deliveries. In Taffell S, editor: Vital and health statistics, Series 21, No 40, DHHS Pub No PHS 84-1918, Washington, DC, 1984, US Government Printing Office.

Neinstein I and Stewart D: Adolescent health care: a practical guide, Baltimore, 1984, Urban & Schwarzenberg Inc.

Nieman L: The progesterone antagonist. RU486: a potential new contraceptive agent, N Engl J Med 316:187, 1987.

Olds S, London M, and Ladewig P: Maternal-newborn nursing: a family-centered approach, ed 2, Menlo Park, Calif, Addison-Wesley Publishing Co Inc.

Public health guidance for enhancing diabetes control through maternal child health programs, MMWR 35:202, 1986.

Roe v Wade citation. Supreme Court of the United States. Jane Roe et al v Henry Wade. Supreme Court of the United States. Opinion No 70-18, January 22, 1973.

Romney S and others: Gynecology and obstetrics: the health care of women, New York, 1981, McGraw-Hill Inc.

Rosso P: A new chart to monitor weight gain during pregnancy, Am J Clin Nutr 41:644, 1985.

Tietze C: Induced abortion. In Barron SK and Thomson AM: Obstetric epidemiology, London, 1983, Academic Press Inc.

Topics in minority health, MMWR 16:4, 1987.

Tyrer L and Duarte J: Guiding adolescents' choice of contraceptives, Contemp Obstet Gynecol 23:172, 1984.

US Bureau of the Census: Statistical abstract of the United States, 1989, ed 109, Washington, DC, 1989, US Government Printing Office.

US National Center for Health Statistics: US Bureau of Census, 1982, US Department of Commerce.

Williams SR and Worthington-Roberts B: Nutrition in pregnancy and lactation, ed 4, St Louis, 1988, CV Mosby Co.

CHAPTER 19

Psychosocial Issues in the Older Adult: Nursing Implications

Mary Anne Neary

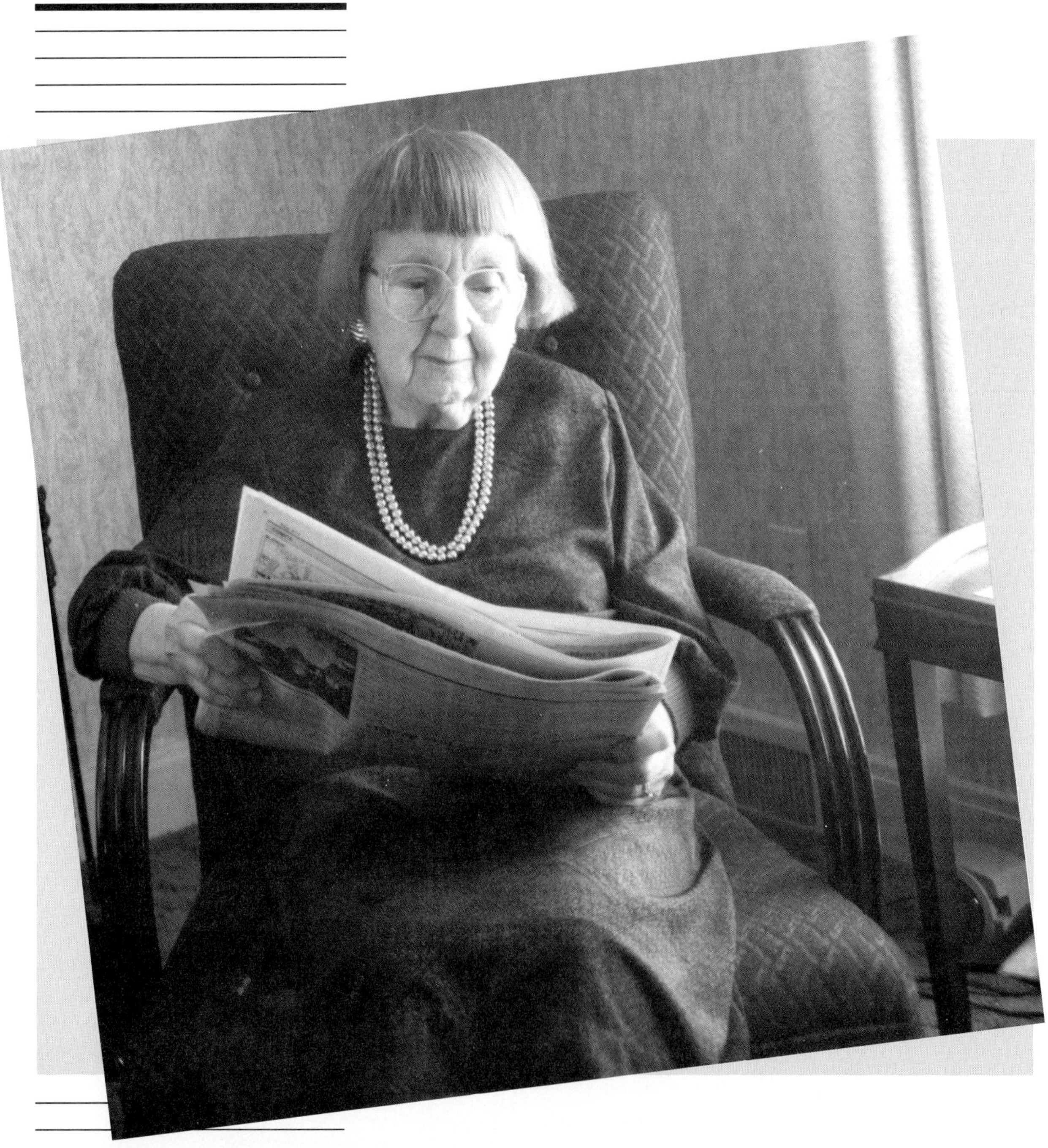

CHAPTER OUTLINE

Theories of aging

Life adjustments associated with aging

- Loneliness
- Retirement
- Role changes
- Health-related issues
- Legal issues
- Poverty
- Community support for in-home living
- Retirement housing alternatives

Depression in elderly people

- Barriers to diagnosis
- Nursing role in the management of depression in elderly people
- Selected behavioral manifestations of depression
- Suicide in elderly people
- Abuse of elderly people

Community nurse as case manager

Role of education and advocacy in community nursing

Summary

OBJECTIVES

After completing this chapter, the reader should be able to:

1. Identify psychosocial theories regarding the aging process.
2. Treat life adjustments associated with the aging process as developmental tasks.
3. List specific areas in which retirement affects the elderly adult.
4. Compare income levels of different ethnic elderly populations.
5. Appraise categories of community support for in-home living for the elderly adult.
6. Distinguish housing alternatives for older adults.
7. Recognize nursing implications regarding maladaptations to the aging process.

THEORIES OF AGING

Since the early 1960s several psychosocial theories have been developed in an attempt to clarify the aging process and find out what constitutes successful aging. Theorists have concentrated on the relationship between life cycle development and aging and person-environment interaction and aging. Although theories about aging lead to a better understanding of certain aspects of adaptation to the aging process, none of them totally captures the multidimensional components of successful aging. However, it is worthwhile to consider these theories to develop one's own perception of the elderly adult.

Havighurst (1968) and his colleagues developed their personality theory of successful aging based on examination of healthy elderly men and women. They determined that eight personality types, which were well established by middle age, determined the level of adaptation to aging. These included the following types:

1. Reorganized—those persons who reorganize their lives by substituting new activities for those they can no longer perform
2. Focused—those persons who are more selective about this substitution process
3. Successfully disengaged—those persons who are content with low levels of activity and interaction
4. Holding on—persons who are satisfied as long as they can continue activities of middle age
5. Constricted—those persons who are holding on but are defensive about their aging
6. Succor-seeking—those persons who depend on others for support
7. Apathetic—those persons who have low levels of both participation and satisfaction
8. Disorganized—those persons who have difficulty maintaining themselves in the community

Erikson (1963) presented the psychosocial theory of ego development, which viewed personality development throughout the life span. His stages included the following:

1. Trust versus mistrust
2. Autonomy versus shame and doubt
3. Initiative versus guilt
4. Industry versus inferiority
5. Identity versus role confusion
6. Intimacy versus isolation
7. Generativity versus stagnation
8. Ego integrity versus despair

The later stages of this theory, although not as well developed as the earlier stages relating to childhood, provided a basis for life span orientation in later theory development. Peck (1968) elaborated on the later developmental stages to better view successful aging and acceptance of mortality.

Levinson (1978) and others divided the life cycle into four areas of approximately 25 years each, including childhood and adolescence, early adulthood, middle adulthood, and late adulthood. Each era is considered a season in a person's life that incorporates identifiable developmental tasks and processes. The primary developmental task of late adulthood is to find a new balance between involvement with society and with self. It is during this era that Erikson's final stage of ego integrity versus despair occurs.

Sheehy (1976) termed these stages "passages" that reflect more a sequencing of stages that individuals pass through than a precise age of transition. The last stage of late adulthood is presented in a positive way that focuses on ego integrity and psychologic renewal.

Person-environment interaction and the aging process are more aptly represented in the theories of activity, disengagement, and continuity. Havighurst (1963) suggested that, to age successfully, individuals should continue their role relationships and activities of middle age. This activity theory holds that, although individuals face inevitable changes related to physiology, anatomy, and health status, their psychosocial needs remain stable. Life satisfaction studies that have tested this theory have found that activity levels, especially informal activity such as social interaction with friends, strongly correlate with life satisfaction (Longino and Kart, 1982).

Contrary to the above theory, Cummings and Henry (1961) saw aging as an inevitable, mutual withdrawal or disengagement of the individual from society and society from the individual. Role losses, seen in widowhood and mandatory retirement, provided these theorists with evidence for decreased interaction between the elderly person and society.

Atchley (1980) recognized the complex nature of personality and adjustment and proposed the continuity theory. The continuity approach to aging assumes that, during the process of becoming an adult, the individual develops such things as habits, commitments, and preferences that contribute to the adaptive process. These lifelong interactions between the individual and the environment unfold into a pattern of routine behavior to which the older adult clings, especially when confronted with new and threatening information.

Viewing the older adult from this theoretic framework is functional for the health care provider. This includes understanding the individual's coping style in stressful situations, such as illness, hospitalization, or institutionalization. An important factor in alleviating some of the stress and facilitating adaptation is the recognition of the person's need for control over the event, whether actual or perceived.

Before applying any of the above theories to the concept of late-life adjustment, one must remember the most significant principle in gerontology—elderly adults represent a highly diverse population. Because of the complex nature of aging human beings, no single theory adequately describes the aging population. Rather, each theory lends to a broader view of aging as a universal process experienced by every individual.

LIFE ADJUSTMENTS ASSOCIATED WITH AGING

The tasks and challenges facing individuals who live to the seventh, eighth, and ninth decades not only are demanding, but also have potential detrimental effects on morbidity and mortality. Elderly adults encounter losses in health, independence, mobility, material possessions, sensory abilities, and memory capacities and are especially vulnerable to loss of their spouses, families, peers, and friends. They lose status related to work roles, family roles, and social roles. Elderly adults also deal with the inevitability of their own death. No one can deny that these losses, including preparation for death, occur. However, many of these elderly survivors not only adjust to such losses, but attempt to live life with acceptable levels of satisfaction and continue to grow within the realities of their lives.

There are at least two major concerns regarding the ability of an elderly person to meet these developmental tasks of aging. First, there is a reduction in the adaptive ability in response to stress that occurs with aging. In old elderly adults (older than 75 years of age) homeostasis has a narrower range, one that is readily compromised by a combination of physical illness and disability, as well as losses of internal and external resources, social roles, and support systems. Physiologic problems, such as anemia or diabetes, compromise the internal resources of elderly people. Psychologic events such as bereavement impose additional stress and can threaten the balance and well-being of the individual.

Second, the intervals between these biopsychosocial assaults become increasingly important to the person's adaptability, since older people require a longer time for homeostasis to occur. Integrating these losses with diminished resources becomes a major task for the elderly population. When losses occur in multiple areas or become cumulative and profound, intervention by the community nurse is necessary for the restoration of an acceptable level of coping, functioning, and quality of life.

The impact of loss is best analyzed by determining its impact on the total person. This includes assessment of the individual's perception of the loss and its significance, the loss's impact on fear of other losses, its effect on the individual's life-style, and the individual's past and present coping style in relation to these losses.

Elderly adults are similar to other age-groups in their need to complete the stages of loss-grief resolution, including acceptance and the search for meaning. However, they differ from younger individuals in that much of the sadness, depression, or guilt caused by the grieving process is often translated into physical symptoms of dysfunction (Carnevali and Patrick, 1986). Some of these symptoms include loss of appetite, insomnia, decreased self-care activity, and intensification of preexisting illnesses.

Although some clients may clearly express concern over losses and their consequences, most frequently the messages are indirect and obscure. For example, "I'm afraid to drive at night" may imply several concerns, such as loss of vision, independence, and control over environment. Some losses are so catastrophic and demoralizing that they are too difficult to share. In such situations only the keen professional observation, communication, and sense of trust established in a genuine nurse-client relationship is adequate to obtain a sufficient database.

Subjective data must be supplemented by clients' medical databases and functional assessment and observation of clients and environmental factors that affect them. In many situations a home visit is an invaluable means of obtaining the necessary information for evaluating a loss and its consequences.

Effective nursing management of the elderly person who is coping with the effects of losses requires a thorough understanding of the aging process, a positive attitude toward elderly people and their worth, and the ability to encourage constructive ways of dealing with those losses. Nurses should be knowledgeable about mechanisms, such as reminiscence and life review, that may facilitate loss resolution. Finally, effective nursing management should be directed at enabling elderly adults to manage daily living despite their diminished resources. This includes mobilization of informal supports, such as family, friends, and neighbors, community resources, and public and financial assistance and recognition of potential crisis situations such as suicide. Active involvement of the elderly client in the management plan is crucial, since compliance depends on the client's acceptance of goals and activities incorporated in the treatment plan.

Observation of patterns of activities of daily living (ADLs) and reinvolvement in the lives of others are the most reliable indices of loss-coping behavior. Only through consistent and committed interaction with and observation of the elderly client can the community health nurse evaluate these indices of loss resolution.

Loneliness

Loneliness, which affects from 12% to 40% of the total population older than 65 years of age, was a problem of elderly persons ranked fourth behind only poor health, financial difficulties, and fear of crime (Harris, 1975). Loss of health, mobility, a spouse, income, or all four may isolate a person from the level of interaction necessary to prevent or delay feelings of loneliness (Creecy, 1985). Loneliness then is the end product of circumstances beyond elderly persons' control that makes it necessary for them to readjust and modify their roles at a time in their lives when their abilities to readjust have decreased.

The effects of loneliness, commonly observed by health care providers, are reflected in psychologic and physical symptoms such as tiredness, anxiety, depression, irritability, backache, palpitations, dizziness, and breathlessness. However, covert messages that reveal patterns of defense against loneliness can be grouped into time-oriented complaints and time-related feelings of familiarity, planlessness, or overplanning, all reflecting life revolved around a series of events instead of people (de la Cruz and Lourdes, 1986).

The first step in developing interventions for loneliness is a careful psychologic assessment. However, since there might be some reluctance to admit to loneliness, health professionals must be alert to clues. Attention-getting behaviors such as dependency and somatic preoccupations may also be evident. Information must be elicited regarding precipitating factors such as death of a spouse, duration of the problem, and usual coping styles. A mental status assessment is also essential to rule out depression or other functional emotional disorders.

Nursing interventions revolve around the dynamics of a nurse's relationship with the elderly adult. Implementation of reminiscence techniques, social-skills training, group counseling, cognitive therapy, pet therapy, touch therapy, and mutual help groups may be successful in resolving loneliness (Page and others, 1985). Community resources, such as volunteer visitors, telephone visitors, transportation services, and adult day care centers, may also be used for lonely elderly people in the home.

Retirement

Retirement is one of the most important events in an American's life at both the societal and individual levels. At the societal level, people are living longer than ever before but they are also retiring, partially or fully, willingly or unwillingly, earlier than ever before.

Before World War I retirement was almost nonexistent. Work was not just a part of life; it was life itself, relinquished only on death or illness. Only 7% of the population at that time was older than 60 years of age (Hornsey, 1982). This number has risen to 15% in the last decade and will rise to about 20% by 2000. Extension of life expectancy to 14 to 15 years beyond retirement for men, and more than 15 years for women, presents a considerable challenge to the United States medical industry.

Retirement is not just a term or phrase; it is a complex process involving work-related variables such as work orientation and job satisfaction, resource-related variables such as income and socioeconomic status of health, and psychosocial variables, including personality, attitude toward retirement, leisure pursuits, and preretirement planning (Howard and others, 1982).

The nurse can play a significant role in providing anticipatory guidance about retirement planning, including income, activities, living arrangements, role changes, health-related issues, and legal issues. Since work is a source of income, it plays a major role in adjustment to retirement. The effect of retirement on financial status often reflects a 50% reduction in income that potentially affects health and life-style, including housing, transportation, social relationships, and leisure activities (Rathbone and Hashimi, 1982). Women are especially penalized by our society because of their low wage base, stop-start work patterns, and duplication of benefits through their spouses. The nurse can facilitate transition by assessment of the individual's level of awareness and preparation for retirement and referral for retirement counseling.

Activity level, often linked to financial resources, is also related to morale and life satisfaction in retirement. Nursing assessment of the client's skills, abilities, and interests, as well as potential for financial remuneration for the client's achievements, should be included for preretirement counseling.

Many retiring individuals consider relocation to a warmer climate, a smaller home, or both for health and financial reasons. The nurse plays an important role in assisting the client during this decision-making process. For example, will the climate be too unbearable for clients or their spouses? Preparation for the move, geographic location, closeness to social contacts, and how the retiree compares the new environment with the previous one are important factors in successful relocation.

Role Changes

Role changes, including more time to spend with a spouse, also need to be addressed in terms of predicting successful adaptation to retirement. Other role changes that are apt to be encountered after retirement include grandparenting, widow(er)hood, and role reversal with adult children. The difficulty encountered by the retiree in adapting to role shifts depends on the flexibility of the individual's personality and the amount of change or the seriousness of changes occurring after retirement. Nursing referral to support groups, preretirement programs, or counseling agencies may be necessary during this adaptation to new roles.

Health-Related Issues

Health-related issues need to be discussed. Will the elderly person have dental, medical, and prescription insurance after retirement? Do health policies provide an acceptable standard of care for both retiree and family? Will retirement affect other biologic needs such as exercise, diet, mental health, and sexuality?

Poor health is more often the cause for early retirement than a negative consequence of retirement. Lower socioeconomic groups exhibit this finding more frequently than do upper or middle socioeconomic groups, who subjectively rate improvement in health status after retirement.

Legal Issues

Legal issues such as wills, inheritance tax, and education regarding community resources for these matters are becoming areas of concern for elderly people. Nurses may not be well versed in these areas but should assume responsibility for appropriate referrals.

Finally, many health professionals, including nurses, persist in their negative attitudes toward aging because the aged clients they see are predominantly ill. It is essential for these negative attitudes to change not only to facilitate the client's transition to postretirement, but also to promote healthy aging at both individual and societal levels.

Poverty

Although elderly persons constitute only 11% of the entire U.S. population, they constitute 13% of those classified as poor. A look at the total elderly population indicates that at least 15% of the elderly are below the poverty line and another 25% are close to that poverty line (Brotman, 1977). Of special concern are selected subpopulations of elderly, including the elderly minority, female, and rural populations. Figure 19-1, which indicates comparative median incomes for the elderly population in 1980, reflects the relative poverty status of minority populations compared with whites.

A close look at these income levels indicates that minority groups of elderly in general and women for all subgroups fall close to or below the poverty line for 1980 ($4954 is the average income for an elderly couple and $3941 for a single person older than 65 years of age). This economic picture also reflects deficits in other areas, such as educational levels, adequate housing, health, and life expectancy (U.S. Department of Health and Human Services, 1980). Limited finances also restrict options for elderly people, both in ability to purchase basic necessities and in ability to make necessary adjustments in response to major life changes associated with old age (Altman, Lawton, and Wohlwill, 1984).

The impact of income on prevention and treatment of illness and disease is multifactorial. In-

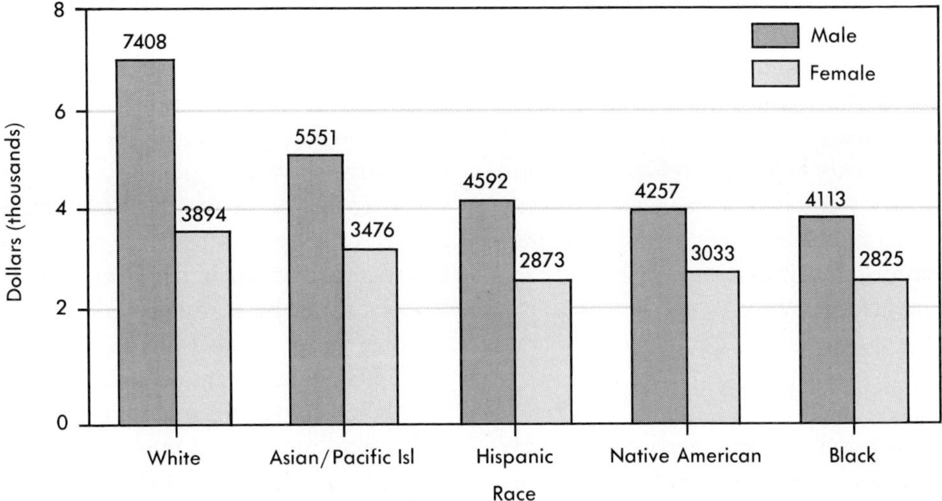

Fig. 19-1 Median income for all elderly, 1980. From US Department of Commerce, Bureau of the Census.

adequate income has a negative effect on nutrition, which in turn leads to greater susceptibility to disease. In addition, inadequate income prevents access to preventive health care. Lack of coverage by government programs, such as Medicare for dental care, prescription drugs, eyeglasses, and other medical supplies, acts as a further deterrent to preventive health care (Berk and Wilensky, 1985).

Inadequate income also affects health care received during illness or disease. It was hoped that Medicare and Medicaid would improve access to health care by elderly people. However, out-of-pocket health costs have risen since the implementation of Medicare and especially since the mid-1970s. Furthermore, although a large percentage of health care expenditures are from public funds, elderly persons generally pay out-of-pocket for more than one half of their medical care costs (Kovar, 1986). This has implications for high-risk groups in the community, such as elderly with poor health and low income.

Elderly poor persons are generally sicker, see the physician more frequently, and require more prescription medications than elderly persons at higher economic levels (Berk and Wilensky, 1985). The lower the socioeconomic status of the individual, the higher is prevalence of disease, age-specific death, confinement to a bed, and restricted activity (McNeely and Colen, 1983).

Rural elderly people, who comprise at least 31% of the elderly population, have poorer health, more disabilities, a higher incidence of chronic conditions, and fewer opportunities to get medical care than their urban counterparts (U.S. House of Representatives, 1973). A larger number of these rural elderly people are predominantly white and poverty stricken because technology has had a negative effect on small farms. Thus their social and geographic isolation puts them at risk particularly for acute, immobilizing illnesses or trauma such as strokes or falls, which may leave them helpless and undiscovered.

It is essential that community nurses explore their roles in promoting health maintenance, providing health information and health care to poor, chronically ill elderly, and facilitating community resource referrals. However, it is even more important that poverty be redefined within a nursing context, which comprehensively views illness within a socioenvironmental framework rather than solely under the medical model. Nurses may then become advocates of this high-risk group and intervene in ways to help poor elderly persons realize their ability to change their environment to improve access to sufficient food, clothing, shelter, education, transportation, and health care (Moccia and Mason, 1986).

Community Support for In-Home Living

Requirements to sustain the elderly person who has multiple chronic problems within the community are both demanding and complex. Organized community supports are often needed to complement such informal social supports as family, neighbors, and friends to maintain an elderly person's independence within the community and delay the need for institutional care. Concern for quality of life within the community involves a wide array of approaches ranging from complex health services that maintain life supports to provision of facilities and resources that promote interaction, high morale, and optimal levels of functioning.

The overall goal of community-based support services for elderly people is to allow the individual the opportunity to live within the community at the highest level of independence possible. This independence involves functional independence—the ability to perform basic ADLs such as dressing, bathing, and toileting—and instrumental independence—the ability to perform complex activities such as managing personal finances, complex housekeeping tasks, and participation in social and recreational events.

Community services are intended to replace neither those activities in which the elderly person is already independent nor the services provided by the older person's natural social network. Community services are intended to complement and replace services that are needed but are either not available or inadequately provided; this keeps the elderly person independent. Ideally, these services reflect a long-term care continuum and are coordinated in a comprehensive manner to accomplish preventive, supportive, rehabilitative, and protective services.

Preventive or facilitative services help competent elderly persons use and retain their existing capacities for productive living after retirement. Senior centers basically provide activities that encourage social interaction, as well as variable extended services such as meals, transportation, health screening and maintenance, and information regarding such things as crime prevention, housing, legal aid, and Social Security. Community organizations supported by local churches and synagogues offer a more extensive array of activities and services that enhance elderly persons' self-concept and provide health maintenance and preventive care for them.

Supportive services help those elderly people who are unable to remain in their own homes without assistance. As older adults become more functionally disabled, they may require increased assistance with light home maintenance, such as household tasks and home repair, or heavy maintenance, such as mowing and snow shoveling. Such services may be provided by a variety of agencies, including volunteer groups, churches, senior centers, or county offices on aging.

Homemaker services, ranging from daily chore services to heavy housecleaning, are provided by a wide range of agencies in the community, including volunteer groups, social services, nonprofit home care agencies, and privately owned homemaker services. Community-based merchants may also provide such assistance as home delivery of groceries and medications and in-home beautician or barber services.

Home-delivered meals, such as the Meals-On-Wheels program, may provide one or two meals daily, five to seven days a week, to older adults who are functionally unable to prepare meals or shop for themselves. Volunteer programs sponsored by local churches and volunteer groups or congregate dining programs at senior centers may be available community resources. Food stamps, a government-sponsored program, may enhance the purchasing power of low-income elderly persons, as well as the quality of foods. Local government-sponsored food distribution centers may also be available at intervals to provide surplus foods such as butter, cheese, honey, rice, and dried milk for low-income elderly people who are willing to wait in food lines for these items.

Social and spiritual needs of older adults may be met by community services such as friendly visitor services, telephone reassurance programs, pastoral counseling services, and companion programs. These programs enhance the individual's well-being, prevent social isolation, and may provide prompt access to emergency services when necessary.

Home health agencies, whether nonprofit, private, or government based, have provided in-home care for homebound elderly persons for many years. However, increasing hospital and nursing home costs have made home nursing a valuable source of care for elderly persons. Hospitals have instituted hospital-based home nursing services to reduce use of hospital services and provide continuity of care to frail elderly persons (Dranove, 1985). Home care on a regular basis is linked to reductions in mortality, the number of hospital admissions, days confined to bed, emergency room calls, and admission to nursing homes (Hendrikson, 1986). Health care clinics, many sponsored by local health departments, also provide chronic and acute care on a walk-in basis to neighborhood residents, especially those with low incomes, diminished health status, and transportation problems. Those ambulatory clinics especially geared toward the geriatric population provide a multidisciplinary approach to elderly client care.

Home health agencies also provide rehabilitative services such as speech pathology, physical therapy, and occupational therapy for elderly clients. These rehabilitative services help restore and maintain a level of functioning consistent with living in the community.

Mental health services are also needed by elderly persons, since they run higher risks for depression than does the general population. As many as 15% to 20% of our nation's elderly people may have significant mental health problems; however, only 1% may seek health services for therapy (Osgood, 1985). Some communities have outreach programs that provide home visits, support groups, family therapy, crisis intervention, and follow-up services.

Protective services are described as services used by the community when it becomes clear that elderly people are mentally incapable of caring for themselves and their own interest (Atchley, 1980). Many times elderly people have a combination of mental health problems that may be complicated by poverty, loss of significant others, social isolation, or abuse by caregivers. Some communities have mental health services targeted specifically to elderly people. Crisis intervention hotlines are also available in many communities on a 24-hour basis for crisis counseling by phone. Some communities also provide follow-up services, including home visits by mental health professionals to provide additional counseling or therapy as needed.

Many communities provide legal aid for senior citizens who have limited financial resources. Some of these legal services also provide advocacy for frail elderly persons.

Communities might also provide support services such as respite care, chore services, and senior day-care centers, which would alleviate some of the pressure of caregiving on family members. Neighborhood watch programs might be expanded so that neighbors would be more concerned about elderly people who have limited social contacts. Active participants in such programs have included meter readers, electric or gas repairpersons, grocery store managers, postal carriers, and delivery persons.

Availability and accessibility of community resources are crucial factors in the long-term community care of elderly people. However, lack of awareness of these services is ascribed as the primary reason for underuse of available programs. It is essential that the nurse, as a member of the health care team, assume an advocacy role as a liaison between the elderly client and the community. Linkage to community services can be facilitated by initially contacting county general information and referral services. However, persistence is needed frequently to negotiate the complexities of the health care system. It may be necessary for the community nurse to assume this responsibility for the elderly person with diminished resources to activate community assistance and facilitate the client's independence and improve quality of life within the community.

Retirement Housing Alternatives

A varicty of housing and living arrangement options are available for the millions of elderly Americans who retire and are functionally independent. Selected relocation options used by the over-65 year age-group include the following (Altman, Lawton, and Wohlwill, 1984):

1. Moving to a smaller home that requires less time, energy, and money for maintenance
2. Moving in with a child, relative, or friend (often for health-related rcasons)
3. Moving to an apartment, retirement community, or other new living arrangement within the same community or elsewhere in the United States

Moves representing the last example are most frequently seen in those persons around 65 years of age who are in relatively good health and who select sites in milder climates for their social attractiveness, that is, for recreational opportunities.

Retirement communities are described as aggregations of housing units with at least a minimal level of service planned for elderly people who are most often retired and healthy. The following are four broad categories of retirement communities:

1. New towns are the largest type of retirement community. These self-contained communities offer a variety of housing options, facilities, and services. They provide recreational, commercial, shopping, dining, financial, and health care facilities.
2. Retirement villages are generally built near larger retirement communities. A variety of housing options, recreational facilities and programs, shopping, and health care are offered, but to a lesser extent than in new towns.
3. Retirement subdivisions are small, bargain-rate subdivisions for independent elderly people. Retirement subdivisions are usually located near cities that provide access to services not contained within the subdivision.
4. Continuing care communities are small retirement communities that provide a medically supportive environment based on the concept of continuing health care. Many require life-care contracts that provide for personal care and skilled nursing as residents become more functionally dependent.

The nurse has a place both in such settings where medical and health care is provided and outside these settings when elderly adults express interest in relocating to a retirement community. Within the retirement community, nurses who have a special interest in continuity care, holistic health, and gerontology can coordinate, initiate, develop, and evaluate creative programs for a select but heterogeneous group of individuals with diverse needs. Community-based nurses can serve as resources for individuals considering such a move. It is strongly recommended that those individuals interested in retirement communities carefully scrutinize the services provided, closely examine the written contract and terms of care, consult with a legal representative before making this commitment, and evaluate the benefits and disadvantages of this type of relocation (Rogers, 1986).

Nursing Homes As Living Alternatives

The home is a particularly important place to the elderly person. It may represent ties to the past, stability in a changing world, and elements of independence and control. Feelings of security and increased morale are also enhanced by familiar surroundings.

As an individual ages and becomes more frail, the decision to stay in the home becomes more complex. Physical and mental impairments increase with age and become more concentrated among persons aged 75 years and older. By the age 75 years, more than 50% of elderly people have limitations in their ADLs, as well as multiple chronic health problems, sensory deficits, and mental impairment (Ebersole and Hess, 1989). Persons with these multiple health deficits require long-term support to maintain optimal levels of functioning so that they can remain at home (Furnkawa, 1982). However, these chronic conditions wear down the elderly person's physical reserve to combat illness, and in time, many elderly people may become homebound and confined to bed. It has been reported that at least 8% of noninstitutionalized elderly persons are in this situation (Brody, 1977).

Cross-sectional studies suggest that nursing home residents, when compared with community residents, are more likely to be old (80 years of age), poor, chronically ill, functionally impaired with respect to ADLs, mentally impaired because of dementia or mental illness, and selectively burdened by multiple medical conditions (Perlman and Ryan-Dylsea, 1986).

Other significant factors related to nursing home admission include recent hospitalization with a debilitating acute illness, lack of a social support network to maintain an elderly person within the home (Brock and O'Sullivan, 1985), and economic factors. In cases where significant home care services are needed, institutionalization may be considered a more cost-effective means of care. In addition, public policy often favors institutional care over home care, depending on the person's income level. Research has suggested that public policy may encourage inappropriate institutionalization for the poor and discourage appropriate institutionalization for the middle class and near poor (Knight and Walker, 1985).

Institutional care should aim at an optimal level of functioning for each resident. To achieve this goal, nurses should take several steps, including the following (Olsen, 1980):

1. Help elderly persons function with remaining capabilities.
2. Help elderly persons compensate for lost skills.
3. Increase elderly persons' abilities to achieve self-care.
4. Improve elderly persons' self-esteem and help them regain a sense of identity.
5. Plan for discharge to home or other community settings.

Dimensions of the nursing home environment that may facilitate these steps include comfort, security, staffing level, and staff quality, service, autonomy, control, and rapport. These indices of quality of care within the nursing home environment address the complex interrelationships between social, mental, emotional, and physical health in elderly people. Environmental influences on health status are also important, since personal territory decreases and amount of space shared with others increases when an elderly person moves to a nursing home.

Nursing Implications

The first option chosen by elderly people and their families when health care needs emerge is a noninstitutional form of care. This is evident from statistics, which indicate that only 5% of elderly people are housed in institutions. However, this 5% represents more than 1 million elderly people who reside in nursing homes in the United States. Negative attitudes toward nursing homes are shared by young and old alike but promote the strongest negative feelings in the population at risk—elderly people. When institutionalization is considered as an option, special attention should be given to the quality of care provided. Literature indicates that quality of care is best provided by small, wealthy, sociable, nonprofit institutions that have a staff with positive attitudes toward residents.

DEPRESSION IN ELDERLY PEOPLE

Depression, the most prevalent psychologic illness of late life, is often overlooked, misdiagnosed, or inadequately treated. Statistics on its prevalence are difficult to ascertain because of the variability of findings. However, it is estimated that anywhere from 5% to 65% of elderly people have a depressive disorder (Blazer, 1982).

Bereavement often simulates depressive illness but is an appropriate grief response to loss of such things as a loved one, a job, and economic security. Elderly people may also experience grief symptoms associated with emotional adjustments to role changes such as retirement and loss of functional ability. These symptoms may include poor self-esteem, feelings of helplessness, hopelessness, dread, sadness, and anxiety, confused thinking, psychophysiologic problems, and perceived poor health (Dohrenwend and others, 1980). Although these symptoms cannot be labeled depression, they should not be ignored in individuals who experience them.

In contrast, depression takes on more severe proportions, lasts longer, and is less easily traced to specific circumstances than bereavement can be. The American Psychiatric Association has facilitated diagnosis of depressive illness through development of certain criteria that include at least four of the following symptoms in addition to a dysphoric (sad or depressed) mood nearly every day for at least two weeks (American Psychiatric Association, 1980):

1. Poor appetite or significant weight loss (when not dieting) or increase appetite or significant weight gain
2. Insomnia or hypersomnia
3. Psychomotor agitation or retardation (but not merely subjective feelings of restlessness or being slowed down)
4. Loss of interest or pleasure in usual activities or decrease in sex drive not limited to periods when the client is delusional or hallucinating
5. Loss of energy, fatigue
6. Feelings of worthlessness, self-reproach, or excessive or inappropriate guilt
7. Evidence of diminished ability to think or concentrate such as slowed thinking or indecisiveness
8. Recurrent thoughts of death, suicidal ideation, death wishes, or a suicide attempt

These symptoms are not listed as a separate entity, but rather under a general category of major affective disorders (mood disorders). The two major mood disorders are bipolar (formerly manic-depressive) and unipolar (also called major depression) (St. Pierre, Craven, and Bruno, 1986). Depressed elderly people most commonly have unipolar mood disorders as a consequence of multiple factors in late life, some of which, such as multiple age-related losses, have already been discussed.

Biologic factors related to endogenous depression include a functional deficit of neurotransmission in the brain (Cunningham, 1984) and the presence of increased amounts of monoamine oxidase in the blood, which further depletes neurotransmitters, especially serotonin and norepinephrine. Other factors that contribute to late-life depression may be exogenous, or related to external factors such as physical illness or environmental stresses. Depression is also linked to physical illness, such as chronic obstructive pulmonary disease, pharmacologic agents, such as antihypertensive and antimicrobial drugs, tranquilizers, alcohol, antiparkinsonian drugs, digitalis, and chemotherapeutic and neuroleptic agents, and age-linked stressors, such as multiplicity of losses of significant others (Cunningham, 1984).

Barriers to Diagnosis

Diagnosis of depression is not difficult when individuals voluntarily admit they are depressed. However, depression may be difficult to diagnose in elderly persons for several reasons, including denial of depressive symptoms or misinterpretation of the client's history by health care providers, resulting in an inaccurate assessment. The latter may especially occur in the case of "masked depression" in which the individual has physical somatic complaints but does not admit having subjective mood changes (Davis, 1985).

Clients with depression tend to have three to six traditional somatic complaints. Complaints most commonly grouped are fatigue, insomnia, upper gastrointestinal distress, anorexia, lower gastrointestinal complaints, and headaches. When elderly people are stereotyped by health care providers, the depressive symptoms of constipation, insomnia, fatigue, irritability, and decreased libido are attributed to old age. Probably the most frequent reason for misdiagnosis by the primary care provider is failure to consider depression as a diagnostic possibility (Chaisson-Stewart, 1985). Even if the diagnosis is a consideration, health professionals often feel hesitant in broaching this subject because of their own fears and misconceptions.

Finally, depression may be misdiagnosed as dementia in elderly persons if the caregiver observes impaired cognition, poor concentration, decreased hearing, poor memory, and loss of interest (Kiloh, 1981). A tragic consequence of this misdiagnosis may be nursing home placement and loss of independence.

Nursing Role in Management of Depression in Elderly People

Elderly people may have multiple problems that demand a holistic nursing approach. Knowledge of the biopsychosocial processes of normal aging provides the framework for nursing management of elderly persons, regardless of the presence or absence of depressive symptoms. Nursing may also contribute to the physical, mental, and functional assessments required at intervals to coordinate care for elderly clients.

Early identification of depression helps identify individuals at risk for suicide. Not only is depression a risk factor for suicide, but it is associated with poorer prognosis in terms of morbidity and mortality when associated with physical illness. Nurses need to become familiar with assessment tools such as the Geriatric Depression Scale (Fig. 19-2), which was developed especially for elderly people (Brink and others, 1982).

Ideally assessments of depressed elderly persons should be done in the home where the nurse can observe home conditions and the client's life-style and habits. This setting also facilitates health education of family, friends, and neighbors who can observe mood changes. This data is invaluable in the management of chronically ill elderly people who are prone to depressive episodes.

Selected Behavioral Manifestations of Depression

Two significant problems associated with depression in elderly people are reactive alcoholism and suicide. Both of these phenomena are attempts made by elderly people to escape the pain associated with living with loneliness, social isolation, and the cumulative losses experienced with aging.

Reactive alcoholism is an overindulgence in alcohol as a late-life adaptive effort to cope with the distress of aging. There are at least 3 million alcoholics older than 55 years of age in the United States with a peak prevalence of alcoholism in this group between 65 and 74 years of age. At least 8% of those who drink heavily are women, most of whom are widows who live alone and without social supports (Calahan, Cisin, and Crossley, 1969). Men, however, come from many settings but have one common characteristic—retirement with associated stress-related loss of

Norms

	m	δ
Normal	5.75	4.34
Mildly depressed	15.05	6.50
Very depressed	22.85	5.07

Choose the best answer for how you felt the past week*

1.	Are you basically satisfied with your life?	YES	NO
2.	Have you dropped many of your activities and interests?	YES	NO
3.	Do you feel that your life is empty?	YES	NO
4.	Do you often get bored?	YES	NO
5.	Are you hopeful about the future?	YES	NO
6.	Are you bothered by thoughts you can't get out of your head?	YES	NO
7.	Are you in good spirits most of the time?	YES	NO
8.	Are you afraid that something bad is going to happen to you?	YES	NO
9.	Do you feel happy most of the time?	YES	NO
10.	Do you often feel helpless?	YES	NO
11.	Do you often get restless and fidgety?	YES	NO
12.	Do you prefer to stay at home, rather than going out and doing new things?	YES	NO
13.	Do you frequently worry about the future?	YES	NO
14.	Do you feel you have more problems with memory than most?	YES	NO
15.	Do you think it is wonderful to be alive now?	YES	NO
16.	Do you often feel downhearted and blue?	YES	NO
17.	Do you feel pretty worthless the way you are now?	YES	NO
18.	Do you worry a lot about the past?	YES	NO
19.	Do you find life very exciting?	YES	NO
20.	Is it hard for you to get started on new projects?	YES	NO
21.	Do you feel full of energy?	YES	NO
22.	Do you feel that your situation is hopeless?	YES	NO
23.	Do you think that most people are better off than you are?	YES	NO
24.	Do you frequently get upset over little things?	YES	NO
25.	Do you frequently feel like crying?	YES	NO
26.	Do you have trouble concentrating?	YES	NO
27.	Do you enjoy getting up in the morning?	YES	NO
28.	Do you prefer to avoid social gatherings?	YES	NO
29.	Is it easy for you to make decisions?	YES	NO
30.	Is your mind as clear as it used to be?	YES	NO

*Each question requires a yes or no answer and each answer is assessed 1 or 0 respectively. The total score varies from 0 to 30.

Fig. 19-2 Brink Geriatric Depression Scale (GDS). From Brink TL and others: Screening tests for geriatric depression, Clin Gerontologist 1:34, 1982.

self-worth and lack of leisure interests. Recently there has been concern about alcohol abuse in retirement communities in the population older than 60 years of age. Hospital and nursing home studies also reveal significant rates of alcoholism, accounting for symptoms of depression, paranoia, organic brain syndrome, or other conditions on admission (Geropsychiatry Report, 1986). Identification of alcoholics requires comprehensive multidisciplinary assessments that include family and significant others. Caregivers must recognize symptoms other than an alcohol odor on the breath, such as personal neglect, anorexia, recurring episodes of confusion and memory loss, confabulation, frequent trips to the emergency room for injuries, a history of frequent falls, an unsteady gait, and episodes of prolonged seclusion including refusal to answer the telephone or door.

Researchers have found that these individuals respond readily when social and emotional supports, such as visiting nurses, transportation services, group or peer counseling, alcohol education, and work with the family, are available (Atkinson, 1981). Development of referral mechanisms between hospital- and community-based alcohol programs such as Alcoholics Anonymous provides continuity of care for elderly alcoholics who are socially isolated and have had many losses associated with aging. If these supports are *not* mobilized, elderly alcoholics, lacking supports and overwhelmed by losses in their lives, are at increased risk of suicide (Osgood, 1985).

Suicide in Elderly People

Suicidologists identify age, gender, race, living arrangements, and life events as important factors in the epidemiology of suicide (Whall, 1985). When these factors are applied to the elderly population, one notes that suicide rate increases in white men 65 years of age and older; the rate increases especially in the eighth decade in persons who live alone, are socially isolated, and suffer from a mild to moderately severe affective disorder that features symptoms of hypochondriasis and sleep disorders with concomitant illness, in persons with recent bereavement, especially in the first year of widow(er)hood, and in persons who attempted suicide in the past 2 to 3 years and who have lethal methods available (Schulman, 1978).

Statistics verify these factors. For example, in 1980 the aged (people older than 65 years of age) constituted 11.3% of the population but accounted for 16.9% of all suicides (Roberts and McFarland, 1986). In addition, attempted suicides in the elderly population are more often successfully completed than in younger populations. Although nonfatal suicide attempts outnumber fatal attempts 200 to 1 in the young, the proportion in the elderly population is 4 to 1 (McIntosh, 1985). Nonfatal attempts by elderly people are attributed to poor planning but rarely to lack of determination. For this reason any threats or attempts should be taken seriously.

Clues to Suicidal Behavior in Elderly People

Individuals who contemplate suicide nearly always display clues to their intentions through their verbal statements, behavior, and life situations. Verbal statements range from clear statements of suicidal intentions to more subtle hints, such as expression of fears and anxieties or increased concern with bodily functions. Hypochondriasis is associated with suicide attempts, but most important, it leads the individual to a health care provider. It has been shown that 70% to 90% of elderly people who commit suicide have seen their physician within three months of their deaths (Barrclough, 1971).

The increased somatic concerns may be misinterpreted, and caregivers may give subsequent prescriptions for symptomatic relief instead of recognizing depression and suicide potential. Unfortunately, prescriptions for barbiturates, analgesics, or antidepressants assume lethal potential in the individual prone to suicide.

Prodromal behaviors suggesting impending suicide attempts include giving away prized possessions or sudden happiness or contentment after a particularly depressing time. However, the most important behavioral clue for potential suicide is a past suicide attempt. Elderly people who fail at a suicide attempt are apt to look for a more effective means of self-destruction.

The health care provider must develop an awareness of suicide potential in any elderly adult who appears depressed and meets the criteria listed earlier for suicide ideation. Communication techniques must be developed to facilitate a therapeutic relationship between health care provider and client. Crisis intervention may be necessary when suicidal thoughts are revealed.

The professional must also be aware of more subtle self-destructive behaviors such as self-starvation, refusal to follow physician orders, medication abuse (not taking medications, taking overdoses, or mixing drugs), or engaging in hazardous, careless actions. Alcohol abuse, especially that of new onset, suggests a desire to destroy oneself.

Family and friends, especially those of recently widowed elderly men, should also be made aware of warning signals of possible suicide. Their close contact lends itself to detection of increasing dependency and hopelessness secondary to bereavement or depression.

Communities must also assume some responsibility for elderly individuals at risk. Elderly people comprise only 1% to 2% of crisis intervention centers' and Samaritan services' caseloads (McIntosh, 1985). Innovative case-finding methods must be considered. Crisis intervention services must be present in facilities most frequented by elderly persons (senior citizens centers) to achieve early identification, establish outreach programs that facilitate early intervention, and increase elderly people's awareness of existing services within the community.

ABUSE OF ELDERLY PEOPLE

A 1981 report on abuse of elderly people indicates that this problem is far from an isolated, localized problem involving a few frail elderly people and their pathologic offspring. Rather it is a full-scale, national problem that occurs slightly less often than child abuse (Caring, 1986). This amounts to about 1 million abused elderly Americans per year (Winter, 1986).

The typical victim is a 75-year-old, ailing female; the typical abuser is a family member. Abuse of elderly people falls into the following four categories:

1. Financial and material
2. Psychologic
3. Physical
4. Neglect

It may also be categorized as active, in which food, medications, and visitors or other social contact is withheld, and passive, where the caregiver is unable to meet or ignorant of the elderly person's needs (Winter, 1986). The most common abuser tends to be a well-intentioned family member, usually a son or daughter, who feels burdened by constant caregiving for a chronically ill, confused, dependent parent.

Signs and symptoms of abuse are readily evident to the knowledgeable nurse. Subjective data may include reports of hours of isolation, expressions of concern over pension checks being used for a caregiver's personal gain, or expressions of fear of a caregiver. Evidence of neglect and abuse may include soiled clothing, persistent body odor, or bruises especially on the head or extremities that are not explained by injury.

The community nurse also has a role in both the assessment and management of real or potential elderly abuse situations to facilitate timely intervention. These resources might include respite for family members who are primary caregivers, physical and homemaker care for the abused elderly person, social interaction measures such as telephone visitors or day-care centers for both the caregiver and elderly person, and counseling measures such as either professional or self-help support groups for primary caregivers. The nurse plays a vital role not only in linking the family with community services, but also in the ongoing evaluation of the therapeutic value of these resources in terms of family and client well-being.

COMMUNITY NURSE AS CASE MANAGER

The case manager who links and coordinates segments of a service delivery system has an important role in the care of elderly clients. Nurses and other health care providers have become "gatekeepers" of the long-term case system (Grau, 1984). The principal functions of case management in long-term care include intake screening, including determining eligibility and need for services, developing and implementing a service plan for care, ranging from coordination of care to provision of care and follow-up services, and monitoring, evaluation, and periodic reevaluation of services in relation to a client's needs (Austin, 1983). Since this process parallels the nursing process, it seems most appropriate that nurses should fill this role with ease and creativity. Intake and screening is the initial process of identifying potential clients through referrals or other means such as nursing home applications. Referrals may come from public agencies, home health services, hospitals, or family members.

Care planning and its implementation is the next step of the case management process. Assessment is a comprehensive data-collection effort designed to provide a database of the client's mental and physical status, functional capacity, emotional status, level of disability, social supports, and economic status (Austin, 1983). The case manager translates this assessment information into a service plan for the client, and decisions are directed to produce a cost-effective package of services and resource allocation. In addition to identification of services to be delivered, the case manager must also periodically determine the frequency, duration, and goals of these services. This may involve meetings with the client and formal caregivers, as well as consultation with specialists.

Evaluation of services, the final step of the case management process, can be considered the reentry phase of the nursing process. Here the nurse case manager monitors the client's health status and the delivery of services, evaluates the outcomes in relation to predetermined goals (mutually developed with client and family), and changes the services as indicated. Interim monitoring, that is, phone calls, provides ongoing contact with both client and family between scheduled services and identifies emerging services needs. Counseling and health education services may also be offered as part of the plan of care or on an emergency basis (Capitman, Haskins, and Bernstein, 1986).

The evaluation phase also provides outcome measures in terms of client function and cost effectiveness, which might serve as indicators for nursing home placement. These data can help clinicians appreciate trends toward improvement or deterioration and can facilitate planned change.

Nurses are actively seeking innovative ways to deliver both high-quality and cost-effective services to homebound elderly people (Maagdengberg, 1983). They have conceptualized community care of the elderly based on a holistic framework and have visualized wellness and self-care as the best level of functioning for a given time. Nurses' comprehensive view and expertise in geriatric care make them well suited for the role of case managers in community elderly care.

ROLE OF EDUCATION AND ADVOCACY IN COMMUNITY NURSING

Establishing sensitive and facilitative community health care services for elderly people is a goal that can be achieved only through an awareness of this population's needs and capabilities. Misconceptions regarding the elderly population and the aging process itself far too frequently stand in the way of attaining this goal. In addition, the high value of youth in American society tends to propagate negative attitudes toward elderly people. Therefore preservation of quality health care and quality of life for this age-group requires the education of all those involved in care-giving, including aged clients and their families, as well as the public sector and legislators who influence this policy of care.

Elderly adults often mistakenly attribute their health problems to the aging process and consequently may fail to seek medical advice and care (Branch and Nemeth, 1985). Elderly people who do not accurately perceive their symptoms or do not initiate contact with the health care system are especially vulnerable to accelerated progression of disease and functional disability.

Elderly people commonly perceive their health in terms of their ability to be active. Health becomes important to them predominantly as it interferes with their independence and daily functioning. Deterioration in self-perception of health in these terms has been strongly associated with poor morale and loss of control over one's environment.

Therefore health education for the elderly adult must be directed at areas that will improve functioning, such as the aging process, self-maintenance, role activity, attitude toward the world and toward self, and negotiating the health care system. Education about community services may reinforce elderly persons' ability to take responsibility for meeting their own health needs.

Families provide ongoing support for the elderly adult in a variety of ways, including the provision of stability, affection, emergency care, economic support, and social interaction. A family's capacity to act as a resource for an elderly adult depends on many factors, including the quality of the relationship with the elderly adult, coping resources, and caregiving skills, and the level of illness and disability in the elderly person, as well as the use of informal or formal services to relieve the burdens that may be involved with caregiving. Nurses within the community can play a significant role in meeting these needs through education, support, and meshing community services with family needs.

Physiologic, sociocultural, and psychologic variables in the community influence the adaptation of the elderly person. Since behavior does not occur in a vacuum, elderly persons affect their environment. Negative attitudes, myths, and stereotyping of elderly people have perpetuated the public image of the aged. The Harris survey (1975) indicated that old people were generally thought of as useless and inactive members of society. These views may indeed affect not only the provision of services, but also policy development. Therefore community nurses have a responsibility to increase public understanding of the aging process and the multidimensional needs of elderly persons. Closely meshed with and not easily separated from this responsibility is that of advocacy for the aged and their families.

Nurses possess the power and potential to plan for and deliver appropriate health care interventions to meet the needs of the elderly population. These efforts refer to not only negotiating within the health care delivery system, but also working to change policies to achieve more humane treatment of elderly people.

As the roles of educator and advocate intertwine, so do the skills of case management and advocacy. Advocacy involves defending and promoting a client's needs. Case management refers to the process of moving a client through the health care system. Both are skills that require a knowledge of private, community, county, state, and federal resources available for the elderly client. Community services are often fragmented and in need of coordination for comprehensive care.

Community nurses have not only the opportunity to serve as advocates of the aged, but also the responsibility of representing frail elderly people with regard to linking services to their needs, protecting their rights, promoting the concepts of health promotion and self-care for them, and elevating their public image. Nurses working with elderly clients should possess professional expertise to intervene on their behalf at both the personal and policy level.

SUMMARY

Elderly people who survive the seventh, eighth, and ninth decades encounter variable losses in health, mobility, independence, material possessions, memory capacities, sensory capabilities, and especially loved ones through death. Yet many of these survivors have adjusted to these losses and live satisfactorily within their capabilities and limitations.

Effective nursing management of the elderly population requires a thorough understanding of the aging process, a positive attitude toward elderly adults, and the ability to facilitate self-care potential and mobilize community supports where necessary. More important, nurses must recognize the importance of their role as advocates for elderly people to preserve health care and quality of life for adults in their later years.

QUESTIONS FOR DISCUSSION

1. Which theory of aging do you feel best explains the social and psychologic processes that take place during the later years of life?
2. Why is depression common among elderly adults?
3. Plan a possible community intervention for abuse of elderly people.
4. Picture a hypothetic situation in which a 60-year-old woman has asked you to help her decide whether to keep her 85-year-old mother at home with her or place her in a nursing home. What variables should be considered in this decision? Describe your nursing role in this situation.

REFERENCES

Altman I, Lawton MP, and Wohlwill JF, editors: Elderly people and the environment, vol 7, New York, 1984, Plenum Publishing Corp.

American Psychiatric Association: Diagnostic and statistical manual, ed 3, Washington, DC, 1980, The Association.

Anderson R and Newman J: Societal and individual determinants of medical care utilization in the U.S., Milbank Q 51:95, 1973.

Atchley R: The social forces in later life, ed 3, Belmont, Calif, 1980, Wadsworth Inc.

Atkinson JH: Alcohol use as a health problem in aging: a psychosocial perspective, Public Health Service Contract 282-78-0163-EJM, Washington, DC, 1981.

Austin CD: Case management in long-term care: options and opportunities, Health Soc Work 8:16, 1983.

Barrclough B: Suicide in the elderly. In Kay DWK and Walk A, editors: Recent developments in psychogeriatrics, Ashford, Kent, 1971, Royal Medico-Psychological Association.

Berk ML and Wilensky GR: Healthcare of the poor elderly: supplementing Medicare, Gerontologist 25:311, 1985.

Blazer D: Depression in later life, St Louis, 1982, CV Mosby Co.

Branch LG and Nemeth KT: When elders fail to visit physicians, Med Care 23:1265, 1985.

Brink TL and others: Screening tests for geriatric depression, Clin Gerontologist 1:37, 1982.

Brock AM and O'Sullivan P: A study to determine what variables predict institutionalization of elderly people, J Adv Nurs 10:533, 1985.

Brody SJ: Resources for long term care in the community. In Brody E, editor: Long term care of older people, New York, 1977, Human Sciences Press, Inc.

Brotman HB: Income and poverty in the older population in 1975, Gerontologist 17:23, 1977.

Calahan D, Cisin J, and Crossley H: American drinking practices: a national study of drinking behaviors and attitudes, Monograph No 6, New Brunswick, NJ, 1969, Rutgers Center of Alcohol Studies.

Capitman JA, Haskins B, and Bernstein J: Case management approaches in coordinated community-oriented long-term care demonstrations, Gerontologist 26:398, 1986.

Carnevali DC and Patrick M, editors: Nursing management for the elderly, Philadelphia, 1986, JB Lippincott Co.

Chaisson-Stewart GM: Depression in the elderly: an interdisciplinary approach, New York, 1985, John Wiley & Sons Inc.

Creecy RF, Berg WE, and Wright R Jr: Loneliness among the elderly: a causal approach, J Gerontology 40:487, 1985.

Cummings E and Henry WH: Growing old, New York, 1961, Basic Books Inc, Publishers.

Cunningham B: Nursing assessment of depression in the aged adult, Home Health Care Nurse 2:9, 1984.

Davis RE: Somatic symptoms as presentations of depression in clinical practice: a review, Physician Assistant 9:97, 1985.

de la Cruz and Lourdes AD: On loneliness and the elderly, J Gerontological Nurs 12:22, 1986.

Dohrenwend BP and others: Measures of nonspecific psychological distress and other dimensions of psychopathology in the general population, Arch Gen Psychiatry 37:1229, 1980.

Dranove D: An empirical study of a hospital based home care program, Inquiry 22:59, 1985.

Ebersole P and Hess P: Toward healthy aging, St Louis, 1989, CV Mosby Co.

Elder abuse: a national disgrace, Caring 5:5, 1986.

Erikson EH: Childhood and society, ed 2, New York, 1963, WW Norton & Co Inc.

Furukawa C: Alternatives to institutionalization. In Furukawa C and Shomaker D, editors: Community health services for the aged, Rockville, Md, 1982, Aspen Systems Corp.

Grau L: Case management and the nurse, Geriatric Nurs 5:372, 1984.

Greene VL: Premature institutionalizations among the rural elderly in Arizona, Public Health Rep 99:58, 1984.

Harris L and others: The myth and realities of aging in America, Washington, DC, 1975, National Council on Aging,

Havighurst R and others: Personality and patterns of aging, Gerontologist 8:20, 1968.

Henrikson C: An intervention study among elderly people, Scand J Prim Health Care 4:39, 1986.

Hornsey E: Health education in pre-retirement education: a question of relevance, Health Educ J 41:107, 1982.

Howard JH and others: Adapting to retirement, J Am Geriatr Soc 30:488, 1982.

Kiloh LG: Depressive illness masquerading as dementia in the elderly, Med J Aust 2:552, 1981.

Knight R and Walker DL: Toward a definition of alternatives to institutionalization for the frail elderly, Gerontologist 25:358, 1985.

Kovar MG: Expenditures for the medical care of elderly people living in the community in 1980, Milbank Q 64:100, 1986.

Levinson DJ and others: The seasons of a man's choice, New York, 1978, Alfred A Knopf Inc.

Longino CF and Kart CS: Explicating activity theory: a formal application, J Gerontol 17:713, 1982.

Maagdengberg AM: A matrix model for geriatric care, Geriatr Nurs 4:310, 1983.

McIntosh JL: Suicide among the elderly: levels and trends, Am J Orthopsychiatry 44:288, 1985.

McNeely RL and Colen JL, editors: Aging in minority groups, Beverly Hills, Calif, 1983, Sage Publications Inc.

Moccia P and Mason DJ: Poverty trends: implications for nursing, Nurs Outlook 34:20, 1986.

Olsen PL: A nurse administered long-term care unit, J Gerontological Nurs 6:616, 1980.

Osgood N: Suicide in the elderly: a practitioner's guide to diagnosis and mental health intervention, Rockville, Md, 1985, Aspen Systems Corp.

Page R, Wrye SW, and Cole GE: The role of loneliness in health and wellness, Home Health Care Nurse 4:6, 1985.

Peck R: Psychological developments in the second half of life. In Neugarten, editor: Middle age and aging: a reader in social psychology, Chicago, 1968, The University of Chicago Press.

Perlman RA and Ryan-Dylsea M: The vulnerable elderly, J Gerontological Nurs 12:14, 1986.

Rathbone ME and Hashimi J: Health and social intervention, Md, 1982, Aspens Systems.

Roberts J and McFarland L: Assessment of suicide risk in the elderly, Caring 5:20, 1986.

Rogers R: Explore life care possibilities, J Gerontological Nurs 12:12, 1986.

Sheehy G: Passages: predictable crises of adult life, New York, 1976, EP Dutton.

Schulman K: Suicide and parasuicide in old age: a review, Age and Aging 7:201, 1978.

St Pierre J, Craven RF, and Bruno P: Late life depression: a guide for assessment, J Gerontological Nurs 12:4, 1986.

US Department of Health and Human Services: National Institute on Aging: Age page: minorities and how they grow old, Washington, DC, 1980, US Government Printing Office.

US House of Representatives Committee on Government Operations: Special problems of the rural aged, Washington, DC, 1973, US Government Printing Office.

Whall A: Geropsychiatry report: alcoholism in older adults, J Gerontologic Nurs 12:36, 1986.

Whall A: Suicide in older adults, J Gerontol Nurs 11:40, 1985.

Winter A: The shame of elder abuse, Mod Maturity, p 51, Oct/Nov 1986.

CHAPTER 20

Chronic Illness in Elderly People

Mary Anne Neary

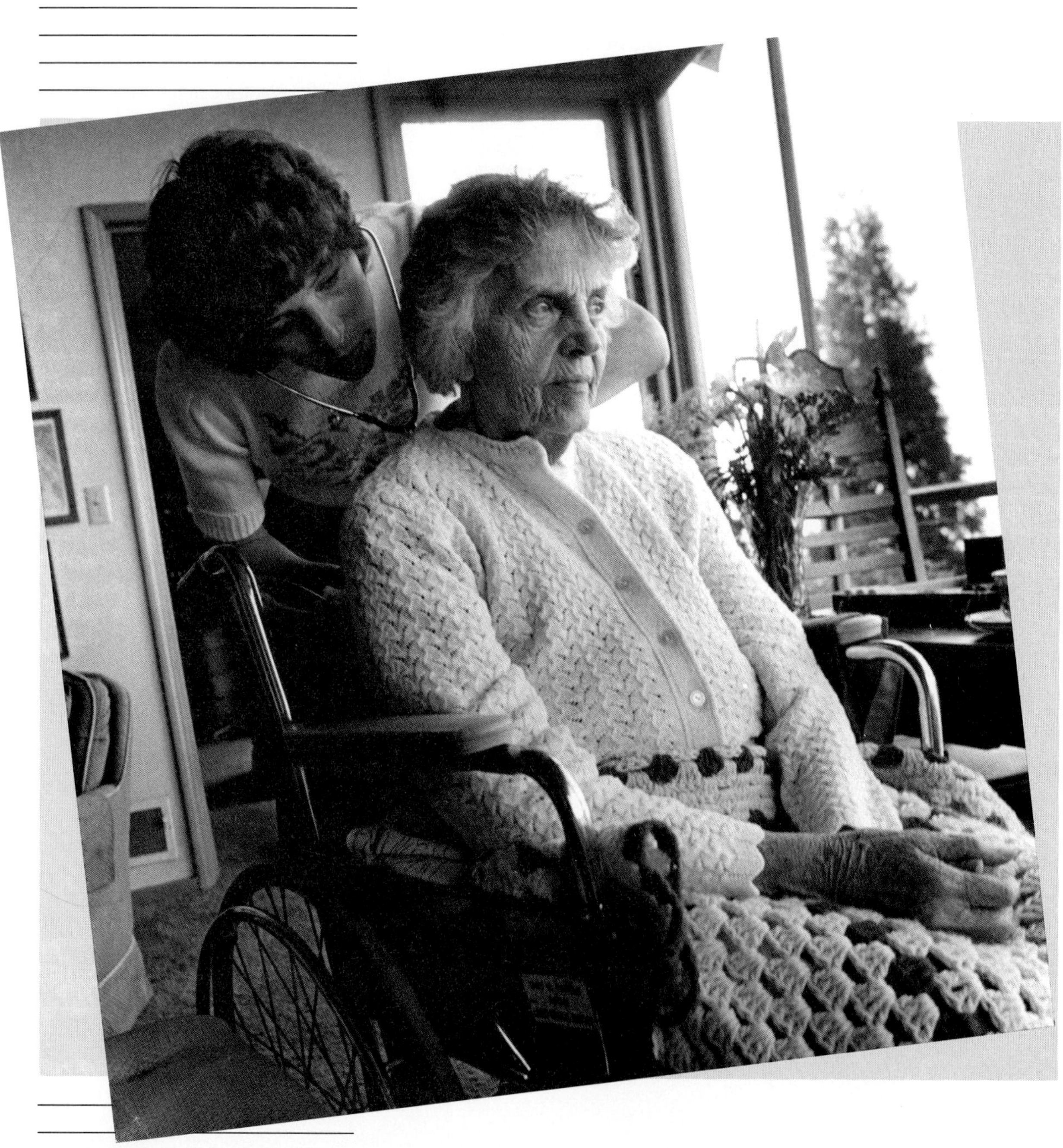

CHAPTER OUTLINE

OBJECTIVES

After completing this chapter, the reader should be able to:

1. Describe the impact of chronic illness on elderly adults and their families.
2. Describe the specific diseases of arthritis, diabetes mellitus, cardiovascular disease, and chronic obstructive lung disease as they affect elderly people.
3. Discuss nursing management of these specific chronic illnesses in the context of special needs of elderly people.

ALTHOUGH aging is not synonymous with disease, incidences of physical health problems do increase with age. For example, individuals 64 to 69 years of age have an average of four chronic health problems, and those 75 years of age and older have an average of five chronic health problems (National Center for Health Statistics, 1983). In general, the number of people with these conditions who report limitations also increases with age (Manton, 1985). More than half the population older than 85 years of age experience major limitations in their activities of daily living (ADLs) secondary to age-related changes, as well as chronic conditions such as heart disease, arthritis, diabetes mellitus, and chronic obstructive lung disease.

The aging process and chronic illness influence each other in many ways. Elderly people are physically, socially, and psychologically more vulnerable to illness and its effects. Although individuals differ in timing and rate of illness, all elderly people face the stresses of physical, social, and environmental changes. Some of these changes, such as retirement, reduction in income, and death of family and friends, come at a time when the elderly person begins to experience some losses in physical and mental capacities. These changes in turn may affect the individual's coping abilities. The onset of illness presents an added crisis that can upset the social and psychologic equilibrium, which in turn may make potential for episodes of illness greater.

The nursing process in the home setting is drawn from many disciplines and targeted at not only elderly people, but also their families and home environment. It is essential to assess the suitability of the client's residence in the following areas:

1. Adequacy of the environment in terms of cleanliness, utilities, sanitation, and food storage
2. Home safety features such as a personal security system and telephone and availability of emergency medical assistance and family supports
3. Availability of supplies and services such as food, financial resources, household supplies, transportation, and social and religious outlets

Environmental assessments should be conducted with respect for the uniqueness of individuals, their chronic health problems, and their informal support system, including assessment of support persons' willingness to provide for the client's identified needs.

In addition to assessing the adequacy of the client's environment, the nurse assesses the elderly person with regard to physical, social, and psychologic functioning. This includes taking a comprehensive client and family health history and a client social and interpersonal health history and conducting physical examinations, including determination of mental status, functional level, and capacity for performance of ADLs. This information serves as an initial database that can be used later as a basis of comparison when determining whether to maintain clients in the home setting or transfer them to alternative levels of care.

Nursing interventions may include client and family counseling, health teaching, medication review, and coordination of services. Nursing management should not substitute for self-care activities of both family and client but instead should emphasize client and family responsibility for an active role in the decision-making process and treatment plan (Schmidt, 1985). In addition, management is an ongoing process because of inevitable, episodic, acute exacerbations of symptoms, which require immediate care.

FINANCIAL ISSUES RELATED TO CHRONIC ILLNESS IN ELDERLY PEOPLE

Many health care costs must be paid out-of-pocket by elderly people, regardless of their medical insurance coverage. These include deductibles from insurance and Medicare, the difference between the maximum allowable Medicare payment and a physician's actual charge for service, and the cost of both private insurance and Medicare premiums (Berk and Wilensky, 1985). There are also many services not covered, including dental care, prescription drugs, eyeglasses, hearing aids, medical supplies, and adaptive equipment. Supportive services, such as social services and homemaker services, and nursing home care are often excluded from health insurance coverage.

Medicaid, funded by both state and federal governments, is an important source of payment of long-term care services. Recipients of Medicaid benefits, however, must meet strict financial eligibility requirements, including having no more than $1500 of liquid assets such as cash savings, stocks, and bonds (Lubkin, 1986). Therefore elderly people find themselves eligible for Medicaid only after they have drained their resources and become members of the aged poor poulation.

As indicated in Chapter 9, both Medicare and Medicaid have pursued changes in long-term care policies that greatly affect care of elderly people. Many states, faced with rising Medicaid expenditures, have instituted policies reducing the growth of nursing home beds (Kavesh, 1986). At the same time, Medicare has instituted two initiatives to reduce expenditures—the prospective payment system (PPS), which encourages early hospital discharges through a classification of clients in one of 470 diagnosis-related groups (DGRs) (Floyd and Buckler, 1987), and home health claims review procedures, which limit the types and length of service reimbursement to homebound elderly people (Home Health Line, 1985). Emphasis is on short-term medical and nursing services and reduction of reimbursement for social services.

These two major policy directions have contributed to concern about hospitalized elderly clients who no longer require acute care and who may be discharged without adequate planning and care, long-term home health services that are not sufficiently available or adequately funded to meet elderly clients' needs, and inadequate home health services that may contribute to avoidable problems that could increase morbidity and necessitate repeat hospitalizations.

Implications for Community Nursing

Community nurses often have firsthand experience with the inadequacies of the health care system. Despite these inadequacies, community nurses' goal is to provide quality care to elderly clients. Direct care is only one step in the nursing process, however. These issues demand that community nurses take an advocacy role on behalf of elderly clients and their families who wish them to remain in the community. This role includes heightening public perception through education of self, consumers, and their families, facilitating continuity of care through the health care system, and continuing to work for change in the care of elderly people toward continuity of care and quality of life (Brody, 1987).

PSYCHOSOCIAL ISSUES IN CHRONIC ILLNESS

Confirmation of a chronic condition at any age often incorporates physicial disability and imposes psychosocial problems on the individual, including intrafamily strain, social isolation, dependency conflicts, self-image consciousness, sexuality issues, and perhaps the threat of death. The threat of institutionalization is an additional concern in the elderly population.

Maintenance of a chronically ill person in the home is often difficult work that requires multiple adjustments on the part of all family members. The illness can have negative physical, emotional, and financial consequences on the entire family. Family relationships change and are accompanied by emotional reactions, such as frustration and anger, to role losses (Crossman and Kaljian, 1984). Offspring struggle with not only caregiving responsibilities, but also the deterioration of a parent's health and the reality of death.

The chronically ill disabled adult also faces redefinition of self in terms of body image, personal losses, social isolation, sexuality, and aging. As mobility declines and the effects of disability becomes more visible, the client is confronted with the realities of these physical defects. Self-esteem may deteriorate, and feelings of helplessness and meaninglessness may lead to depression. Decreased mobility, fatigue, pain, or all three may predispose an elderly person to isolation when physical limitations inhibit involvement in social activities and relationships.

Chronic progressive diseases cause emotional responses like those expressed in the grieving process, especially anger and the feeling of being punished. Sorrow accompanies losses of physical function, social status, employment, and familiar life-style (Lubkin, 1986).

Sexuality is often negatively affected by chronic disease. Loss of mobility and decreased range of motion set limitations on sexual position. Pain and fatigue may impede sexual interest or arousal. In addition, many medications induce variable degrees of inability to have sex particularly in male clients. Guilt or fear may result from inability to satisfy self or partner (Lubkin, 1986).

The aging process interacts with chronic disease in presenting greater challenges to adaptation. For example, visual or hearing impairments associated with aging limit ability to interact with one's environment. Elderly people become more vulnerable to these compounded losses in terms of ability, desire, or encouragement to maintain previous levels of activity and social interactions. Deterioration of cognitive ability further affects the elderly person's ability to maintain self in the community setting.

Implications for Community Nursing

The major portion of health care for the chronically ill takes place in the community setting. Therefore ongoing communication between client, family, and health care provider is essential in facilitating continuity of care. Nurses can play a key role in filling the gaps between care requirements and service alternatives.

Consideration must be given to how well the family as a whole is coping with and managing chronic illness needs. Chronically ill individuals may not require nursing assistance if their families are compensating for these deficits (Eliopoulos, 1982). However, the nurse is in a key position to recognize the physical and emotional strains of caregiving and to problem solve creatively to relieve these burdens. Thus the management plan may include education, ongoing support and encouragement, linkage with community resources, especially respite services and self-help groups, and advocacy activities.

Sometimes a family cannot continue to care for an elderly member, despite use of community resources. Nursing home placement is always a difficult decision for the family, since it can produce feelings of failure on the part of family members and feelings of abandonment on the part of the elderly person. The nurse can serve both as an adjunct to the family undergoing this process and as a resource person, providing necessary information and guidance. More important, the nurse can encourage family members to become more knowledgeable and determined in their search for the best facility before placement is mandatory.

Ideally, elderly clients should also be as involved as possible in this decision-making process. Every effort should be made to include the elderly client's thoughts, preferences, and fears related to relocation. The nurse can play a significant role in stabilizing support systems during the waiting period and after institutionalization. Communication and counseling skills provide aged clients and their families an opportunity to resolve conflicts precipitated by the nursing home decision.

Nursing interventions on the community-based level can best be demonstrated by addressing the most common chronic illnesses in elderly people—chronic obstructive lung diseases, diabetes mellitus, cardiovascular disease, and arthritis.

Nursing interventions for these health problems involve the education of both client and family on an ongoing basis to sustain community-based living at quality levels. The generalized issues addressed above are applied to these specific illnesses to demonstrate personalization of nursing care.

CHRONIC OBSTRUCTIVE LUNG DISEASE

Chronic obstructive lung disease (COLD) is the most common cause of pulmonary dysfunction symptoms in elderly people and the leading cause of disability that affects both clients and their families. COLD is a condition in which there is a chronic airflow obstruction caused by chronic bronchitis, emphysema, or both. Chronic bronchitis is a condition associated with excessive tracheobronchial mucus production and characterized by a productive cough for at least three months of the year for two consecutive years (Oregon Thoracic Society, 1981). Emphysema is characterized by permanent, abnormal enlargement of the peripheral airways beyond the terminal bronchioles, destruction of the alveolar walls, and loss of elastic recoil of the lungs (Brodoff, 1984).

Breakdown of the alveolar walls leads to less surface area available for gas exchange. Loss of elastic recoil causes instability and collapse of distal airways during expiration, a major mechanism in increased airflow resistance.

There are predominantly two factors that predispose an individual to COLD—genetic factors and cigarette smoking (Patrick, 1986). The genetic form of emphysema is seen in younger individuals, even those who do not smoke.

Cigarette smoking, however, is the primary cause of chronic bronchitis and emphysema. Studies have shown that individuals who smoke 25 or more cigarettes per day are about 20 times more likely to develop bronchitis or emphysema than are nonsmokers, with disease severity increasing proportionally to the amount of cigarettes smoked (U.S. Department of Health, Education, and Welfare, 1979).

TABLE 20-1 Functional Classification of Dyspnea

Level	Description
I	Can keep pace when walking on a level surface with a healthy person of same age and build, but unable to do so on stairs and hills
II	Can walk 1 mile at own pace without dyspnea but cannot keep pace with a healthy person when walking on a level surface
III	Becomes breathless after walking 100 yards or a few minutes on a level surface
IV	Becomes breathless when dressing or talking

Nursing Management of Chronic Obstructive Lung Disease

An initial health assessment is necessary to determine the level of adaptation to airway obstruction in clients with COLD. Many elderly clients are in the advanced stage of this disease and have gradually and insidiously adapted to its limitations. In addition, they may attribute decreased exercise tolerance and breathlessness to old age and delay seeking health care until advanced stages or complications evolve (Gioiella and Bevil, 1985).

Dyspnea is the foremost symptom of airway obstruction. It is present at variable levels depending on the disease process and factors such as infection, sputum production, weather, altitude, and exertion. It is useful to classify dyspnea functionally as shown in Table 20-1.

Other symptoms of COLD are fatigue from the effort of breathing, chronic cough, and inability to sleep at night. Clients with predominant emphysema, also called "pink puffers," are generally thin, undernourished, and debilitated. On the other hand, clients with bronchitis, also called "blue bloaters," are generally overweight, edematous, and drowsy because of hypoxia, carbon dioxide retention, polycythemia, and pulmonary hypertension. Since individuals often have both bronchitis and emphysema, many clients fall somewhere between these two descriptions. Individuals with bronchitis and emphysema also have a barrel-shaped chest and show increased use of accessory muscles and labored breathing. Lung sounds are distant, and wheezes and rhonchi are present.

Elements of a comprehensive program for a client with COLD include client education, medication management, bronchial hygiene, oxygen therapy, nutrition, progressive exercise, and life-style modification, including coping with stress (Gioiella and Bevil, 1985).

Client and family education is probably the most crucial aspect of care, since it should facilitate cooperation in the management plan. Areas of educational need include anatomy of the respiratory system, the disease process and its prognosis, and all aspects of the treatment plan and their rationale. The nurse has the opportunity to reinforce and reevaluate learning needs as necessary and to refer the family to community resources such as the American Lung Association for educational material.

Most clients with COLD take a large number of medications, including bronchodilators, antibiotics, and steroids. These agents help control symptoms but do not halt the disease process. These drugs have numerous side effects that are potentially dangerous for the elderly client. Therefore it is important that both the client and family be educated so that the client can benefit from the drug regimen (see box).

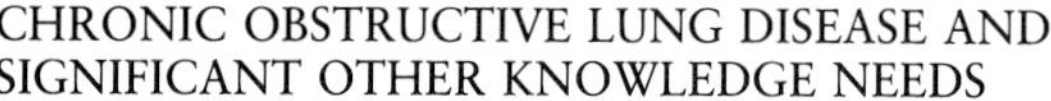

CHRONIC OBSTRUCTIVE LUNG DISEASE AND SIGNIFICANT OTHER KNOWLEDGE NEEDS

1. The name, purpose, and side effects of each medication.
2. A schedule of self-administration that is compatible with life-style.
3. Proper drug administration techniques, especially inhaler use. This includes special help such as large-print directions on medicine bottles for elderly clients with vision deficits.
4. Which symptoms to report to the health care provider.

Bronchial hygiene includes measures that maximize airflow and prevent bronchial irritation. Every COLD client must be urged to stop smoking cigarettes since cigarette smoke is the single most important source of respiratory irritation. Elderly clients with this lifelong habit have difficulty quitting. To quit smoking they need support and encouragement, as well ideas for ways to cut down during the process of smoking cessation such as switching to a brand lower in tar and nicotine. Other irritants should also be identified and avoided. Clients should be advised to accommodate for temperature changes with an air conditioner in hot weather and a humidifier in winter.

Increasing hydration, the most effective way to liquify bronchial secretions, may improve airflow. Elderly clients without cardiac disease may benefit from a daily intake of 2 to 3 liters of fluids. However, to prevent nocturia they should be cautioned to take in fluids throughout the day rather than just at bedtime.

Inefficient air exchange is the primary consequence of COLD. Whenever COLD clients breathe rapidly, as they would during stress or exercise, air trapping becomes more significant, since rapid breathing prevents adequate exhalation. The COLD client needs instruction, observation, and support to minimize the number and severity of these episodes. Helpful techniques include slowing of breathing pattern and prolongation of exhalation, the pursed lip breathing technique, to occupy two thirds of the total breathing cycle. These clients also need to be made aware of the dangers of breath-holding activities, such as prolonged talking and physical exertion, since these activities aggravate breathlessness (Acee, 1984).

Special equipment such as nebulizers may also help clear the airway. Clients should be observed for proper technique to ensure effectiveness. Physical limitations such as muscle weakness and poor coordination may limit use of special equipment. Instructions should be written in large print if the client has vision problems. Proper cleaning must be ensured to prevent recurrent lung infections.

Portable oxygen systems have enabled clients with COLD to stay in the home setting in advanced stages of the disease. Although oxygen therapy does not affect the disease, it can improve exercise tolerance, facilitate performance of ADLs, and enable the client to sleep more easily at night. The nurse is often involved in instruction and monitoring of equipment use to ensure client safety.

Lung infection is a significant factor in the morbidity and mortality of clients with COLD. Pneumonia, a risk for elderly people in general, is a special concern for those with COLD. Both clients and their families need to be aware of signs and symptoms of lung infection, including increasing cough frequency and sputum production, change in color of sputum from clear or white to yellow, green, or gray, increased shortness of breath, decreased exercise tolerance, and fever and chills (Patrick, 1986). Frequently the COLD client has a standing prescription for a broad-spectrum antibiotic to be initiated at the first sign of infection. Preventive measures, such as influenza virus vaccine, are of utmost importance in protecting an elderly person with COLD from complications that can lead to respiratory failure. The nurse becomes a key factor in detecting symptoms of respiratory failure, such as agitation, clouded sensorium, insomnia, tachycardia, and increasing dyspnea. Lack of recognition of these symptoms of respiratory failure can lead to mistreatment with sedatives, which further precipitate respiratory failure.

Although COLD clients may have a reduced activity tolerance caused by respiratory effort, they should still be encouraged to maintain some level of exercise, especially walking. Careful supervision and monitoring is necessary to ensure activity within the limits of fatigue and dyspnea. Clients are more apt to maintain a regular exercise program if close follow-up and support are given. Clients must be taught to walk slowly, rest intermittently, keep breathing controlled, and use abdominal breathing to minimize fatigue or dyspnea.

Nutrition and weight maintenance are special challenges to nurses caring for clients with COLD. The client may be fatigued secondary to the effort of eating or have fullness related to air swallowing or increased fluid intake. Fullness itself affects diaphragmatic movement and may induce dyspnea. Medications may adversely affect appetite. Support and education may be needed in terms of high-protein diets, increase in caloric intake, vitamin supplementation, and spacing of meals.

Besides the physiologic consequences of COLD, the individual must also go through enormous psychologic adaptation to this illness. The disabling effects of COLD often occur in the fifth to sixth decades of life. When symptoms increase, the individual is often forced to retire early; this in turn may precipitate loss of self-esteem (Burk, 1982).

A client's adaptation to COLD may be accompanied by several emotional responses, such as denial, anger, and blame, before final resignation and acceptance of dependence on others. At first the individual may continue smoking and blame dyspnea on lack of exercise or the aging process itself. Anxiety related to both dyspnea and fear of the unknown becomes a predominant emotional response of the person with COLD.

Family members also experience stages in the adjustment to the client's illness and dependency. Both client and family experience negative emotions, such as grief, loneliness, anger, and guilt, in response to this illness. Coping with these emotions is improved with education and support. It is also vitally important that clients be educated so that they can become full participants in their own care (Michaels and Stephenson, 1985).

Community support groups are available for both COLD clients and their families. Regular sessions provide them with opportunities to meet other people with COLD and learn how they cope with problems caused by this illness. These sessions also feature talks to experts who discuss new treatments, equipment, and ways of improving quality of life.

ARTHRITIS IN ELDERLY ADULTS

Arthritis, although not a cause of mortality in any age group, does affect the health care system, especially in terms of economy and disability. More than 7 million individuals are disabled from arthritis, and a total of $14.5 billion per year is spent on medical care, taxes, and lost wages (Arthritis Foundation, 1979).

Elderly adults often have various forms of this disease, especially osteoarthritis and rheumatoid arthritis. Although only 4% of all young adults are afflicted, 50% of people older than 65 years of age have some type of arthritis and at least 85% of people older than 75 years of age are afflicted with arthritis in one or more joints. Rheumatoid arthritis, which has a relatively small prevalence (0.3%) relatively in young adults, has a prevalence of 10% in people older than 65 years of age (Fries, 1980). These statistics have tremendous implications for care of elderly people, especially in terms of long-term community management.

Osteoarthritis

Osteoarthritis (OA), or degenerative joint disease, is a common, nonsystemic, generally noninflammatory condition characterized by breakdown of cartilage, subsequent changes in underlying bone, and development of bony spurs (osteophytes) at the joint edges. OA may be idiopathic, or it may be secondary to trauma of the joints, immobility, or neuropathic disorders such as diabetes mellitus. Recent data suggest that the inflammatory stages are due to deposits of hydroxypatite crystals (Calin, 1981). Obesity, although not causative, contributes to OA's severity.

OA most commonly affects joints that are subjected to the greatest stresses—the lumbar spine, hips, and knees. Pain in the early stages occurs only after the joint is aggravated by prolonged activity and is relieved by rest. As the disease progresses, pain may occur at rest or awaken the client at night.

Stiffness after inactivity or sleep usually lasts only minutes and is relieved by activity. As the disease progresses, however, motion becomes more limited and weight-bearing joints may give way. Muscle weakness may occur secondary to increased stiffness, leading to abnormalities of posture and gait.

Rheumatoid Arthritis

Rheumatoid arthritis is a chronic, extremely disabling, systematic disorder characterized by bilateral and symmetric joint inflammation and erosion. Typically, it involves the hands, wrists, and feet but may also involve elbow, shoulder, hip, knee, and ankle joints, as well as the cervical spine.

The disease usually begins as an inflammation of a synovial membrane (synovitis), which causes edema and vascular congestion and eventually results in irreversible joint damage. Persistent and progressive joint involvement leads to disorganized joints, with pain, swelling, and discomfort being the most common characteristics. Systematic symptoms, such as malaise, fatigue, weight loss, and fever, and systemic involvement of the heart, lungs, kidneys, eyes, skin, and peripheral nerves also occur.

This disease is marked by acute episodes and

remissions; within 10 to 15 years these clients experience a moderate to marked decline in functional capacity.

The cause of rheumatoid arthritis is not fully understood. Currently, it is viewed as an autoimmune disease in which rheumatoid factor, a serum antibody, perpetuates the inflammatory process.

Unlike that in clients with OA, morning stiffness in clients with rheumatoid arthritis lasts longer (one half to several hours). Pain is greatest in the morning, accompanied by tenderness and swelling in variable degrees. Symmetric joint involvement, as well as the systemic symptoms mentioned earlier, is common. Contracture deformities are common in this disease.

TABLE 20-2 Functional Classification of Arthritis

Class	Description
1	Client can carry out all usual duties completely without handicap
2	Client can perform normal activities despite handicap of discomfort or limited motion of one or more joints
3	Client is limited to few or none of duties pertaining to usual occupation or self-care
4	Client is bedridden or confined to wheelchair with little or no self-care

From Elkowitz EB: Geriatric medicine for the primary care practitioner, New York, 1981, Springer Publishing Co Inc.

Assessing the Arthritic Client's Adaptations

It is not uncommon for elderly clients to have manifestations of both rheumatoid arthritis and degenerative joint disease. When such conditions are suspected, it is important to focus on the adaptations required in arthritis and how these affect the client's ability to function. The initial assessment becomes a database for comparison with future changes in symptoms, manifestations, function, and response to therapy. Therefore a thorough history and physical examination with special emphasis on the musculoskeletal system are important. This should also include measurement of active and passive ranges of motion of all joints and observation and palpation of each joint for pain, tenderness, heat, redness, effusions, osteophytic formation, subluxation, and deformity (Gioiella and Bevil, 1985). Joints should also be assessed for crepitus and instability.

Muscle strength, especially grip assessment, must also be determined, since losses affect ability to perform ADLs. It is especially important to assess the client's ability to ambulate and perform certain activities in the home setting, including stair climbing, ability to get in and out of a chair, dressing, eating, cooking, and washing clothes. A functional classification of arthritis is also helpful in the baseline assessment, as well as in periodic reevaluations (Table 20-2). One example of such a tool is suggested by Elkowitz (1981).

Systemic adaptation to arthritis should also be assessed. Clients with rheumatoid arthritis are especially limited by symptoms of fatigue and malaise, which in turn may negatively affect activity tolerance.

Nursing Intervention in Arthritis

Goals of nursing management of the arthritic adult include the following:

1. Reduction of pain, stiffness, and inflammation
2. Prevention of crippling deformities
3. Maintenance of optimal functional ability
4. Education of client and family regarding the disease and its management
5. Fostering of adjustment to chronic illness

To achieve these goals, nurses need to be aware of the role they play in the treatment plan. Continued education and support, as well as observation of negative changes, are crucial in helping the client not only adapt to the chronic aspects of this disease, but also maintain optimal function. Close cooperation between the client and nurse is vital.

Medication Therapy

Medications play an integral role in the treatment plan at every stage of arthritis. The first agents used in drug management of arthritis, especially in rheumatoid arthritis, are salicylates, or aspirin, which have analgesic and antiinflammatory properties.

The side effects of aspirin are a special consideration when managing an elderly arthritic client. Tinnitus, hearing loss, gastrointestinal upset, and occult blood loss secondary to insidious peptic ulcer formation resulting from treatment with aspirin are serious concerns in the elderly population. It is therefore appropriate to monitor salicylate levels on a regular basis in individuals who take a lot of aspirin. This not only evaluates therapeutic effect, but also alerts the health care provider to approaching toxic salicylate levels. Salicylate intoxication results in severe symptoms such as respiratory depression, hyperpyrexia, and convulsions (Bruce, 1985).

Nonsteroidal antiinflammatory drugs (NSAIDs) may be substituted in place of aspirin for the drug treatment of arthritis, since they have lower gastrointestinal side effects, may be administered once or twice a day, and have a therapeutic effect comparable with aspirin. Side effects of NSAIDs include gastrointestinal irritation, headaches, and fluid retention. Fluid retention is a special concern in individuals with a history of congestive heart failure (Braun, 1981). NSAIDs can also affect renal function and cause liver toxicity. Therefore NSAIDs must be used with great care in elderly and debilitated individuals.

Corticosteroids are used for acute flare-ups in both OA and rheumatoid arthritis. Intraarticular injection of steroids may provide temporary relief of severe joint pain while a client waits for other medications to take effect. Individuals with rheumatoid arthritis may require oral administration of steroids to suppress acute systemic inflammation. The lowest effective dose is most desirable, with short-term use preferred to reduce the risk of toxicity. Use of steroids may be especially helpful for elderly clients, who may experience improvement in mobility within 48 hours of steroid administration.

A number of other potent medications may be considered, especially for the client with rheumatoid arthritis who is not responsive to the preceding regimens. These medications include gold salts, antimalarial drugs, cytotoxic agents, immunosuppressive drugs, and penicillamine. The severity of adverse effects secondary to any of these medications warrants caution and close monitoring, especially with elderly clients.

There are two areas of concern regarding medications and arthritis—fads and quackery and compliance. Chronicity, pain, and failure to respond to therapy frustrate clients and lead to a search for a miracle cure. Remission, which may occur incidentally after use of a fad cure, serves only to reinforce faith in would-be cures. Such fad remedies, including grapefruit, beets, and copper bracelets, may provoke more problems. The fad may be harmful, arthritic clients may abandon prescribed medical regimens for the fad, and they may not tell the health care provider about the fad for fear of being ridiculed or reprimanded. The nurse has the responsibility to determine whether the fad is harmful, gain the client's confidence to facilitate communication regarding these treatments, and be nonjudgmental to help clients make wise choices.

Multiple chronic health problems often warrant multiple medications. Multiple medications, in turn, predispose clients to noncompliance or drug interactions, which are especially dangerous in the elderly adult. The nurse must make special note of evidence for noncompliance. Some reasons for noncompliance include cost of prescribed medications, unawareness of potential problems related to overmedication or undermedication, misattribution of adverse effects of medication to age-related changes, and fear of ridicule or reprimands from health care providers, which may prompt clients to file false reports. Nonjudgmental evaluation of the problems of noncompliance or use of fads is therefore essential in this phase of management.

Mobility Problems in Arthritis

Physiologic changes associated with aging and physical limitations induced by arthritis affect elderly arthritic clients' independence greatly. Therefore a nursing goal should emphasize a balance between rest and exercise that would maintain joint mobility and prevent further disability. Once clients return home from the hospital or physician's office, they may become so discouraged that they fail to follow their regimen, no matter how well the health care provider explained it. The nurse becomes the focal point in reeducating both client and family. Elderly people may not only have negative feelings about exercise in general, but may also be afraid to exercise because of pain and stiffness. The nurse can facilitate change by educating the elderly person about the safety and the physiologic and psychologic benefits of exercise in moderation.

Physical disability secondary to arthritis has serious implications for self-care and independence. Assistive devices, such as canes, walkers, braces, and knee supports, may provide stability and prevent falls. Initial reluctance to use such devices may be due to a sense of pride and embarrassment. Consultation with a physical therapist is invaluable in identifying and managing the client's retraining needs.

Environmental structuring may be necessary to facilitate safety and maneuverability. Areas that need to be evaluated include bathrooms, where nonskid strips must be installed in the tubs or showers, stairwells, where railings must be secure, high-hazard areas, where lighting must be adequate, and walkways, where obstructions such as extension cords must be removed.

Psychosocial Problems Related to Arthritis

However physically limited individuals with arthritis are, they can still have improved quality of life. A social evaluation reveals areas of concern and fear that could lead to social isolation and depression in turn. This should include assessment of the client's and family's coping skills, communication patterns, and means of problem solving before a therapeutic plan is developed. The nurse must also try to imagine life with daily pain and accept the significance pain has for each individual. Only then can a program of daily goals be developed for an arthritis client. Nursing assessment identifies areas in which the client and family need support, further teaching, or both. Since denial often interferes with acceptance of diagnosis, reevaluation of the client's knowledge base is essential. Use of interviewing techniques enables the nurse to detect the client's level of understanding and acceptance and provide clarification of myths and misconceptions.

The cost of health care, especially for arthritis, is a constant problem. Inability to work, mounting bills, cost of medicines, and health care visits all add to a strained home environment. Coordination of community services, such as homemaker services, Meals on Wheels, or the Arthritis Foundation, is an essential part of counseling.

Evaluation of the effectiveness of the treatment plan focuses on the degree of successful adaptation to life-style, relative control of pain and stiffness, maintenance of mobility, a balance between rest and activity, and a realistic expression of desired outcomes that are compatible with the individual's age, functional ability, and interests.

CHRONIC CARDIOVASCULAR DISEASES IN ELDERLY PEOPLE

Cardiovascular disease is the most prevalent cause of death in the United States; it accounts for 44% of deaths in individuals older than 65 years of age (Yurick, Robb, and Spier, 1980). Atherosclerosis, a disorder of the larger arteries, is the cause of most coronary artery disease, cerebrovascular disease, peripheral vascular disease, and diseases of the aorta.

The pathogenesis of atherosclerosis is not completely understood. It appears that atherosclerosis is a multifactorial disease related to a combination of intrinsic aging processes and such factors as diet that over time are superimposed on certain genetic factors to produce the disorder.

A number of risk factors are present more frequently in people with atherosclerosis than in the general population. Therefore the assessment of cardiovascular risk factors, especially diabetes, obesity, and hypertension, is pertinent even in elderly people.

Coronary Artery Disease

Coronary artery disease is by far the most important category of cardiovascular disease in the elderly population; it is a factor in approximately three fourths of the deaths of elderly people. Ischemic heart disease is also a source of significant morbidity and mortality in the elderly population.

Elderly adults have symptoms of cardiac ischemia similar to those in younger persons with less frequency and less intensity. Although angina, chest pain of cardiac origin, tends to be the classic symptom younger adults complain about on examination, elderly people most frequently have painless syndromes, such as sudden death, pulmonary edema, chronic congestive heart failure, or nonspecific complaints. Instead of angina, they may report shortness of breath, gastrointestinal complaints, or mental and neurologic symptoms associated with cerebrovascular insufficiency (Wild, 1986).

In elderly people who do experience anginal pain, episodes are precipitated by any stresses that impose increased myocardial need for oxygen. These stresses include eating a meal, physical exercise, extremes in weather such as cold, wind, heat, and humidity, emotional stress, nightmares, or even normal activities such as stair climbing or walking. Additional stresses may exacerbate angina in the elderly person. For example, anemia, hyperthyroidism, obesity, tachyarrhythmias, and hypoglycemia may precipitate severe angina, which in turn may result in congestive heart failure (Gioiella and Bevil, 1985).

Peripheral Vascular Disease

Atherosclerosis affects not only the heart, as seen in ischemic heart disease, but also the peripheral vessels. Peripheral vascular disease, which commonly affects the femoral artery, the distal aorta just below the renal arteries, and the carotid arteries, may result in occlusion of the artery, aneurysmal dilatation of the arterial wall, or embolization in distal arteries (Rubin and Goldstone, 1985).

Although all elderly people are at risk, peripheral vascular disease is most likely to occur in men who smoke, have a history of coronary artery or cerebrovascular disease, and have diabetes mellitus.

Intermittent claudication, a cramplike pain in the affected leg, is a feature of peripheral vascular disease and represents inadequate blood flow to sustain muscular movement during activity. The most common complaint is a walk-pain-rest cycle that has a consistent pattern at some level of activity. Other signs of occlusive disease include cool skin temperature, pale or mottled appearance of skin, sparse growth of hair on the affected extremity, thin shiny skin, thickened toenails, reducing sensation, and ulcerations. Pain at rest signals advancement of disease. The client with advanced peripheral vascular disease wakes up from sound sleep because of pain in the foot and finds it necessary to lower the extremity to reduce the pain. Extremities can become gangrenous if obstruction is prolonged.

Hypertension

It is predicted that, by 1990, 29 million people in the United States will be 65 years of age or older. Of these, 45% will have a systolic blood pressure (SBP) of 160 mm Hg or greater or a diastolic blood pressure (DBP) of 95 mm Hg or greater (1988 Joint National Committee, 1988). Evaluations of SBP and DBP increase the risk for cardiovascular morbidity and mortality in elderly adults just as in younger adults. According to the

U.S. Department of Health and Human Services (1980), hypertension may also contribute to senile dementia of vascular origin.

According to the U.S. Department of Health and Human Services' Third Joint National Committee on Hypertension, hypertension in an individual 65 years of age or older exists primarily in two forms. Combined type hypertension exists when SBP is greater than 160 mm Hg with a DBP greater than or equal to 90 mm Hg. Isolated systolic hypertension generally exists in elderly people who have a long history of elevated blood pressures. SBP greater than 160 mm Hg with a DBP less than 90 mm Hg constitutes isolated systolic hypertension.

There are a number of physiologic changes associated with the aging process that contribute to arterial pressure elevations. These include aortic rigidity secondary to arteriosclerosis, decreased glomerular filtration rate, and a sluggish renin-angiotensin system. The net result of these age-related physiologic changes is a normal increase in baseline blood pressure readings.

Extrinsic factors affecting blood pressure in elderly people include obesity, diet, and to a lesser extent smoking and alcohol consumption. Other variables, such as stress and medication-induced high blood pressure, are more prevalent in the young population.

Dietary sodium is the most important nutrient considered in the causation and control of hypertension (Dairy Council Digest, 1981). Preference for adding salt to foods may be culturally determined and often begins at an early age. Elderly adults, in addition, may use more salt for flavoring because of diminished taste and reduced ability to perceive salty flavors with aging.

Obesity is strongly correlated with elevated blood pressure, particularly in children and young to middle-aged adults (U.S. Department of Health, Education, and Welfare, 1979). Weight reduction by caloric restriction often results in a substantial decrease in blood pressure even if ideal body weight is not achieved.

Congestive Heart Failure

Congestive heart failure (CHF) is a syndrome that has a variety of causes and is manifest as several symptoms. Simply stated, CHF is the inability of the heart to deliver sufficient blood to the peripheral tissues to meet their metabolic demands (Parmley, 1985). CHF in turn affects the functioning of the central nervous, gastrointestinal, excretory, and musculoskeletal systems.

In elderly people, heart failure is often a physiologic response to stress, especially in the presence of underlying hypertensive or ischemic heart disease. The stress most often underlying CHF is cardiac disease such as hypertension or ischemic heart disease. A sudden onset of another health problem, such as pneumonia, thyrotoxicosis, diabetes mellitus, or anemia, can precipitate or aggravate heart failure in elderly people who have little cardiac reserve (Gioiella and Bevil, 1985).

Medications may also precipitate heart failure in elderly adults. Toxic reactions to digitalis may cause arrhythmias, which in turn may precipitate heart failure. Less commonly prescribed medications include corticosteroids and antiinflammatory agents that may cause heart failure secondary to sodium and water retention.

Excessive dietary intake of sodium has also precipitated failure symptoms. Likewise, obesity, which increases cardiac workload, may be a causative factor.

The elderly client does not necessarily have the usual signs and symptoms of CHF such as dyspnea and orthopnea or nocturia. Rather, the major complaint may be a chronic, nonproductive cough, which may be CHF misdiagnosed as a lingering viral infection. Symptoms of right-sided failure such as right upper abdominal discomfort, anorexia, or nausea and vomiting might be mistakenly attributed to CHF instead of a gastrointestinal problem caused by hepatic engorgement. Fatigue, edema, and shortness of breath might be considered noncardiac symptoms and overlooked as symptoms of CHF. Therefore the community health nurse must be especially aware of the systemic consequences of CHF in the elderly adult.

Cerebrovascular Insufficiency

Cerebrovascular disease is a broad term that encompasses all types of occlusive processes in the cerebral blood vessels, including the carotid arteries. Transient ischemic attacks (TIAs) are often forerunners of strokes and may simulate strokes but result in complete recovery. Completed strokes, on the other hand, leave residual damage and affect the client, family, and community.

The main predisposing factors for development of a stroke include the following (Petrowski and Tyzenhouse, 1984):

1. Hypertension—blood pressure more than 140/90 mm Hg
2. History of TIAs especially within one year
3. Cardiac disorders, such as atherosclerosis and atrial fibrillation, that predispose clients to cerebral emboli or thrombosis
4. Advancing age

Risk factors of lesser importance include family history of strokes, physical inactivity, cigarette smoking, obesity, and elevations in blood cholesterol or glucose levels.

A TIA or a series of TIAs, which suggests an impending stroke, is a symptom of cerebral insufficiency. Transient losses of central nervous system function reverse completely within two to 15 minutes but in some cases may last up to a day or two. Among clients who have a TIA, one third will never have a recurrence, one third continue to experience the attacks without progression to a stroke, and one third develop a stroke within a year of the TIA (Petrowski and Tyzenhouse, 1984).

Strokes, depending on their location, may result in varying degrees of permanent problems such as hemiparesis, aphasia, dysarthria, apraxia, bladder and bowel incontinence, mental impairment, emotional lability, dysphagia, and visual impairment. Recovery from a stroke occurs on two levels—neurologic recovery and improvement in functional abilities. Neurologic recovery depends on the mechanism and location of the lesion and generally peaks at about three months after a stroke (Anderson, 1981). Functional improvement depends on many factors, including the rehabilitative environment, degree of mobility training, and client motivation.

NURSING ROLE IN CARDIOVASCULAR DISEASE IN ELDERLY PEOPLE

General Considerations

Health appraisal of an elderly client with any cardiovascular problem is essential in maintaining stable health and preventing further complications. Since multiple systems are affected by these diseases, a thorough history and physical examination is recommended as a baseline for comparison at regular intervals. Historical data should include family history, past medical history, cardiovascular risk factor analysis, medication history including over-the-counter drugs, inquiry into significant life changes during the past year, and a thorough inquiry into initial symptoms, as well as review of systems pertinent to secondary involvement such as the urinary, central nervous, musculoskeletal, respiratory, and digestive systems. A psychosocial history is also necessary, especially with regard to the client's available support systems.

A complete physical examination of the elderly person with cardiovascular disease must also be performed, with special considerations of changes associated with the aging process, as well as those that are disease related. For example, special considerations in obtaining a blood pressure in an elderly adult include bilateral blood pressure readings in sitting, supine, and standing positions and palpation of the artery before and during the procedure to prevent misinterpretation of the findings. Full cardiopulmonary, peripheral vascular and neuromuscular, thyroid, and mental status evaluations must be given special attention to obtain all pertinent data. Only then can the community nurse formulate the nursing diagnosis and management plan specific to an individual client.

Management Goals for Elderly Clients with Coronary Artery Disease

The goals of home management of elderly people with coronary insufficiency include an increased myocardial supply and a reduced myocardial demand. Commensurate with these goals are the identification of aggravating and precipitating factors and facilitation of ADLs that are self-gratifying for the client but do not produce angina.

Angina brings with it more than accompanying symptoms. It is associated with a high-level anxiety and fear of myocardial infarction and death. That angina is precipitated by exertion or stress greatly affects and often controls an elderly person's daily living. Education and support enable elderly people with angina to learn how to prevent an anginal episode, treat an anginal attack, and have an acceptable life-style.

Prevention of anginal attacks entails recognition of precipitating factors, including exercise, stress, temperature changes, meals, or strong emotions. Review of recent attacks may facilitate more awareness of these factors; this awareness in turn can contribute to the development of an activity plan that is safe for the client. Both client and family also need to become more aware of stress- or anxiety-producing situations and be assisted with improvement of coping skills. Emotional support for elderly clients is most important, since fear of precipitating angina can provoke overcautiousness and preoccupation with cardiac status.

There are times when an anginal episode is inevitable. At a point when chest pain occurs, the elderly person must stop activity immediately, rest, and self-administer nitroglycerine tablets as ordered. Special instructions should be given regarding nitroglycerine to facilitate its prompt effectiveness in relief of angina.

Nursing Management of Peripheral Vascular Disease

Nursing care for the elderly person with peripheral vascular disease (PVD) is directed at retarding disease progression, increasing collateral circulation in the affected area, and maintaining skin integrity. Progression of PVD can be delayed by control of cardiovascular factors, especially smoking and diabetes mellitus. Certain pharmacologic agents, including aspirin, dipyridamole, nifedipine, and pentoxifylline, may be used singly or in combination to improve circulation in the affected extremity.

Collateral circulation, muscle tone, and blood flow are enhanced by a program of graduated walking. Even clients with pain on minimal activity should be encouraged to walk at least four times daily. Special instructions include making a record of the distance that produces pain, walking 80% to 90% of the distance that produced pain, stopping and resting until the incipient pain subsides, and continuing the walk, but for a distance that does not reproduce calf pain. Consistent practice should result in increased walking time before onset of pain and faster recovery from pain between walks (Rubin and Goldstone, 1985).

Hygienic and safety measures are extremely important in preserving skin integrity of the affected extremities. These measures include caring for the skin meticulously, wearing well-fitting shoes, using support hose, and avoiding trauma.

Other measures to prevent trauma include evaluation of environment to be sure that lighting is adequate, passageways are clear and free of obstacles, furniture is not too soft, which predisposes clients to vascular constriction because they must bend their legs more than with firm furniture; and evaluation of the client's sensory abilities including ability to detect water temperature before bathing to prevent scalding.

Management of Hypertension in Elderly People

Once hypertension is diagnosed, compliance can be ensured only by active client participation in the therapeutic plan. Nurses can be especially helpful in this process.

Hypertensive clients must at least understand the following:

1. Their blood pressure exceeds normal values.
2. Long-term, follow-up therapy is necessary.
3. Hypertension is known as the "silent killer" because hypertensive clients are asymptomatic until major organs are damaged enough to produce symptoms.
4. Therapy controls but does not cure hypertension.
5. A consistently followed regimen should reduce risk.

Successful therapeutic intervention, whether nonpharmacologic or combined with medication, requires client readiness to control blood pressure and adopt a life-style compatible with blood pressure control.

Since there are considerable risks for elderly people taking medications, nonpharmacologic approaches, such as diet modification, weight reduction, sodium restriction, smoking cessation, moderation of alcohol intake, exercise, and behavioral techniques, are treatments of choice and should be attempted on a trial basis before progression to medications. However, if blood pressure readings are extremely high, medications may be prescribed immediately to prevent a stroke or other complications. If drugs are prescribed, the elderly client should be examined carefully and at frequent intervals. The SBP should be lowered cautiously to 140 to 160 mm Hg. Since elderly persons are more sensitive to volume depletion and sympathetic inhibition than younger people, they are more susceptible to hypotensive problems. All drugs should be initiated in small doses, spaced at longer-than-usual intervals, and increased gradually over weeks instead of days unless the blood pressure is extremely high.

Elderly people need to become involved in their own treatment program to facilitate its integration into their life-style, whether they live at home or in an institution. They need to become aware of hypertension, its organ complications, management options, and the myths, such as hypertension means "too nervous," that interfere with adherence to a treatment regimen. The National High Blood Pressure Education Program recommends some special considerations for interaction with a hypertensive elderly person. Early sessions with the client should be task oriented, simplified, and repeated to ensure comprehension. Written material and memory aids may be used for clients with sight and hearing limitations as long as their educational background and current mental status are considered. One such example is called the "Age Page," a large-print client education guide for hypertensive people with vision problems. The medication schedule should be as simplified and inexpensive as possible to encourage adherence. The complexity of the therapeutic program is an important factor in compliance, since multiple changes in life-style make it more difficult to comply.

Congestive Heart Failure Management

Management goals of CHF include reduction of cardiac workload, improvement of cardiac contractility, and reduction of sodium and water retention. Reduction of cardiac workload is best facilitated by careful regulation of activities, including frequent rest periods as needed during exercise. Weight reduction in an obese elderly person would also relieve cardiac workload. Supportive nutritional counseling might be appropriate in this situation to maintain adequate nutrition within a cultural-ethnic context during weight reduction efforts.

Dietary sodium reduction to 2 g per day is generally the mode of management for control of water retention. Elderly persons need to be educated about hidden salt content in canned foods, ready-to-eat fast foods, or processed foods. Frozen and fresh foods are preferred choices for dietary selection, since they contain only primarily inherent sodium.

Medications must also be closely monitored in clients with CHF. Pharmacologic agents may include vasodilators such as nitroglycerine, which reduce cardiac workload, digitalis derivatives to improve cardiac contractility, and diuretics to reduce fluid retention. Potentially lethal adverse effects of these agents when used singly or in combination warrant close observation for such things as signs of fluid-electrolyte imbalance and potentially lethal arrhythmias.

Client education regarding the detection of early signs of recurrent CHF must be directed at both the client and significant others. Education includes some simple instructions, such as call the nurse or physician if any of the following occur (McGurn, 1981):

1. Shoes become too tight.
2. ADLs become too tiring.
3. Need for sleep increases.
4. Nocturia occurs or increases in frequency.
5. Severe dyspnea, a precursor of pulmonary edema, occurs.

Routine follow-up on a regular basis (every three to four weeks) is of great importance in maintaining clients who have chronic CHF within the community. Such close follow-up on an outpatient basis proves both cost effective and beneficial to client satisfaction. In addition, such follow-up decreases hospital time secondary to complications of CHF exacerbation (Cintron and others, 1983).

Prognosis of CHF is dependent on the ability of elderly people to accept the limitations imposed on them secondary to cardiac dysfunction and to comply with the treatment plan. Quality of life is variable for each client and depends on individual expectations and previous life-styles (Wild, 1986).

Nursing Management of Cerebrovascular Problems

TIAs are forerunners of strokes and must be recognized and evaluated promptly. Caution must be taken not to attribute TIA symptoms to normal signs of aging and thereby delay medical treatment. Nursing activity in this area is primarily educative and directed at education of family, the client, and significant others regarding the significance of the disease, possible manifestations and immediate management of TIAs, control of risk factors, and caution in sudden change of position, which could provoke syptoms. Nurses must also assist with environmental adaptations. The elderly person who lives alone is isolated from assistance and may need a more systematic method of observation by family members, neighbors, friends, or health care providers. A telephone at the client's bedside and in other accessible areas facilitates prompt contact with potential helpers. Environmental safety should also be secured to prevent falls and subsequent complications.

Once a stroke has occurred, nursing care in the home setting is guided by the physiologic, psychologic, social, and spiritual concerns associated with the stroke. Physiologic care is a first priority, since rehabilitation must be reinitiated immediately on arrival from the hospital. Environmental adaptations are also necessary to facilitate the process. Physical restoration includes positioning, exercise for range of motion and strengthening, progressive mobility training, and ambulation with or without assistive devices.

Passive and active exercises are necessary to maintain and build muscle strength, maintain joint function, prevent deformities, stimulate circulation, and build endurance. Both client and family should be involved in the process so that the exercises are incorporated in the client's

ADLs. The client should be encouraged to perform self-care activities, such as combing hair and eating, as much as possible to facilitate independence and functional improvement.

The need for adaptive equipment must be assessed on an individual basis and used selectively to improve quality of life and safety in the home environment. Numerous adaptive accessories are available to facilitate self-care, including long-handled combs, soap mitts, playing card holders, grab bars, and bathtub seats.

Adaptive appliances, such as slings, braces, walkers, wheelchairs, or canes, may also be needed to protect weakened muscles and facilitate independent ambulation. Use of such equipment requires special precautions including routine equipment maintenance to ensure optimal functioning, meticulous skin care to prevent pressure sores, and environmental modification to remove environmental barriers such as furniture or rugs.

Bowel and bladder retraining may also be a necessary component of the rehabilitative process. Both client and family should be actively involved in the retraining program, which should include regular physical exercise, sufficient dietary roughage and bulk, and simple measures such as hot liquids to stimulate continence and adequate liquid intake to prevent constipation. Stool softeners, laxatives, and suppositories may be prescribed by the physician to promote regularity. However, enemas should not be recommended on a regular basis.

Bladder retraining may require close supervision and management. A close record of drinking and urinating patterns, as well as activities, should assist the nurse in formulating a plan for retraining the client. Fluids should be maintained at an adequate and consistent level to facilitate regularity. Special considerations include family education regarding the benefits of rewarding elderly people and avoiding scolding them.

Stroke-induced aphasia does not generally resolve spontaneously; therefore communication is a difficult problem for both client and family. Speech evaluation and therapy should begin early in the client's rehabilitation. However, the nurse can help the client and family adapt to this difficult problem in several ways. Communication techniques include speaking clearly and slowly, using short simple sentences, repeating and rephrasing, reducing environmental distractions, and, if possible, using communication aids such as notebooks, pencils, chalkboards, and picture cards. Family members should be encouraged to speak with the person, be patient when clients respond, and avoid anticipating needs, which limits clients' opportunity for self-expression.

Nurses also play a special role in helping the client and family deal with the psychosocial aspects of disability and rehabilitation. Depression often accompanies stroke recovery and on a temporary basis is part of the readjustment process. Prolonged depression and apathy may require mental health interventions. Emotional support and nursing skill are important in managing emotional lability, loss of confidence, or lack of motivation. Short-term realistic goals that encourage independence and may improve morale and motivation must be established. Clients should neither view themselves nor be viewed by family members as hopeless, pathetic, and helpless. Continued social interaction must be encouraged. Stable clients should take part in family activities and decision making and remain as active in family as their capabilities permit.

Stroke rehabilitation is a long-term process that often requires the input of a team of health care providers. The family caregiver must be recognized as part of that team. Most important, caregiver needs should be addressed, not only in terms of professional assistance but in terms of respite and social support.

DIABETES MELLITUS IN ELDERLY PEOPLE

It has been estimated that at least 20% of all people with diabetes are 60 years of age or older. In the elderly population, women are more prone to diabetes, and diabetes develops in nonwhite women twice as often as it does in white women (Graves, 1985).

The elderly adult is in danger of delayed diagnosis of diabetes mellitus for two significant reasons. The aging process, which normally reduces the glomerular filtration rate in the kidney, causes a delay in urine glucose level elevations until the blood glucose level is elevated to 280 to 300 μg/dl. As many as 50% of elderly people in a hyperglycemic, hyperosmolar, nonketotic coma die from this complication even before diagnosis of diabetes mellitus is made (Graves, 1985). In addition, elderly clients may not complain of the usual signs and symptoms of diabetes mellitus—polydipsia, polyphagia, polyuria, or weight loss. The only symptom may be fatigue until severe complications of diabetes occur. In fact, initial detection of diabetes is often incidental, either during a routine office visit or during hospitalization for another problem.

It is important for the health care provider to be able to differentiate between diabetes and the normal aging process. A misdiagnosis of diabetes can be physically, psychologically, and functionally detrimental to elderly people.

Treatment of Elderly Diabetics

Treatment for diabetes begins with the collection of baseline data obtained at the initial health assessment when diabetes is suspected. During the initial appraisal of an elderly client with diabetes the community nurse's foremost responsibility is to evaluate the client's readiness and willingness to learn and capacity for engaging in self-care activities. At the same time there is a need to identify barriers to effective self-care, such as inadequate motivation, physical or mental dysfunction, or lack of social or financial resources. After this nursing assessment is made, the health care provider must develop strategies for teaching the diabetic client and primary caregiver the day-to-day skills, routines, and dietary patterns needed to live with diabetes.

Once baseline data are obtained, management of the elderly diabetic is directed at the following goals:

1. Achieving normoglycemia
2. Preventing or delaying vascular and neurologic complications
3. Assessing clients physically, mentally, and functionally so that they can self-manage diabetes
4. Helping the elderly diabetic client cope with the disease and subsequent life-style changes

To achieve and maintain normoglycemia, one must consider four variables—diet, exercise, stress, and insulin regulation.

Modification of the diet is the most important component of the therapeutic plan for clients with diabetes mellitus. In fact, for some individuals an appropriate diet may be the only therapeutic intervention required to achieve normoglycemia. Dietary management is directed at maintenance of proper nutrition, distribution of calories throughout the day to prevent wide swings of blood glucose, achievement and maintenance of ideal body weight, and distribution of carbohydrates, protein, and fat as required for dietary control.

In addition, the dietary regimen should be developed around clients' ethnic, cultural or religious needs, as well as their particular life-styles and economic constraints. An elderly diabetic may have coexisting health problems that also require dietary restriction. This individual needs special guidance regarding foods that are compatible with each special diet.

Elderly adults may eat some of their meals at a senior center or local fast-food restaurant and consider these meals a vital part of their social life. The health care provider can also consider favorite items on these menus as part of the exchange equivalents. Often fast-food chains have lists of the food items the chains serve and their nutrient information and exchange equivalents (Kloster, 1982).

Elderly diabetics may also have age-related deficits. Visual impairments may limit the ability to read food labels and dietary instructions. Functional limitations can reduce the elderly person's ability to shop for foods or prepare them. Resolution of these problems may require coordination of services and supports to facilitate dietary compliance.

Obesity and inactivity contribute to glucose intolerance in a genetically predisposed individual. For this reason exercise is an important component in the therapeutic program for the diabetic. Special considerations must be given to the elderly diabetic who has concomitant atherosclerotic heart disease such as exercise-induced arrhythmia, angina, or myocardial infarction, arthritis, or other musculoskeletal limitations that are aggravated by certain types of exercise. The potential hazards of exercise can be minimized if previous medical clearance is obtained and the client progresses gradually to higher levels of activity. The exercise program should be designed with individualization depending on the client's interests, physical condition, and motivation (American Diabetes Association, 1984).

Psychologic or physical stress such as trauma, inflammation, or infection can raise antiinsulin hormone levels, which in turn can induce hyperglycemia if body insulin levels are inadequate (Jovanovic and Peterson, 1986). Health professionals must be knowledgeable about the deleterious effects of both acute and long-standing stress on the diabetic client; health professionals must develop strategies that help clients improve their coping techniques and encourage clients to participate in self-care activities.

Insulin Regulation in Diabetes

When dietary control is inadequate to maintain normoglycemia, two pharmacologic methods are considered—oral hypoglycemic agents or insulin administration.

Oral hypoglycemic agents are indicated for the client whose pancreas is capable of producing insulin. These agents are most effective in clients who had the onset of diabetes after 40 years of age, have had diabetes for less than five years, are of normal weight or obese, and have never received insulin or have been well controlled on less than 40 units per day (American Diabetes Association, 1984).

Elderly diabetic clients tend to have decreased renal and hepatic function (secondary to aging) and cardiovascular problems, as well as a tendency to skip meals and snacks. For these reasons an agent with shorter duration of action is preferred, since it is less likely to cause profound hypoglycemia. In addition, the medication should be started at the lowest effective dose, with small increments every one to two weeks until satisfactory glycemic control is achieved. If this is not effective, the client may be a candidate for another hypoglycemic agent or insulin therapy.

According to the American Diabetics Association, approximately 60% to 70% of clients with type II diabetes initially demonstrate a satisfactory response to oral sulfonylurea compounds. Initial success with subsequent drug failure may be due to dietary indiscretion, progression of diabetes, or the development of another condition such as infection or heart disease. Those controllable factors should be considered by the community nurse before the client is switched to insulin therapy.

Insulin is required for 20% of elderly clients who have diabetes mellitus. Selection of insulin by the primary care provider requires knowledge of onset, peak, and duration of action of selected insulin(s), regulation of meals and snacks in accordance with the insulin's mechanism of action, and calculation of the client's ideal body weight (American Diabetes Association, 1984).

Characteristics of the elderly diabetic, such as significant decline in physical activity, occurrence of acute or chronic illness, excessive weight gain or loss, or behavioral changes representing depression or dementia, may affect caloric requirements and insulin administration. Close supervision is necessary to ensure client compliance, efficacy of insulin dosage, and ability of the elderly diabetic to self-administer insulin.

Efficacy of therapy for diabetes is determined by measuring the degree of glucose control using a variety of techniques. Blood glucose monitoring, done by extracting a small amount of blood usually by finger prick, is more reliable than urine glucose tests, especially for elderly people, whose age-related impairment of renal function may result in misleading urine glucose levels.

Age-related changes can affect the efficacy of testing by the elderly diabetic. Vision changes cause a reduction in accommodation and color discrimination, with subsequent decrease in accuracy of reading the results. Reduced finger and hand mobility secondary to aging may cause difficulty with both grasping reagent strips required for urine glucose evaluation, and also using the glucometer for blood glucose evaluation. Incomplete emptying of the bladder secondary to loss of bladder muscle tone may cause false high or low urine glucose level readings. Consequently, an assessment of the elderly diabetic's self-care abilities is necessary before methods of testing for presence of glucose are selected.

Community Nursing Implications

Chronic management of diabetes requires that the client assume primary responsibility for day-to-day care. If the elderly people have difficulty accepting the diagnosis and its implications or have difficulty learning or integrating diabetic health care into their life-styles, promotion of self-care is impeded.

Periodic review, reinforcement, and evaluation of instruction is a necessary component of a teaching plan. In the case of elderly diabetics, the ideal method of instruction is one-to-one in the home setting, where clients can be evaluated and instructed in the context of their own environments. Group instruction and support groups may also be considered for diabetics who prefer a group setting for the sharing of ideas, concerns, and coping strategies.

Other areas of concern in the care of an elderly diabetic include recognition and treatment of hyperglycemia or hypoglycemia, management during illness, foot care, and early detection and treatment of the complications of diabetes.

Recognition and Management of Hyperglycemia and Hypoglycemia

Persistent hyperglycemia is linked to the development of severe complications such as cardiovascular, renal, and neuropathic diseases. Recurrent hypoglycemic reactions are known to cause brain cell damage and decrease intellectual ability. Diabetics and their families need to learn signs, symptoms, and prompt treatment of either condition to prevent irreversible effects in the diabetic. Clients and family should be advised of the importance of maintaining a regular schedule, including diet, exercise, and medication, daily record keeping, and notification of the primary health care provider when illness is apparent.

Generally speaking, oral hypoglycemic agents produce less severe symptoms than does insulin. However, elderly people are prone to frequent hypoglycemic reactions, especially if they use long-acting oral agents such as chlorpropamide. Clients should also be warned not to mix alcohol with sulfonylureas because of the "antabuse" effect. This reaction, most common in clients who take chlorpropamide, includes headaches, nausea, flushing of the face, tachycardia, and shortness of breath.

Treatment of hypoglycemia is directed at increasing blood glucose by immediate oral ingestion of a rapidly absorbing refined carbohydrate such as honey, a soft drink, orange juice, or sugar cubes. Symptoms should abate within 10 minutes, or administration of more refined carbohydrates is necessary. Chocolate bars or hard candies are not recommended; chocolate contains fat, which delays absorption, whereas hard candy takes time to dissolve.

It is of utmost importance to advise the client to wear diabetes identification and to carry a sugar source at all times; this should be stressed regularly by the health care provider.

Care During Acute Illness

The body has an increased need for insulin during stress and times of illness as a result of increased glyconeogenesis and elevated blood glucose levels. Gastrointestinal upset and vomiting interferes with dietary intake and provokes excessive loss of fluid and nutrients. This presents a potential crisis, especially for elderly diabetics, even if the illness is mild or short. Special instructions from the physician are mandatory to prevent serious consequences. In general the primary care provider must be notified when urine examination reveals acetone, urine tests show a 2% glucose level or blood glucose is elevated, nutritional intake is inadequate, frequent urination persists, an illness lasts more than 72 hours or an elderly client cannot eat after two or three meals (American Diabetes Association, 1984). During these times, elderly people should remain in bed, keep warm, and have someone near them in case a hypoglycemic reaction occurs or illness progresses.

Foot Care

Elderly diabetics are at high risk of decreased circulation secondary to vascular disease and decreased sensation secondary to neuropathy in the feet and legs. They are subsequently susceptible to infection and injury and need to be instructed about routine foot care. Daily foot care and inspection is essential, and special attention should be given to keeping skin moist with lanolin or petroleum jelly and managing signs of infection promptly. The client should be instructed to avoid constricting footwear, going barefoot, and foot injury. Podiatry should be considered for the client who has difficulty keeping nails manicured because of reduced mobility or vision.

Early Detection and Treatment of Complications of Diabetes

The major chronic complications of diabetes include accelerated macrovascular disease (premature atherosclerosis in heart, brain, and peripheral vascular system), diabetic retinopathy, diabetic renal disease, and selected neuropathic conditions. Diabetics and their families need regular reinforcement regarding diet and exercise to maintain weight and glycemic control. Periodic ophthalmologic examinations, preferably with dilated pupils, are extremely important to the early detection of retinopathy and prevention of serious sequelae that cause blindness. There may also be a relationship between lack of glycemic control and progression of the disease.

Certain predisposing factors, such as infection, hypertension, neurogenic bladder, urinary obstruction, and nephrotoxic drugs like analgesics and dye contrast used in radiographic studies, precipitate diabetic renal disease (American Diabetes Association, 1984). Prompt treatment of urinary tract infections, maintenance of normoglycemia, and normalization of blood pressure are also necessary to prevent renal complications.

Little is known about the development and treatment of diabetic neuropathy. However, it is believed that sorbitol accumulation in the Schwann cells of nerve tissue is responsible for peripheral nerve tissue damage. The sensory nerves are more often involved than the motor nerves, causing significant paresthesia and pain, especially in the lower extremities. Male diabetics with autonomic neuropathy may have symptoms of a neurogenic bladder or sexual impotence. Voiding every four hours, using the Valsalva maneuver if necessary, may serve as a preventive measure for neurogenic bladder. A sexual history with intermittent reassessment of baseline data is important for detection and management of sexual dysfunction secondary to diabetic neuropathy.

Diabetes mellitus is a complex disorder of relative insulin insufficiency resulting in abnormal metabolism of carbohydrates, fats, and protein. Although no cure for diabetes exists yet, serious complications secondary to poor glucose control can be delayed or prevented with normoglycemia. Diet, weight control, exercise, and medical management are used to balance the metabolic state in the diabetic. The elderly diabetic is at high risk for development of complications unless proper health education, supervision, and support are given. The nurse remains a primary figure in the elderly diabetic's adjustment to a chronic disease, which requires many restrictions and life-style changes.

SUMMARY

The complex interaction of biopsychosocial factors related to both the aging process and chronic illness represents important reasons for monitoring chronic health problems in the community setting. To provide this care, the nurse must have a basic knowledge of rehabilitation nursing and prevention and management of common chronic diseases, as well as public health nursing skills. More important, with the increasing elderly population, the nurse must understand the normal aging process and the vulnerability of elderly adults to biopsychosocial stresses in terms of coping in health and illness.

QUESTIONS FOR DISCUSSION

1. What is meant by chronic obstructive lung disease (COLD)? Describe the nursing process as it relates to COLD.
2. In what ways might arthritis change the life-style of an elderly adult?
3. An elderly client who has peripheral vascular disease has said that he does not understand why he should be expected to take long walks. Outline your explanation to him of the value of walking.
4. Outline a teaching program for a group of elderly diabetics whose disease can be managed without medication. Include dietary advice, recognition of hyperglycemia, foot care, and other important aspects of the knowledge base needed by the members of this group.

REFERENCES

Acee S: Helping patients breathe more easily, Geriatr Nurs 84:230, 1984.

American Diabetes Association: Physician's guide to type II diabetes (NIDDM): diagnosis and treatment, 1984, The Association.

Anderson TP: Principles of rehabilitation: cerebrovascular accident. In Anderson SV and Bauwens EE, editors: Chronic health problems: concepts and application, St. Louis, 1981, CV Mosby Co.

Arthritis Foundation: Arthritis alert #1: message to Congress, Washington, DC, 1979, The Foundation.

Berk ML and Wilensky GR: Health care of the poor elderly: supplementing Medicare, Gerontologist 25:311, 1985.

Braun J: Arthritis in the ages, New York, 1981, Upjohn Co.

Brodoff A: Diagnosing COPD earlier, Patient Care 18:128, 1984.

Brody SJ: Strategic planning: the catastrophic approach, Gerontologist 27:131, 1987.

Bruce MF: Arthritis and osteoporosis. In Hogstel MD, editor: Home nursing care for the elderly, Bowie, Md, 1985, Brady Communications Co Inc.

Burk NK: Pulmonary diseases, New Hyde Park, NY, 1982, Medical Examination Publishing Co.

Calin A: Gerontology—aspects of rheumatology. In Ebaugh FO, editor: Management of common problems in geriatric medicine, Menlo Park, Calif, 1981, Addison-Wesley Publishing Co Inc.

Cintron G and others: Nurse practitioner role in a chronic congestive heart failure clinic: in-hospital time, costs and patient satisfaction, Heart Lung 12:237, 1983.

Crossman L and Kaljian D: The family: cornerstone of care, Generations 8:44, 1984.

Dietary factors and blood pressure, Dairy Council Digest 52:5, 1981.

Eliopoulos C: Chronic care and the elderly: impact on the client, the family and the nurse. In Wells T, editor: Aging and health promotion, Rockville, Md, 1982, Aspen Publishers Inc.

Elkowitz EB: Geriatric medicine for the primary care practitioner, New York, 1981, Springer Publishing Co Inc.

Floyd J and Buckler J: Nursing care of the elderly: the DRG influence, J Gerontol Nurs 13:20, 1987.

Fries JF: Aging, natural death and the compression of morbidity, N Engl J Med 303:130, 1980.

Gioiella EV and Bevil CW: Nursing care of the aging client: promoting healthy adaptation, East Norwalk, Conn, 1985, Appleton & Lange.

Graves M: Metabolic disorders. In Hogstel MO, editor: Home nursing care for the elderly, Bowie, Md, 1985, Brady Communications Co Inc.

Health Care Financing Administration: Long-term care: background and future directions, Washington, DC, 1981, Department of Health and Human Services.

Home Health Line. (11/25/85). Washington, D.C.

1988 Joint National Committee: 1988 Report of the Joint National Committee on Detection, Evaluation, and Treatment of High Blood Pressure, Arch Intern Med 148:1023, 1988.

Jovanovic L and Peterson CM: Update of diabetes, Physician Assistant 2:43, 1986.

Kavesh WN: Home care process, outcome, cost. In Eisdorfer C, editor: Annual review of gerontology and geriatrics 6, New York, 1986, Springer Publishing Co Inc.

Kloster P: Nutrition—fast food, is it junk? Geriatr Nurs 3:184, 1982.

Lubkin IM: Chronic illness: impact and interventions, Monterey, Calif, 1986, Jones & Bartlett Publishers Inc.

Manton KG: Future patterns of chronic disease incidence, disability and mortality among the elderly, NY State J Med 313:623, 1985.

McGurn W: People with cardiac problems: nursing concepts, Philadelphia, 1981, JB Lippincott Co.

Messerli F: Osler's maneuver and pseudohypertension, N Engl J Med 312:1548, 1985.

Michaels D and Stephenson C: Pulmonary problems. In Hogstel MO, editor: Home nursing care for the elderly, Bowie, Md, 1985, Brady Communications Co Inc.

National Center for Health Statistics: Health statistics of Medicare beneficiaries, series B. Descriptive Report #2 (NMLVES), Hyatsville, Md, 1983, The Center.

Oregon Thoracic Society (COPD Manual Committee): Chronic obstructive pulmonary disease, New York, 1981, American Lung Association.

Parmley WW: Pathophysiology of congestive heart failure, Am J Cardiol 56:7A, 1985.

Patrick, M: Respiratory problems. In Carnevale DL and Patrick M, editors: Nursing management for the elderly, ed 2, Philadelphia, 1986, JB Lippincott Co.

Petrowski DD and Tyzenhouse P: The elderly at home, in clinics, and in nursing homes. In Petrowski D, editor: Handbook of community health nursing: essentials for clinical practice, New York, 1984, Springer Publishing Co Inc.

Rubin JR and Goldstone J: Peripheral vascular disease: treatment and referral of elderly. Part I. Geriatrics 40:34, 1985.

Schmidt MD: Meet the health care needs of older adults by using a chronic care model, J Gerontol Nurs 11:30, 1985.

Tuck ML and Sowers JR: Hypertension and aging. In Karenman SG, editor: Endocrine aspects of aging, Amsterdam, 1982, Elsevier Publishing Co Inc.

US Department of Health and Human Services. 1980. Statement of hypertension in the elderly: revised data. Washington, DC, 1980, The Department.

US Department of Health, Education, and Welfare: Smoking and health: a report of the surgeon general, Washington, DC, 1979, US Government Printing Office.

Wild L: Cardiovascular problems. In Carnevale DL and Patrick M, editors: Nursing management for the elderly, Philadelphia, 1986, JB Lippincott Co.

Yurick AG, Robb SS, and Spier BE: The aged person and the aging process, New York, 1980, Appleton & Lange.

One of the most interesting aspects of the nursing role in the community is the wide variety of clients community nurses can see and help. In the preceding unit clients were separated by age. However, there are other ways in which people can be grouped for study. In this section selected groups of people who are of special interest to nurses are described. Some of these groups represent populations at risk for health problems and in need of extra care and attention from nurses. These populations include people with mental health problems that can be managed in the community rather than an institution, families of mentally retarded persons, families with abusive patterns, and people with handicapping conditions and their families. The focused material in this section is designed to help nurses cope more effectively with members of these groups.

Rural health and sexual health are two topics in this section that are ordinarily neglected in community-oriented textbooks. It is being recognized that the rural population is in need of attention. The chapter on sexual health is included because we have done research in this area for years and think that a better understanding of clients' sexual problems and concerns could add an important dimension to both the preventive and curative health care that is delivered by nurses. The need for this understanding increases each day as the AIDS epidemic spreads.

The concepts of culture and poverty are covered because they are important in most community settings. The hallmark of good community nurses is a sensitivity to cultural differences and an ability to work with people whose norms and value systems are different from their own. This sensitivity grows with experience, but a beginning knowledge base helps lay the groundwork for a lifetime of growth.

Nursing Care for Special Populations

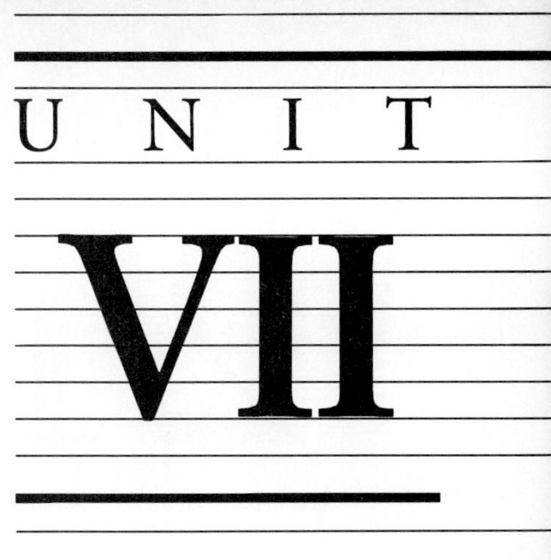

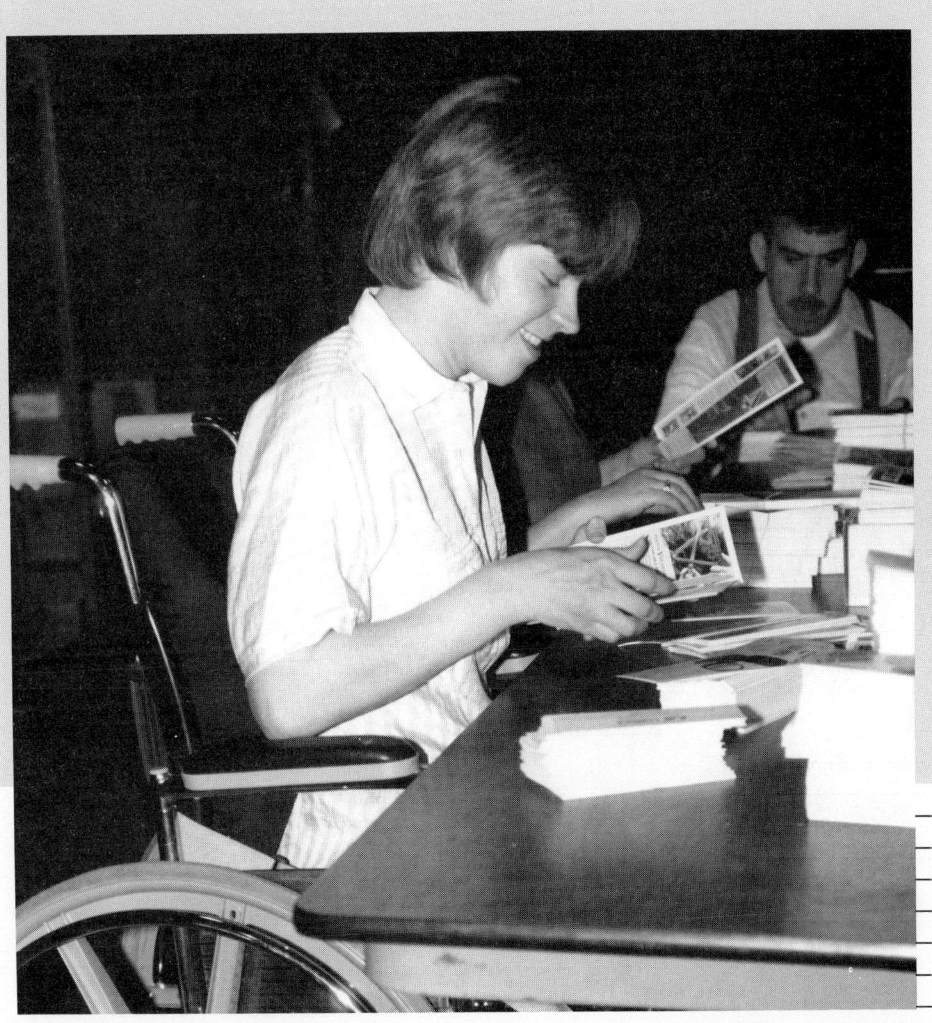

CHAPTER 21

Culture and Poverty as Variables in Care

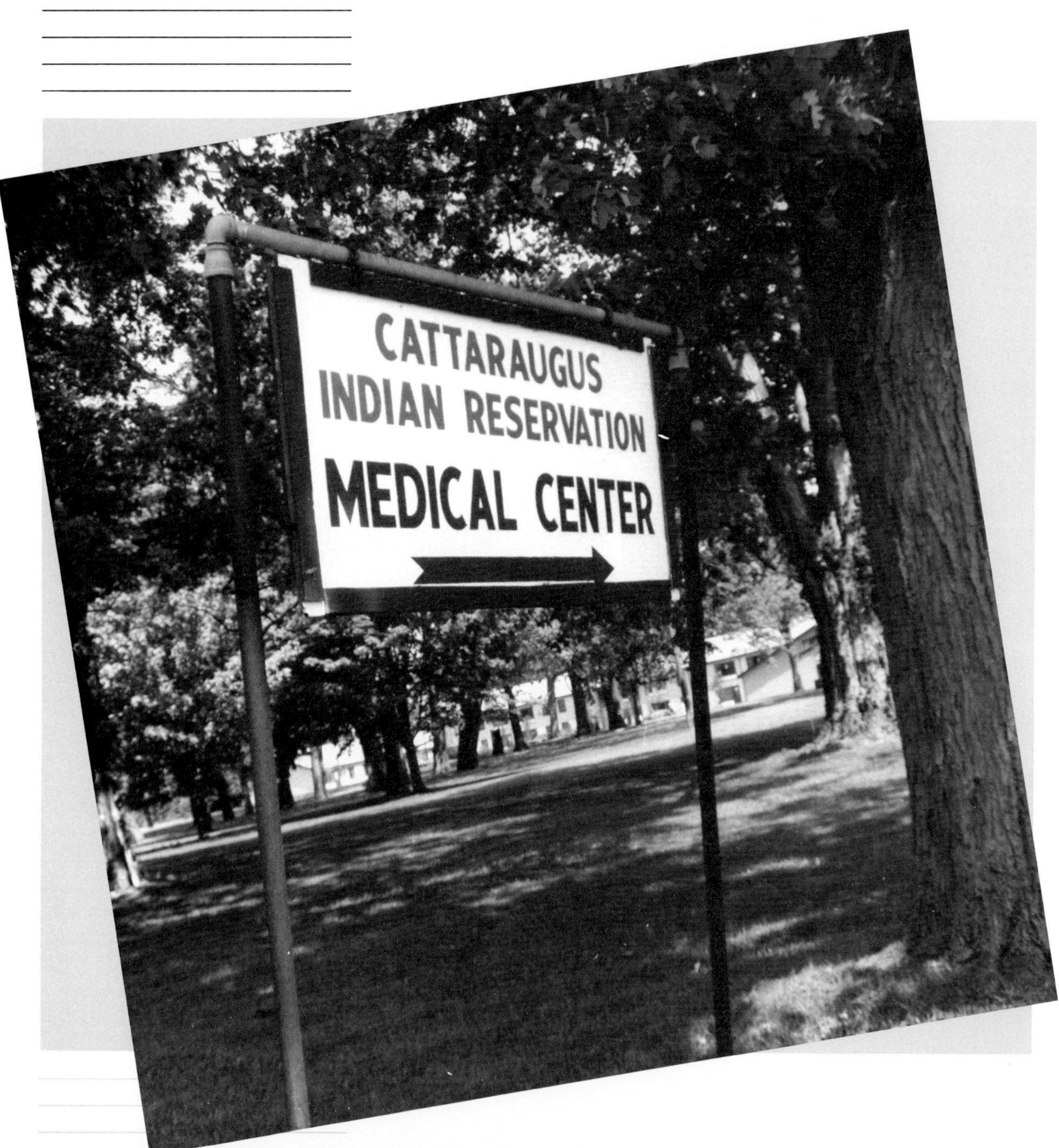

CHAPTER OUTLINE

Culture and illness

Varieties of culture in the United States

- Asian Americans
- Gypsies
- Black Americans
- Spanish-speaking minority groups
- Native Americans

Effect of religion on health practices

Culture of poverty

- The homeless

Summary

OBJECTIVES

After completing this chapter, the reader should be able to:

1. Define the concept of culture within the context of community nursing.
2. Describe the importance of folk medicine and give examples of it among different cultural groups.
3. Describe the process of acculturation.
4. Discuss the impact of the culture of poverty on health behavior.
5. Assess the problems of the homeless population.

HUMAN behavior is not isolated from the culture in which it occurs, and this is as true of health-related behaviors as of other aspects of life. Although there is a broadly defined American culture, every American also belongs to other cultural groups. A person raised in a southern Texas rural area is part of a culture that is different from someone raised in New York City.

Culture provides a set of norms, values, and behaviors that are common to a group, but these attitudes and behaviors are not always consciously acknowledged as being aspects of the culture. Cultural patterns are learned through a process of socialization, most of which takes place during childhood. Therefore people tend not to question their culture, but to accept it as a given. Sometimes life circumstances, such as marriage or job relocation, force people to adapt to a different culture. Still, certain aspects of the culture of childhood remain and provide the initial responses to such major life events as birth, death, childrearing, and illness. Cultural patterns also often determine the trivial aspects of behavior. For example, personal space seems to be culturally set. Americans seem to want a great deal of personal space and stand apart from one another. In Japan, as in Italy, people seem to bunch together more closely. It is interesting to watch members of two cultures with differing views of personal space in conversation; they do a kind of dance as each unconsciously seeks a comfortable amount of space.

Because much of what constitutes culture is unconscious, people have a tendency to look on their way of doing things as the correct way. Technically this is termed "ethnocentrism," since many people are so enmeshed in their own culture that they either fail to realize or forget that other people have different values.

Cultural shock, the feeling of helplessness, discomfort, and even anger at what people from other cultures do when they are ill, what they eat, or how they eat, is something that most nurses go through at some time in their life. But as nurses suffer cultural shock when they first encounter the culture of a barrio or ghetto, clients also do when they come into contact with the health care system. The nurse must keep in mind that members of nondominant cultural groups view the traditional health care system and illness in general from a different perspective.

People usually belong not just to one culture, but to two or more. The term "bicultural" is sometimes used to describe people who have competing values, life-styles, and cultures, but it is somewhat limiting because "bi" suggests only two competing cultures, whereas people often belong to many different cultures at the same time. Within American society, for example, cultural groups vary by age, as well as other factors. Tastes in music, movies, clothes, and style are different from one age-group to another. There is also a gay culture, that is, a culture based on sexual desire toward others of the same sex; although the gay culture may be thought to comprise only men, lesbians are also members. The list of cultural groupings could go on, but the point is that nurses must be prepared to deal with various cultures and subcultures and respond to them as effectively as they can. The box defines various terms used when discussing concepts related to culture.

CULTURE AND ILLNESS

Cultural background has an effect on illness. One of the early demonstrations of this took place in Chicago in 1939 when Robert E.L. Faris and H. Warren Dunham found that people in whom schizophrenia was diagnosed were most likely to live in the slum and rooming-house neighborhoods near the central part of the city, whereas people in whom manic depression was diagnosed (a diagnosis that is no longer used) were scattered throughout the city. Since schizophrenia was the most common type of functional psychosis, the high rate of this disease found in poverty neigh-

DEFINITIONS OF CONCEPTS RELATED TO CULTURE AND POVERTY

Culture: The ideas, values, and behavior that are learned by members of a social group constitute culture. Culture acts as a guide to interpreting the actions of other people and behaving in ways that make sense. It can be defined as a set of rules that guides individuals, although they might not always be conscious of these rules.

Ethnicity: The term "ethnicity" is derived from a Greek word that could be literally transplanted as nation or people. In modern terminology, however, the term is used to describe large groups of people classed according to their common traits and customs, usually derived from a common geographic, racial, or religious origin, shared standards of behavior, and a sense of identity. Polish Americans, for example, have an ethnic identity based on national origins, whereas the ethnic identity of Mormons is based on religion.

Ethnocentrism: Regarding one's own race or cultural group as superior to others is the literal meaning of ethnocentrism. As used here it means a tendency to judge others in terms of one's own assumptions, regardless of their scientific validity.

Race: Race is a biologic term. Members of a racial group share some common biologic characteristics such as skin color, genetic traits, and bone structure. Ethnic and racial groups sometimes overlap, but ethnicity is a smaller subgrouping than race.

Cultural shock: Leininger (1976) described cultural shock as "the feeling of disorientation experienced by an outsider attempting to comprehend or effectively adapt to a different cultural group because of differences in cultural practices, values, and beliefs."

Minority: Minority is defined as a part of a population differing from others in some characteristics and often subjected to differential treatment. A minority may be a racial, religious, ethnic, occupational, or interest group. In effect everyone is a minority group member in some way. Male nurses, for example, are a minority group within nursing, whereas nurses are a minority group in the general population.

Culture of poverty: A set of norms, values, and world views learned by members of a society who grow up in poverty neighborhoods constitutes the culture of poverty. As described by the anthropologist, Oscar Lewis (1966), the culture of poverty is marked by a fatalistic attitude, a sense of helplessness, and a present (rather than future) time orientation.

Index of poverty: The index of poverty is an index developed by the Social Security Administration that periodically assesses the economic well-being of the country and defines families in poverty. The poverty level in 1986 for a family of four was $11,203. There were 32.4 million people below the poverty line (Statistical Abstract, 1986).

borhoods helped account for the correlation between hospitalization and low socioeconomic status. In trying to explain their findings, Faris and Dunham hypothesized that schizophrenia might be more common in poverty neighborhoods because people in such locations felt a greater sense of isolation, owing to the social disintegration of their neighborhood (Faris and Dunham, 1939).

The Faris and Dunham thesis set off a lively debate that is still taking place. Researchers have found that slums are not particularly disorganized, but their social structure is different from that of more affluent neighborhoods (Suttles, 1968). On the other hand, the interpretation has been challenged because it implies a causal chain between poverty and schizophrenia. Later researchers, including Dunham himself, argued that poverty might be a consequence rather than a cause of schizophrenia. Schizophrenic individuals may drift down to live in a poor neighborhood because of the socially debilitating symptoms of their illness (Dunham, 1965).

The link between poverty and mental illness has been the subject of much subsequent research. A summary of the research linking income with mental illness done by Bruce and Barbara Dohrenwend stated that psychologic problems including drug addiction are more common among people with low incomes (1969). The physiologic component of psychoses, including the depressive illnesses and schizophrenia, is probably the same across socioeconomic lines, but the life experiences add to the physiologic problems. Poor nutrition, lack of schooling, and personality damage from unfavorable life changes create situations that affect mental health negatively (Rhoades and others, 1980; Roberts, 1980).

Culture is also related to mental health and mental illness, although the relationship is even more complex than the relationship of mental illness to poverty. To understand the cultural variable it is necessary to first note the differences between illness and disease. Disease is a biologic entity and is diagnosed by determining that the body condition deviates from the norms of contemporary medical standards. Illness, on the other hand, is what the individual experiences. Kleinman, Eisenberg, and Good (1978) define illness as "culturally shaped in the sense that how we perceive, experience, and cope with disease is based upon our explanations of sickness." This definition of illness also recognizes that people may be ill even in the absence of disease, an important factor to emphasize, since a significant percentage of visits to health care providers (some estimates go as high as 50%) are not due to biologic causes. That people often visit health care providers for nonbiologic causes is most evident in looking at the use of services for mental health. Proportionately, Asian Americans use mental health services less frequently than white Americans do. Those Asian Americans who do seek mental health services have more severe forms of mental disorders that do white, black, Hispanic, and Native Americans (Flaskerud, 1986a, 1986b, and 1987; Sue, 1977; Sue and McKinney, 1975). One explanation for this discrepancy is Asian Americans' practice of using mental health services only after many years of caring for disturbed persons within the family. It is only when symptoms become so severe that family members cannot cope that Asian Americans finally come to a mental health center.

VARIETIES OF CULTURE IN THE UNITED STATES

Although the United States has always had a variety of different peoples and cultures, the nature of this mix has changed drastically in the last two decades. This is due in large part to the change in the United States immigration policy and the establishment of special refugee categories. From 1921 until 1968 the United States operated on the basis of quotas; these quotas were filled based on nationality. Europeans were favored, and people from other areas, particularly Asia, were discriminated against. The Immigration Act of 1965, which became fully effective in 1968, abolished the old quota system, permitted the entrance of at least 170,000 immigrants from Eastern countries to the United States each year, and gave residents of all Western countries an equal chance to enter the United States. In addition, special groups are allowed to enter the United States with refugee status, which was given to Cubans in 1966, to Vietnamese in 1977, and to all who met the United Nations' definition of refugee in 1980. The result has been the admission of more than 2 million individuals from Asian countries since 1970 under regular immigrant status and nearly 1 million more under special refugee status. Most Asian immigrants have been from China (including Formosa), Hong Kong, Korea, Vietnam, Laos, and Cambodia, but many have come from Thailand, Afghanistan, Indonesia, India, Iran, Iraq, and Japan. There also have been numerous people from South America and Central America admitted with special status (Statistical, 1986). Immigrants to the United States rarely contact a community nurse, but refugees, who are ill more often, are more likely to have contact with nurses. One of the major areas of public health concern with refugees from Southeast Asia is that many have chronic hepatitis B, and this infection can be spread from mothers to their newborn infants (Poss, 1987).

The following sections describe the characteristics of five different cultural groups found in the United States. Although similarities exist within every cultural group, it is important to remember that cultural groups cannot be stereotyped, since every person is different. For example, rural blacks have different attitudes and assumptions than do urban blacks. Middle-class blacks have different attitudes and assumptions than welfare mothers. Similarly, Native Americans who grew up on Navajo reservations have different attitudes and assumptions than Native Americans born and raised in Buffalo, New York. Although all blacks and all Native Americans are different, they share a common heritage of past and present discrimination.

Asian Americans

The Asian population in the United States has increased dramatically in the last two decades with two rather distinct waves of immigration. Before 1979 the immigrant group included many highly educated and professional people; since 1979 Asian immigrants have primarily been refugees from Vietnam, Cambodia, and Laos who were generally not well educated. Some were illiterate in their own language (Muecke, 1983). Many had experienced great hardship before they left; some were beaten or tortured by soldiers or attacked by pirates if they tried to escape in small boats. Some spent many years in crowded resettlement camps before they came to the United States (Poss, 1989).

Although Western medical concepts are accepted by affluent and well-educated Asian Americans, folk medical beliefs are still important to many Asians including elderly people and the new refugees. There are three major folk medical belief systems in Far Eastern countries—the Chinese system, the Indian system, and the hot and cold balance system.

The Chinese system originated several thousand years ago. It is probably the dominant system because of the large Chinese immigrant communities found in most other Asian countries. The system is based on the concept of yin and yang, with yin representing the male, light, positive force and yang representing the female, dark, negative force. If yin and yang are out of balance, a person becomes ill; the key to good health is a balance between yin and yang. One way of maintaining the balance is through acupuncture, which is based on the theory that the body has hollow points that close up. The needles open these 365 points on the skin and keep the person healthy (Wallnofer and von Rottauscher, 1965).

The Indian folk tradition is as old as that of China, and increasing numbers of Indians are also coming to the United States. Many Americans have also converted to Indian religions. Traditional Indian medicine relies heavily on a wide-ranging pharmacopoeia with ingredients being derived from almost every natural substance available. Taste is an important part of the treatment because each taste is believed to have special properties. Sweet supposedly increases phlegm, appeases hunger and thirst, and causes flatulence, worms, and goiter. Acid increases salivation and appetite, improves digestion, and causes heartburn. Salt is said to purify the blood and stimulate digestion but causes headaches and results in convulsions when taken in excess. In Indian medicine pungent provokes the appetite and lessens corpulence, bitter stimulates the appetite and clears the complexion, and astringent augments the action of any of the above if it is taken with them. Within each of these categories there are also hot and cold, heavy and light, sticky and dry, energizing and sluggish, stationary and fluid, soft and hard, clear and slimy, smooth and rough, coarse and subtle, and dense and liquid qualities that have special effects (Walker, 1968).

Separate and distinct from other Asian cultures is that of the Philippines. Based primarily on Malayan culture, the Philippine culture has been influenced by Chinese, Arabic, Indian, Spanish, and American beliefs and represents a combination of different medical traditions, including sophisticated beliefs of the Filipino health practitioner who comes to the United States and the less sophisticated beliefs of poor immigrants. An acceptance of the ancient Hippocratic theory, which calls for a balance between the four humours of blood, phlegm, black bile, and yellow bile, underlies Filipino-American folk beliefs. Each humour originates in a different part of the body—the heart, brain, spleen, or liver. The theory has often been operationalized as an attempt to balance hot and cold, as well as wet and dry. At other times three basic concepts are emphasized—flushing, heating, and protection. Flushing keeps the body free from debris; heating maintains a balanced internal temperature; and protection guards the body from outside influences. Flushing is more than simply purgings of the body, since it also involves rubbing the skin with lemons, taking special care during menstruation, and limiting activities after giving birth. For example, women are not supposed to read after giving birth because it is believed that their eyes will be strained seriously and ultimately they will go blind. Heat involves not only local application, but also rubbing and massage. Protection is providing a gatekeeping system against the invasion of both natural and supernatural forces into the body (McKenzie and Chrisman, 1977). Protection can be accomplished by wearing a charm, by not washing the face of a baby and thus preventing the "evil eye," or by avoiding certain behaviors such as stepping on a crack in the sidewalk.

Although the Vietnamese had much contact with American military forces during the Vietnam War and were thus exposed to American health practices, there are unique Vietnamese health care concepts that are important. Like the Filipinos, the Vietnamese subscribe to the humoral theory and focus on balancing humors to prevent illness. In most Asian cultures the preservation of social and familial harmony takes priority over individual rights and needs and there is a major effort to suppress conflict. Some illnesses are particularly stigmatized. Among Vietnamese, for example, unmistakable mental disorder is usually attributed to the bad luck of familial inheritance, possession by spirits of malicious intent, or accumulated misdeeds in past lives (Muecke, 1983; Sutherland and others, 1983).

Gypsies

Some cultural groups pose greater health care problems than others because their cultural traditions are hostile to institutionalization. Gypsies constitute one group that requires special knowledge by health care workers. Gypsies came to the United States primarily before World War I from various parts of Europe, although they probably originated in India. In Europe they were a migratory people, often ignoring national boundaries. Accustomed to existing independently of other people, as a general rule gypsies have remained far less integrated in U.S. culture than other groups that arrived in America at the same time. As a group American Gypsies have a characteristic tribal structure, with four main tribes and extended family groups, or vitsas, in each tribe. Each vitsa, ranging in size from 25 to 50 people, has a chief or king whose responsibilities include directing the people's economic opportunity, hiring lawyers to represent them, and protecting their political, economic, and social interests.

Gypsies believe that the source of disease can be traced to demons, the evil eye, breaking taboos, and the fear of disease itself. Cutting one's fingernails on Tuesday or Friday, for example, is unlucky and might cause illness. Many Gypsy treatments involve symbolic transference of disease to another person or object. The Gypsy attitude toward health care seems different depending on the nature of the problem. Generally, Gypsies turn to hospitals and Western medicine for a crisis, but preventive and follow-up care is not used much. Medicine is regarded as curative, not preventive, so serious problems such as diabetes or high blood pressure go either undetected or untreated until they are far advanced (Anderson and Tiche, 1973).

Black Americans

Race does not divide groups, especially blacks and whites, in contemporary American society as much as it used to. Still the inequalities of the past discriminatory practices, repression, and suspicion have left their marks on the health of black Americans. Life expectancies for blacks are less than those for whites; the incidence of infant mortality is higher—19.6 deaths per 1000 black births compared with 10.1 deaths per 1000 white births (Statistical, 1987); and there are more low–birth weight infants (David, 1986) and more delays in prenatal care for blacks (Ingram, Makuc, and Kleinman, 1986). Part of the explanation for these problems is that blacks are still found disproportionately in the lower economic class. A major cause of this is past patterns of discrimination.

Many blacks, especially those in large cities, still live in urban ghettos where traditional folk medicine continues to play an important role. This is also the case among some of the southern rural blacks, many of whom are poor and uneducated. Much of the culture of the ghetto, however, is more a poverty culture than a black culture. There are, however, some folk medical concepts that represent an amalgam of African traditions and rural, Southern black traditions (Puckette, 1979) and that are important for the community health nurse to understand. Some of the folk beliefs are purely superstition, whereas others have been empirically tested over generations and seem to be logical and reasonable treatments. Many treatments seem harmless, and the nurse dealing with poor, uneducated black clients should be prepared to encounter such folk practices as placing a knife under a bed to "cut" the pain of labor and delivery or wearing a variety of amulets and charms to ward off disease. Some customs, however, pose great difficulty. This is particularly true of *pica,* the ingestion of items normally considered inedible, particularly during pregnancy. In the case of blacks it often takes the form of geophagia, or the eating of dirt or clay (Hertz, 1957; Neumann, 1970).

Clay eating is practiced in much of West Africa, perhaps to get a feeling of fullness when food is scarce. Whatever the reason, it is hypothesized that black slaves brought this custom with them to the United States. In the major cities of the South, clay can be purchased in large sacks or simply dug from favorite clay banks in many areas. Blacks who move north into the urban ghettos sometimes have clay mailed to them. If this is not possible, they may turn to eating laundry starch. The starch, which is perhaps reminiscent of the clay they knew in the South, is worse than clay, since it is high in calories and its ingestion leads not only to the neglect of other, more nutritious foods, but also to obesity, deficiency diseases, and possibly poor fetal development. Since the custom has been handed down for generations, it is difficult to deal with unless it can be brought out in the open. Probably the most effective way for nurses to handle this when they encounter clients who eat starch is to counsel clients about the dangers of starch eating and to make certain that clients have an adequate nutritional intake and enough filling food that they no longer crave starch.

Much of folk medicine, such as massage, heat, and baths for rheumatism or the use of various herb teas and poultices for colds, is associated with empiric evidence of results or relief. These practices suggest a rich cultural heritage and should be supported by the nurse unless they interfere with well-being. Such practices not only give comfort, but also help sustain clients through difficult times. The chief repositories of folk remedies in the black community today, as in many other societies, are elderly women who have gained their wisdom through long experience.

The problem the health professional has is in updating the skills and knowledge of such women without threatening them or forcing the client to choose between modern and folk medicine. If clients are forced to make a choice, there is a real danger that they will not choose modern medicine or at the least their recovery will be delayed.

The genetic makeup of blacks is different from that of people of European descent. The result is that blacks are likely to suffer from somewhat different illnesses than whites. Sometimes this affects dietary intake. For example, a significant percentage of blacks, perhaps as many as 60% are lactose intolerant. In these individuals, drinking milk can result in unpleasant gastrointestinal symptoms. Nurses must be careful not to push milk on a child who rejects it until they are certain that milk will not unduly irritate the child's bowel. Since the decrease in milk intake might contribute to rickets in a child, alternative dietary supplements of protein and vitamin D should be considered (Hongladarom and Russell, 1976) Blacks are more likely to have sickle-cell trait or actual sickle-cell anemia than whites. A history of complaints of weakness or pain in the large joints, anorexia and vomiting, or signs of retarded growth should arouse suspicion, and an appropriate referral for testing, treatment, and genetic counseling should be made (Marlow and Redding, 1988).

Additionally, nurses unaccustomed to caring for blacks or other dark-skinned individuals, will need to sharpen their observation skills. For example, one of the major problems among poor ghetto children is iron deficiency anemia (Gutelius, 1969), but a white nurse must acquire special skills of observation, since the signs of fever, rash, and cyanosis in a white person do not apply to black skin. Color changes in both black adults and children are best observed in the sclera, conjunctiva, nail beds, lips, buccal mucosa, tongue, palms, and soles of the feet, where pigmentation for melanin, melanoid, and carotene is least. Pallor in a dark-skinned individual is observable by the absence of the underlying red tones that normally give the brown and black skin its "glow" or "living color." The brown-skinned person with pallor therefore appears more yellowish brown, and the black-skinned person appears ashen gray. Admittedly it takes an experienced eye to identify the change, but those health professionals who are not acquainted with black clients can quickly learn the techniques. Obviously, skin observation must be supplemented by sickle-cell anemia laboratory tests and other means of detection until the caregiver acquires expertise. Sometimes the best consultant for the novice is the mother, who can identify a "pale" appearance in her child long before the inexperienced professional can see it.

Some diagnoses more common in blacks than others might be not so much because of genetic inheritance as because of the problems of living as a minority. This is the case with hypertension, which is higher among blacks than whites. There is a probability of a genetic component, but high-salt, high-carbohydrate diets (generally the least expensive kinds of food), and stress (from discrimination) are also implicated (Bullough and Bullough, 1982). Some other diseases are not so much genetically related as a result of lack of effective education or an ineffective use of the health care delivery system. Such diseases result from lack of immunization against poliomyelitis and measles, lack of treatment for parasitic diseases, lack of fluoridated community water supplies that would prevent dental caries, and failure to give vision tests to children to identify myopia. Better prenatal care would also reduce infant and perinatal mortality (Goldstein, 1963; Kitagawa and Hauser, 1973). Clearly many of the differences are associated with economic status rather than with race. The effect of poverty on health care is discussed in greater detail later in this chapter.

Spanish-Speaking Minority Groups

One of the fastest growing minority groups in the United States is the Spanish-speaking population from various parts of the Western Hemisphere, particularly Mexico, Puerto Rico, and Cuba. Spanish-speaking minority groups have been augmented by the recent immigration of large numbers of refugees from Central America. As in the black community, there is wide variation in social class and economic conditions among the Spanish-speaking population. Many Cuban refugees came from the middle or upper class, and in much of the Southwest there are important and powerful families descended from the original Spanish-speaking settlers in these areas. Still, a disproportionate share of recent immigrants have come from the poor and impoverished population. In the Southwest many crossed the border to work as farm laborers. Many Puerto Ricans, who are U.S. citizens, come to the eastern part of the continental United States from rural areas with little education. Although there are greater concentrations in some areas than others, almost every section of the United States has a community made up of people whose native language is Spanish.

In the larger cities of the Southwest, many of the poor, recent immigrants from Mexico, are concentrated in *barrios,* a section of the city where Spanish is often spoken and where there are many touches of Mexico. Most studies show that neonatal deaths are much higher among Spanish-speaking groups than among Anglos, a catchall term Hispanics use to refer to white English-speaking people regardless of their ethnic background. This is due not to any genetic inheritance, but to a lack of prenatal care, poor nutrition, and generally less healthy mothers—all signs of poverty more than anything else.

In dealing with the people in the barrio, the nurse faces not only a language problem, but also a cultural problem. Mexican cultural tradition tends to hold that bad health, although unpleasant, is something that one endures. Men tend to be particularly Spartan in their attitude toward illness, and there is a belief that a man who admits to illness is not *macho,* or tough and rugged. Sickliness is thought to reflect moral and physical weakness. Often an ill person is commended by friends and relatives for endurance. Women and children are allowed to show more "weakness" during illness than men, although women who work outside the home show much the same stoicism about pain. Also complicating treatment is the traditional Mexican concern with privacy, something that demonstrates itself in what many Anglos would regard as extremes of modesty. Natural functions such as urinating, defecating, and bathing are considered private activities, not to be observed by others. It is somewhat difficult for many Mexican-Americans, even men, to visit male physicians who probe, examine, and inspect bodily areas that Mexican-Americans feel are private. In women such attitudes serve as a deterrent to prenatal care. Undoubtedly all clients, regardless of culture, have some of these feelings but they are accentuated in people who were raised in a *barrio culture* or who have recently arrived from Mexico.

When a person becomes ill, it is often regarded as a family affair. The client in the hospital is likely to be visited by next of kin, as well as far distant relatives, and if the client is ill at home, the same support group visits. Nurses must be considerate of the custom so that the client does not feel slighted, but at the same time nurses must emphasize the welfare of the client who might need long periods of rest and quiet. Sick clients from the barrios also have a low expectation of what can be done for them and are often reluctant to ask for medications that are used on an as-needed basis without the nurse's suggestion.

What is true of the Mexican-Americans in the barrio is also true of many of the recent emigrants from Puerto Rico, which has its own unique culture even though it is a part of the United States. Recent emigrants from Puerto Rico may have a variety of parasitic diseases not common in the continental United States, such as dysentery, filariasis, which is caused by a small worm that lives in the lymphatic channels of the body and is spread by the mosquito, schistosomiasis mansoni, which is dependent on a snail carrier, and hookworm, which is occasionally still found in the southern United States. However, these parasitic diseases have been overcome for the most part in Puerto Rico and thus are less likely to appear, although some elderly immigrants still have aftereffects of these parasitic diseases.

Widespread malnutrition caused primarily by diets consisting mainly of rice and beans, the standard fare of the poor in Puerto Rico, also influences the general health of Puerto Rican emigrants. Traditionally Puerto Ricans eat few green or leafy vegetables and only occasionally use milk and eggs; beans serve as the main source of protein. Bread is still not used in some parts of the island. To this starchy diet, Puerto Ricans add fats in liberal quantities. When a Puerto Rican is transplanted to New York or elsewhere in the Northeast, deficiencies in the diet, such as lack of Vitamin D, are made worse by the lack of sunshine.

As the Puerto Rican communities have grown in the United States, some of the trauma of emigration, common among early emigrants from the island, has lessened. The family patterns in both Puerto Rico and Mexico tend to be extended, and the individual can call for and expect help from many relatives in times of illness or other crises. Initially the move to the United States broke up some of these units, and they have only recently reestablished themselves. Some common customs in Puerto Rico are still weakened by the different life-styles in the United States. Consensual marriages are common in Puerto Rico (Goode, 1960), and although many of these unions are fairly stable when the couples are in Puerto Rico, the impact of urbanization and emigration tends to break them down (Otterbein, 1965). This means that many women are left as heads of households in the continental United States (Wakefield, 1960).

Common both to the Mexican-American and Puerto Rican culture is a folk practitioner known as the *curandero* (*curandera* in the case of a woman). The role is not as institutionalized in Puerto Rican culture as in Mexican-American culture. The curandero not only has acquired considerable empiric knowledge, but also possesses the charismatic qualities associated with the more spiritual aspects of the role. Good curanderos show great warmth and concern for both clients and their families; curanderos offer advice and give treatment with little overt attention to fees. Special prayers are often part of the therapy. If the treatment is successful, the family is expected to give an offering. On the other hand, if treatment fails, no payment is expected. This means that the curandero, simply because there is no fee involved, will refuse to treat a client with a bad prognosis. The implications of this are not lost on the client and emphasize the need to turn to the Anglo medical system, which is associated with serious illness or death, a heavy psychologic burden that further inhibits the chance for recovery.

The curandero is not the only folk practitioner common in Mexican-American culture. In fact, before this folk specialist is sought out, a number of home remedies are tried. Most probably a neighborhood *senora* (elderly woman) is consulted. The line between the senora and the curandero is not clear because elderly women usually start out helping their friends and family during times of illness, and if they gain a reputation for success, they then become known as healers. A male healer may start as a *sovador,* a person who specializes in giving massages, and move on to become a full curandero. The *partera,* or midwife, is also an important practitioner but to a lesser extent in the barrios of the United States than in Mexico (Rubel, 1966).

Mexican-American folk medicine also accepts the Hippocratic theory of the four humours common among some of the recent immigrants from the Philippines. Disease is often thought to be caused by too much hot, an imbalance between "hot" foods and "cold" foods. Other folk diagnoses not recognized by the scientific community include *mollera ciada,* or fallen fontanel. This is the most common type of organ displacement believed to take place, and folk caregivers usually attribute it to withdrawing the infant's mouth from the nipple too suddenly (Martinez and Martin, 1966). Symptoms of the ailment include diarrhea and vomiting. When balancing the four humours in folk medicine, it is not taken into account that infant diarrhea is accompanied by severe dehydration. Therefore the nurse must somehow convince the parents to give liquids even to infants with a "depressed fontanel."

Mal ojo (the evil eye) is also part of *barrio culture,* and the nurse must take into account such beliefs when trying to give effective nursing care (Kosko and Flaskerud, 1986). There are other beliefs unique to particular Mexican-American subcultures besides those listed here, and the nurse has to somehow figure out ways to use these beliefs to aid effective health care.

Native Americans

There are millions of people in the United States who have Indian ancestors, that is, who have an ancestor who might be classified as an indigenous Native American. Even in the 1980s there are still nearly 1 million individuals who live under some kind of control of the Bureau of Indian Affairs. Although Native Americans are popularly thought of as living in the West, large numbers of Indians live in most states of the union.

Life expectancy rates for Native Americans are lower than for whites, and with diseases that must be reported to the Public Health Service, such as amebic and bacillary dysentery, gonorrhea, hepatitis, measles, mumps, syphilis, and tuberculosis, the incidence in Native Americans is higher than in any other subgroup in the United States. The Native American mortality figures reflect not only the conditions of poverty, but also the stresses on Native Americans, especially tribal Native Americans, since they are not well integrated in mainstream American culture, often by choice. Evidence of cultural stress comes also from figures on accident rates, which are higher for Native Americans than for other groups, and suicide, homicide, and cirrhosis of the liver rates, all of which are higher, sometimes four times as high as in the 1960s, among reservation Native Americans than among other Americans (Bashshur, Steeler, and Murphy, 1987; U.S. Department of Health, Trends and Services, 1969).

In sociologic terms, Native Americans might be described as living under the conditions of *anomie,* a concept developed by the sociologist Emile Durkheim at the beginning of this century. Although Durkheim made his generalizations on the basis of rapid social changes created by industrialization, they apply to any society undergoing the kind of social change that causes old norms to lose their saliency without the rules being replaced with functional new rules. According to Durkheim (1951) all kinds of stressors come into play when two competing populations that are different in outlook and technologically unequal encounter each other. The extent of stress imposed by the conflict is not always predictable, if only because it varies from group to group. Anthropologists have developed various terms to describe the types and degrees of contact between two life-styles. These terms are helpful in trying to understand the differences in Native American adjustment, since stresses vary according to the nature of contact. One type of contact is called *diffusion,* the process of a people borrowing an idea, a piece of equipment, or a type of food from another people and incorporating it into their own life-style.

Another type of contact is termed *acculturation.* This implies intense and continuous contact between two previously autonomous cultural traditions, with extensive change in one or both systems. Many American Indians have become acculturated, but the exchange has usually been one sided, with the Native Americans giving up their own culture. *Assimilation,* a third type of contact, occurs when one group changes so completely that it becomes fully integrated into the dominant society or when two groups merge into a new cultural system. Most immigrants to the United States have eventually assimilated into American society, but large numbers of Indians have not done so. One of the reasons for not assimilating is the preservation of Indian culture through the reservation system; this can give young Native Americans a strong grounding in traditional Indian culture. The effect of American culture as a whole, however, has been to undermine much of the traditional Indian culture. Since many Indians do not want to give up and assimilate totally into American culture, this has resulted in stress.

When racial or class barriers to assimilation deter total changes in life-style or when people become disillusioned and frustrated in their attempt to adjust to a powerful foreign culture, one of the most effective coping mechanisms is to revitalize old systems in slightly new forms. Both of these things have happened to Indians in dealing with American culture. In a sense this is a stage in the assimilation process, since at each level of contact and acculturation, some individuals look to traditional, ritual, or political mechanisms to regain a sense of control, revitalize their culture, and attempt to restore equilibrium. It is important in any process of cultural exchange that the less technologically efficient culture not be entirely submerged. In a positive sense the rise of Native American consciousness and Native Americans' assertion that their own heritage is something about which they can be proud will result in a more effective health care delivery system, since the Native Americans not only will be the recipients but will have an effective voice in the planning and delivery of health care.

More than 300 tribal groupings exist in the United States, each with its own language, religion, folkways, mores, and patterns of interpersonal relationships. It is therefore difficult to generalize about Native American medical traditions. Generally before contact with Western medical and health practices, Native Americans tended to attribute inexplicable ailments to the anger of the gods of malevolent spirits. Medicine as such was not only a herb or a drug, but also some supernatural article or agency that might aid in curing. Most tribes had special persons known as medicine men, who in some tribes were organized into societies, whereas in others they practiced as individuals.

Among the Navajos, the most populous of American tribes, the "hand trembler" is an important healer. The name is derived from the fact that the diagnosis is made through intervention of the deities who take over diagnosticians' hands as they draw a picture interpreting the cause of illness. When the drawing is complete, the hand trembler informs the client of the diagnosis and gives recommended actions that might include such things as medications, sweat baths, bed rest, isolation, and special diets. Many Native American clients possess an item they believe has special curative powers; the nurse who encounters this situation must make sure that Native American customs are observed (Primeaux, 1977).

EFFECT OF RELIGION ON HEALTH PRACTICES

Probably the dominant factor influencing the health of vast numbers of people born in the United States is not their nationality, background, or racial composition but their religious beliefs. The United States has a religious variety that is perhaps bigger than in any other country.

Religion is important to most Americans, and this is particularly true in the treatment of illness as distinct from disease. For example, Bertholf (1979) found in a sample of 139 cancer clients that prayer was a major coping mechanism for 20% of the group. Some groups, such as the Greek Orthodox and the Roman Catholics, give Holy Communion to those who desire it, and many Christians believe it helps them recover. Roman Catholics and other groups, including Lutherans and Mormons, believe in a special anointing of the sick. Many Baptists practice "laying on of hands," as do Armenian Christians, Nazarenes, and others. Some groups, such as Christian Scientists, refuse most traditional medical intervention and have their own practitioners who are recognized by Medicare and Medicaid.

Religious beliefs are an important factor in diets, a subject of particular interest to community health nurses. Mormons do not drink coffee or tea, and Seventh Day Adventists not only abstain from coffee and tea, but also are often vegetarians, as are other large segments of the American population. Orthodox Jews, as well as many Conservative Jews, eat only kosher food. Keeping kosher includes not only avoiding pork, pork products, and shellfish, but also not mixing meat and milk products, killing animals in a special way, and even using special methods of preparation. Muslims also do not eat pork and observe other dietary restrictions similar to Jews; Muslims also prohibit the use of alcohol except for medicinal purposes. Many religious groups advocate special diets during certain parts of the year, as most Christians during Lent and Muslims during Ramadan do.

Childbirth and infant care is another area where the community health nurse might encounter religious practices of which she should be aware ranging from infant baptism (as among Catholics) to circumcision for males (as among Jews). Some religious groups such as Christian Scientists oppose giving immunizations to infants, and Jehovah's Witnesses oppose blood transfusions.

One of the more rapidly growing religions in this country is that of Islam. This population includes immigrants and converts, as well as members of the Black Muslim movement in the United States. Many Christians from Arabic countries are also influenced by Islamic medical tradition. Traditional Islamic medicine is more like Western medicine than Hindu, Chinese, or Filipino medicine, since it was also based on the assumptions of the ancient Greeks. In fact, much of the surviving knowledge of Greek medicine and science came to use through Arabic editions, and Islamic medical publications were part of the standard medical curriculum in the West until almost the beginning of the nineteenth century.

Uneducated Muslim immigrants and converts may believe in the existence of the evil eye. Sometimes this means that parents keep a child encrusted with filth so that the child does not attract the attention of the evil eye. Stating publicly, as a health professional might do, that a particular child is a beautiful child or a beautiful baby is regarded as inviting the attention of the evil eye, the same as putting a curse on the child. To help overcome evil spirits and fight off illness, Muslims often recite passages from the Koran and call out *bismillah a-rahman a-rahim* (in the name of God the merciful, the compassionate) for help.

A particularly difficult time for many Muslims is the monthlong fast associated with Ramadan, and since Muslims use a lunar instead of a solar calendar, the fast is not at the same time every year. No food or drink is consumed from dawn to sunset, and in the summer such abstinence is difficult and can cause dehydration. The sick, the aged, and the very young can be exempted from the fast, and the community health nurse should be aware of this. If problems arise, the nurse should consult with the proper religious officials, since often the religious leader of a particular Islamic group can make sure clients know they can be exempted from the fast (Chilungu, 1974).

CULTURE OF POVERTY

Not all poor people are the same. They come from different cultural groups, and the nature of their poverty might be different. One of the differences is between acute and chronic poverty. John Kosa (1969) defined the acutely poor as those who have lived much of their lives with an adequate income by the standards of the society in which they live but then either suddenly become unemployed or gradually become old and have to live in reduced circumstances. Acutely poor people face severe problems of adjustment because they must find ways of coping with their new economic status. Acutely poor people are more likley to attempt to find ways to modify their conditions than chronically poor people who have spent their whole lives in poverty. In some families, chronic poverty is a multigenerational condition. The chronically poor, accustomed to poverty as they are, have developed a whole pattern of life for coping with their condition.

The anthropologist Oscar Lewis (1966) studied poor people in Mexico City, New York, and San Juan, Puerto Rico, and from these studies he argued that there was a culture of poverty passed on from one generation to another that transcends racial and nationality lines. This means that at least some of the characteristics attributed to a particular nationality or race are actually common to all people caught in the condition of poverty.

The culture of poverty must necessarily exist inside of another more affluent culture because the perception of being poor depends partly on knowing there are others who are more affluent. The poverty culture is marked by low levels of political power and participation in the decision-making processes of society. In the families he studied, Lewis also found a low marriage rate, a high rate of illegitimacy, and many families headed by women, all of which are now accepted as common characteristics among American groups whose socioeconomic status is low.

It is the psychologic characteristics of the culture of poverty that seem most important for health care. Lewis found that fatalism, helplessness, dependence, and feelings of inferiority were common. He also found that the time orientation tends to be on the present instead of the future, as is the case with middle-class society. There is a sense of powerlessness about controlling the future, so planning is not likely (Lewis, 1961, 1965, and 1966). Such a world view acts as a deterrent to seeking preventive health care, higher education, or other future-oriented activities.

Although Lewis was careful to emphasize that basic structural changes in society may alter some aspects of the characteristics of the poor, conservative critics of welfare programs focused almost exclusively on Lewis's interconnection between cultural traditions, family history, individual character, and poverty. From this they argued that a ghetto family with a history of welfare dependence would tend to bear offspring who lack ambition, a work ethic, and a sense of self-reliance (Auletta, 1982; Banfield, 1970). Some critics (Murray, 1984) went so far as to argue that the federal government was a major factor in perpetuating poverty because of its policies designed to relieve it.

Such use of the concept of a culture of poverty is misleading, since the culture stems from social and economic conditions. Changes in social and economic conditions can lead to radical changes, just as moving from one cultural group to another forces people to examine their assumptions. One of the difficulties with being poor is that the gap between behavior norms and aspirations is wider than among more well-to-do people. Thus if people of relative affluence fail to fulfill all their occupational aspirations, for example, they can still satisfy other aspirations. For the poor, however, so much depends on their economic conditions that if they fail economically, their other aspirations also fail (Gans, 1968; Wilson, 1987).

Understanding the existence of a culture of poverty leads to the realization that overcoming poverty is not a simple matter of giving the poor more short-term economic opportunities, but something that can be overcome only by treating it as a culture and going through the assimilation, diffusion, and acculturation processes as with any other culture.

Poverty is also both absolute and relative. An absolute standard defines poverty in terms of the necessary basic resources for an adequate existence. The U.S. government issues these standards periodically for both urban and rural poor. Relative poverty is relative to what others have and is usually defined in terms of the median standard of society. Thus relative standards for a family of four might be 50% of the median income for four-person families. To give even more precise information, in recent years the government has also defined poverty for a single individual or a family of two differently than for a family of four, as well as for other sizes of families. In 1984 the poverty level for a family of four was $10,609, whereas for a single individual it was $5400 and for people older than 65 it was $4979. Over the years as inflation has caused the cost of living to increase, the poverty level income has risen. In 1970, for example, the poverty level for a family of four was $3968.

By 1984 13.6% of the population was classed as living below the poverty level (Statistical, 1986). There were differences in groups, however. Only 11% of those classed as white lived below the poverty level, whereas 31.1% of those classed as black and 27.3% of those classed as Spanish, which includes blacks who are Spanish speaking, were below the poverty level. More than 43 million Americans (18.2% of the population) were living at 125% ($14,000 for a family of four) of the poverty level (Statistical, 1987).

The Homeless

A new poverty-related crisis in health care is emerging with the appearance of many homeless people in the United States. Estimates vary as to their number, depending on the person or agency doing the estimates and what definition of homeless is used. Minimum figures start at 350,000, whereas maximum figures go as high as 3 million (Bassuk, 1984; Brickner and others, 1985; Newsweek, 1988; Robertson and Cousineau, 1985). Although there have probably always been homeless people in the United States, their numbers have escalated in the past few years because of inflation, the rising cost of housing, the demise of low-rent rooming houses, the insufficient supply of publicly subsidized, low-rent housing, and the increase in absolute poverty that has taken place since 1980.

The homeless comprise mostly three large subgroups—the chronic, or traditionally homeless, the deinstitutionalized, and the "dishoused," or temporary, homeless. Although drug addicts, alcoholics, and the severely mentally ill make up the hardest core of the homeless, most studies indicate that they are less than half of the total homeless (Doolin, 1980; Haugland and others, 1983). The existence of the large number of homeless people raises serious public health issues, since homelessness is associated with excess morbidity and mortality, probable increases the risk of communicable diseases, injuries, hypothermia, and malnutrition, and exacerbation of other existing conditions. Since the homeless also have special problems gaining access to the health care system because of their poverty and unemployment, there is greater need for intervention by community health nurses (Abdellah, Chamberlain, and Levine, 1986).

There are some innovative nursing projects that deliver health care to the homeless. One of the pioneers in this effort was the Pine Street Clinic in Boston established in 1972 by a group of nurses from Boston City Hospital. Originally the clinic was restricted to men, but in 1980, as the number of homeless women increased, women were also accepted (Lenahan and others, 1985; Slavinsky and Cousins, 1982). The clinic began originally with volunteers, but the nurses soon proved so valuable that they were paid by Pine Street Inn and are supplemented by a Boston public health nurse and two nurses from the Massachusetts Department of Mental Health.

Emphasis is put on gradually developing a one-to-one relationship, since many of the potential clients are wary of anything that smacks of institutional care or even of compulsion. Particularly helpful is the use of what the staff calls foot soaks. A foot soak is a therapeutic soaking of feet and legs and treatment for ulcers, calluses, and blisters. Since these require the client to sit for a while, the nurse can establish communication and relationships, The nurses found that clients unwilling to address major problems such as hypertension would soak their feet, and this proved the entry point to offering more effective health care both in the clinic and where necessary in affiliated hospitals (Lenahan and others, 1985; Reilly and McInnis, 1985).

Similar clinics have sprung up in other areas of the country including Buffalo, New York, and Los Angeles. The school of nursing at the State University of New York at Buffalo and UCLA have established clinics for street people. A nurse practitioner and a community health nurse are aided by faculty and students who can learn first-hand about some of the problems of street people. Most large cities and many smaller ones where homelessness is a problem have similar clinics, and many of them are staffed by nurse practitioners. Some shelters are only for women (Slavinsky and Cousins, 1982), some are only for men, and some for both men and women.

When nurses first encounter the problems of the homeless, they often experience a culture shock. They are unaccustomed to serving the homeless outside of a hospital or clinic. Researchers have found that the reaction of most health care professionals when first working with a group like the homeless is to distance themselves from the group and to perceive members as unclean. Many of them do not have a stable or self-sufficient life-style, and most are subject to diseases such as tuberculosis, which are increasingly rare in the general population (Center, 1985). This emphasizes the need for effective nursing care and regular testing of clients for infectious diseases.

GUIDELINES FOR PROVIDING CULTURALLY RELEVANT NURSING CARE

The key to successful nursing care of clients from different cultures is for nurses to be aware of their own cultural, ethnic, and racial backgrounds, as well as the attitudes of their own social class. The following list of six "alerts" is something all nurses should keep in mind and to which they might add other alerts as they gain experience.

1. Be alert that a large proportion of the clients come from radically different cultural settings and with different notions of what constitutes illness and health than you have.
2. Be alert that there is often a language barrier between the client and the nurse. This is obvious when the client speaks a foreign language, but even among those who speak the same language, words have different meanings to different groups. Nurses should strive to use jargon-free language and make sure that their message is understood.
3. Be alert that different cultural groups often have different diets. At one time community health nurses spent a considerable amount of their time trying to persuade Italian-Americans to eat less garlic, pasta, and cheese and more meat and potatoes. Nurses today need to avoid making the same mistake. Kim chi, a fermented cabbage dish, for example, may not be appealing to non-Koreans when they first encounter it, but it is the Koreans' national dish.
4. Be alert that major differences in life-styles exist and that they include such things as child rearing, response to illness and stress, reaction to pain, and any number of similar aspects of life.
5. Be alert that different genetic inheritances of different cultural, ethnic, and racial groups can cause problems. Lactose intolerance, sickle-cell anemia, thalassemia, and other conditions are related to genetic factors.
6. Be alert that the most effective health care takes into account the cultural and genetic background of the client.

SUMMARY

To be effective, the nurses who work in the community must be aware of the impact of sociocultural variables on clients' readiness to accept proffered health care. In addition, nurses need to be aware of their own natural tendency to ethnocentrism but be willing to rise above that tendency and deliver culturally relevant health care.

Among the many cultural groups the community health nurse may encounter are Asian-Americans, Gypsies, black Americans, Spanish-speaking Americans, and Native Americans. Although many differences exist within each group, nurses should be aware of similarities that they may encounter in practice. In addition to the factors listed above, religion and economic status influences an individual's health practices.

QUESTIONS FOR DISCUSSION

1. List several ethnic groups other than those discussed in the chapter. Are there special folk medicine practices common among those ethnic groups? (An interview study of grandmothers is a good data source for folk remedies.)
2. Why might ethnocentrism be a deterrent to good nursing practice in the community?
3. Why might a Mexican-American woman from Los Angeles prefer to visit a *curandera* rather than an Anglo physician?
4. What is Ramadan? Why might the celebration of Ramadan create special health problems for aged persons, diabetics, and small children?

REFERENCES

Abdellah F, Chamberlain JG, and Levine IS: Role of nurses in meeting needs of homeless, Public Health Rep 101:494, 1986.

Anderson G and Tiche B: Gypsy culture and health care, Am J Nurs 73:282, 1973.

Auletta K: The underclass, New York, 1982, Random House Inc.

Banfield E: The unheavenly city, ed 2, Boston, 1970, Little, Brown & Co Inc.

Bashshur R, Steeler W, and Murphy T: On changing Indian eligibility for health care, Am J Public Health 77:690, 1987.

Bassuk E: The homeless problem, Sci Am 252:40, 1984.

Bertholf C: Prayer as a coping mechanism among mastectomy patients, Unpublished manuscript, 1979.

Brickner PW and others, editors: Health care of homeless people, New York, 1985, Springer Publishing Co Inc.

Bullough VL and Bullough B: Health care for the other Americans, New York, 1982, Appleton & Lange.

Center for Disease Control, MMWR 34:28, 1985.

Chilungu SWA: A study of health and cultural variants in an industrial community, Unpublished manuscript, 1974.

David RJ: Did low birthweight among U.S. blacks really increase, Am J Public Health 76:415, 1986.

Dohrenwend BP and Dohrenwend BS: Social status and psychological disorder: a causal inquiry, New York, 1969.

Doolin J: Planning for the special needs of the homeless elderly, Gerontologist 26:3, 1986.

Dunham HW: Community and schizophrenia: an epidemiological analysis, Detroit, 1965, Wayne State University Press.

Durkheim E: Suicide: a study in sociology. Translated from the French by JA Spaulding and G Simpson, Glencoe, Ill, 1951, Free Press.

Faris REL and Dunham HW: Mental disorders in urban areas: an ecological study of schizophrenia and other psychoses, Chicago, 1939, University of Chicago Press.

Flaskerud JH: Diagnostic and treatment differences among five ethnic groups, Psychol Rep 58:219, 1986a.

Flaskerud JH: The effects of culture-compatible intervention on utilization of mental health services, Community Ment Health J 20:127, 1986b.

Flaskerud JH: A proposed protocol for culturally relevant nursing psychotherapy, Clin Nurse Specialist 1:150, 1987.

Gans HJ: Culture and class in the study of poverty: an approach to anti-poverty research. In Moynihan DP, editor: Understanding poverty: perspectives from the social sciences, New York, 1988, Basic Books Inc, Publishers.

Goldstein MS: Longevity and health status of the Negro American, J Negro Education 32:337, 1963.

Goode ME: Illegitimacy in the Caribbean social structure, ASR 25:21, 1960.

Gutelius MF: The problem of iron deficiency anemia in preschool Negro Children, Am J Public Health 59:290, 1969.

Haugland G and others: Mortality in the era of deinstitutionalization, Am J Psychiatry 140:848, 1983.

Hertz H: Notes on clay and starch eating among Negros in a southern community, Soc Forces 25:343, 1957.

Hongladarom GC and Russell M: An ethnic difference—lactose intolerance, Nurs Outlook 24:764, 1976.

Ingram DD, Makuc D, and Kleinman JC: National and state trends in use of prenatal care, 1970-83, Am J Public Health 76:415, 1986.

Kitagawa EM and Hauser PM: Differential mortality in the United States: a study of socioeconomic epidemiology, Cambridge, Mass, 1973, Harvard University Press.

Kleinman A, Eisenberg L, and Good B: Culture, illness, and care, Ann Intern Med 88:251, 1978.

Kosa J, Antonovsky A, and Zola IK, editors: Poverty and health: a sociological analysis, Cambridge, Mass, 1969, Commonwealth Fund Book, Harvard University Press.

Kosko DA and Flaskerud JH: Mexican American, nurse practitioners, and lay control of group beliefs about cause and treatment of chest pain, Nurs Res 36:226, 1986.

Leininger MM: Nursing and anthropology: two worlds to blend, New York, 1970, John Wiley & Sons Inc.

Lieninger MM: Transcultural health care issues and conditions, Philadelphia, 1976, FA Davis Co.

Leininger MM: Transcultural nursing 1979, St Paul, Minn, 1980, Masson Publishing.

Lenahan GP and others: A nurses' clinic for the homeless, Am J Nurs 85:1237, 1985.

Lewis O: The children of Sanchez, New York, 1961, Vintage Books.

Lewis O: La vida: a Puerto Rican family in the culture of poverty, New York, 1965, Random House Inc.

Lewis O: The culture of poverty, Sci Am 215:19, 1966.

Marlow DR and Redding BA: Textbook of pediatric nursing, Philadelphia, 1988, Harcourt Brace Jovanovich Inc.

Martinez C and Martin HW: Folk diseases among urban Mexican-Americans, JAMA 196:147, 1966.

McKenzie JL and Chrisman NJ: Healing herbs, gods, and magic: folk beliefs among Filipino-Americans, Nurs Outlook 25:326, 1977.

Muecke MA: In search of healers: Southeast Asian refugees in the American health care system, West J Med 139:835, 1983.

Murray CA: Losing ground: American social policy, 1950-1980, New York, 1984, Basic Books.

Neuman HH: Pica—symptom or vestigal instinct? Pediatrics 46:441, 1970.

Office of the Surgeon General, US Department of Health, Education and Welfare: Health services for American Indians, Public Health Service Publication No 531, Washington, DC, 1957, US Government Printing Office.

Otterbein KF: Caribbean family organization: a comparative analysis, Am Anthropologist 67:66, 1965.

Poss JE: Protocol for hepatitis screening and follow-up of Southeast Asian refugees, Nurse Pract 12:8, 1987.

Poss JE: Providing health care for southeast Asian refugees, J New York Nurses Assoc 20:4, 1989.

Primeaux M: Caring for the Indian patient, Am J Nurs 77:95, 1977.

Reilly E and McInnis B: The Pine Street Inn Nurses' Clinic and Tuberculosis Program. In Brickner and others, editors: Health care of homeless people, New York, 1985, Springer Publishing Co Inc.

Rhoades ER and others: Mental health problems of American Indians seen in outpatient facilities of the Indian health services, Public Health Rep 95:329, 1980.

Roberts RE: Prevalence of psychological distress among Mexican Americans, J Health Soc Behav 21:135, 1980.

Robertson M and Cousineau MR: Health status and access to health services among the urban homeless, Am J Public Health 75:561, 1985.

Rubel AJ: Across the tracks: Mexican-Americans in a Texas city, Austin, Tex, 1966, University of Texas Press.

Slavinsky AT and Cousins A: Homeless women, Nurs Outlook 30:358, 1982.

Statistical Abstract of the United States, 1988: Washington, DC, 1987, US Government Printing Office.

Stamler J, Stamler R, and Curry CL: Hypertension in the inner city, Minneapolis, 1974, Proforum Modern Medical Publications.

Sue S: Community mental health services to minority groups, Am Psychologist 32:616, 1977.

Sue S and McKinney H: Asian Americans in the community mental health care system, Am J Orthopsychiatry 45:111, 1975.

Sutherland and others: Indochinese refugee health assessment and treatment, J Fam Pract 16:61, 1983.

Suttles GD: The social order of the slum: ethnicity and territory in the inner city, Chicago, 1968, University of Chicago Press.

US Department of Health, Education and Welfare, Health Services and Mental Health Administration: health service use: national trends and variations—1953-1971, Publication No HSM 73-3004, Rockville, Md, 1972, Health Services and Mental Health Administration.

Wakefield D: Island in the city: Puerto Ricans in New York. New York, 1960, Corinth Books.

Walker B: The Hindu world, New York, 1968, Praeger Publishers.

Wallnofer H and von Rottauscher A: Chinese folk medicine, New York, 1965, Crown Publishers Inc (Translated by Marion Palmedo).

What can be done: homeless in America, Newsweek, p 57, March 21, 1988.

Wilson WJ: The truly disadvantaged: the inner city, the underclass, and public policy, Chicago, 1987, University of Chicago Press.

CHAPTER

22

Rural Community Health Nursing

Jeri L. Bigbee

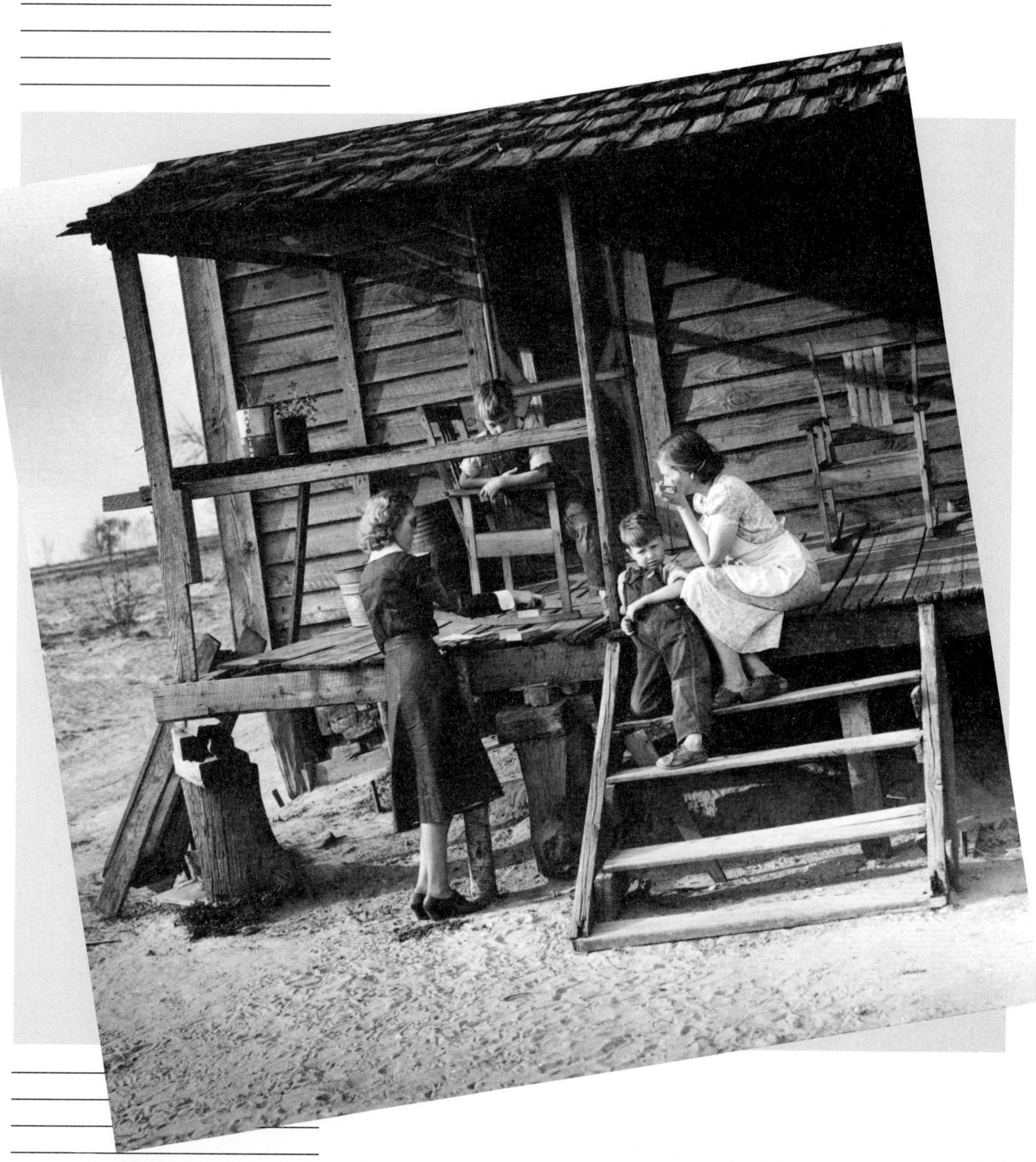

CHAPTER OUTLINE

- Historical background
- Rural nursing as a specialty
- Rural community nursing practice
- Characteristics of rural communities
  - Rural families
  - Health characteristics
- Specific nursing concerns in rural community practice
  - Parent-child nursing
  - Environmental and occupational nursing
  - Nursing care of rural elderly people
- Case study
  - Assessment
  - Diagnoses
  - Planning
  - Implementation
  - Evaluation
- Summary

OBJECTIVES

After completing this chapter, the reader should be able to:

1. Describe three unique aspects of rural community health nursing.
2. Identify five health characteristics of rural populations.
3. Discuss the historical tradition of rural community health nursing in America.

RURAL HEALTH CARE in the United States is an area of health service that is often neglected even though it is essential. In the last decade increasing attention has been given to the specific needs of rural communities in terms of primary, secondary, and tertiary care. Nursing has been directly involved in this process, especially in relation to primary care and community health nursing. Unfortunately, most rural residents, health care providers, politicians, and scholars would agree that the provision of high-quality, accessible rural health services throughout America has progressed slowly. Too often rural concerns in nursing and other fields have been neglected. Rural nursing is a unique practice specialty, particularly in the area of community health.

In this chapter rural community health nursing is explored from historical, conceptual, and practice perspectives. Specifically, the history of rural community nursing is presented and a conceptual view of rural nursing as a specialty is discussed. The characteristics of rural communities are reviewed, and specific nursing practice concerns related to serving rural communities are presented.

HISTORICAL BACKGROUND

Rural public health nursing first developed and progressed in Europe and British colonies in the late 1800s. Perhaps the earliest and most significant development was the establishment of the Queen's Jubilee Institute in 1887 by Queen Victoria of Britain. The "Queen's nurses" established a nationwide system designed specifically to provide public health nursing services to rural communities and served as models for the development of similar programs in countries associated with Great Britain. In Canada the Victorian Order of Nurses for Canada was founded in 1897. The Order developed into a nationwide plan that has no parallel in the United States. It provides public health nursing services to cities, rural areas, and Native American settlements and supports small rural hospitals throughout Canada (Stewart and Austin, 1962). At about the same time, Australia began developing a similar system of "bush nursing" that began in the state of Victoria but failed to extend nationwide as originally intended. Later the Australian Inland Mission was established to provide nursing services to the hinterlands and isolated islands.

In the United States, as public health nursing began to develop in the late 1800s and early 1900s, a few isolated rural projects were initiated. Ellen M. Wood established a pioneer rural nursing program in 1896 serving Westchester County, New York. This highly successful model program grew to serve more than 20 villages by 1920 and later served as a training site for rural nurses (Dock, 1922). In 1911 Lydia Holman established an independent nursing service in the Appalachian mountains with the intention of extending the program nationwide eventually. This ambitious project provided rural nursing, sanitation, and social services; however, it terminated within a few years (Clement, 1913). Mary Breckinridge established the Frontier Nursing Service in Kentucky in 1925. This innovative program focused primarily on midwifery and public health nursing services for three counties in southeastern Kentucky. All nurses were required to be prepared in midwifery, as well as general nursing and public health. Traveling by horses and mules, and later in jeeps, the nurses provided maternal and child health care to approximately 200 families. Evaluation of the service indicated that as a result of the nursing care provided, the perinatal complication rate and maternal and infant mortality were reduced (Kalisch and Kalisch, 1978). This historically significant local project still exists and serves as a major education facility for nurse-midwives.

These early flickerings of the development of organized rural health nursing in America were set in a social environment of change and reform. The U.S. rural population was rapidly declining because of rural-urban migration associated with industrial development. In 1900, 60% of the U.S. population was rural, and by 1920 the U.S. rural population had declined to 49% (Carlson, 1981). Thus this period is highly significant in that within 20 years America moved from a predominantly rural to a predominantly urban society. Health problems affecting rural communities during this time included high infant and maternal mortality and high rates of malnutrition and communicable diseases. These problems were similar to those in the urban areas, but the magnitude of the problems was often greater in rural areas.

In 1912 the first and only nationwide rural public health nursing service was established by the American Red Cross. The Rural Nursing Service, later known as the Town and Country Nursing Service, supported the establishment of rural nursing services throughout the country. These nurses had a broad scope of practice. The majority of their time was spent providing bedside visiting nursing to the ill; however, health promotion services, including maternal-child health care, infectious disease prevention, detection, and treatment, sanitation, and health education, were also provided (Clement, 1917). In many areas the rural nurse was the only health care provider besides lay midwives, who were often supervised by the rural public health nurse. Many of these early rural nurses were country bred and their characteristics included love of the open country, good health, knowledge of handicrafts, cheerfulness, enthusiasm, good judgment, patience, firmness, courage, an even temperament, love of work, a sense of humor, a discreet and silent tongue, a knowledge of country traditions, sympathy toward country people, willingness to give up city comforts when necessary, interest in everyday affairs and topics of the times, the broadest intelligence and best training, a well-balanced, broad-minded, womanly character, an ability to teach, experience in managing a horse, and a never-ending charity for the shortcomings of human beings (Clement, 1914).

By 1917, 70 Red Cross rural nurses were employed in 22 states, primarily in the East. Recruitment of adequate numbers of qualified nurses willing to work in rural settings, especially in the West and South, was a continuing problem. Following World War I the Red Cross rural nursing service, known then as the Bureau of Public Health Nursing, was greatly expanded. However, it was no longer solely rurally oriented. By 1921 the Bureau reached a peak of 1032 full-time nursing services (American National Red Cross Public Health Nursing, 1944). During this period of expansion the Red Cross program was often in conflict with state and local agencies, especially health departments that were developing their own public health nursing services. Public health nursing moved from a nationwide, voluntary agency–sponsored program to state-sponsored, state-administered services. Federal support and the Works Progress Administration programs as a result of the Social Security Act of 1935 enhanced the growth of state and local health agencies. By 1939 Red Cross nursing services had declined to less than 500; all services were formally terminated in 1947. Between 1913 and 1947, 3109 local nursing services were established in 1800 counties, one half of all the counties in America (Flagg, 1851).

The development of rural nursing services under official agencies has been slow. According to a 1940 report, in that year 857 rural counties still had no public health services (More Nurses in Rural Areas, 1940). Nurses functioning in the state-administered rural nursing services typically had minimal preparation in nursing and public health. This is still the case in many rural counties. Critics argue that the movement of rural community nursing from voluntary agency control (Red Cross) to state control compromised standards and autonomy.

The early models of rural community health nursing played a vital role in the development of public health nursing in general. The philosophies and standards established during the early years or rural nursing serve as the basis and inspiration of contemporary rural community health nursing practice.

RURAL NURSING AS A SPECIALTY

Rural nursing is being recognized as a specialty in nursing, with rural community health nursing representing a subspecialty (Benson, Sweeney, and Nicolls, 1982; Fletcher, 1981; Hester, 1986; and Thobaden and Weingard, 1983). Rural nursing is defined as the practice of professional nursing within the physical and sociocultural context of rural America. It involves the continual interaction of the rural environment, nurses, and their practices. This specialty area is characterized by a unique style and approach to practice that requires an innovative, truly generalist perspective. Rural nursing thus is not just a weaker or more primitive brand of mainstream urban nursing. The unique aspects of rural practice require specific preparation and personal qualities in nurses. Some say that rural nursing requires a different breed of nurses—one who is committed to generalist practice. Rural nursing is seen as nursing as it was intended to be, with a strong connection between all aspects of the community and the nurse who functions independently in primary, secondary, and tertiary levels of care with a generalist approach. In essence, as one rural nurse stated, "Rural nursing is more than a job; it's a way of life" (Hester, 1986).

A definition of rural is required before the concept of rural nursing is explored further. Currently there is no agreement on the definition of rural; it has been the subject of debate among rural scholars for years. Depending on one's orientation, the definition of rural and urban are highly relative. The New York City resident may see suburbs as rural. To the isolated ranch family, a small town might be considered urban. Gilford (1981) says, "Rural-urban is clearly a continuum, not a dichotomy." However, convention has focused on defining rural in terms of population density. Most simply the U.S. Census delineates rural people as individuals living in open country or in a town with a population of less than 2500 (U.S. Department of Commerce, 1983). Rural scholars debate this definition as being too limited, preferring a more flexible definition such as "people and communities in the nation's nonmetropolitan counties—counties that have no cities with as many as 50,000 people" (Dillman and Hobbs, 1982). On a more theoretic level, Ferdinand Tonnies has defined rural in relation to the characteristics of individuals (Murdock and Sutton, 1974). Rural communities are described by the term "gemeinschaft," whereas urban is often considered synonymous with the term "gesellschaft." In a gemeinschaft social organization the individual is the primary unit of interaction, bound by close, personal, long-term relationships with family and friends. In contrast gesellschaft social environments have shorter, less intense interpersonal relationships, more formal relationships, and less family involvement. Rural nursing reflects the gemeinschaft orientation, including long-term, complex relationships with clients. A family-oriented approach to care is essential to effective care. Urban nursing, in contrast, reflects the gesellschaft concept. Care is more specialized, formalized, and institutionalized.

Emile Durkheim applies a similar typology of mechanical versus organic types to the definition of rural (Murdock and Sutton, 1974). A generality common to most all of the definitions and theories related to rurality is low population density. This definitional debate is not a problem for the discussion of rural community nursing, since all the perspectives hold value in relation to rural practice. A strict delineation of what is rural is not necessary for the purposes of this chapter. Problems do arise, however, in relation to research and theory development related to rural practice, and thus nursing must ultimately acknowledge the definitional ambiguity.

RURAL COMMUNITY NURSING PRACTICE

Characteristics of rural nursing practice include diversity of function, flexibility, greater personal involvement with clients, and greater professional responsibility and autonomy. In many rural areas the functional lines between community and institutional nursing are blurred because of the diversity of roles and expectations. For example, a rural nurse might well work a shift at the local 20-bed hospital (including emergency, maternity, and nursing home clients), make a home visit on the way home, and teach a childbirth preparation class in the evening. Thus greater continuity of care is characteristic of rural nursing practice (Cummings, 1978; Diers, 1982; Elder, 1978; Hadbavny, Smith, and Griffith, 1980; Stuart-Burchardt, 1982). Because of this, Stricklin (1980) contends that rural nursing is the essence of what nursing should be.

The rural nurse often occupies multiple statuses within the community, including professional, co-worker, employee, family member, community member, neighbor, and friend (Hester, 1986). Perception of the appropriate roles and responsibilities of these various statuses may differ throughout the community, and often expectations may overlap or conflict. Thus differences in perception between the nurses and others can lead to role confusion and conflict. Inability to deal with these role dynamics can lead to inability to perform optimally in the rural environment. Fletcher (1981) specifically describes the professional roles of the rural nurse as shaper of health policy, epidemiologist with strong community ties, and program developer and initiator of change. These roles clearly fall within the scope of practice of community nursing.

The limited research and literature related to rural nursing suggest that this specialty area requires a broadly prepared generalist. Data collected among rural nurses indicate that the following capabilities were integral to rural nursing practice: strong technical and clinical skills, adaptability and flexibility, assessment skills, organization, independence, positive attitudes toward continuing education, decision-making skills, leadership, self-confidence, teaching skills, and public relations (Benson, Sweeney, and Nicolls, 1982; Cummings, 1978; Hadbavny, Smith, and Griffith, 1980; Leonard and Rogers, 1978; and Stuart-Burchardt, 1982). The rural community nurse must possess a strong commitment to confidentiality. A comprehensive knowledge of sociocultural and economic community dynamics is also a requirement of effective rural practice (Cummings, 1978; Fletcher, 1981). Hester (1985) states, "The rural nurse is an ethnoscientist, who learns how the local culture perceives and practices caring." This approach is particularly relevant to rural community nursing.

Rural practice certainly has its pluses and minuses. Based on research with Arizona rural nurses, Benson, Sweeney, and Nicolls (1982) suggest that the benefits of rural nursing include close client-nurse relationships, professional challenge, variety, rural life-style, and professional autonomy. Problems associated with rural practice include limited shopping, limited educational opportunities, personal, professional, and geographic isolation, restricted social life, lack of personnel, cultural difference, workload, responsibility to function in diverse areas, and low professional demands and stimulation. The factors that attract and promote retention of nurses to rural areas have received some attention. In the Arizona study 29% of the nurses lived in a rural area because of their spouse, whereas employment opportunities caused 24% of the respondents to live in a rural area (Benson, Sweeney, and Nicolls, 1982). Growing up in a rural area is also a positive factor when nurses decide to live in a rural area. Too often nurses are unprepared for the culture shock and demands of rural practice. Colorado data suggest that nurses leave rural areas because of "inhospitable" communities, limited social activities, difficult working conditions, and job stress (Fletcher, 1981). The motivators and demotivators surrounding rural nursing reflect both personal and professional dynamics that interact with the rural environment.

In relation to rural community health nursing in particular, the American Public Health Association published a position paper on rural health in 1982. The Association acknowledged the nursing shortage as a tradition in rural areas that results in overreliance on the least skilled nurses. Unique problems cited for rural nurses included the lack of variety in available nursing positions, long distances to travel, often in inclement weather, low pay and few benefits, limited educational opportunity for career mobility, lack of in-service education, and the need for flexible scheduling and part-time employment. Recommendations to alleviate these problems included the establishment of nursing scholarships that include rural service requirements, promotion of baccalaureate-prepared nurses in rural settings, and increased use of nurses in expanded roles in rural areas.

Nursing education has addressed the concerns of rural nursing by attempting to better prepare nurses for rural practice through rural clinical experiences (Fletcher, 1981). Schools of nursing have developed independent rural nursing clinics that focus largely on community practice (Thornton, 1983). Graduate programs specifically designed to prepare rural nursing specialists have recently been developed in various parts of the country. Nevertheless, rural nursing has for the most part been ignored by most of the dominant urban-based institutions of nursing education. Greater efforts are needed to correct the situation.

CHARACTERISTICS OF RURAL COMMUNITIES

In drawing a profile of rural America in the 1980s, one must constantly remember that diversity is by far the most common trait. However, overall demographic trends can provide insights to the present and future dynamics of rural America.

Currently approximately 66 million people live in rural America. There has been a fairly consistent decline in the proportion of rural population during the last 200 years because of urban migration. In 1790, 95% of the U.S. population was rural, but by 1970 only 27% was rural (Carlson, Lassey, and Lassey, 1981). However, the most dramatic demographic trend affecting rural America today is the rural to urban migration turnaround. Since 1970 rural areas have grown at a faster rate (15.4%) than metropolitan areas (9.1%). The young, middle-aged, and elderly groups were those showing the greatest increases. Ploch (1981) characterizes these in-migrants as back-to-the-land social isolates, rural pragmatists, and middle-aged or other urbanites turned rural romanticists. The most significant commonality of these in-migrants is that their motivation is voluntary, not economic. Rural in-migrants move primarily to seek quality-of-life attributes they find lacking in urban society. The social, economic, and cultural impact of this turnaround has been minimally addressed in research literature.

Concurrently there has been a shift in the age demographics of rural areas. The average age in rural communities is increasing, resulting largely from the in-migration of retirees and out-migration of the young. Carlson (1981) cites the following seven major factors causing the growth of rural populations:

1. Growth of rural-based recreational activities
2. Increased location of students from higher education institutions in rural areas
3. Dispersion of manufacturing, business activity, and services
4. Rural residential development adjacent to metropolitan areas
5. New resource developments, often energy related
6. Continuing higher birth rates in rural areas
7. Retirement of elderly people in rural areas

The rural occupational structure has also changed markedly. Traditionally, primary industries in rural areas have been largely extractive (agriculture, mining, and lumbering), but there has been a recent shift away from these industries. Currently less than 5% of the U.S. rural population is engaged directly in farming (Carlson,

1981). Unfortunately, much of the rural-oriented research has focused solely on the farm family, thereby neglecting the unique aspects of 95% of rural residents. Today rural workers, including many women, are increasingly involved in manufacturing, trade, and professional services.

Other demographic characteristics demonstrate persistent rural-urban differences. Some argue that these differences have blurred considerably because of the increased mobility of the population and electronic communication as a carrier of urban culture. Nevertheless, statistically and culturally rural areas consistently differ from urban areas. Average rural incomes are consistently lower than urban incomes in the United States. The states with large concentrations of persons falling below the poverty line ($11,203 for a family of four in 1986) tend to be either those states with large urban poverty areas or rural states such as South Dakota, Maine, New Mexico, Idaho, Arizona, and the Southern states (U.S. Statistical Abstract, 1987). Similarly, rural housing is of lower average quality. Educationally, the white nonmetropolitan population is comparable with urban populations, averaging 12.2 school years completed. Rural women tend to have slightly higher levels of education than rural men. However, rural women have been unable to turn their educational achievements into comparable incomes and job status as have their rural male or urban female counterparts (Dunne, 1980). Another rural-urban difference is that the proportion of "dependent" groups (younger than 18 years and older than 65 years) is consistently higher in rural areas. As a result the demand for already scarce health and human services is greater.

Most scholars agree that rural peoples differ culturally from their urban counterparts to some degree. From a community perspective, rural communities fit closer to a gemeinschaft type of social organization, emphasizing close, long-term personal relationships and traditionalist value systems (Carlson, 1981). Rural residents tend to be more work oriented, morally and politically conservative, self-sufficient, individualistic, and community and family oriented than do their urban counterparts (Glenn and Alston, 1982; Larson, 1977).

An additional common factor affecting rural communities and their residents is social and cultural isolation. This isolation in varying degrees enhances the development of a rural culture distinct from the dominant urban culture. Willits, Bealer, and Crider's (1974) research showed that the farther people are from an urban center, the more traditional are their values and attitudes. Community nurses must interpret all these generalizations carefully, however, in light of the increasing blending of value systems between rural and urban cultures and the inherent diversity of rural America.

Rural families

In keeping with larger societal changes, families in rural America are also changing. Historically, rural families have been characterized by younger average age at marriage, lower rates of divorce, and higher fertility rates than urban families. Recent changes, however, indicate that some new trends may be emerging with a narrowing of these rural-urban differences. The percentage of single women and divorce rates have increased, whereas fertility rates and household size have decreased in both rural and urban areas (Brown, 1981). Of particular importance is the dramatic increase in the female labor force in rural areas in recent decades.

The family holds a central place in the social system, value structure, and economic dynamics of rural cultures. This familism functions to maintain nuclear and extended family ties but may also produce stress caused by the multiple expectations within family roles and the subjugation of individual goals for those of the family (Rosenblatt and Anderson, 1981; Schumm, 1981). Rural families tend to maintain fairly traditional roles among members. In relation to family and marital satisfaction, most recent studies show negligible differences between rural and urban couples (Schumm and Ballman, 1981). These findings may indicate differences in marital and family expectations in light of the lower divorce rates among rural families.

The role of women in rural families reflects the traditional value system along with changing social trends. Because of the scarcity of out-of-home child socialization opportunities along with traditional familism, women in rural families assume a dominant role in child care. The rural mother's child socialization role also includes components of "keepers of the culture" and transmitters of traditional values to the young (Clarenbach, 1977; Dunne, 1979). Similarly, in keeping with traditional sex-role task delegation, rural women and girls assume the majority of home management, including food preparation and preservation, clothing construction, cleaning, laundry, and shopping. These activities are often more involved and time consuming in rural homes because of fewer technologic conveniences along with traditional patterns of rural homemaking. In addition to her domestic responsibilities, the rural woman also maintains the links between the community and the family through involvement in community groups. Battenfeld (1981) discusses an additional family role of rural women as "the carriers of the collective healing experience." Out of necessity, self-care strategies have developed over generations in rural families, with women assuming the major responsibility for the implementation and transmission of care.

Health Characteristics

Specifically addressing the health characteristics of rural America presents problems because of lack of complete information. The data related to the distribution of health professionals and services in rural areas are abundant, whereas concrete data on the actual health status of rural populations are minimal. Clearly "virtually all rural Americans are at a locational disadvantage with regard to professional health services" (Miller, 1982). Rural areas consistently have suboptimal population/ professional ratios and fewer hospital beds and health care facilities than urban areas. Emergency care represents a continuing need in many rural areas and often is accomplished largely through voluntary efforts (Rosenblatt and Moscovice, 1982). Unfortunately, emergency and trauma concerns are addressed only at a secondary or tertiary level and rarely on a primary prevention basis. In recent years, family planning services have become increasingly available to rural families, with 80% of rural counties having an organized family planning program as of 1975 (Proceedings, 1977). With the conservative political and economic policies that have predominated in the past decade, however, these services have undoubtedly been reduced.

Data related to the distribution of nurses reflect health care needs in rural areas. According to the Report to the Congress on Nursing (1986), there is a consistent shortage of rural nurses. A higher percentage of nurses in rural areas are engaged in community settings than are nurses in urban areas, and thus rural nursing shortages particularly affect community health practice. In a statewide study of community health nursing staffing in Wyoming, a predominantly rural state, Kennedy and Taheri (1981) found that a shortage of community health nurses existed in every county. Miller (1975) studied "medically underserved" areas and found that infant mortality and the age-sex adjusted death rate increased consistently as the availability of physicians and hospital beds increased. However, this relationship was reversed in the case of nurses. Miller suggests that nurses, particularly public health nurses, through their educative and counseling functions "seem to have a genuine positive impact on health."

Based on information regarding health services it is not surprising that rural people report lower use of health resources. Since access is a primary determinant in seeking care, factors such as distance, cost, isolation, and transportation, as well as cultural factors such as a philosophy of self-sufficiency and self-care, must be considered. Particularly lacking in rural areas are preventive health services aimed at health promotion. For example, dental visits are nearly 50% higher in urban areas than in rural areas (Ahearn, 1979). Data related to preventive health services for women and children also suggest inadequate well care. Among women older than 17 years of age, 24% of nonmetropolitan women report never having had a Papanicolaou test or breast examination as opposed to 17% and 19%, respectively, for urban women (Proceedings, 1977). Prenatally, 20% of rural women say they do not see a physician before four months of gestation as compared with 15% of urban women. In 1973, 14% of rural children as opposed to 7.8% of urban children had never received a well-child examination (Proceedings, 1977).

Several government attempts at improving access and distribution have met with limited success. Federal efforts, initiated mainly in the 1970s, included the National Health Service Corps, Health Underserved Rural Areas Program, Rural Health Initiative, Community Health Centers Program, Appalachian Health Program, Migrant Health Program, Farmers' Home Administration rural health facility loan program, and the Rural Health Services Clinic Act. The Rural Health Services Clinic Act is of particular importance to community nursing in that it provides for direct reimbursement for primary care and home nursing services in rural areas. The act was an attempt to facilitate the rural practice of nonphysician providers, including nurse practitioners and nurse-midwives. Unfortunately, the implementation of this law has been slow, with only a small proportion of rural clinics participating. The main barriers to implementation have been restrictive state laws, lack of promotion and support of the program at state and federal levels, inadequate information, reimbursement problems, and excessive reporting requirements (Bigbee, 1984).

Many rural residents have limited or no health insurance because of their unemployed or self-employed status (Ahearn, 1980). Most importantly, it must be remembered that the delivery of health services alone is a "necessary but not sufficient condition to improve the health status of the rural population" (Miller, 1982).

Attempting to evaluate the other half of the health question, health status, demonstrates the lack of data. It is known that using the combined indices of infant mortality, the age-standardized mortality, and the age-standardized mortality caused by influenza and pneumonia, rural populations have the poorest overall health status nationally (Ahearn, 1979). In the past, maternal and infant mortality has been higher in rural areas, but in recent years little rural-urban difference has been found. The higher concentration of low-income and ethnic populations in rural areas must also be considered. These subgroups may experience infant mortality as high as twice the national average, lower life expectancies, higher mortality from infectious diseases, higher accident rates, and disproportionately higher rates of disability (Mutel and Donham, 1983). The prevalence of chronic illness is higher, whereas the incidence of acute conditions is lower among rural people, perhaps in part because of age distributions (Gilford, Nelson, and Ingram, 1981). The problems of chronically ill rural residents, particularly elderly rural residents, are compounded by limited support services, poverty, inadequate transportation, and cultural reluctance to accept assistance. Motor vehicle accidents and occupationally related injuries are particularly common in rural areas (Carlson, Lassey, and Lassey, 1981). Approximately two thirds of all the deaths caused by motor vehicle accidents nationally occur in rural areas.

The available data on rural mental health are incomplete. Some studies suggest that rural areas may have higher rates of psychosis, depression, suicide, family violence, incest, and alcoholism because of the effects of isolation and limited options and services; however, the results are conflicting (Dunne, 1979; Flax, 1978). With the recent economic crises affecting rural communities, concerns regarding mental health status have increased. In agricultural communities, the farm crisis has produced considerable financial stress for families as reported by Rowe and others (1985) and the popular media. Energy-based (coal, oil, and natural gas) rural communities during the same period of the mid-1980s have experienced similar economic stress resulting in increased need for community health and human services but declining revenues. Periods of economic stress are characteristic of many rural communities but may affect the long-term mental health status of the population.

Thus these basic health data demonstrate that rural areas certainly represent potential at-risk populations with a need for health promotion intervention as provided by community health nurses. Community nursing diagnoses based on general, rural community characteristics could include the following:

1. Potential for increased mortality and morbidity because of inadequate emergency care systems.
2. Increased rates of teenage pregnancy because of inadequate community education and family planning services.
3. Community stress because of economic decline and social isolation.

SPECIFIC NURSING CONCERNS IN RURAL COMMUNITY PRACTICE

What is practice like for rural community health nurses today? Typically the rural community nurse is employed by a county health department. Health departments with one to five nurses and perhaps one support clerical person to serve an entire county are common. The health officer is often a community physician (or perhaps a veterinarian) who has little involvement with the day-to-day functioning of the agency. The agency is typically housed in cramped facilities that are often shared with other county offices. Rural county health departments often seem to be located in the basement of an aging courthouse with few windows and no handicap access. Services provided are usually varied and include maternal and child health promotion (immunization clinics, well-child clinics, prenatal classes, and women, infants, and children programs), adult health promotion (well-elderly clinics, influenza immunization, and sexually transmitted disease clinics), and home visitation for home health clients and high-risk families. Thus the agencies provide a full range of community nursing services, with most nurses engaged in all aspects. Travel to clients' homes and clinics is often long and problematic because of poor roads, inclement weather, or both. Based on this profile of rural community health nurse practice, some of the specific health concerns related to rural areas are considered here.

Parent-Child Nursing

In the area of parent-child nursing the needs for creative community health nursing practice in rural areas are great. As previously discussed, rural women and children receive significantly less preventive health care than do their urban counterparts. Because of the higher birth rates, particularly among rural teenagers, family planning and perinatal services are critical. The higher density of low-income families in rural areas often necessitates that public health agencies assume leadership in advocating or providing maternal child health services. Because of the limited resources in rural areas, the rural nurse must often be an advocate for clients in areas such as birthing alternatives and childcare options. The provision of health promotion services for women and children is well within the scope of the rural community health nurse.

Family planning in a rural community is a necessary but often highly sensitive community nursing service. The conservative political and religious values of the community affect the acceptance and visibility of the services. Problems of confidentiality are particularly applicable to rural teenagers who seek contraceptive services. Many teenagers seek these services outside their community rather than risk someone seeing their car outside the public health nurse's office on family planning day. Confidentiality must be strictly maintained in all aspects of rural community nursing practice, especially in relation to reproductive health.

A controversial area in which rural community nurses must often assume leadership is sex education and the prevention of teenage pregnancy. Rural schools often reflect the conservative value structure of the community but are increasingly acknowledging their role in sex education and value formation. Providing school nursing services is often within the general duties of rural community health nurses, and thus they need to be actively involved in sex education, as well as the support of teenage parents. The children of teenagers are of course at higher physiologic and psychosocial risk and thus need close nursing follow-up. The rural nurse should also be a strong advocate of constructive recreational programs and facilities for rural teenagers who often see drinking and sex as the only options for social activity.

The rural nurse must also often deal with family violence among clients. Prevention, early detection, and intervention in this area is often difficult because of the conservative nature of many rural communities and the limited social and health services available. Greater emphasis on the prevention of family violence is needed through such strategies as parents' groups and stress management programs that are tailored to the rural environment and culture.

With the increasing frequency of both parents working outside the home in rural areas, the rural community health nurse needs to address the childcare needs in the community. Many rural communities lack high-quality childcare facilities. The nurse should be actively involved in the promotion of a variety of high-quality childcare options for families, as well as the monitoring and advising of childcare facilities in terms of health concerns.

Environmental and Occupational Nursing

A commonly held misconception of rural living is the presence of a "clean, healthy environment." In fact, many rural communities face significant environmental health risks. Rural water quality is a concern to rural residents. Most rural families depend on wells that may be easily contaminated or unsophisticated, underfunded public water systems (Mutel and Donham, 1983). Agricultural pollutants, including nitrates, pesticides, infectious agents such as *Giardia lamblia,* and particulates from soil erosion are major threats to rural water systems and to the long-term health of the population. Air pollution also concerns some rural communities because of "urban drift," as well as odors and particulate matter from rural agricultural or industrial operations. The rural community must also address the risks of hazardous waste disposal, since most dump sites are located in areas of low population density. The rural community nurse must work closely with environmental specialists in monitoring potential environmental health risks, particularly water quality, and be an advocate for environmental safety. Rural community nurses also need to be aware of naturally occurring environmental health concerns related to infectious agents found primarily in the rural environment. These include Rocky Mountain spotted fever, Colorado tick fever, plague, tularemia, and arthropod-borne viral encephalitis (Mutel and Donham, 1983).

Occupationally the extractive industries, including agriculture, mining, fishing, and forestry, predominate in most rural areas and present serious health threats. Agriculture and mining rank first and second as the most dangerous of all occupations, with respective mortalities of 61 and 50 deaths per 100,000 workers, compared with an average mortality of 13 deaths per 100,000 for all occupations (Accident Facts, 1981). Agricultural workers suffer from high rates of accidents, sun- and heat-related problems, vibration-related problems, hearing loss, acute and chronic respiratory diseases including asthma, farmer's lung, grain fever, byssinosis, and silo-filler's disease, zoonotic diseases such as tetanus from livestock, skin problems, cancer (especially leukemia and cancer of the skin), and pesticide-related problems (Mutel and Donham, 1983). In the lumber and wood products industry hazards include accidents, hearing loss, vibrational injury such as Raynaud's phenomenon, and higher rates of various cancers. Among miners greater risk of accidents, respiratory problems including pulmonary embolism, emphysema, asthma, and tuberculosis and pneumoconiosis (black lung), hearing loss, exposure to hazardous gaseous vapors, and various cancers predominate (Mutel and Donham, 1983).

Significant occupational health threats to rural workers and their families exist. The rural community health nurse, again reflecting the generalist role, must assume leadership in promoting occupational health and safety. Education for workers and employers related to occupational safety practices should be provided along with ongoing monitoring of occupational health threats in the community. From a health promotive perspective the rural nurse needs to become involved in "wellness in the workplace" strategies and address general issues such as stress management, mental health, and fitness. Immunization programs for adults, including tetanus protection and influenza and pneumonia vaccination for at-risk workers, are also important.

Rural Elderly People

As previously discussed, there is a high concentration of elderly people in rural communities (13%). This subgroup of the rural population is beginning to receive greater attention (Coward and Lee, 1985; Krout, 1983). According to the 1980 census, 43% of Americans older than 65 years of age live in rural areas. Rural elderly people are generally younger, more likely to be married, and less educated than urban elderly people (Rosenblatt, 1982). Health statistics indicate that the rural elderly people are less physically healthy than their urban counterparts even after the effects of age, sex, race, and income are removed (Coward and Lee, 1985, Rosenblatt, 1982). The effects of poverty compound the problems of the rural elderly people, since higher proportions of poor elderly people live in rural areas. Coward and Lee (1985) suggest that "improved health status of rural older people can best be achieved by strategies involving health promotion and health maintenance, rather than greater investments in the curative components of the health care system associated with advanced medical skills, technology, and high-cost facilities." This statement has direct applicability to community health nursing practice, which is on the forefront of health promotion services for elderly people.

Specific nursing interventions needed for elderly rural residents must be multifaceted. Because of the lower incomes of many rural elderly people, the provision of affordable, accessible, preventive care is a priority. Well-elderly clinics that provide holistic wellness care for rural elderly people have been successful in many areas. Mental health services for the rural elderly population, particularly depression and substance abuse services, need much greater attention. Home health services and creative alternatives for residential care of chronically ill rural elderly people that will maintain clients in their home communities are also needed (Rosenber and Pomeranz, 1984).

Community nurses could also include rural elderly people more actively in the delivery of nursing services. Since older women in particular often assume the role of family healer, they could be used as volunteers or staff members in home visitation programs, well-child clinics, and self-care programs. This use of indigenous persons in health care delivery would certainly strengthen the community nursing program and tie it even more closely with the community.

The rural community health nurse must address other health-related concerns of elderly people including food programs to provide adequate nutrition especially to isolated rural elderly, improved housing that is safe and culturally acceptable, opportunities for socialization and continued learning through senior centers, agricultural extension services, rural libraries, and creative public transportation alternatives for the elderly both within the community and to more populous areas for health care services and socialization (Talbot, 1981). Because of the generalist role of rural community nurses they must be actively involved in advocating health and social services for the elderly community.

CASE STUDY

The following case study exemplifies the unique dynamics inherent in rural community health nursing practice. The nursing process, including assessment, diagnosis, planning, intervention, and evaluation, is applied.

Assessment

The Jones family lives in a three-room cabin in the mountains 30 miles from the nearest town. Mr. Jones is a 62-year-old retired logger with emphysema and Mrs. Jones, 61, is severely disabled with multiple sclerosis. Their physician has recommended nursing home placement for Mrs. Jones, but the couple refuses, insisting they can make it on their own. The nearest nursing home is 50 miles away, and only limited home health services are available in the county. The Joneses' extended family consists of one married son and his family who live 40 miles away. The Joneses' home is heated only with wood, and in winter it is often inaccessible without a four-wheel drive vehicle. The family does not have a telephone, and the nearest neighbor is 3 miles away.

Diagnoses

Based on the preceding information the nurse formulates the following nursing diagnoses:

1. Altered family processes related to an ill family member
2. Altered health maintenance
3. Self-care deficits in feeding, bathing and hygiene, dressing and grooming, and toileting
4. Social isolation

Planning

With the family, including the Joneses' son, the following goals are established.

1. Mrs. Jones will be maintained in the home as long as possible.
2. Assistance for the Joneses' will be maximized using formal and informal resources.
3. The health of the family will be maintained through support services, health maintenance, and promotion of communication.

Implementation

To implement the above goals the community health nurse and the family agreed on an initial implementation plan. The nurse will visit weekly (weather permitting). During these visits the nurse will assess the physical and emotional status of both Mr. and Mrs. Jones and discuss with them how they are coping and any new concerns. The nurse will communicate with the family's physician on a regular basis and update her on the status of the family. The family will ask a neighbor to relieve Mr. Jones for three hours each week so that he can get away and have time to himself. The nurse will also contact local church volunteers and ask them to help the family chop wood and to provide a meal once a week. The nurse will communicate with the Joneses' son regularly and he and his family will visit monthly. An emergency plan will be established with the family and a neighbor in the event of the family needing immediate assistance, particularly during bad weather.

Evaluation

The above plan was implementated over a three-month period. At that time the nurse met with the entire family to evaluate how things were going. She noted that Mrs. Jones's physical status was stable and her emotional status had improved. Mr. Jones's emphysema was also stable, and he had finally been able to stop smoking after 42 years because he was feeling less stressed. The son was pleased with the care his parents were receiving and expressed feeling closer to them since he had been more involved. The nurse and the family agreed to continue with the plan of care and reevaluate in another three months.

This case study demonstrates several of the unique aspects of rural practice. The barriers of isolation and limited resources, as well as the strengths of family and community cohesion, are apparent. The nurse provided creative sensitive care using the appropriate informal and formal resources. She worked in partnership with the family, maximizing their sense of control while motivating them to achieve a higher state of wellness as a family.

SUMMARY

Rural community nursing is a unique specialty area of practice characterized by a truly generalist approach. Many challenges exist in this area of nursing practice. Rural community health nursing practice in the United States has a rich tradition of progressive approaches to the promotion of health through nursing services tailored to the needs and character of rural communities. Although disagreement exists regarding the precise definition of rural, scholars agree that rural communities have unique characteristics, including greater isolation, a dominance of traditional values, and fewer services, particularly in relation to health promotion. Rural community health nursing practice reflects the community characteristics, including a closer, more autonomous relationship with clients and families in addition to professional isolation and overload, the need to maintain confidentiality, and limited resources. Specific clinical rural community nursing concerns include adolescent pregnancy, family violence, water quality, occupational safety, and meeting the needs of rural elderly people. The rural community health nurse must indeed be a special breed with a commitment to professional nursing and all aspects of community health within the unique context of rural living.

QUESTIONS FOR DISCUSSION

1. Describe the role of the Red Cross in the history of rural nursing.
2. How does the role of the rural community-based nurse differ from that of an urban nurse who works in the community?
3. What are the barriers to the implementation of the Rural Health Services Clinic Act?
4. What special problems might the nurse who cares for rural elderly people encounter?

REFERENCES

Accident-facts, Chicago, 1981, National Safety Council.

Ahearn MC: Health-care in rural America, Agriculture Information Bulletin No. 428, Washington, DC, 1979, Economic Development Division; Economics, Statistics and Cooperatives Service.

Ahearn MC: Health care needed for rural children, Rur Dev Persp 3:26, 1980.

The American National Red Cross public health nursing, 1944. Excerpts from American Red Cross National Headquarters, DO 10, Supplement No 2.

Babich K, editor: Mental health issues in rural nursing, Boulder, Colo, 1982, Western Interstate Commission on Higher Education.

Barker V: Baccalaureate education in a rural setting, Nurs Outlook 20:335, 1972.

Battenfeld DE, Clift EG, and Graubarth RP: Patterns for change: rural women organizing for health, Washington, DC, 1981, National Women's Health Network.

Benson A, Sweeney M, and Nicolls R: A faculty learns about rural nursing, Nurs Health Care 4:78, 1982.

Bigbee JL: The implementation of the rural health clinic services act, P.L. 95-210, Tex J Rural Health, p 44, Jan 1984.

Brown DL: A quarter century of trends and changes in the demographic structure of American families. In Coward R and Smith W, editors: The family in rural society, Boulder, Colo, 1981, Westview Press Inc.

Carlson JE, Lassey ML, and Lassey WR: Rural society and environment in America, New York, 1981, McGraw-Hill Inc.

Clarenbach KF: Educational needs of rural women and girls, Report of the National Advisory Council on Women's Educational Programs, 1977.

Clement FE: Rural nursing, Am J Nurs 13:520, 1913.

Clement FE: American Red Cross town and country nursing service. Am J Nurs 14:1074, 1914.

Clement FE: Town and country nursing service, Am J Nurs 17:515, 1917.

Coward RT and Lee GR, editors: The elderly in rural society, New York, 1985, Springer Publishing Co.

Cummings D: What a rural FNP needs to know, Am J Nurs 78:1332, 1978.

Diers D: Nursing reclaims its role, Nurs Outlook 30:459, 1982.

Dillman DA and Hobbs DJ, editors: Rural society in the US: issues for the 1980's, Boulder, Colo, 1982, Westview Press Inc.

Dock LL and others: History of American Red Cross nursing, New York, 1922, Putnam's Sons.

Dunne F: Occupational sex-stereotyping among rural young women and men, Rural Sociology 45:396, 1980.

Dunne F: Traditional values/contemporary pressures: The conflicting needs of America's rural women. Paper presented at the Rural Education Seminar, 1979.

Elder N: The expanded role in nursing, Mo Nurse 47:13, 1978.

Fayey P: A small town nurse is still a nurse—and a lot more, RN 41:60, 1978.

Feldbaum EG: Will nurses alleviate health service maldistribution problems? Nurs Admin Q 4:61, 1979.

Flagg M: They showed the way, Red Cross Mag 1:27, 1851.

Flax JW and others: Mental health and rural America: an overview, Community Ment Health Rev 3:1, 1978.

Fletcher DF: Report on rural nursing, Denver, 1981, Colorado Office of Rural Health.

Ford T: Rural U.S.A.: persistence and change, Ames, 1978, Iowa State University Press.

Gilford DM, Nelson GL, and Ingram L: Rural America in passage: statistics for policy, Washington, DC, 1981, National Academy Press.

Glenn N and Alston J: Rural-urban differences in reported attitudes and behaviors, Soc Sci Q 47:381, 1982.

Glenn NO and Hill L: Rural-urban differences in attitudes and behavior in the United States, Ann Am Acad Politic Soc Science 429:36, 1977.

Hadbavny N, Smith E, and Griffith K: An interview with a rural nurse practitioner, Oregon Nurse 45:8, 1980.

Hassinger E: Rural health organization, Ames, 1982, Iowa State University Press.

Hester S: A descriptive study of the professional and community roles of the hospital-employed registered nurse in rural Wyoming settings, master's thesis, Laramie, 1986, University of Wyoming.

Heuther SE and Fritz JN: Assessing rural community practice potential, Nurs Pract 3:12, 1978.

Kalisch PA and Kalisch BJ: The advance of American nursing, Boston, 1978, Little, Brown & Co Inc.

Kelly D: One town's one-nurse service, Am J Nurs 73:1536, 1973.

Kennedy D and Taheri B: Methods for estimating staffing needs for the public health nursing program in Wyoming, Cheyenne, 1981, Department of Health and Social Services, State of Wyoming.

Krout JA: The rural elderly: an annotated bibliography of social science research, Westport, Conn, 1983, Greenwood Press Inc.

Larson OF: Values and beliefs of rural people. In Ford TR, editor, Rural USA persistence and change, Ames, 1977, Iowa State University Press.

Lassiter PG: Education for rural health professionals. . . nurses, J Rural Health 1:23, 1985.

Leonard A and Rogers I: Role imagery: a delicate balance, J Nurs Educ 17:42, 1978.

MacAbee O: Rural parenting classes: beginning to meet the need, MCN 2:315, 1977.

McAtee P: Rural health care, Pediatr Nurs. 4:14, 1978.

Miller MK: Health and medical care. In Dillmen DA and Hobbs DJ, editors: Rural society in the U.S.: issues for the 1980's, Boulder, Colo, 1982, Westview Press Inc.

Miller MK: Health status, health resources and consolidated structural parameters: implications for public health care policy, doctoral dissertation, University Park, 1975, The Pennsylvania State University.

More nurses in rural areas, Am J Nurs 40:1217, 1940.

Moscovice I and Nestegard M: The influence of values and background on the location decision of nurse practitioners, J Community Health 5:244, 1980.

Murdock S and Sutton W: The new ecology and community theory: similarities, differences and convergencies, Rural Society 39:319, 1974.

Mutel CF and Donham KJ: Medical practice in rural communities, New York, 1983 Springer-Verlag, New York Inc.

Nicoll J: A nurse-owned rural health clinic, Nurse Pract 4:29, 1979.

Oseasohn R and others: Primary care by a nurse practitioner in a rural clinic, Am J Nurs 75:267, 1975.

Ploch LA: Family aspects of the new wave of immigrants to rural communities. In Coward R and Smith W, editors: The family in rural society, Boulder, Colo, 1981, Westview Press Inc.

Proceedings of the national conference on the delivery of family planning services in rural America, New York, 1977, Alan Guttmacher Institute.

Report on nursing: fifth report to the president and Congress on the status of health personnel in the United States, Rockville, Md, 1986, US Department of Health and Human Services.

Rolshoven R: Rural nursing, Nurs Careers 3:10, 1982.

Rosenber S and Pomeranz W: Developing home health services in rural communities—an innovative solution to a thorny problem, Rural Health Care 6:8, 1984.

Rosenblatt PC and Anderson RM; Interaction in farm families: tension and stress. In Coward RT and Smith WM, editors: The family in rural society, Boulder, Colo, 1981, Westview Press Inc.

Rosenblatt RA and Huard B: The nurse practitioner as a physician substitute in a remote rural community: a case study, Public Health Report 94:571, 1979.

Rosenblatt RA and Moscovice IS: Rural health care, New York, 1982, John Wiley and Sons Inc.

Rowe G and others: The impact of economic stressors on rural and urban family relationships. In Williams R and others, editors: Family strengths: enhancement of interaction, Lincoln, 1985, University of Nebraska Press.

Schumm WR and Bollman SR: Interpersonal processes in rural families. In Coward RT and Smith WM, editors: The family in rural society, Boulder, Colo, 1981, Westview Press Inc.

Stewart IM and Austin AL: A history of nursing, ed 5, New York, 1962, Putnam's Sons.

Stricklin R: The rural ED nurse: an expanded role, J Emerg Nurs 6:5, 1980.

Stuart-Burchardt S: Rural nursing, Am J Nurs 82:616, 1982.

Stuart-Siddall S: Backwoods nursing, Nurse Educ 6:14, 1981.

Talbot DM: Assessing needs of the rural elderly, J. Gerontol Nurs 11:39, 1981.

Thobaden M and Weigard M: Rural nursing clinic, Nurse Educ 6:24, 1983.

Thorton J: Developing a rural nursing clinic, Nurse Educ 6:24, 1983.

US Bureau of the Census: Statistical abstract of the United States, 1986, Washington DC, 1987, US Government Printing Office.

US Department of Commerce, Bureau of the Census: 1980 census of the population: general population characteristics, United States summary, Washington, DC, 1983, US Government Printing Office.

Wallace SS and Kretz SE: Rural medicine, Lexington, Mass, 1981, Lexington Books.

Warner AR, editor: Innovations in community health nursing: health care delivery in shortage areas, St Louis, 1978, CV Mosby Co.

Weinback RW: Health care needs of rural residents, Hum Serv Rural Envir 5:12, 1980.

Weinstein P and Demers JL: Rural nurse practitioner clinic, Am J Nurs 74:2022, 1974.

Willits FK, Bealer RC, and Crider DM: The ecology of social traditionalism in a rural hinterland, Rural Soc 39:334, 1974.

CHAPTER 23

Community Mental Health

Mary Anne Noble

RESOURCES
We support licensing of social workers in Missouri.
National Association of Social Workers
BECAUSE WE CARE.
HELP IS AVAILABLE. CALL:
421-INFO
FIRST CALL FOR HELP
It brings out the best in all of us.
Community Resources for Single-Parents
Divorce Therapy Group; Wed. 7-8:30pm
Support Group for Separated, Divorced Women
Mondays 7-9pm
Mother's Hotline
call 965-KIDS
Single-Support Group
PARENTS OF HYPERACTIVE CHILDREN SUPPORT GROUPS
Divorce Support Group

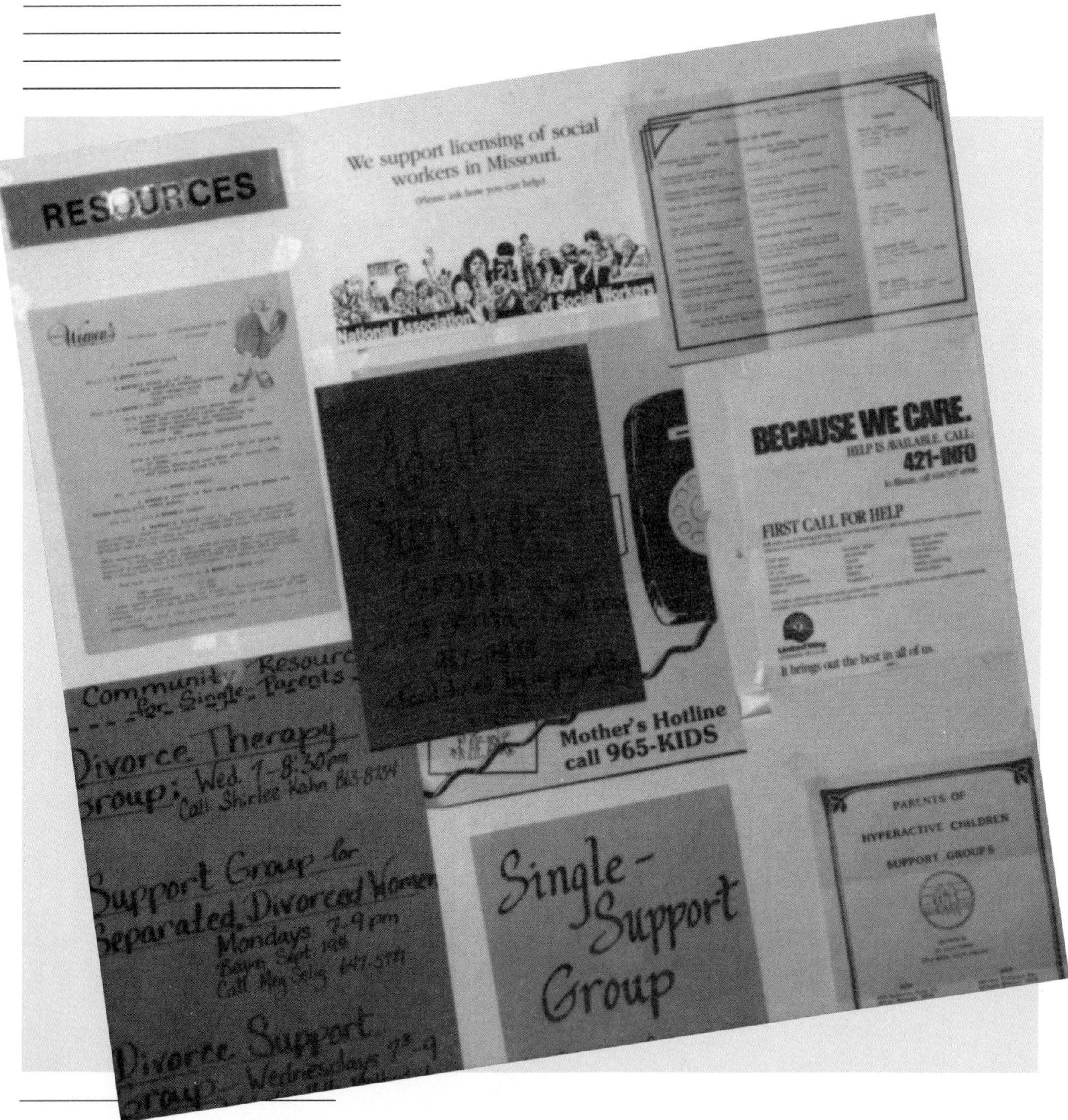

CHAPTER OUTLINE

Definition

Historical perspective

Deinstitutionalization effort

Mental health problems or disorders and their management in the community

- Schizophrenia
- Depression
- Anxiety disorders
- Personality disorders
- Mental retardation

Aging

Theories of causation

Role of nurses in community mental health

Summary

OBJECTIVES

After completing this chapter, the reader should be able to:

1. Describe the relationship of health and illness to the concept of mental health and mental illness in a holistic and comprehensive sense.
2. Develop an understanding of psychiatric nursing theory and skill in the community.
3. Gain a perspective of community mental health and the community treatment of mental illness in the past, present, and idealistically the future.
4. Appreciate the complexity and diversity of mental health problems and treatment in the community.
5. Appreciate the overlapping and blurring of roles among mental health professionals, yet recognize the unique contribution of the nurse.

WHAT IS COMMUNITY MENTAL HEALTH? Community nurses who work in the mental health field are involved in a variety of psychiatric mental health activities including primary prevention, secondary prevention, and tertiary prevention with emphasis on practice in the community as opposed to practice in institutional settings (Koldjeski, 1984).

Primary prevention in this field includes activities focusing on the prevention of mental and emotional disorders. Mental health education and mental health counseling in schools or in youth centers are examples of primary prevention. The objective is to help people develop constructive attitudes and behaviors so that they are less likely to become ill later in life. Drug counseling, sex education, and stress management education are more specific types of primary prevention. Many community agencies and facilities lend themselves to primary prevention. These activities are valued by our society because medical researchers believe mental illness can be prevented.

Secondary prevention in community mental health refers to activities aimed at preventing mental illness from developing in people at risk. Examples of such activities include counseling or education of people experiencing a traumatic loss or counseling or education of children in poverty-stricken areas. Although it is not absolutely known who is at risk of mental illness, it is theorized that poverty, unemployment, loss of a loved one, and physical illness are related to mental health problems and that counseling these people is a sound prevention strategy. Both primary and secondary preventive mental health activities are sufficiently broad that one may wonder how different these are from general community health preventive activities. There is considerable overlap between these two areas of community health; general health embraces many of the concepts and practices of the community mental health field.

Tertiary prevention is more specific and addresses the care and management of clients who experience serious or long-term psychiatric problems in the community. These clients may need periodic hospitalization. Current belief is that treatment and especially hospitalization should be community based, that hospitalization should be as short as possible, and that institutionalization results in a poor prognosis. Even clients who are dangerous to themselves or others are candidates for community mental health services. Thus today we see severely mentally ill or psychotic clients being treated in community mental health centers.

Since increasing emphasis is placed on the biopsychosocial approach to health and illness, community mental health is subsumed under the concept of community health. Health is a holistic phenomenon, and it is more than the sum of biologic, psychologic, and social wellness. Furthermore, when one dimension is affected, other dimensions are also affected. In other words people who have physiologic problems frequently develop mental problems. In addition, people with mental or psychologic problems frequently develop physical problems. Both physical and psychologic problems affect what can be defined as social health of persons or communities. There is increasing evidence in medical and nursing literature supporting the interaction of the mind and the body, or the psyche and the soma (Shaver, 1985).

Nurses seem to have had intuition about this for many years. Even old nursing texts refer to the need to care for the whole person. How this approach was to be operationalized was never discussed in old texts; however, today we are beginning to make some progress in this area. For instance, today we recognize that a client recovering from a myocardial infarction must adhere to treatment consisting of medication, diet, exercise, and also reduction of stress, usually with a change of life-style. We recognize that such things as emotional problems, family problems, and financial problems may influence the course of diseases and are crucial factors in recovery.

Community health nurses, as well as nurses in

other settings, must be cognizant and skilled in this biopsychosocial approach to health and illness. A broad base of knowledge, skills, and attitudes is necessary for community health nurses to meet the needs of the people they must serve.

HISTORICAL PERSPECTIVE

Psychiatric mental health nursing, as well as the other mental health professions, was launched in the community with the advent of the community mental health movement. The beginnings of this movement can be traced to the early 1960s with the final report of the Joint Commission on Mental Illness and Health titled *Action for Mental Health*. This famous document was published in 1961, and it set the stage for a new era.

The community mental health movement is sometimes referred to as the third revolution in psychiatry. Before the movement mentally ill clients were treated or cared for primarily in institutions on a long-term basis. Inpatient treatment was considered appropriate and legitimate. New thinking, however, considered outpatient community treatment appropriate. It was believed that communities should be responsible for client care and that clients should recover in small social groups near or even within their homes. The community was to become the locus and focus of treatment.

Among the recommendations of the commission were the following. No more state mental hospitals with more than 1000 beds should be built, since large institutions where psychiatric clients were warehoused and cared for in large groups were viewed as unnatural and nonconducive to personal growth, a sense of identity, and ultimate recovery. Community mental health centers should be built in sufficient quantity and proximity to serve the population. It was believed that if clients were treated in these centers, the need for repeated and prolonged hospitalizations would be reduced. If hospitalization was necessary, it was considered preferable to hospitalize a client in the psychiatric unit of a general hospital instead of a state mental hospital because of general hospitals' emphasis on short-term therapy and because general hospitals were more likely to be located closer to the client's home.

Other services the committee considered necessary to the community health movement were day hospitals, night hospitals, after-care clinics, public health nursing services, foster family care, convalescent nursing homes, rehabilitation centers, work services, and former-client groups. The emphasis in these services was to be to keep clients in the mainstream of society and ultimately to enable them to function as productive members of society. It was hoped a changing attitude toward the mentally ill would accompany the recommendations for mental health services. Acceptance, not rejection, would become the norm, and people would begin viewing mental illness in the same way that physical illness was viewed. Last there were to be national recruitment and training programs for all categories of mental health personnel (Joint Commission on Mental Illness and Health, 1961).

President Kennedy appointed a committee to study the recommendations of the committee. Congress responded with the Community Mental Health Centers Act in 1963. Much federal money went into the recommended services, research, and training programs for mental health personnel. At this time psychiatry and mental health became popular fields for all health professions, including medicine, nursing, social work, and mental health counselors.

Psychiatric nursing was at its peak in the mid-1960s. Assistance in the form of traineeships for nurses pursuing a master's degree was available to almost anyone who applied for it. Furthermore, at that time psychiatric nursing was undergoing an expanded role. Nurses were being prepared to function in a variety of settings and in a variety of therapeutic roles with the major emphasis on short-term treatment intervention geared to individual clients, groups of clients, and families. Nursing psychotherapy, or nursing therapy, as a technique and intervention was taught and practiced. Nursing therapy, although it was never well defined, was actually not much different from the psychotherapy practiced by psychiatrists, psychologists, and social workers. Because the emphasis was to make therapy available to more clients in many settings, there was a true blurring of roles among the mental health professions. This blurring or overlapping of roles still exists.

The 1960s were exciting times for those in the mental health field. It was believed that a real contribution to a forgotten segment of society would finally be made. Many professionals who had long been in the mental health field were extremely committed to the mentally ill, but they had worked in isolation and without recognition from the rest of the professional world. Now, however, services to the mentally ill were held in high esteem, and mental health professionals were recognized. In addition, because of the efforts of expanded treatment modalities and increased research, it was believed that a cure for mental illness was not far distant. It was also believed that prevention was possible, chronic mental illness would no longer exist, and the demise of institutionalization would be witnessed.

Despite legislative efforts through the years, including the Community Mental Health Systems Act of 1980, the community mental health movement has failed. The movement has not helped the mentally ill significantly. Although much federal money has been spent, most states could not or would not pay the difference between the federal money given and the actual cost to provide the necessary community services. Many clients were discharged from institutions during the deinstitutionalization movement and clients are still being discharged. However, the adequacy of community mental health centers leaves much to be desired. Clients are discharged without support, monitoring, supervision, therapy, attention, and often the basic necessities of life. Many of the homeless in the United States are former mental clients who must now live on the streets, since they are forgotten and abandoned. Frequently they stay on the streets until they cause a disturbance, and then they are shuttled back to the institution. Some clients who could do well in the community seek to return to the institution because it provides food, shelter, and medical attention. For some, home is equated with the institution. Sometimes we speak of the "revolving door phenomenon" to describe the process of discharging clients from an institution without adequate support and readmitting them when a crisis occurs.

THE DEINSTITUTIONALIZATION EFFORT

As discussed previously, deinstitutionalization was a crucial part of the community mental health movement. Although deinstitutionalization is a vague term for a process that has been under way for 25 years, it refers to the planned effort to discharge clients from the large state mental hospitals, reduce the institutions in size and scope of function, and, most important, prevent new clients from becoming dependent on institutions for survival.

Evaluation of this effort is difficult because of many factors, not the least of which is the attempt to assess the quality of life for clients both in and out of institutions. Today the concept of deinstitutionalization is still viewed as ideal, good, and desirable, since it approximates the normal state for human beings. There is the belief that people, regardless of their mental ability, are happier in small, family-like settings close to support groups and in situations with conventional interpersonal roles and relationships. It is also believed that these people can achieve their potential and contribute to society in noninstitutional settings with adequate support and supervision.

However, many experts believe that this good

idea was executed poorly and that the pendulum has swung too far in the direction of community care; that is, institutions have either emptied out too quickly or, in some cases, closed prematurely. Many clients discharged from institutions fell between the cracks of the various agencies or community services, and they were lost or ignored until a crisis occurred and they were returned to a state hospital or other restrictive setting such as a jail. There were many problems in defining agency and staff roles and in the communication between the various agencies designed to monitor clients away from the institution (Halpern and others, 1980).

Another significant problem with the deinstitutionalization effort is the continuing opposition by families, communities, and the mental institutions to community placement of mentally ill clients. Some of this opposition is warranted. Families frequently are overburdened with the care of their loved ones because adequate support is not available. Some clients need 24-hour supervision, and families simply do not have the resources for this. Not only is the task physically and psychologically exhausting with no opportunity for respite, but it also often means a family member must give up outside employment to care for the client.

Communities have difficulty tolerating and accepting deviance. Although former clients may not be dangerous to themselves or others, their peculiar appearance and behavior is frowned on in shopping areas, recreational facilities, restaurants, churches, and even on the streets. It is a rare community that has citizens who tolerate a group home for the mentally ill or are not upset by their real or imagined fears that these homes will interfere with their routine and ultimately affect the value of their homes.

Even the staffs of institutions have opposed the deinstitutionalization effort because they viewed the effort as taking away their jobs, which, in fact, it did and still is doing. Since many state hospitals are located in or near small towns, a sizeable percentage of these populations was employed at the institutions. Thus the deinstitutionalization effort is seen as a gigantic threat to the livelihood of large numbers of residents. Even though there exists a need for skill and services in these communities, the means, education, and support for this transition have not been available.

The economic factor may be the greatest threat to the deinstitutionalization effort and the ultimate welfare of the mentally ill. Economic funding patterns, resource constraints, financial incentives, federal versus state and local participation, and cost effectiveness of benefits and policies are all factors that must be resolved before the value of deinstitutionalization can be realized (Noble and Conley, 1981; and Noble, 1981).

MENTAL HEALTH PROBLEMS OR DISORDERS AND THEIR MANAGEMENT IN THE COMMUNITY

In the community it is possible to manage almost any type of emotional problem or disorder, ranging from mild to severe and acute to chronic. Of course, adequate support, supervision, and evaluation are necessary to manage these clients successfully, and, as previously discussed, the community mental health movement has failed in this regard. It is possible, however, to discuss ideal management and the nurse's role in this management.

Schizophrenia

Schizophrenia is a broad term to describe a wide range of thought disorders. Clients with schizophrenia are psychotic, and they have difficulty distinguishing between fantasy and reality. Schizophrenia may be manifest as anxiety, fear, hostility, paranoia, withdrawal, or catatonia. These clients may be dangerous to themselves or others, and frequently they are unable to care for themselves or satisfy even basic survival needs. People with schizophrenia commonly experience hallucinations and delusions, and they have major problems with interpersonal relationships. Schizophrenic episodes may be acute and transient, or the disease may develop into a long-term chronic condition. Some clients are not so sick that they cannot live a relatively normal life (with management), and other clients are so sick that they need constant treatment and confinement. It is difficult to talk about these clients as a single group because they are extremely variable. However, it is the acutely ill, wild, raving lunatic schizophrenic client whom society associates with the term "mental illness." Only a small percentage of schizophrenic clients fit this stereotype.

Until the 1950s with the advent of the psychotropic medications, specifically phenothiazines, treatment or control of schizophrenia was almost impossible; institutionalization was usually a necessity. These drugs have revolutionized the entire field of psychiatry and have made it possible to control the symptoms of many clients. Control is the concept to keep in mind because antipsychotics do not cure schizophrenia. They do not change the basic disease process, but they do control psychotic thoughts, affect, anxiety, and disturbed behavior.

Drug treatment of schizophrenia is complicated. There are many side effects and contraindications. There is also a lot of guesswork, trial and error, and dosage uncertainty in prescriptions. It is not known why these drugs work and to what extent they will work with different clients. Also, some of these drugs interact adversely with other medications. Yet treatment of schizophrenia with antipsychotic medications is the cheapest, primary, and most successful treatment to date despite the many and varied other therapies that have been tried through the years, including psychotherapy, electric shock therapy, and insulin therapy. Thus nursing management of schizophrenics in the community usually involves drug management.

Noncompliance, that is, not following the prescribed medication routine, is the greatest problem in management of clients in the community, and it is the reason why symptoms develop suddenly in many controlled clients, forcing them to be readmitted to a hospital. Clients may begin to feel better and then suddenly decide they no longer need medication. Their paranoid ideation may also contribute to their noncompliance. Fluphenazene decanoate (Prolixin) and haloperidol (Haldol) are available in intramuscular preparations that can be given every two to four weeks; this regimen reduces the possibility of noncompliance of some clients. It allows nurses at clinics or centers to be confident that clients will not become disturbed at home unless they fail to appear for their periodic injections. If this happens, nurses can take more active approaches such as visiting clients at home in an attempt to persuade them to comply. With oral medications compliance is more difficult.

Drug supervision and management of the schizophrenic client is a big responsibility for community mental health nurses. Nurses must be familiar with the antipsychotic medications, including dosages, side effects, and contraindications. Important considerations in general management include the following (Hervey, 1984):

1. There is no tolerance to the therapeutic effects of these medications. In other words, clients do not become resistant to the medications, and can be treated for many years.
2. Overdoses usually are not fatal, except in young and old clients, because there is a wide therapeutic index with no maximum at any reasonable dose. The exception is thioridazine (Mellaril); thioridazine may cause blindness if a daily dose of 800 mg is exceeded. Combining these medications with alcohol is potentially dangerous.
3. Antipsychotic agents have a long half-life, making daily administration feasible. Administration at bedtime is a good strategy, since maximum drowsiness or sedation will

occur at night and thus enable the client to function better during the day. Daily administration also increases client compliance and decreases side effects and cost.

4. There is a wide range of client response to the antipsychotic drugs, so the nurse must be aware of the multitude of behaviors and symptoms that could indicate effectiveness or dangerous side effects. Nurses must be astute in their observation of both physical and psychologic symptoms, and they must report these frequently to the prescribing physician, who is usually not in a position to observe the client regularly. Polypharmacy, or the simultaneous prescription of two or more antipsychotics, is not considered a good policy because it makes it difficult to determine a client's reaction to any one medication.

It is impossible to discuss the complex subject of antipsychotics completely here. Therefore the nurse working with schizophrenic clients needs to be familiar with the Physician's Desk Reference (PDR) and other psychiatric drug literature (Hervey, 1984; Wilson and Kneisl, 1983). The most common and important side effects and complications of antipsychotic medications are presented in the following list:

1. Tardive dyskinesia is a severe irreversible condition characterized by involuntary movements of the face, jaw, and tongue. Lip smacking, tongue protrusion, and facial grimaces are common symptoms. Early recognition of beginning symptoms is the key to prevention because it makes it possible to reverse the condition. In this case medication should be discontinued, reduced, or changed. Although tardive dyskinesia usually occurs after clients have been receiving antipsychotics for years, it can occur soon after antipsychotics are initiated.
2. Extrapyramidal syndrome (EPS) is common among clients taking antipsychotic medications and occurs early in treatment. Symptoms include acute dystonic reactions, a parkinsonian syndrome, and akathisia. Muscle spasm, restlessness, rigidity, and tremor are commonly observed. This syndrome can be controlled with the anticholinergic or antiparkinsonian drugs of which the more common are trihexyphenidyl (Artane), benztropine mesylate (Cogentin), and diphenhydramine (Benadryl). These drugs should be used only to control the EPS symptoms and only when clearly indicated. Again there are many unknown reactions of these drugs, and they have a toxicity of their own.
3. Allergic reactions to the antipsychotics include agranulocytosis, dermatitis, and jaundice. These reactions are acute but rare. Agranulocytosis can be fatal; a high fever and a sore throat with ulceration are symptoms that should make the nurse suspicious. Dermatitis or skin problems may be mild or severe. Clients receiving chlorpromazine (Thorazine) are apt to be photosensitive and to sunburn easily. These clients should use extreme precaution when exposed to the sun, and they should use a sunscreen agent. Jaundice is usually a benign, self-limited, transient condition.
4. Phenothiazines interfere with the ability of the body to regulate heat, and the antiparkinsonian drugs interfere with perspiration. Consequently these clients are at special risk for heat stroke, hyperthermia, and resulting sudden death. Although this condition is rare, it is malignant once the process starts. Clients in hot climates who do not have access to air conditioning are susceptible. Education and advocacy for these clients is an important nursing role. Where do the clients live? Where do they work or spend their days? Do they have adequate fluids and shade to cool themselves? Client teaching alone may not be sufficient if the means for survival are not present. Advocacy therefore must go hand in hand with client education.

TABLE 23-1 Commonly Used Antipsychotic Medications

Trade name	Generic name
Thorazine	Chlorpromazine
Mellaril	Thioridazine
Stelazine	Trifluoperazine
Prolixin	Fluphenazine decanoate (oral and intramuscular preparations)
Trilafon	Perphenazine
Taractan	Chlorprothixene
Navane	Thiothixene
Haldol	Haloperidol
Moban	Molindone

5. Antipsychotics are known to interact with medications used for other conditions such as cardiovascular disease, hypertension, diabetes, and renal disease. Consequently, clients receiving these medications, especially elderly clients who usually have at least one chronic condition, need to be monitored carefully. Also the safety of antipsychotics has not been established in pregnancy, lactation, and childhood.

6. Common annoying reactions to antipsychotics include drowsiness, blurred vision, constipation, and a dry mouth. These problems are not serious and are easily managed. Nurses can do much to counsel and educate clients about these issues. Clients should use caution when driving or doing other dangerous or exacting activities.

The more commonly used antipsychotic medications are listed in Table 23-1. Both generic and trade names are given. Since dosages are extremely variable, the nurse is referred to the PDR and other psychiatric medication literature for further information (Hervey, 1984).

Although medication maintenance and management are probably the most important roles of the community nurse working with schizophrenic clients, there are other crucial roles and skills. Interpersonal communication and the ability to relate to these clients are particularly important. Typically they have not been able to enter into meaningful relationships throughout their lives. Interacting with families is important too because families who can support these clients are more likely to be successful in keeping them happily and productively in the community. Communication with other professionals is also important. Often it is difficult for the psychiatric mental health team to obtain a total picture of clients because the clients lack communication skills. Consequently a closely knit team is vital for the schizophrenic client's welfare.

Depression

Probably depression is the most commonly occurring mental disorder in the population. Depression can range from a mild or acute condition to a chronic or long term and severe form of illness. In its more benign form it can be defined as a sadness or a state of being "blue." In its most severe form the clients are withdrawn, self-deprecatory, guilt ridden, energy deficient, unable to care for themselves, and suicidal. Depression frequently accompanies physical illness, loss of a loved one, or loss of a job. Nurses working in all aspects of community health come in contact with clients who have depression and should therefore be prepared to deal with them.

Treatment of depression can include simple counseling, electric shock therapy (EST), or treatment with the antidepressant drugs. Sometimes people who have experienced a significant loss need only support and time to work through their depression and come to a healthy resolution. Other people become severely depressed to the point of psychosis and suicide. There is increasing research that some depressions are unrelated to loss and may have an organic basis, although as with all mental illness the evidence is nonconclusive. Also depression accompanies a number of physical illnesses and hormonal disorders. Some medications, such as hypertensives and corticosteroids, can induce depression (Field, 1985). Depression is truly a complex problem in society.

EST can be used to treat some depressions. A short course of eight or 10 treatments can help some clients return to their families, jobs, and communities quickly. Often the result of this treatment is dramatic, and clients demonstrate nearly normal behavior; some clients appear cured, at least for a period. However, EST is not used as much as it was some years ago. Many experts frown on the use of EST because it is not known why EST is effective or if there are any long-term ill effects. Also it is considered by many professionals and laypersons to be a barbaric form of treatment. Consequently, the nurse working in a community mental health center will probably encounter few clients receiving EST even on an outpatient basis. Working with depressed clients demands primarily a familiarity with the antidepressant medications and the assessment of suicide potential.

Suicide is a risk with any client who is depressed. The first rule that nurses (or any other professionals) must follow is that no suicide threat should be taken lightly. Most people who kill themselves have made threats to family, friends, or health personnel. A threat can be viewed as a desperate plea for help. It is as if these people are trying to say that they really want to live but need assistance to keep from acting impulsively. People who make frequent suicide attempts and antagonize others but are ignored and not taken seriously are apt to become more depressed and ultimately succeed in ending their lives. It is better to be safe than sorry, and if nurses have doubts about clients' intentions, they should arrange for hospitalization and immediately involve other members of the health team and family members.

Statistics show that suicide is prevalent among adolescents and young adults in the throes of life change or turmoil. It is also prevalent among elderly people. Women make more suicide attempts, but men are more likely to succeed in their attempts. When suicidal people made sudden plans to put their lives in order or give away many of their precious belongings, the nurse should interpret these actions as intent to attempt suicide. Indirect suicide attempts, such as taking unnecessary risks with machinery, participating in dangerous sports, or not taking necessary medications, are also significant. Thus a diabetic who purposely does not take insulin or a cardiac client who does not take digoxin may be suicide prone. Nurses must be perceptive of behavior changes and watch for them at every interaction.

Perhaps the most commonly used treatment for depression is the antidepressant medications. There are two classes of medications, the monoamine oxidase (MAO) inhibitors and tricyclic compounds. Today MAO inhibitors are used less frequently and primarily for clients who do not respond to or cannot tolerate tricyclics. Although MAO inhibitors work well in relieving the symptoms of depression and do not promote addiction, they are contraindicated with a long list of food and drugs, including over-the-counter drugs and alcohol. Reactions from tyramine-containing drugs and food can be so severe that they can be fatal. Therefore the MAO inhibitors should be used only with highly motivated and compliant clients who, nonetheless, require a great deal of monitoring. Nurses must be well aware of contraindicated food and drugs so that they can advise both clients and families. Other less serious reactions to these medications are postural hypotension, daytime sleepiness, and dry mouth.

Tricyclic compounds are given much more often than are MAO inhibitors. Many clients function well while receiving these medications and lead near normal lives. Important considerations include the following (Hervey, 1984):

1. The antidepressive effect takes several weeks to develop. Therefore suicidal clients must be observed and supervised closely until the medication takes effect.
2. There is no tolerance or physical addiction.
3. Treatment failure is frequently related to inadequate dosage.

TABLE 23-2 Commonly Used Antidepressant Medications

Medication class	Trade name	Generic name
Monoamine oxidase inhibitors	Marplan	Isocarboxazid
	Nardil	Phenelzine sulfate
	Parnate	Tranylcypromine sulfate
Tricyclic antidepressants	Elavil, Endep	Amitriptyline
	Asendin	Amoxepine
	Adapin, Sinequan	Doxepin
	Tofranil, Presamine	Imipramine
	Surmontil	Trimipramine maleate
	Norpramin, Pertofrane	Desipramine
	Aventyl, Pamelor	Nortriptyline
	Vivactil	Protriptyline

4. These medications have a long half-life and can be administered once a day. Daily administration increases compliance.
5. Overdoses may result in fatalities. Therefore it is important for the nurse to be aware of safe ranges.
6. Tricyclics are not recommended for children.
7. Caution must be used in prescribing these drugs if the client has certain physical disorders such as seizures and cardiac disease.
8. Common side effects include constipation, orthostatic hypotension, dry mouth, blurred vision, and sedation.
9. If medication is to be decreased or discontinued, it should be done slowly.
10. As with the antipsychotics, polypharmacy or concurrent use of more than one antidepressant should be discouraged.

The more commonly used antidepressant medications are listed in Table 23-2. Both generic and trade names are given. The nurse is referred to the PDR and other psychiatric medication literature for dosage and other information (Hervey, 1984).

The type of depression that is observed in manic-depressive disease, now commonly referred to as bipolar or unipolar affective disorders, is generally not treated with the antidepressant medications but with lithium therapy. The discovery of lithium in 1970 has made it possible for clients with manic-depressive disease to live useful and nearly normal lives. Lithium is effective for clients who exhibit both mania and depression or either mania or depression in a cyclic pattern. The primary problem with lithium therapy is that the therapeutic dose, which is highly individualized, is close to the toxic dose. In other words, the therapeutic range is extremely narrow. Consequently, the client must be monitored carefully for serum lithium levels. Normal serum blood level ranges from 0.9 to 1.5 mEq/L. Maximum therapeutic serum concentration is 2 mEq/L. Lithium toxicity develops gradually, and it may be fatal. Tremors, vomiting, diarrhea, sluggishness, confusion, and ataxia are suspicious symptoms. In addition, lithium substitutes for sodium ions, sometimes causing sodium depletion. Clients may have to increase their fluid and salt intake to prevent this condition. The symptoms of minor lithium toxicity include transient nausea, fatigue, thirst, polyuria, diarrhea, and muscle weakness. These symptoms usually disappear after the first few weeks of therapy. Clients with manic-depressive disorders receiving lithium therapy can lead productive lives if they are managed and monitored closely while receiving lithium therapy (Kreigh and Perko, 1983).

Fluoxetine (Prozac), a completely new and different antidepressant came on the market in early 1988. Some practitioners believe it is the miracle drug for which everyone has been waiting. Fluoxetine relieves symptoms of depression well, and it has relatively few side effects. One such side effect is a slight weight loss, which of course is desirable for many depressed clients. Unfortunately, the generic form of Prozac is not available, and it probably will not be for several years. It is dispensed in 20 mg capsules ranging in cost from $1.40 to $1.50 per capsule. Some clients must take three to five capsules a day, which makes treatment with this new drug too costly for many clients.

It cannot be emphasized strongly enough that nurses must be familiar with the medications their clients are taking. With such diverse individual client response, variability in physician preference, numerous contraindications, and serious side effects, antidepressant medication supervision is a task that requires a skilled nurse.

Anxiety Disorders

People with anxiety disorders are seldom hospitalized. A certain amount of anxiety is therapeutic for healthy development because it fosters learning and achievement and it helps one exercise caution and deliberation in life. Only when anxiety causes clients to become incapacitated or immobilized and interferes with daily routine do they need treatment. Short-term anxiety precipitated by a crisis or traumatic life event can often be easily managed by support, counseling, and education. Long-term, pervasive anxiety needs more intensive psychotherapy or treatment with antianxiety medications.

Sometimes we refer to clients with severe anxiety as being neurotic. Neurotic people are in touch with reality. Usually clients have a great deal of insight to their anxious behavior, and intellectually they know that it is not normal, but they are unable to control their feelings of uneasiness, dread, fear, and panic. These clients truly suffer, and for some of them life is a continuous nightmare.

There is speculation that some of the classic anxiety disorders in our society are disappearing. These include dissociative reactions, obsessive-compulsive neuroses, conversion reactions, and phobias. It is beyond the scope of this chapter to explore the many theoretic positions on anxiety disorders, but it must be noted that nurses working in community settings of any sort should be able to recognize manifestations of anxiety, have some beginning skills in counseling, and of course be familiar with antianxiety medications.

Most nurses have some background in anxiety assessment because of their own experiences and because anxiety is associated with surgery, acute illness, pain, and imminent death. Symptoms of severe anxiety include tachycardia, hyperventilation, dilated pupils, muscle tension, perspiration, and trembling. In panic states these clients are immobilized and have a sense of impending doom. They cannot respond to stimuli in their environment, and they seem to have a decreased ability to see, hear, and comprehend.

Psychotherapy, group therapy, and other nonbiologic therapies have been helpful in treating some anxiety disorders. Even supportive counseling has been beneficial. However, many clients, if not most, cannot afford this long process of therapy even though theory may dictate its efficacy. It is simply not practical for the average person. Yet the nurse who deals with clients who have anxiety disorders should be skilled in counseling and interpersonal relations. Nurses should know that the client cannot be "talked out" of this anxiety. They should attempt to protect clients as much as possible, especially if clients are experiencing a panic attack. It is difficult for nurses (and other professionals) to do this because most of these clients appear normal and they have considerable insight into their behavior. For instance, a client who is phobic and afraid of being in crowds will state that the fear is silly and ir-

TABLE 23-3 Commonly Used Antianxiety Medications

Medication class	Trade name	Generic name
Benzodiazepines	Librium	Chlordiazepoxide
	Valium	Diazepam
	Tranxene	Chlorazepate
	Ativan	Lorazepam
	Vestran	Prazepam
	Serax	Oxazepam
Diphenylmethanes	Vistaril, Atarax	Hydroxyzine pamoate
	Benadryl	Diphenhydramine
Barbiturates	Luminal	Phenobarbital
	Nembutal	Sodium pentobarbital
	Amytal	Amobarbital
	Seconal	Secobarbital sodium

rational. Yet clients may be so incapacitated that they cannot function in their jobs. Nurses must recognize the powerful dynamics inherent in this phobia. They may need to refer clients to affordable counselors or therapists or find self-help groups. In other words, community health nurses must be skilled in referring clients to other community services that can help change client behavior.

Antianxiety medications are used for clients suffering from anxiety disorders, as well as for people who are transiently anxious at various stages in life. These medications are overused; it has been estimated that 20% of the adult population takes one of the benzodiazepines on a regular basis. The most commonly prescribed ones are chlordiazepoxide (Librium) and diazepam (Valium). As with the other psychotropic medications, there are many side effects and complications. The greatest dangers are that most of these agents produce tolerance and physical dependency and discontinuation produces a withdrawal syndrome. Central nervous system depression is enhanced if the client also takes alcohol, and overdoses of the medications result in coma. Therefore accidental overdoses are not infrequent occurrences, and of course intentional suicide with one of these agents is possible. Benzodiazepines are considered the safest group of antianxiety medications; barbiturates are considered the most dangerous. A list of commonly used antianxiety medications is presented in Table 23-3 (Hervey, 1984).

Nurses should educate clients and families concerning the uses and risks of these medications. If relief from anxiety can be obtained through a change in routine, job, interpersonal relationships, or exercises, such alternatives should be explored first. Antianxiety agents should not be considered a desirable long-term treatment for anxiety disorders.

Personality Disorders

In the personality disorder category of mental disorders are people who abuse drugs or alcohol or who exhibit antisocial or criminal behavior. Usually people with personality disorders come into conflict with others, for example, family, friends, teachers, law-enforcement officials, and society at large. Interpersonal relationships of people who have personality disorders are usually manipulative, shallow, and superficial, and the true antisocial personality rarely experiences anxiety, guilt, or depression. Because the behavior of people with personality disorders adversely affects society, they frequently come into contact with health, social, and legal agencies.

Community health nurses see these clients in a wide variety of settings. In addition, nurses see distraught families of clients and can involve the families in care plans. School nurses, for example, may assess and assist students using drugs or alcohol; they may also involve families. Clinic nurses may help women who are physically abused by their husbands. The children of abused mothers are likely to have emotional problems as a result of living in a combative environment and may need nursing support. Visiting nurses detect these persons in families of clients they visit for a physical illness or for health teaching. Nurses working in a crisis center encounter spouses or children of alcoholics or addicts who are desperately seeking assistance with their problems.

People with personality disorders are often members of multiproblem families. Because their relationships are superficial and their life-styles are disruptive, they create problems for all members of their families. This situation, in turn, causes them more frustration, and they become more problematic; perhaps they begin to drink, fight, or abuse more than ever. These dynamics are not always the case, however. Some multiproblem families are the victims of external circumstances such as poverty, unemployment, illness, or tragedy. Coping becomes impossible, and such people engage in disruptive behavior simply to survive. In this case we cannot assume these people have personality disorders. A classic example of this latter behavior is a father who shoplifts or cheats to provide food for his family.

Assessment is probably the greatest skill nurses must possess for working with people with personality disorders. Assessment includes physical and mental dimensions, as well as family and environmental dynamics. Nurses must be aware of their own values, attitudes, and stereotypes. Nurses reared in middle-class families valuing achievement, upward mobility, and the work ethic may have difficulty accepting and dealing with people who have different values, particularly people from low socioeconomic classes who live only for today. Sometimes these people plan only for today because they are not sure tomorrow will come. Successful health professionals who work with these people often develop their expertise only after many years of experience.

A second skill in working with people with personality disorders and their families is referral. Since many community agencies could be involved with the same problem, it is important for the nurse to be able to speak intelligently for clients and their families, to be aware of available resources, and to act as an advocate. Alcoholics may first need detoxification in a hospital and then rehabilitation and support from an organization such as Alcoholics Anonymous. The spouse may need counseling or even job training. Children may need school counseling for learning problems and physical health care. Families may need health education and financial assistance.

As with other mental disorders, personality disorders can range from mild to severe. People with mild disorders can be educated, counseled, or supported in more healthy life-styles. People with severe personality disorders are seldom if ever cured. No medicine, treatment, or intervention seems effective. Many criminals fall into this category, and, as hopeless as it seems, often the only strategy is to prevent these people from affecting the lives of others. Therefore the best solution may be removal from family or society and incarceration in jails, correctional institutions, or forensic mental hospitals. Health professionals and particularly nurses have difficulty giving up on these people. However, the community has a responsibility to protect others, and nurses are an important and pivotal part of the community.

Mental Retardation

In some agencies and programs the services for the mentally retarded are organized with services for the mentally ill. There has been and still is confusion among the public regarding differences between mental retardation and mental illness; they are not the same. It is beyond the scope of this chapter to discuss retardation as a condition, but mental health implications of care for retarded persons and their families are discussed.

Mental retardation is sometimes called a developmental disability. The birth of a retarded child is a true crisis for a family, and it is a heavy burden that often lasts a lifetime for parents. Current thinking is that mentally retarded people should be kept in the community and in their homes throughout their lives if possible. The belief is that normalization enables these people to achieve their potential and contributes to their emotional health. However, families can care and support these persons only if adequate social, educational, health, vocational, recreational, and financial services are available and affordable. Mentally retarded persons need services from birth to death. Obviously these services have not been available, and many families have to institutionalize mentally retarded family members or drain their resources trying to keep them in the home. Because mental retardation is a significant crisis for families, they need comprehensive mental health services, as well as other health and social services. Community mental health nurses must work closely with members of the entire health team to provide services such as mental health assessment, counseling, therapy, referral, and advocacy. An extensive discussion of these families, their needs, and nurses' roles in providing services is given in Chapter 24.

Mildly retarded persons or mentally retarded people who are educable and capable of learning and being productive and employed have a difficult time surviving in most communities. The gifted child is valued; the retarded child is not. These children frequently experience rejection by their peers in school and later in life in their jobs. Mentally retarded people often cannot compete in today's job market, even in the most unskilled jobs. They need assistance and, most of all, support for this stigmatizing disability. The future of employment for these persons, as for people with other types of developmental disabilities, is uncertain (Kiernan and Stark, 1986). Good training and supervision is necessary for success and emotional adjustment. Nurses need to be skilled team workers in this important venture.

Primary and secondary preventive mental health activities for mentally retarded people and their families are pervasive throughout their life span. When a mental illness develops in mentally retarded people and they require tertiary prevention, their care and treatment in the community become more complicated. In some areas these people are referred to as the dually diagnosed. Also, if mentally ill people become ill as children and remain ill throughout their lives, they may appear retarded because they have never been able to attend school and become literate. In that case the question of mental retardation versus mental illness becomes somewhat academic. Some of these people have been institutionalized since childhood, and with the deinstitutionalization effort they have been forced to make a community adjustment. These forgotten people are often regarded as hopeless, and they present a true challenge to the health professionals in the community.

AGING

Growing old in this society is not pleasant. We live in a youth-oriented society; we value good health, beauty, activity, and productivity. All of these attributes diminish with aging, leaving little except memories for many individuals. The aging process is fraught with mental health problems. The nurse working in community health encounters these problems in almost any setting.

Depression associated with loss is one of the most common emotional problems of the elderly client. Loss of physical health, loved ones, productive capacity, and financial resources is normal; sadness or depression is a natural response. How people cope with these losses determines their mental health. People who can maintain their activities or stay involved with others usually make a better adjustment. Nurses need to expect depression in their elderly clients. They should attempt to involve family and friends in their care; they should prevent isolation; and they should seek ways to maintain the client's self-concept. Nursing measures for dealing with depression in general are relevant for the elderly person.

Organic mental disorder, previously known as organic brain syndrome, is a frequent mental disorder of aging. It occurs in about 10% of people older than 65 years of age. The diagnosis of Alzheimer's disease is given to many of these clients, although this diagnosis can never be confirmed until autopsy. Sometimes "senility" and "dementia" are terms that are used to define the client's mental state. Whatever the cause or defined condition, the client is one whose dysfunctional behavior is caused by organic brain changes. These changes are irreversible, and the behavior is characterized by progressive memory loss, progressive loss of intellectual and judgmental ability, and ultimately the impairment of the ability to care for one's physical needs.

A family history is critically important in assisting the health professional make the initial assessment. Sometimes a pseudodementia, which is a depressive reaction, mimics a true organic mental disorder. Misdiagnosis may lead to mismanagement and institutionalization. Pseudodementia is characterized by rapid onset in contrast to the usual insidious onset of true organic disease. Loss is frequently associated with pseudodementia, and clients appear genuinely concerned about their failing memory. This is not the case in true dementia where clients are not aware of their impairment. Misdiagnosis of this condition and failure to treat it predisposes clients to becoming genuinely senile (Fopma-Loy, 1986).

In true organic impairment nurses have a supportive role. Clients should be kept in familiar surroundings and in familiar routines. Their loss of functioning should be minimized, and their current level of functioning should be maximized with as many prompts, cues, and aids as possible. Consistency and a calm, quiet environment are beneficial. Nurses need to instruct and counsel families in this regard. The longer clients can be kept at home, the better they will be. Sometimes clients with severe impairment engage in meaningful activities such as cleaning, cooking, sewing, yard work, and hobbies if they have supervision and support. Sometimes these clients have lucid moments when they seem to realize how deteriorated they have become. This realization makes clients with organic impairment sad and anxious, but usually they can be distracted and diverted into activity.

Caring for elderly clients can be stressful for their families. In our society with its emphasis on the nuclear family, the supports of extended family living are missing, and the burden of care often falls to the daughter or daughter-in-law. Day centers and home nursing care can help the client, as well as provide respite for the family. These families desperately need respite and assistance for their own emotional health. When the situation becomes impossible, family members themselves become sick. Abuse of elderly people is increasing and appears to be an outgrowth of an intolerable arrangement. This abuse can be physical or mental, and it can include neglect. Recent studies suggest that this problem has been around for a long time, but it has not been recognized or reported. It is thought to be common and related to a combination of problematic behavior in the client and personal life disarray of the caretaker (Hirst and Miller, 1986). Community nurses come into contact with this problem in many settings. They must use physical and psychologic assessment skills with both client and family. Above all community health nurses must work with other professionals to find ways of providing quality care for elderly people.

THEORIES OF CAUSATION

Throughout this chapter reference is made to some theories of causation for psychiatric mental health problems and disorders. In actuality, however, no cause or causes are known despite many years of research. Yet we have countless theories. There is perhaps no other field of medicine where there are as many conflicting theories. Research is difficult in part because classification of mental disorders is difficult.

For instance, it is hard to present a textbook definition of schizophrenia. There are almost as many different scenarios as there are clients. This makes schizophrenia difficult for the student and even the expert to understand. Schizophrenia is defined as a thought disorder. Yet a thought disorder cannot be seen as a cancerous tumor can. One can observe only behavioral manifestations of a thought disorder, and these manifestations may vary from client to client, may not be observable at all times, and may be subject to interpretations of different observers. It is interesting to review records of long-term clients who have been institutionalized for many years. The written diagnosis or impression can change depending on who observed the client or what the current thinking or theory was at the time the diagnosis was written. A client might be described as "hebephrenic" one year, "paranoid" the next, and "manic" the next. The situation is common even though nurses and aids related that the client's behavior has changed little over the years.

For many years in the United States we were influenced by the psychoanalytic theory of Sigmund Freud. This theory stated that mental disorder was largely due to the influence of the unconscious and the conflicts and events of a child's first few years. Psychoanalysis and long-term psychotherapy as treatment modalities were built on this theory. Today, however, psychoanalytic theory and psychotherapy have lost credibility because this treatment is far too expensive, energy consuming, and time consuming for the average person and because it simply has not cured mental illness, although it has helped some people, particularly those suffering from neurosis.

The most effective treatments for mental illness are the psychotropic medications. These medications cannot be considered a cure but only a control. Usually clients who are severely ill must take these medications for the rest of their lives, and as discussed previously, these treatments have many drawbacks. There are a number of biologic or physiologic theories behind these medications, but we really do not know why they are effective. There are many other biologic theories and therapies such as nutrition therapy and electrosleep therapy, and they are used in some settings. Yet the fact remains that to date the most inexpensive and accessible treatment based on largely vague theories is psychotropic medications.

It is popular to speak of mental illness today as multidetermined. By this we mean that there are a number of factors that probably cause mental illness, usually both physiologic and psychologic. In addition, we recognize that physical illness itself may have psychologic determinants and that the interaction of the psyche and the soma may be the ultimate key to the discovery of causative factors for every illness. No illness is simple, every person is complex, and health, however one defines it, has many unknowns. Yet health—physical, mental, and holistic—is recognized as vital to humans' happiness and well-being, and we must find the cause before we can find the cure.

ROLE OF NURSES IN COMMUNITY MENTAL HEALTH

So pervasive is the need for community mental health nursing that such nurses could and should function in any community health setting. These settings include crisis centers, schools, clinics, day-care centers, hot lines, and clients' homes. In other words community health nurses should have mental health skills because mental health is a part of health and cannot be separated from it. Community health nurses must have broad, generalized skills, and in a sense they must be jacks-of-all-trades.

Mastery of mental health skills is usually attained by graduate education in psychiatric nursing. Here nurses learn individual, family, and group therapy, and they can diagnose mental health problems, plan and prescribe interventions, and engage in research. However, community mental health nurses prepared at the baccalaureate level must have basic knowledge and basic skill in all these areas.

Probably the most important skill is the knowledge of psychotropic medications as is discussed throughout this chapter. New drugs are constantly appearing on the market, and drug companies advertise them heavily, always downplaying side effects and contraindications. Because clients are likely to receive these medications for extended periods, it is imperative that nurses be knowledgeable and accurately relate client behavior and symptoms to physicians and the rest of the health team. Nurses are in a position to observe clients more closely than are physicians; nurses spend more time with clients. In other words nurses might be considered the first line of defense for clients. Sometimes clients continue taking the same medication until the nurse brings a physician's attention to the need for change or reassessment. Although social workers, psychologists, and counselors may see clients frequently, they are neither educated in drug therapy nor expected to know anything about these medications. In addition, because noncompliance is the main reason that psychiatric clients must be rehospitalized, nurses are needed to monitor compliance and instruct clients and families. Sometimes nurses need to find creative ways of promoting compliance such as color-coding bottles or establishing a contract with clients. A therapeutic interpersonal relationship with both clients and families is also helpful in promoting compliance.

Nurses working with clients who are mentally ill or mentally disturbed need to have well-developed physical health assessment skills. One reason these skills are important is that disturbed clients may be so preoccupied with their psychologic concerns that they neglect their bodies and their daily hygiene, predisposing them to illness and infection. They may be unaware of warning signs of illness such as dizziness, headaches, and blurred vision because of this preoccupation or because they believe the symptoms are side effects of their medications. Usually mentally ill clients are not reliable historians regarding health history and risk factors. For them life has been a crisis for so long that a history may be too complicated or simply irrelevant at present. Also, these clients may not respond to pain or discomfort in usual ways; frequently they have high pain thresholds, probably focusing their attention on inner concerns. Nurses working with these clients must keep good health records and compare one client encounter with another. When nurses notice signs of injury or illness, they must be skilled at getting clients to talk about physical problems. ("How long have you had that rash?" "I notice you are limping; how did you hurt yourself?" "You seem out of breath?" "You are perspiring!" "Do you realize you are bleeding?") It is the rare client who is concerned with physical health problems. Therefore nurses must be concerned for them, and nurses must have the health assessment skills to detect physical problems.

Health education is another important skill and role for community health nurses working with mentally ill clients. This education is especially important for certain clients; only a few kinds of health education can be discussed here. One prime example is the education of the mentally ill mother. If mothering can be viewed as stressful for a healthy person, it is doubly stressful for someone who is mentally ill. Nurses must teach mentally ill mothers safe, nurturing, and stimulating childcare practices. At the same time they must understand that these mothers also have needs that make it difficult for them to focus on their children. These clients demand a great deal of time and energy from health care providers. Also necessary is the need for sexual education and family planning for mentally ill persons. Female clients in particular can be victims of sexual exploitation. Experience indicates that recently discharged clients are easy targets for exploitation as they seek adjustment to an anonymous and sometimes uncaring community. With the advent of acquired immunodeficiency syndrome (AIDS), the need for education becomes even greater not only for clients but for society at large. Last, health teaching in nutrition is vitally needed for the mentally ill. Many clients in the community shop and cook for themselves. Poverty, lack of energy, and confusion can contribute to poor eating habits. In addition clients who have been mentally ill for a long time are likely to have decayed and missing teeth because of poor dental hygiene, making good nutrition difficult.

Interpersonal skills and the therapeutic use of self are crucial for working with mentally ill clients and their families in the community. The foundations of these skills are learned in nurses' basic educational programs, but these skills need development and practice. For some nurses learning these skills is much easier than for others. Experience and role modeling can help new nurses learn, but in-service and continuing education are probably the best methods for development. Nurses want to help clients improve their self-concept and develop insight into behavior. Nurses need to establish a trusting relationship with mentally ill clients; they need to understand how their own behavior and feelings affect clients; they need to know where to show sympathy and when to set limits. These skills are the traditional skills of the psychiatric mental health nurse.

No discussion of the role of the community mental health nurse can be complete without incorporating the nursing process. Assessment, diagnosis, planning, intervention, and evaluation constitute the process. However, as the reader may realize, the nursing process that is applied to mentally ill clients may be different or varied from that applied to clients with primarily physical problems or illness. Assessment, for example, must include not only the client's symptoms and behavior, but also a complete client history, family perceptions, and the assessments of other team members. Nursing diagnoses may be variable or controversial as is the case with many psychiatric diagnoses. In addition, diagnosis is complicated because there are large gaps in categories of diagnoses in the current work of the North American Nursing Diagnosis Association (NANDA) for psychiatric clients (McFarland and Wasli, 1986). In making both the assessment and the diagnosis the nurse must ask, "Is this client dangerous to himself or herself or to others?" "Does this client need treatment or care to protect his or her physical, mental, or social welfare?" "How is this client's family affected, and is the community or group of his or her associates affected?" All these factors influence the assessment and diagnosis, which in turn guide planning, intervention, and evaluation. Nursing intervention varies with the individual nurse and is influenced by the interventions of the team. For instance, the team may decide that the client needs education to control aggressive behavior. One nurse may use a system of rewards for appropriate behavior, whereas another nurse may use role playing to teach the client to control aggression. Finally the evaluation in the nursing process must be done in conjunction with other team members, the family, and consideration of the client's community.

Last, all professionals working with mental illness and mental problems in the community must develop the skills of advocacy. This skill does not come easy for nurses because it demands aggressiveness, strong oral and written abilities, unrelenting persistence, and hope. Schwartz (1986) discusses this skill well. Nurses must ask, "Can anything else be done for this client?" "Could another person or another agency provide assistance?" "How can this problem be solved?" "How can the rules be changed; what are the loopholes; what are the exceptions?" In a society that does not value its old, weak, sick, or unproductive members, advocacy is vital to the survival of all people with mental health problems, as well as those with severe mental illness. Advocacy is vital to the success of the community mental health movement itself.

SUMMARY

Community mental health practice includes both preventive care and the management of those mental health problems that can be handled in the community rather than an institutional setting. The preventive component of care includes primary, secondary, and tertiary levels of prevention, and it is linked to physical health promotion because physical and mental health are likely to interact with each other.

The community health movement is a relatively recent development. Its beginnings can be traced to a 1961 report published by the Joint Commission on Mental Illness and Health, which recommended that clients be moved out of large psychiatric hospitals and into their homes or small community facilities where they could be supported by staff from community mental health centers. Massive deinstitutionalization of clients followed, and state mental hospitals were downsized. The movement has not been completely successful because the local facilities and community mental health centers have not grown to support the deinstitutionalized clients. This has placed a significant burden on the few existing community facilities.

Nurses who work in community mental health have a challenging role. Their knowledge base includes an understanding of the theories of causality of mental illness, familiarity with the properties of the major psychotropic medications, and an ability to work within a diverse group of mental health professionals.

QUESTIONS FOR DISCUSSION

1. Evaluate the movement to deinstitutionalize mental patients. Was it a good idea? What have been the barriers to its full and effective implementation?
2. How did the development of the phenothiazines and other psychotropic medications in the 1950s influence the treatment of mental illness?
3. What are the symptoms of tardive dyskinesia? What is its cause?
4. Why must the client who is taking lithium be monitored closely?
5. Why is a knowledge of physical health and illness important to professionals who care for persons with mental illness?

REFERENCES

Field W: Physical causes of depression, Nurs Ment Health Serv 23:10, 1985.

Fopna-Loy J: Depression and dementia: differential diagnosis, J Psychosoc Nurs 24:2, 1986.

Halpern J and others: The myths of deinstitutionalization: policies for the mentally disabled, Boulder, Colo, 1980, Westview Press Inc.

Hervey V: Inservice on psychotherapeutic medications, unpublished manuscript,1984.

Hirst S and Miller J: The abused elderly, 24:10, 1986.

Joint Commission on Mental Illness and Health: Action for mental health, New York, 1961, Basic Books Inc, Publishers.

Kiernan W and Stark J: The adult with developmental disabilities. In Kiernan W and Stark J, editors: Pathways to employment for adults with developmental disabilities, Baltimore, 1986, Paul H. Brooks Publishing Co.

Koldjeski D: Community mental health nursing; new directions in theory and practice, New York, 1984, John Wiley & Sons Inc.

Kreigh H and Perko J: Psychiatric and mental health nursing: a commitment to care and concern, Reston, Va, 1983, Reston Publishing Co Inc.

McFarland G and Wasli E: Nursing diagnoses and process in psychiatric mental health nursing, Philadelphia, 1986, JB Lippincott Co.

Noble J: New directions for public policies affecting the mentally disabled. In Bevilacqua J, editor: Changing government policies for the mentally disabled. Cambridge, Mass, 1981, Ballinger Publishing Co.

Noble J and Conley R: Fact and conjecture in the policy of deinstitutionalization, Health Policy Q 8:1, 1981.

Schwartz L: The day I felt most like a nurse, Image 18:4, 1986.

Shaver J: A biopsychosocial view of human health, Nurs Outlook 33:4, 1985.

Wilson H and Kneisl C: Psychiatric Nursing, ed 2, Menlo Park, Calif, 1983, Addison Wesley Publishing Co Inc.

CHAPTER

24

Families of Mentally Retarded Children

Althea Glenister

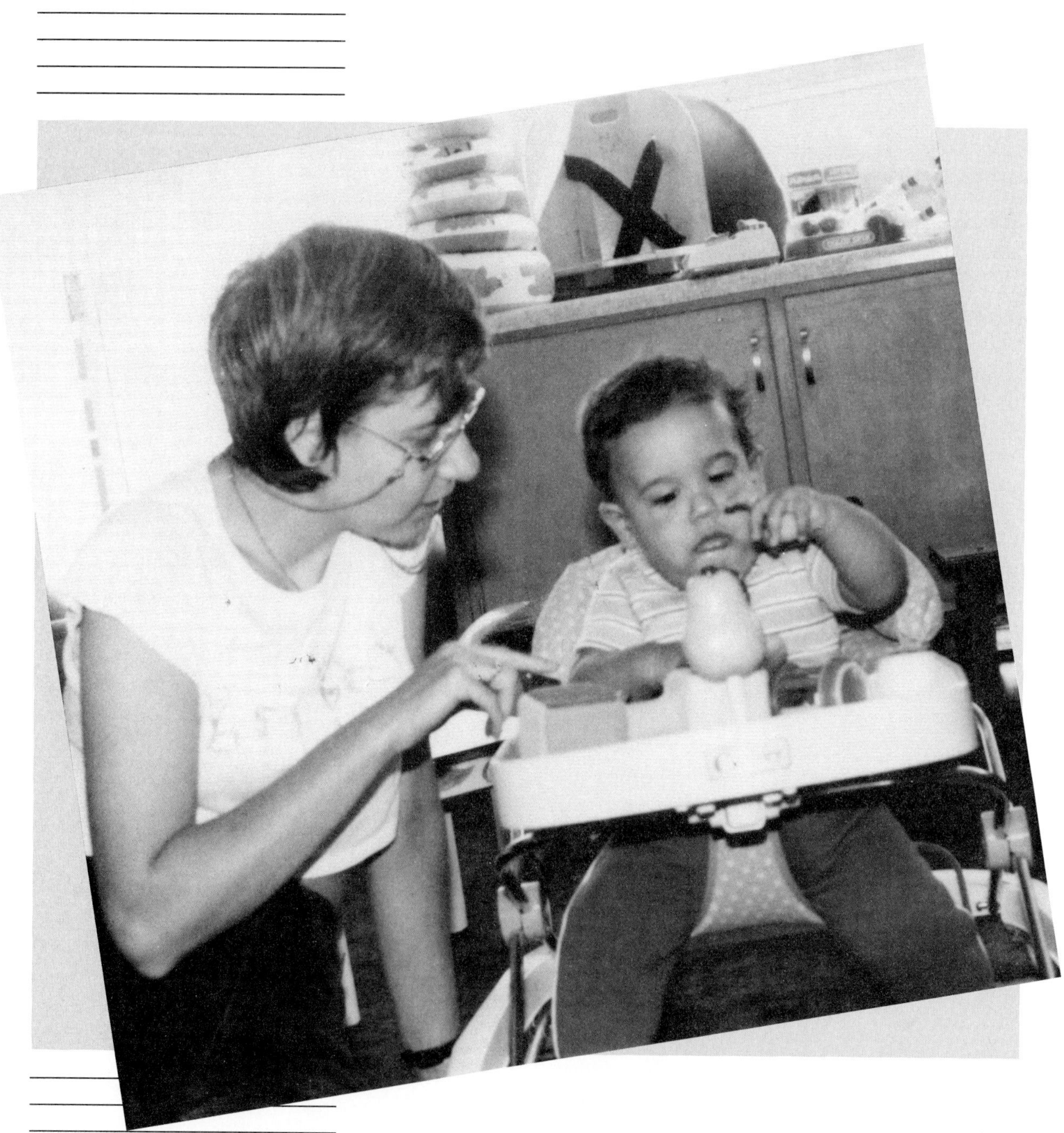

CHAPTER OUTLINE

Historical perspective

Family as the primary caregiver

Heterogeneity of mentally retarded people

Characteristics of families of mentally retarded people

Impact of mental retardation on the family

- Psychologic stress
- Social stress
- Economic stress

Community support services

Community health nurses' role

Summary

OBJECTIVES

After completing this chapter, the reader should be able to:

1. Describe the heterogeneity of both families and their retarded children.
2. Identify sources of stress in families of retarded children.
3. Discuss the community support needs of families.
4. Identify planning and implementation strategies for working with families of retarded children.
5. Discuss the importance of evaluation of nursing approaches in working with families.

HISTORICAL PERSPECTIVE

In the 1950s and early 1960s the following developments resulted in a major change in the way mentally retarded individuals were viewed and treated:

1. New treatment methods and philosophies
2. Establishment of Medicare, Medicaid, and other federal programs that provided direct and indirect aid to the mentally retarded
3. Court decisions that protected the constitutional rights of mentally disabled persons to liberty, treatment, due process, equal protection under the law, and freedom from cruel and unusual punishment (Willer, Scheerenberger, and Intagliata, 1978)
4. Adoption of the normalization principle, which in essence advocates making available to all mentally retarded persons patterns of life and conditions of everyday living that are as close as possible to life in society (Nirje, 1976; Maloney and Ward, 1979)

These and other developments resulted in a movement and philosophy known as deinstitutionalization. This approach to the care of the mentally disabled has several dimensions including the following (USGAO, 1977):

(1) Prevention of unnecessary admission to and retention in institutions
(2) Development of appropriate alternatives in the community for housing, treatment, training, education, and rehabilitation of the mentally disabled
(3) Improvement of conditions, care, and treatment for those who need institutional care

This meant that people who had previously been cared for in institutions of various types and sizes would be returned to the community for care and supervision. It also meant that mentally retarded individuals living in the community could not be admitted to institutions except under specific circumstances. The care and supervision of these deinstitutionalized people shifted from institutional personnel to communities and often the families of the disabled people. The costs of this care in terms of time and money also shifted to families and communities.

By the mid-1970s it was apparent that the policy of discharging the mentally disabled from the stable, long-term residences in state mental hospitals to sometimes transient existences in the community was in need of reassessment. Some communities were not prepared to receive the discharged people because of a lack of appropriate housing or treatment programs. Many discharged mentally retarded people were placed in nursing homes, some of which were not prepared to deal with the needs of this group. Others were placed in group homes, foster care homes, halfway houses, room and board facilities, and single-room occupancy hotels, which also lacked provision for needed services. Residents of some neighborhoods resisted the presence of the mentally disabled in the community (Stedman, 1977), and many clients drifted to substandard housing that was overcrowded, unsafe, dirty, and isolated, creating a new kind of ghetto subpopulation (Bassuk and Gerson, 1978). Families who had previously gone through the difficult and stressful process of institutionalizing their members, usually children, found themselves confronted with the painful reversal of an earlier decision to separate the child from the family (Stedman, 1977). The return of a retarded family member represented a crisis situation that had been faced earlier when the member was insitutionalized, and the family was again faced with the responsibility of caring for that individual (Willer, Intagliata, and Atkinson, 1979). Those families considering institutionalizing a family member for the first time found this option removed because of changes in admission policies. Furthermore, these families were found to have been ignored with respect to assessment of needs and provision of services (Willer and Intagliata, 1980). Some admissions to institutions did occur for the mentally retarded, but 64% of these admissions were actually readmissions (Braddock, 1981). The primary reason given for readmissions was lack of community services, such as living accommodations and comprehensive and follow-up services.

Halpern and others (1980) interviewed 279 individuals in seven states who were associated with the caregiving system or were otherwise involved in the desinstitutionalization process. Specific problems identified by this group included implicit messages from staff members to clients that they were not expected to survive in the community, opposition to deinstitutionalization by communities and some families, and difficulty in accessing medical, dental, vocational, transportational, and recreational services.

Critics of the deinstitutionalization policy in the 1970s and early 1980s and even today say that, although this was a well-intentioned reform, it lacked a comprehensive plan for implementation or consideration of the possible consequences to the mentally disabled, their families, and the community (Cruickshank, 1977; Newburgh, 1978; Talbott, 1980; and USGAO, 1977). The movement to retain and maintain the mentally retarded in a more natural setting requires that attention be given to factors that may assist mentally retarded people and their caregivers, especially their families, in living as normal a life as possible. The focus of this chapter is on the family of the mentally retarded individual with special emphasis on families of moderately and profoundly mentally retarded children.

FAMILY AS THE PRIMARY CARE PROVIDER

During the 1970s the philosophy and concepts of primary care emerged and became an established and visible part of the health care system. Primary care was classified as a level of care distinct from secondary and tertiary care, and health personnel who practiced this level of care became known as primary care practitioners. Primary care evolved because of recognized lacks in health care and a rekindling of interest in the generalist as a first-level provider of care for a large part of the population's health needs. First-care contact, comprehensive personal care, and continuity of care for individuals were identified as major functions of primary care.

Much has been written about primary care in the health care system. Few, however, have noted that the family is an important resource of care even though families have always contributed comprehensive and continuous care to their ill members. In mental retardation the family is the primary locus of care for many individuals; the majority of mentally retarded persons in the United States live with their natural or adoptive families (O'Connor, 1983). Even when institutionalization was at a peak, only 10% of mentally retarded people were in institutions (MacMillan, 1977); the other 90% with few exceptions lived with their natural families (Willer and Intagliata, 1984). For the mentally retarded child, as well as all developmentally disabled children, the majority of care continues to be rendered by family members in homes (Kornblatt and Heinrich, 1985). Families differ in their abilities to manage the care of their retarded children and cope with the stress that these children's presence imposes on them. Studies have documented a variety of sources of stress including the need for continuous care and supervision of the child, marital conflict, economic burden, and social isolation (Willer and Intagliata, 1984). It has been suggested that the family be recognized as the primary provider and caregiver of services for its members (National Commission of Families and Public Policies, 1978). However, public policy should be shaped differently to help families carry out their functions to minimize any sense of stress or burden.

The family has been viewed as the basic social institution (Suelzhe and Keenan, 1981), yet many of the functions and services the family provided have been taken over by other societal institutions such as schools and health and social agencies. In the past, families assumed they were responsible for their disabled members and did all they could to provide the care and support needed. With the growth of public programs and the changing nature of society, families became more dependent on the public and others to provide more and more of their needs. Despite these developments the family remains as a resource for the care and rehabilitation of its affected members. With help and support from nurses and others in the care systems, families could be even more effective.

HETEROGENEITY OF MENTALLY RETARDED PEOPLE

Mentally retarded people, contrary to stereotypic images, are a heterogeneous group with members whose disabilities range from mild learning disabilities to total deficiencies in learning abilities and knowledge, gross social maladaptations, and often serious physical problems. Approximately 86% of mentally retarded people are only mildly retarded. Moderate retardation is thought to involve approximately 10% of all mentally retarded people, and only 3% to 4% of all mentally retarded people are severely and profoundly retarded (Chinn, Drew, and Logan, 1979). Mildly retarded as a group tend to do well, since they are capable of learning basic academic skills and can be self-sufficient as adults and live independently in society (MacMillan, 1977). A disproportionate number of mildly retarded come from families in lower socioeconomic classes, which suggests that incidence may be sensitive to environmental influences (Munro, 1986).

In contrast, individuals who are more severely impaired come from all social, ethnic, racial, and economic groups throughout the general population (Craft, 1979; Gearheart and Litter, 1979; Munro, 1986; and Taft, 1980). Moderately and severely mentally retarded people also tend to have a physical or psychiatric disability (Munro, 1986). Some moderately mentally retarded people can learn self-help skills and other aspects of daily living and cause little burden to their families. Others need considerable assistance throughout their lives and may create a heavy burden for their families. Moderately mentally retarded people were often institutionalized as children in the past, but now they generally remain with their natural families until they can be appropriately placed in an out-of-home setting, which may not occur for many years, if ever.

CHARACTERISTICS OF FAMILIES OF RETARDED PEOPLE

Since the families of moderately or severely retarded persons are not indigenous to any particular social class or geographic area, they show the same structural differences as all families. They vary in size, ages of parents and children, presence of parents in the home, extent of informal support networks, and caretaking and earning functions. These differences in structure and function may mean there are also differences in their knowledge, ability, and resources to cope with the needs of their affected members.

Most public policy is built around the image of the family that has both parents present (Family Impact Seminar, 1978). However, since 1960 a significant increase has occurred in the number of families headed by women. By 1986 the number of families headed by women increased to 10.2 million compared with 4.5 million in 1960, 5.6 million in 1970, and 8.7 million in 1980 (U.S. Bureau of the Census, 1986). The number of households headed by a single man has also increased consistently since 1960 from 1.3 million to 2.4 million in 1986. There has been little research done on the needs of single parents of mentally retarded children. Divorce rates among parents of mentally retarded children are no higher than those of parents of nonretarded children when social class is controlled (Roesel and Lawlis,

1983; Schufiet and Wurster, 1976). However, when divorce occurs, the burdens on the single parent of a retarded child outweigh those of the single parent of a normal child (Wikler, 1981). MacMillan (1977) reports that studies consistently show that institutionalization is highly related to divorce in the family. The data, however, do not indicate causation; that is, they do not indicate whether the divorce leads to the decision to institutionalize the child or whether the decision to institutionalize the child precipitates the divorce. The lack of family integration is a problem that is less obvious than family breakup. The mentally retarded child frequently has a disrupting influence on family relations that varies with the social class of the family, the sex of the retarded child, and the age and sex of the siblings (Farber, Jenne, and Targo, 1960).

How the size of the family of the retarded child affects economic costs has not been fully explored in medical and nursing literature. Only one study could be found that specifically addressed one aspect of this area. Piachaud, Bradshaw, and Weale (1981) discussed data from the 1974 General Household Survey in Great Britain in which families with and without a disabled child were compared with respect to such factors as work participation rates, hours worked, earning, and net incomes. They found no significant difference between families with disabled children and families without disabled children with regard to the father's labor force participation, hours worked weekly, and hourly or annual earnings. The mother's participation rates and earnings were highly related to the age of the youngest child. When their analysis of the survey was limited to families whose youngest child was 6 years of age or older, there were indications that in families with a disabled child, participation in the labor force and hours worked increased with family size. Piachaud, Bradshaw, and Weale suggested three possible explanations for this. First, if there are other children in the home to care for the child, it may be easier for the mother to work. Second, the need for an increased income in a larger family makes it essential that the mother work. Finally, mothers may be more inclined to work to gain respite from home life.

There is a growing body of literature that recognizes the importance of informal social support networks in shaping responses to stress in both individuals and families (Beavers and others, 1986; Caplan, 1974; Horwitz, 1978; and Pattison and others, 1975). In fact, Hill (1958) states that families become increasingly vulnerable as they lose kin, neighbors, and friends. His study of families during the crisis of wartime separation found that families who were most successful in meeting this crisis made frequent mention of the accessibility of relatives, neighbors, and friends.

Extended family networks in families with a retarded child are positively correlated with successful coping (Wikler, 1979). "The ability of a family to maintain some degree of normal socialization may be partly a function of the degree of acceptance by the extended family and by the neighbors within the community" (Chinn, Drew, and Logan, 1979). The family network is viewed as the first line of support, with friends and neighbors serving as supplements rather than substitutions (Croog, Lipson, and Levine, 1972).

IMPACT OF MENTAL RETARDATION ON THE FAMILY

The addition of any new child to a family may cause complications, inconveniences, expenses, changes in life-style, and worries. That a child might also be mentally retarded does not mean that other family members do not experience the joy and pleasure the child brings. However, mental retardation is a peculiarly pervasive disability of lifelong duration and usually requires special interventions in many areas such as care, health, and education (Boggs, 1975). The care and maintenance of a mentally retarded child in the family setting affects all the other members of the family.

The effect of mental retardation is never restricted to the mentally retarded individual (Crnic, Friedrich, and Greenberg, 1983). Furthermore, the problems and demands faced by these families do not disappear as the child matures. New concerns arise that relate to such factors as the child's behavior, learning capacities, dependence, developmental lags, and socialization. That the child may never be able to live independently creates increasing anxiety, especially as the parents age. Parents of mentally retarded children must plan on behalf of their child well beyond the point that other parents must. Siblings of the mentally retarded child may find that later in life the responsibility for their mentally retarded brother or sister shifts from their parents to themselves. Thus care and supervision may be needed throughout the mentally retarded individual's life, and it is the family who assumes most of this burden.

In the past several years medical and nursing literature documents a growing interest in the effect of mental retardation on the family. Nurses need to be aware of this literature on family stress, since it is relevant for their understanding and actions.

Families of mentally retarded children are more likely to experience stress than families who have normal children (Gallagher, Beckman, and Cross, 1983; Wikler, 1981). Some families can cope successfully with this stress, but for other families it can seriously disrupt their ability to function.

> The physical and emotional stress of 24-hour care, the anxiety and guilt in giving birth to an "imperfect" child, the sense of hopelessness about the future, the neglect of normal children and their consequent disturbance, the exacerbation of marital frictions, all of these reactions make difficult the retarded child's retention in the home (Begab and Richardson, 1975).

Without some form of intervention this stress may lead to family dysfunction, and the family may eventually turn to out-of-home placement as a way of coping with the stress (Eyman and others, 1972; Fotheringham, Skelton, and Hoddinott, 1972; and Saenger, 1960). Delineating the types of stresses and identifying high-risk periods for families increases the possibilities for preventing family problems (Wikler, 1981).

Psychologic Stress

Psychologic stress of family members differs according to their expectations of the mentally retarded child and the effect of the child on their roles and relationships.

Wikler and others (1981) describe the concept of chronic sorrow experienced by parents of retarded children. This is a chronic, recurring event triggered by developmental and transitional stages in a mentally retarded child's life. Chronic sorrow begins at the child's birth and occurs at nine other critical developmental milestones or transitions in the life of an affected child. The child's deviance from normal performance at these stages precipitates an intensity of emotions that does not decrease over time. Instead the level of intensity seems to be a function of the particular developmental stage, as well as the individual coping strengths of the family. These developmental or transitional stages include when the child is expected to walk, talk, and enter school and at puberty. These stages create anxiety and grieving for the parents regardless of their adjustment level.

Psychologic stress is experienced somewhat differently by the various members of the family. In her study of parents of mentally retarded and emotionally disturbed children, Holroyd (1974) found that mothers had a less cheerful humor and were less able to experience personal development or freedom, more sensitive to how the child might not fit into the community, and more aware of disharmony in the family than were fathers. Cummings, Bayley, and Rie (1966) studied mothers of mentally retarded, chronically ill, and neurotic children in terms of psychologic stress. They found that mothers of mentally retarded children carry a greater psychologic burden than do the other mothers studied. These mothers experienced a greater degree of anxiety, depression, and conflict. A later report of a similar study on the fathers found that they too experience psychologic stress and that many of these fathers undergo long-term personality changes that resemble a pattern of "neurotic-like constriction" (Cummings, 1976). Cummings also found differences between the parents, with the mothers experiencing greater stress than the fathers, especially in the areas of self-esteem and interpersonal satisfactions.

The ill effects of having a mentally retarded sibling are shared unequally among the children in a family. Sisters, especially those who are the oldest child, are more vulnerable to psychologic stress than the other children (Cleveland and Miller, 1977; Gath, 1974). Middle-born girls are at risk only when they come from large families. Both male and female siblings younger than the retarded child have not been shown to be adversely affected. Both Fowle (1968) and Farber (1959) also found that the oldest female sibling appeared to manifest more role tension than did the oldest male sibling.

Social Stress

As the mentally retarded child approaches adolescence, new worries may arise in families. Parents may express concerns about the welfare of the child in the event of parental death. Parents also worry about sexual behavior, social behavior, social maladjustment, antisocial behavior, lack of self-sufficiency, and need for dependence (Kotsopoulos and Matathia, 1980).

Uncomfortable social situations can arise with outsiders, especially if there is a large discrepancy between the child's size and mental age. Neighbors and friends may show mixed reactions to the families and the child. Some may be warm and supporting, whereas others may be aloof and disinterested (Carver and Carver, 1972). Families may report diminished contacts with extended families and friends and find themselves socially isolated. Disapproval from others can be destructive to the family's coping efforts (Berger and Foster, 1976).

Economic Stress

In addition to psychologic and social stress, there is stress that emanates from the economic impairment of the family because of the presence of a mentally retarded child. In 1974 the British government published a white paper on social security provisions for the disabled. This paper noted that the presence of a disabled child in a family can create financial needs in the following four ways (Piachaud, Bradshaw, and Weale, 1981):

1. It can eliminate or reduce parents' earnings.
2. It can involve payments for services that the parents might normally provide themselves.
3. It can involve extra costs in providing for the child.
4. It can make additional physical and emotional demands on the parents that might be partially compensated for by cash.

In examining the economic burden on families then, several types of costs need to be considered. First, there are the direct, out-of-pocket expenditures or those amounts paid directly by the family for such things as food, clothing, health care, and recreation. Families of nonretarded children share many of the same costs as families of mentally retarded children. However, the care of a handicapped member costs more than it would if the member had no handicap (Boggs, 1979; Glenister, 1984). These expenses may be considered extraordinary, since they occur because of the child's special needs.

A second form of cost to the family is indirect costs of caring for an impaired member. These costs may be viewed as what family members might have done differently had there not been a mentally retarded child present. It also includes the cost of the time devoted by family members to the care and raising of the child. Studies indicate that effects on the family include the mother's inability to take an outside job and the curtailment of social activities such as vacations, social visits, and eating out (Baldwin, 1976; Glenister, 1984). The increase in single-parent families and the increase in the number of women who work outside the home suggest that these indirect costs may be assuming even greater importance for the mother.

COMMUNITY SUPPORT SERVICES

The concepts of normalization and least restrictive environment are the major philosophic bases for the promotion of care of mentally retarded people in more natural yet viable settings. The natural home is generally viewed as the least restrictive and most normal setting for a mentally retarded person.

Underlying these concepts is the belief that wherever the mentally retarded person lives, he or she should be supported. Building on this approach, when the handicapped person lives within a family setting, both the handicapped person and the family require supportive services (Maroney, 1980).

A variety of services are available, especially in urban settings, that can provide support and other forms of assistance to families in caring for their mentally retarded children.

Bruininks and Warfield (1978) identify the following essential services for retarded and other handicapped persons:

1. Developmental programs including day activities, education, and training
2. Residential services including special living arrangements
3. Employment services including employment preparation, provision of sheltered workplaces, and competitive job situations
4. Identification services including diagnosis and evaluation
5. Facilitating services including information and referral, counseling, and protective, sociolegal, follow-along, and case management services
6. Medical and dental treatment services
7. Transportation
8. Leisure and recreation opportunities

In addition to these specialized community functions are generic services that provide health, educational, social, rehabilitative, and vocational assistance to a broad spectrum of people, including the mentally retarded. Community organizations such as the Association for Retarded Children publish directories of services as a resource for both professionals and families in locating and initiating contact with specific organizations.

The mere existence of services and programs does not give clear indications of their use or effectiveness, nor does their existence indicate the degree of knowledge or satisfaction that families have toward them. Some parents may lack the skills and energies to obtain the services they need. Many parents are simply unaware of the services that are available to them (Ayer, 1984; Glenister, 1984). Occasionally service systems have been problematic to those parents who sought their assistance (Anderson and Gardner, 1973; Berger and Foster, 1976; and Bruininks, Williams, and Morreau, 1979). Families in rural areas may be in greater need of services than those in urban areas because of the lack of resources and the greater distances they must travel to reach needed services.

Families can be helpful in indicating the kinds of services they need. This information is essential for program planning. A needs assessment of community services for the mentally retarded and their families is incomplete without the input of the recipient of these services. For example, some parents in Minnesota were asked what types of services they would need to keep a developmentally disabled child at home (Bruininks, 1979). Services listed in order of importance to the parents included the following:

1. Medical (professional availability and funds)

2. Supplemental assistance
3. Home assistance
4. Special school programs
5. Respite care
6. Social activities for the child
7. Transportation for the child
8. Home tutors
9. Parent guidance
10. Day activity centers

In general, the needs of families for community services should be made more explicit, and the community service support system needs to be made more visible to both families and to those responsible, including nurses, for providing the guidance and support for them. Families must be linked with the services they need. A concentrated effort is needed to inform families of what is available to them and what application procedures are for the services.

Since resources to a community are limited, they should be concentrated on those services that directly assist the family by providing some relief from the day-to-day, 24-hour care and supervision that many retarded children require. Respite services have been recognized for their value in preventing crises or problems (Moroney, 1980). Families who are experiencing physical or psychologic stress and find that their social and recreational outlets are curtailed can seek these services for relief. The concept of normalization applies to familes, as well as their retarded children, and they need the opportunity to function as someone other than a caregiver from time to time. Nurses' sensitivity to these families' needs and their understanding and support may be essential for relieving some of the burden families have and enhancing their quality of life, as well as that of the families' retarded children.

Community Health Nurses' Role

In the field of mental retardation, interest in the concept of social support for the individual and the family is growing (O'Connor, 1983). Those supplying this support include friends, relatives, and neighbors. Another major segment of the support network includes the care providers of whom nurses constitute an important part.

Before the deinstitutionalization movement the contact the community health nurse had with mentally retarded children and their families was limited and infrequent. However, since these children, especially the more severely mentally retarded children, are being kept in the home and community, and with the implementation of such policy directives as mainstreaming, the probability of a community health nurse working with retarded children and their families has increased. School nurses especially have become more involved with the supervision and care of retarded children since the implementation of the Education For All Handicapped Act in 1975. This act mandated special education services such as health care that would help the child benefit from special education (Learner, 1979).

The community health nurse most typically works with families in the home setting, although contact occurs in other setting such as clinics, schools, and health centers. Much information can be gained from observing the family in their natural setting, and work with the families may be more effective than in other settings. The nursing process is used by the community health nurse in working with families of mentally retarded children and encompasses a variety of dimensions including assessing, planning, implementation, such as counseling, education, linking, and coordinating, advocacy, and evaluation. Each of these dimensions is directed at helping and supporting the family in providing an optimal environment for not only the retarded child but themselves as well. Each dimension is covered separately in the following discussion.

Assessment and Planning

Assessment and planning are essential first steps for the community health nurse regardless of the mentally retarded child's stage of development or the degree of contact the family has had with the service system. Information about the family's needs and their coping mechanisms is necessary to plan and implement care. A lot of information which the nurse should try to obtain, may already be available from outside sources. Occasionally this information must be validated, and in most cases it must be updated as needs and family circumstances change. When information is not already available, every effort should be made to get as complete a data base as possible.

Data generated from the assessment of the mentally retarded child should not serve as the sole basis for the plan of care for the family. One must also assess such important factors as the impact of the child's diagnosis, behavior, abilities, and care requirements on each member of the family, the family's ability to cope with problems and responsibilities, the particular needs expressed by family members, and the overall functioning of the family as a unit. The family should not be viewed only as a resource or a factor to be considered when planning and implementing care for the mentally retarded child. The family *is* the client. Their needs, concerns, and problems become the focus of the nursing care plan.

Important information can be gained from an interview with family members. Their knowledge of the child's condition, developmental and functional status, and future expectations is basic data for the nurse to obtain. Contacts with community agencies, as well as the family's knowledge of the services that are available to assist them in the care of their child, should be identified.

As the nurse's contact with the family increases, other information can be obtained through interview and observation. The behaviors of the child and the family's reaction to them should be noted. The behaviors of each member of the family, especially their interactions with each other and the affected child, are also important to observe. Questions about roles and functions of each family member, as well as their coping abilities and mechanisms, are necessary to pursue to determine whether the family is experiencing an undue burden of care. Family problems related to the retarded child's condition can become so overwhelming that the family may become dysfunctional. Emotional, social, and economic problems are frequently seen in these families, and the nurse must be sensitive to their nonverbal, as well as their verbal behavior. Even in the strongest and most well-adjusted families, the continuous need for care and supervision of their disabled children can create stress and tension.

As needs and problems are identified by the nurse, they should be validated with the family to make sure they are accurately perceived and there are no omissions. As in any other area of nursing care, planning should be done jointly *with* the family and not *for* them. The nurse's focus throughout the relationship with the family should be to help families help themselves, rather than substitute for them. Family members are the major and primary caregivers and therefore have the right to make decisions that affect them and their mentally retarded child. Nurses, as well as all caregivers, have the responsibility of providing the data needed to make decisions and can use their expertise to guide the family in this process. It may also be necessary to validate initial impressions and plans with others in the caregiving system who have knowledge regarding the family and who may have treatment plans set up for either the child or the family. Collaboration with interdisciplinary team members in establishing plans is necessary in many instances in identifying priorities and establishing goals. Otherwise there exists the possibility of multiple plans that are not only in conflict but may also cause confusion and frustration for the family. In addition, some needs cannot be met by the nurse alone, or the nurse may not have the appropriate expertise to deal with them.

Counseling and Education

A major role of the community health nurse in working with families of mentally retarded children is to listen to concerns expressed by the family, to give information when needed, and to provide advice and support. The mere presence of someone who conveys an interest in them can be a tremendous source of support. Parents should be encouraged to freely verbalize their feelings and concerns about their retarded child. The nurse should be accepting of parental feelings of anger and frustration, which may be expressed occasionally, and should indicate to them that areas of concern such as a lack of progress with the child does not reflect negatively on them or their abilities as parents. Often, parents just need reassurance and the recognition that they are doing a good job. A nurse who is attentive and conveys genuine interest in the family provides a supportive milieu for the expression of feelings, concerns, and needs that might otherwise remain hidden. As these are revealed, the nurse can offer advice that provides direction for the family in how to deal with a particular concern. Other forms of intervention, such as demonstration of care, individual counseling of a family member, referral to a community service, and teaching about a specific content area may be needed.

Families may have many learning needs in regard to the care of their mentally retarded child. Teaching plans should not focus solely on the mother; fathers and older siblings should also be included (Fig. 24-1). Gallagher and others (1983) note that counseling activities tend to be mother oriented, which may discourage the participation of fathers who are seeking a role different from mother-surrogate. Friends and other relatives who show an interest in the child can also be included in teaching plans. Teaching topics vary depending on the needs and expressed interest of the family and the age of the mentally retarded child. In general, families should be knowledgeable about the following:

1. Growth and development, both normal and for the child who is functioning below chronologic age
2. Parenting skills, which can be adapted to the special needs of the child

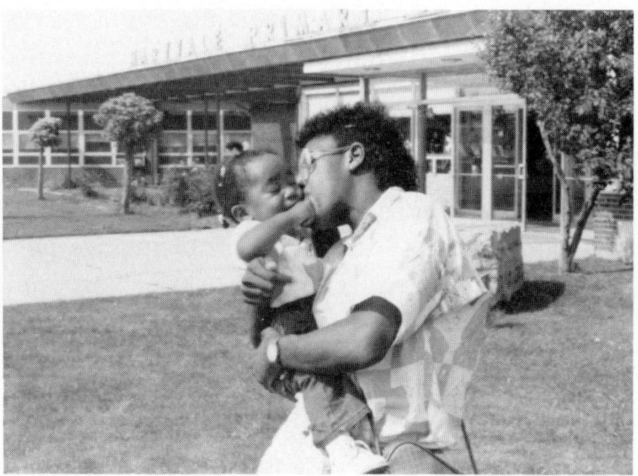

Fig. 24-1. Older sister is important to mentally retarded child.

3. Basic health needs including nutrition, sleep, elimination, and safety
4. Management of the mentally retarded child including behavior modification, discipline, and activities of daily living
5. Social and recreational activities, for both the retarded child and the family
6. Economic, social, medical, and educational resources available to the family

Families not only have the right to be informed about the preceding general content areas, but, in fact, must also have possession of these data if they are to be successful in providing a warm and supportive home environment for both the mentally retarded child and themselves and in functioning as independently as possible. Nurses can spend only a fraction of time during any 24-hour period with the child and family. For the remainder of the time families assume decision-making responsibility as it relates to the care of the mentally retarded child. Teaching and counseling take on a special significance with this in mind.

Linking and Coordinating

A variety of helping professions may be needed by the family of a mentally retarded child, beginning with the birth of the child and extending through the child's development into young adulthood and beyond. Many families can successfully cope with the responsibilities of raising a mentally retarded child and can independently seek out needed services. Other families have multiple problems that they may be reluctant to broach in the clinical setting unless the problems are perceived as emergency situations (Kornblatt and Heinrich, 1985). In addition, research has documented that mentally retarded children who live with their families receive fewer specialized services than those who live in out-of-home settings (Seltzer and Krauss, 1984). The family's need for a variety of services coupled with an often bewildering array of agencies, organizations, and private entrepreneurs in their community underscores the need for assistance to link families with appropriate services and coordinate the work of those who are involved with the family.

They not uncommonly need a range of health, mental health, and social services provided by many different agencies, but the agencies may have conflicting and incompatible goals that make coordinated care difficult (Platman and others, 1982).

What is needed is a knowledgeable person who can link families with those services they need and coordinate the efforts of the providers to maximize effectiveness and efficiency of services and promote continuity of care for families.

The community health nurse has traditionally functioned in the role of coordinator for families with health problems and needs. In mental health this role is referred to as case management. As Platman and others (1982) have commented, community health nurses are one group that would make exceptional case managers for the mentally disabled and their families. Their knowledged of the community and the resources available, as well as their experience in the coordinating role, make this a natural function of the community health nurse.

As a first step, nurses can inform families of the services available to them. A description of each service should be provided, which could include the nature of the services offered, what is involved for the child and the parents, expectations, requirements, length of service, and potential results. Equally important information includes cost, how to apply for services, where to go, and whom to contact at a service agency. The nurse should encourage the families of mentally retarded individuals to make their own arrangements if possible. If not, the nurse provides the assistance needed to link the family with the service. Most services are directed toward the mentally retarded child, but some may also include specific guidance, education, and other activities for family members, especially the parents. These are services that are designed to assist the parents directly. Parent support groups are one example of these services. These groups generally encourage the verbalization of experiences and the sharing of information, as well as support and encouragement of parents. Parent groups have also historically served as strong advocates for mentally retarded people and their families.

Other important resources for families include respite services, which are mentioned earlier in the chapter. These services provide relief from the day-to-day, 24-hour care and supervision that many mentally retarded children require. Comprehensive respite care services range from babysitting services in the home during the day to longer periods of out-of-home care. These services can help increase the family's social activities and alleviate physical and emotional strains (Joyce and others, 1983).

The identification of community services for the family is a vital first step in the linkage process. Unfortunately, in many rural communities, services are few and usually limited to those mandated by law. The community health nurse may be instrumental in organizing such services as parent support groups, outreach programs from nearby urban areas, and respite services if there are sufficient numbers of interested and eligible families. In addition, many small communities have resource people who can provide support and assistance to families. These people include school personnel, the clergy, social workers, nurses, physicians, and psychologists.

Once families have been linked to services, the nurse can serve in an important coordinating role between services, as well as between families and the services. Agencies are not always aware of other organizations that serve the family, or if they are, they may not communicate on a regular basis. The community health nurse may need to meet with key people within the service agencies to inform them of family needs, progress, and concerns, as well as the kinds of services the family is receiving. The nurse can ask to attend case conferences both to provide input and to receive information.

The coordinating function also includes helping the family through the process of interacting with the various agencies. Explanation and interpretation of treatments, evaluation, and recommendations are frequently needed. The nurse can also reinforce any teaching that takes place. Finally the nurse can monitor the progress of the family and the child to be sure that needs are being met, families are receiving the support that they need, and community services complement family care rather than substitute for it (Ayer, 1984).

Advocacy

Another major role of the community health nurse in working with families of mentally retarded children is advocacy, or specific activity or support provided on behalf of others. There are two aspects to the advocacy role—activity on behalf of a particular family of a mentally retarded child and activity on behalf of families of mentally retarded children in general.

Advocacy for a particular family includes the linkage-coordinating functions previously discussed, whereby a nurse may speak or act on behalf of the family in getting into a service network and keep people informed of the family's needs, concerns, and problems, as well as their progress. Involvement in committees, case conferences, and staff meetings that are concerned with the family provides the nurse with opportunities to represent the family point of view and circumstance. Meetings with individual care providers may also be necessary if communication breakdowns have occurred or if families feel too stressed or overwhelmed to absorb and follow through with treatment plans.

Advocacy of families of mentally retarded children in general relates to those activities of the nurse that help the public and the helping professions realize the needs of this group. Advocacy also involves the promotion of policies and services that assist families and their retarded children. Advocacy also means that one monitors legislation and policy in terms of their impact on families and examines whether the well-being of the family, as well as the child, is addressed. Finally advocacy means supporting and promoting educational programs for both the public and the helping professions to dispel misconceptions about the mentally retarded and to provide accurate information about the needs of mentally retarded people and their families.

Evaluation

Evaluation is the final dimension of the community health nurse's role. This is an ongoing activity that begins during the planning phase of the nursing process and continues through implementation of activities and finally back to the assessment phase via feedback. In the assessment and planning phases a determination of family needs and how they can be met is made. Goals and objectives are established in the nursing care plan based on family input, and specific interventions are outlined. Evaluation strategies should also be identified at this point. If the objectives are written in terms of the results to be achieved, they can be used to indicate not only what to evaluate, but also how to evaluate. In addition, the nurse can build into the implementation plan specific points where evaluation can occur. During implementation the nurse should monitor nursing activities to determine family members' reactions and responses to nursing approaches, behaviors, and actions in working with their child and other indicators that provide information on the process of care itself.

Techniques for evaluating the success of nursing interventions might range from observation of family interactions to noting specific behaviors of the family such as initiatives taken by them to obtain services from other community agencies. Families need to be involved in the evaluation phase, as well as the planning phase. Although the nurse observes and questions the family to determine progress toward meeting the objectives, the family needs to assess progress from their own perspective. Decisions can then be made jointly as to whether objectives have been met or whether reassessment is needed, and plans can be altered to increase the nurse's effectiveness in helping families meet the objectives. Evaluation may also show that the objectives were unrealistic or otherwise inappropriate, in which case they need to be rewritten.

SUMMARY

Meeting the health and social needs of all people is basic to the nation's welfare, and society has the responsibility to meet these needs. The well-being of the family is intertwined with the well-being of society, but the reverse of this is also true. If society is committed to helping mentally retarded people live the most normal and productive lives they can, and there are indications that society is committed, the helping professions, including nursing, have a responsibility for helping these individuals and their families meet this goal.

Community health nurses are in a special position to help the families of mentally retarded children, since their work is community based and community focused. Family-centered care, long a recognized concept in community health nursing, is critical to the health and well-being of this special group. In the multidimensional role the community health nurse serves as a major instrument of society in reaching out and assisting both mentally retarded children and their families.

QUESTIONS FOR DISCUSSION

1. How has the deinstitutionalization movement affected the families of mentally retarded people?
2. Describe the stressors in the lives of these families.
3. What support sources are available in your community for these families?
4. Invent a case study of a teenager who is mildly retarded in a family setting in your community. List the sources of stress for the teenager and family. Outline the nursing process as you would follow it to assist this family.

REFERENCES

Anderson KA and Gardner AM: Mothers of retarded children: satisfactions with visits to professional people, Ment Retard 11:36, 1973.

Ayer S: Community Care: failure of professionals to meet family needs, Child Care Health Dev 10:127, 1984.

Baldwin S: Families with handicapped children. In Jones K and Baldwin S, editors: The yearbook of social policy in Britain 1975, London, 1976, Routledge & Kegan Paul Inc.

Bassuk EL and Gerson S: Deinstitutionalization and mental health services, Sci Am 238:46, 1978.

Beavers J and others: Coping in families with a retarded child, Fam Process 25:365, 1986.

Begab MJ and Richardson SA, editors: The mentally retarded and society: a social science perspective, Baltimore, 1975, University Park Press.

Berger M and Foster M: Family-level interventions for retarded children: a multivariate approach to issues and strategies, Multivariate Exp Clin Res 2:1, 1976.

Boggs E: Legal, legislative, and bureaucratic factors affecting planned and unplanned change in the delivery of service to the mentally retarded. In Begab MJ and Richardson SA, editors: The mentally retarded and society: a social science perspective, Baltimore, 1975, University Park Press.

Boggs EM: Economic factors in family care. In Bruininks RH and Krantz GC, editors: Family care of developmentally disabled members: conference proceedings, Minneapolis, 1979, University of Minnesota.

Braddock D: Deinstitutionalization of the retarded: trends in public policy, Hosp Community Psychiatry 32:607,1981.

Bruininks RH: The needs of families. In Bruininks RH and Krantz GC, editors: Family care of developmentally disabled members: conference proceedings, Minneapolis, 1979, University of Minnesota.

Bruininks R and Warfield G: The mentally retarded. In Meyen EL, editor: Exceptional children and youth, Denver, 1978, Love Publishing Co.

Bruininks RH, Williams SM, and Monian LE: Issues and problems of deinstitutionalization in HEW Region V (Project Report No 2), Information and Technical Assistance Project on Deinstitutionalization, Minneapolis, 1979, University of Minnesota.

Caplan G: Support systems and community health, New York, 1974, Behavioral Publications.

Carver JN and Carver NE: The family of the retarded child, Syracuse, NY, 1972, Syracuse University Press.

Chinn PC, Drew CJ, and Logan DR: Mental retardation: a life cycle approach, St. Louis, 1979, CV Mosby Co.

Cleveland DW and Miller N: Attitudes and life commitments of older siblings of mentally retarded adults: an exploratory study, Men Retard 15:38, 1977.

Craft M: Classification, criteria, epidemiology and causation. In Craft M, editor: Tredgold's mental retardation, London, 1979, Bailliere Tindall.

Crnic KA, Friedrich WN, and Greenberg MT: Adaptation of families with mentally retarded children: a model of stress, coping, and family ecology, Am J Ment Defic 88:125, 1983.

Croog SH, Lipson A, and Levine S: Help patterns in severe illness: the roles of kin network, non-family resources, and institutions, J Marriage Fam 34:32, 1972.

Cruickshank WM: Forward. In Paul JL, Stedman DJ, and Neufeld GR, editors: Deinstitutionalization: program and policy development, Syracuse, NY, 1977, Syracuse University Press.

Cummings ST: The impact of the child's deficiency on the father: a study of fathers of mentally retarded and of chronically ill children, Am J Orthopsychiatry 46:246, 1976.

Cummings ST, Bayley HC, and Rie HE: Effects of the child's deficiency on the mother: a study of mothers of mentally retarded, chronically ill and neurotic children, Am J Orthopsychiatry 36:595,1966.

Eyman RK and others: Factors determining residential placement of mentally retarded children, Am J Ment Defic 76:692, 1972.

Family Impact Seminar: Toward an inventory of federal programs with direct impact on families, Washington, DC, 1978, George Washington University.

Farber B: Effects of a severely mentally retarded child on family integration, Monographs of the society for research in child development 24:5, 1959.

Farber B, Jenne WC, and Toigo R: Family crisis and the decision to institutionalize the retarded child, Council for Exceptional Children, Monograph Series A, Issue 1, 1960.

Fotheringham JB, Skelton M, and Hoddinott BA: The effects on the family of the presence of a mentally retarded child, Can Psychiatr Assoc J 17:283, 1972.

Fowle CM: The effect of the severely mentally retarded child on his family, Am J Ment Defic 73:468, 1968.

Gallagher JJ, Beckman P, and Cross AH: Families of handicapped children: sources of stress and its amelioration, Except Child 50:10,1983.

Gath A: Sibling reactions to mental handicap: a comparison of the brothers and sisters of mongol children, J Child Psychol Psychiatry 15:187, 1974.

Gearheart BR and Litton FW: The trainable retarded, St Louis, 1979, CV Mosby Co.

Glenister AM: Economic impact of mental retardation policy on the natural family of the mentally retarded child, Unpublished manuscript, 1984.

Halpern J and others: The myths of deinstitutionalization: policies for the mentally disabled, Boulder, Colo, 1980, Westview Press Inc.

Hill R: Generic features of families under stress, Soc Casework 39:139, 1958.

Holroyd J: The questionnaire on resources and stress: an instrument to measure family response to a handicapped family member, J Community Psychol 2:92, 1974.

Horwitz A: Family, kin and friend networks in psychiatric help seeking, Soc Sci Med 12:297, 1978.

Joyce K, Singer M, and Isralowitz R: Impact of respite care on parents' perceptions of quality of life, Ment Retard 21:153, 1983.

Kornblatt ES and Heinrich J: Needs and coping abilities in families of children with developmental disabilities, Ment Retard, 23:13, 1983.

Kotsopoulas S and Matathia P: Worries of parents regarding the future of their mentally retarded adolescent children, Int J Soc Psychiatry 26:53, 1980.

Learner S: PL 94-142: Related federal legislation for handicapped children and implications for coordination, Washington, DC, 1978, National Education Association.

MacMillan DL: Mental retardation in school and society, Boston, 1977, Little, Brown & Co Inc.

Maloney MP and Ward MP: Mental retardation and modern society, New York, 1979, Oxford University Press.

Moroney RM: Families, social services, and social policy: the issue of shared responsibility, US Department of Health and Human Services, DHHS Publication No (ADM) 80-846, Washington, DC, 1980, US Government Printing Office.

Munro JD: Epidemiology and the extent of mental retardation, Psychiatr Clin North Am 9:591, 1986.

National Commission of Families and Public Policies: Families and public policies in the United States, Columbus, Ohio, 1978, National Conference on Social Welfare.

Newburgh JR: Policy values in community mental health program planning, J Community Psychol 6:48, 1978.

Nirje B: The normalization principle. In Kuzel RB and Shearer A, editors: Changing patterns in residential services for the mentally retarded, Washington DC, 1976, President's Committee on Mental Retardation.

O'Conner G: Social support of mentally retarded persons, Ment Retard 21:187, 1983.

Pattison EM and others: A psychosocial kinship model for family therapy, Am J Psychiatry 132:1246, 1975.

Piachaud D, Bradshaw J, and Weale J: The income effect of a disabled child, J Epidemiol Community Health, :123, 1981.

Platman SR and others: Case management of the mentally disabled, J Public Health Policy 3:302, 1982.

Roesel R and Lawlis GF: Divorce in families of genetically handicapped/mentally retarded individuals, Am J Fam Therapy 11:45, 1983.

Saenger G: Factors influencing the institutionalization of mentally retarded individuals in New York City, New York, 1960, New York University.

Schufeit LJ and Wurster SR: Frequency of divorce among parents of handicapped children, Resources Education 11:71, 1976.

Seltzer MM and Krauss MW: Family community residence, and institutional placements of a sample of mentally retarded children, Am J Ment Defic 89:257, 1984.

Stedman DJ: Introduction. In Paul JL, Stedman DJ, and Neufeld GR, editors: Deinstitutionalization: program and policy development, Syracuse, NY, 1977, Syracuse University Press.

Suelzhe M and Keenan V: Changes in family support networks over the life cycle of mentally retarded persons, Am J Ment Defic 86:267, 1981.

Taft LT: An overview of the etiology of mental retardation and developmental disabilities. In McCormack MK, editor: Prevention of mental retardation and other developmental disabilities, New York, 1980, Marcel Dekker Inc.

Talbott JA: Toward a public policy on the chronically mentally ill patient, Am J Orthopsychiatry 50:43, 1980.

US Bureau of the Census: Statistical abstract of the United States: 1987, ed 107, Washington, DC, 1986, US Government Printing Office.

US General Accounting Office, Comptroller General of the United States: Returning the mentally disabled to the community: government needs to do more, Washington, DC, 1977, US Government Printing Office.

Wikler L: Chronic stresses of families of mentally retarded children, Fam Relations 30:281, 1981.

Wikler L: Stress in families of mentally retarded children, Unpublished manuscript, 1979.

Wikler L, Wasow M, and Hatfield E: Chronic sorrow revisited: parent vs. professional depiction of the adjustment of parents of mentally retarded children, Am J Orthopsychiatry 51:63, 1981.

Willer B and Intagliata JC: Deinstitutionalization of mentally retarded persons in New York state: final report. Submitted to DHEW Region II, Office of Human Development, Developmental Disabilities Office, June 30, 1980.

Willer BS, Intagliata JC, and Atkinson AC: Crises for families of mentally retarded persons including the crisis of deinstitutionalization, Br J Ment Subnormality 25:38, 1979.

Willer B, Scheerenberger RC, and Intagliata JC: Deinstitutionalization and mentally retarded persons, Community Ment Health Rev 3:2, 1978.

CHAPTER

25

Physical Disabilities and Rehabilitation: The Role of the Nurse in the Community

Anne Herrstrom Skelly

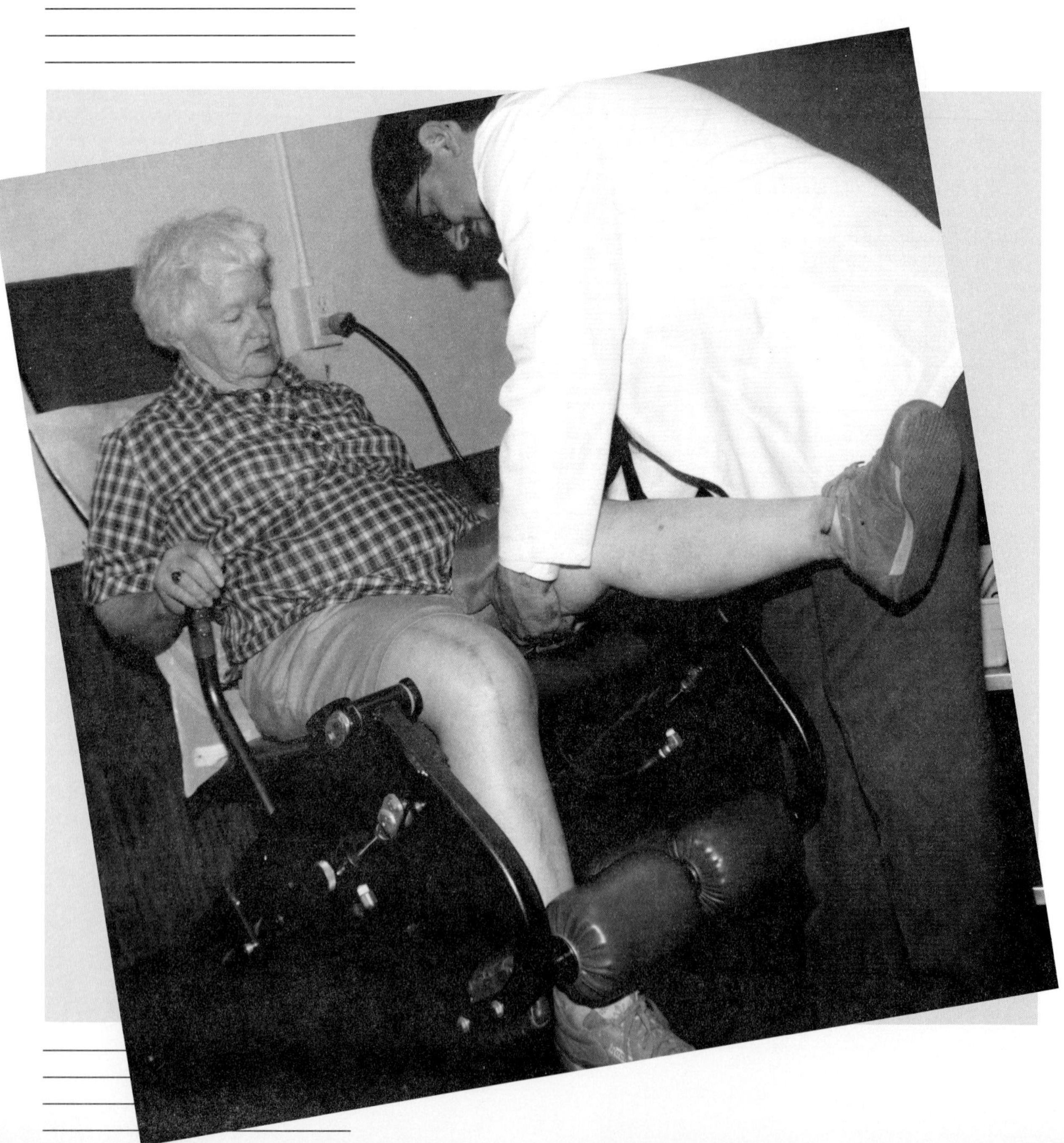

CHAPTER OUTLINE

Historical perspective

Terminology

- Habilitation
- Rehabilitation
- Disability
- Handicap
- Rehabilitative nursing

Role of the nurse in work with individuals with disabilities

Disability and crises

Barriers to disabled people

Incidence and prevalance of disability and chronic disease

Applying the nursing process to disabled individuals and their families

- Assessment
- Diagnosis
- Planning
- Implementation
- Evaluation

Physical disorders seen in the community

- Cerebral palsy
- Visual impairment
- Hearing impairment

Summary

OBJECTIVES

After completing this chapter, the reader should be able to:

1. Discuss the role of the nurse in the community in working with individuals with disabilities.
2. Describe the barriers that exist in the community that prevent disabled individuals from fully participating in society.
3. Apply the nursing process to develop a nursing care plan for disabled individuals and their families:
   a. Discuss the four major components of assessment—a complete health history and physical assessment, environmental assessment, and family assessment of the client.
   b. List nursing diagnoses that may be applicable to clinical situations involving disabled individuals.
   c. List the pertinent factors involved in planning care for disabled individuals and families in the community.
   d. Discuss the implementation of nursing interventions for disabled individuals using a multidisciplinary approach in a community-based setting.
   e. Describe how evaluations of the nursing care plan might be accomplished in the community.
4. Discuss how nurses in the community might apply the nursing process to deliver health care to individuals with cerebral palsy and vision and hearing deficits.
5. Describe how community resources can be used by the nurse in the community to enhance the effectiveness of the nursing care plan.

Disabilities can affect individuals at any time in their lives and can result from congenital or traumatic causes, illness, or the aging process. As a result individuals and families are often faced with overwhelming challenges to their physical, emotional, and financial resources as they attempt to deal with varying degrees of disability. The nurse in the community, functioning as a primary care provider, a case manager, or a home health care nurse, plays a critical role in not only the provision of direct care services and client and family education, but also support of clients and their families.

HISTORICAL PERSPECTIVE

Throughout history societies have responded to their sick and disabled in a variety of ways. In ancient Hebrew cultures disability was thought to reflect a sin committed by individuals or their families. The early Greeks equated physical disability with social inferiority (Diamond and Jones, 1983). During the fifth and sixth centuries the disabled were often treated with cruelty or persecuted. The increase in importance of Christianity in the Middle Ages brought with it more emphasis on religious and ethical concepts. The attitude toward the disabled became more charitable, although the mechanism of delivery of this charity, institutionalization of the disabled, remains an ethical problem. Use of the scientific method resulted in the discovery that illness arose from factors beyond the control of individuals. For the first time the hypothesis that a disabled individual was not to blame for infirmity was advanced. Various combinations of these historical perspectives can be seen in contemporary societal views of disability (Diamond and Jones, 1983).

The factors influencing a society's response to the disabled have been described by Safilios-Rothschild (1970). These factors include a society's belief about the cause of the disability; the status of a society's economy, including the rate of unemployment and whether the society is agrarian or more technologically oriented; the attitudes of a society in regard to poverty and the role of government in regard to the poor, since the disabled and chronically ill are often poor; and the stigma of disability—whether it is visible or causes others to be uncomfortable. All these factors also contribute to the misinformation and stereotyping that have traditionally been associated with disabled people and chronically ill people.

TERMINOLOGY

There are a variety of terms used commonly in regard to care of individuals with chronic illnesses and disabilities. Often a precise definition of a concept is elusive. However, it is important to remember that these definitions influence how a specific condition is perceived by affected individuals, their families, nurses, and society in general. Perceptions influence actions, and in a given situation whether a physical condition is defined as a disability or a handicap provides the basis for how disabled individuals interact. Following are discussions of commonly used terms in the nursing care of individuals with disabilities.

Habilitation

Habilitation refers to the development of individuals to their fullest physical, mental, social, vocational, and economic capacities (Stryker, 1977). This term is used when a new functional ability is developed by an individual.

Rehabilitation

Rehabilitation refers to the restoration of individuals to their fullest physical, mental, social, vocational, and economic capacities (Stryker, 1977). This term is used when a functional ability has been lost because of accident or disease.

Disability

A disability is a condition in which there is an impairment of structure or function, but this impairment is not perceived as causing limitations. Disabilities may be classified as congenital or acquired, and they can be stable or progressive. Disabilities may be visible or invisible to the observer.

Handicap

A handicap is a condition in which there is an impairment of structure or function that is perceived as limiting a person's ability to perform certain activities (Jarvis, 1981).

Many definitions of disability and handicap exist in current medical and nursing literature. Nagi and Haber discuss an additional concept—functional limitations in regard to individuals with disability. Nagi defines a functional limitation as a reduction in an individual's ability to carry out daily activities or to perform certain roles (Nagi, 1966). Haber defines the same concept as a loss in an individual's capacity for activity (Haber, 1967). This term appears to parallel disability; both reflect impairment of functional ability without additional perception of limitation.

Rehabilitative Nursing

Rehabilitative nursing is a creative process beginning with immediate preventive care, continuing through the restorative phase of care, and involving the adaptation of the whole being (Stryker, 1977). It is holistic, views the individual in totality and aims to encourage a sense of dignity, personal worth, and power in all functionally disabled people.

ROLE OF THE NURSE IN WORKING WITH INDIVIDUALS WITH DISABILITY

Nurses working in a community-based role come into contact with disabled individuals and their families in a variety of situations. Because of their generalized nursing background, assessment techniques, and knowledge of community resources, community nurses are invaluable in assessing, planning, implementing, and evaluating the care necessary to maintain disabled individuals in the community and restore them to an optimum level of functioning.

Primary, secondary, and tertiary levels of prevention are also a part of the nursing role. Primary prevention of disability includes education of the community in regard to adequate nutrition, rest, and exercise to prevent illness; proper sanitation; environmental surveillance, use of seat belts to prevent injury; home safety to prevent accidents; early and regular prenatal care; proper immunization of children and at-risk populations; and maternal and child health to prevent birth defects. The goal of primary prevention is to reduce the risk factors associated with the occurrence of a specific disability.

Secondary prevention of disability has as its goal the early identification and treatment of individuals so that normal functioning can be regained as soon as possible. Nursing activities related to secondary prevention include case finding, counseling, and referral. Examples of secondary prevention include preschool screening clinics to identify children with visual, hearing, or developmental impairments; vision and hearing screening clinics for adults; and referrals of families with children who have cystic fibrosis, Down syndrome, or muscular dystrophy for genetic counseling.

Tertiary prevention of disability has as its goal the restoration of a person to optimal levels of functioning. At this level the physical or mental condition has become irreversible, and the major nursing focus is directed towards habilitation and rehabilitation. Examples of tertiary prevention include teaching of relaxation techniques, stress management, educational, social, recreational, and nutritional counseling, energy conservation, exercise, use of adaptive equipment, and referral for vocational rehabilitation.

DISABILITY AND CRISES

The effectiveness of interactions with disabled people depends to a large part on nurses' attitude toward disability and their feelings about working with the disabled. The occurrence of a disability creates a situational crisis. Individuals and families react to a crisis situation in unique ways depending on their perception of the disability and its meaning to them, coping mechanisms, and the amount of available support (Barrell, 1974). Individuals dealing with a disability often pass through the same stages as individuals dealing with death and dying. These stages may overlap, and clients may either skip a stage or regress to an earlier stage. The stages are summarized in the following box. For most disabled people the denial stage is the longest. In some cases it lasts several years. Spradley defines the term "crisis" as a temporary state of severe disequilibrium for which people are unable to achieve a solution with their usual coping abilities. She states further that crises are too important and threatening not to be dealt with (Spradley, 1985). A crisis often represents a turning point in an individual's life, with the potential for restoration of health existing concurrently with the threat of permanent loss of physical or cognitive functioning.

Community health nurses should also be aware that caring for a disabled individual may create a crisis situation for themselves. Janken has described behaviors seen in nurses under stress that limit the effectiveness of the nurse-client interaction (Janken, 1974). These include positive or negative stereotyping of the disabled individual or family; partisanship, that is, seeing the individual as all good or all bad; withdrawal from the stressor, which may increase the impact of the problem for both the nurse and the client; and projection, in which nurses incorporate their own feelings and assumptions in the case of disabled individuals or their families. In working with the disabled, nurses should be aware of their own responses to the situation.

STAGES OF GRIEVING IN REGARD TO DISABILITY

1. Denial. At this stage the individual is unable to deal with the reality of the disability and does not think about it consciously.
2. Anger. As the individual begins to confront the reality of the disability, negative feelings about the disability and its effects are expressed.
3. Bargaining. An attempt is made by the individual to change the reality of the disability by making deals with God or others.
4. Depression. As acceptance of the nature of the situation begins, the individual experiences periods of depression with or without physical and psychologic immobilization.
5. Acceptance. The individual can now deal with the reality of the disability with new understanding, evidencing new strength and ability to cope with its ramifications.

Modified from Kubler-Ross E: Death: The final stage of growth, Englewood Cliffs, NJ, 1975, Prentice Hall, Prentice Hall Press.

People in crises seek assistance, and the nurse is often in a unique position to intervene and help clients and their families to reestablish the equilibrium that has been lost. Goals during the initial period of stress include resolution of the immediate crisis and restoration of functioning to the precrisis level if possible. Ultimately nurses should direct their interventions toward strengthening the client's coping mechanisms so that future crises might be prevented or dealt with more effectively. A paradigm showing how the presence or absence of balancing factors can predict the development of crises is shown in Fig. 25-1. Honest, open client-nurse communication is essential for success. Spradley (1985) proposes the following guidelines to assist nurses in intervening with clients and families during crisis:

1. Encourage clients to accept assistance.
2. Show acceptance and support of clients.
3. Provide information for clients.
4. Help clients express their concerns.
5. Help clients face and discuss crises.
6. Help clients develop effective coping skills.

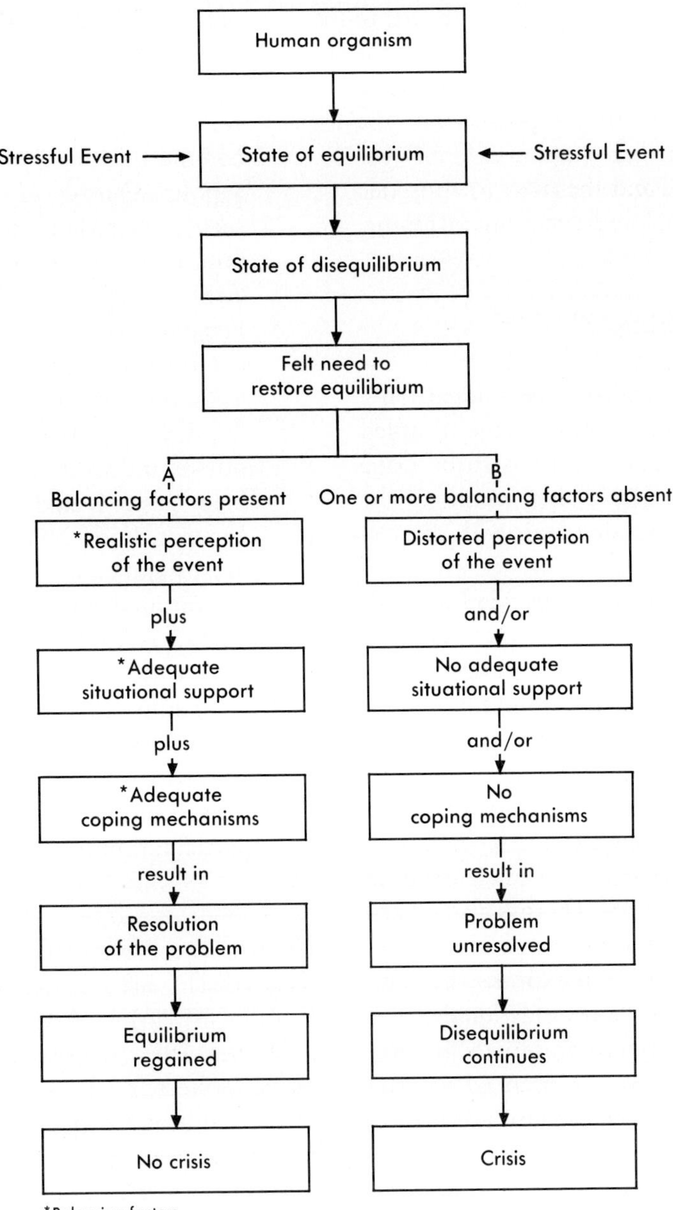

Fig. 25-1. Development of crisis can be predicted with the presence or absence of balancing factors. From Aguilera D and Messick J: Crisis intervention: theory and methodology, ed 5, St Louis, 1986, CV Mosby Co.

7. Promote the development of new positive relationships.

As the crisis is resolved, the nurse and client should evaluate the outcome of the interventions used and discuss which interventions were effective and how they might be used in future situations. This evaluation conference provides an excellent opportunity for the community health nurse to help the client establish new goals for the future and means to implement them. Ideas could also be exchanged at this time in regard to how the client and family perceive the role of the nurse, what services the family needs to maintain the client as independently as possible in the home, the need for further client and family education or counseling, and the need for possible referrals for educational and vocational training.

BARRIERS TO DISABLED PEOPLE

Although progress has been made in identifying and addressing the special needs of the disabled population, much more work needs to be done in several areas. Bowe (1978) has identified the following six barriers to individuals with disabilities.

1. Architectural barriers. As disabled individuals move into the community they confront a variety of obstacles in buildings, transportation facilities, and community accessibility.
2. Educational barriers. Although advances have been made in securing the legal rights of the disabled to education, barriers still exist in the form of educational attitudes toward disabled people. There is also a need to develop new methodologies and environmental adaptations to maximize the educational potential of these individuals.
3. Occupational barriers. Employment provides not only a source of financial security for the disabled person, but also a source of satisfaction and self-esteem. Although some disabled workers might require special environments, such as sheltered workshops, many jobs can be done well by the disabled with or without special vocational rehabilitation. Misconceptions regarding employing the disabled, such as the belief that they are high-risk employees who use a lot of sick time, contribute to the barriers found in the workplace.
4. Legal barriers. Although legislation exists to prevent architectural, transportational, and educational barriers and to protect the civil rights of the disabled, enforcement is usually slow or minimal. It remains for the disabled community to unite and represent itself as a political force in the legislative arena to secure their rights further. Legislation pertaining to the disabled is summarized in Table 25-1.
5. Personal barriers. Disabilities can be congenital or acquired. Individuals who acquire a disability or are born with a disability are faced with many challenges not faced by others. Individuals who acquire a disability may be subjected to threats to their self-concept, body image, and self-esteem. The most significant potential personal barrier to the optimal rehabilitation of disabled individuals is how they perceive and choose to deal with disability and the amount and availability of support.
6. Attitudinal barriers. Stereotyped attitudes toward disabled people often lead to discrimination, which serves as a barrier to full participation in society by disabled people.

INCIDENCE AND PREVALENCE OF DISABILITY AND CHRONIC DISEASE

During 1977 the National Health Interview Survey collected data on the prevalence and effect of certain selected physical impairments among noninstitutionalized people in the United States (Prevalence, 1981). The types of impairments chosen for study were visual, hearing, and speech impairments, absence of extremities, paralysis, and four types of nonparalytic orthopedic impairments affecting the back and spine, upper extremity or shoulder, lower extremity or hip, or other areas of orthopedic impairment not covered by the foregoing categories. The prevalence and incidence of these impairments in 1977 is summarized in Table 25-2. For this survey prevalence

TABLE 25-1 Overview of Legislation Pertaining to the Disabled

Date	Law	Effect
1943	Barden-LaFollette Act of 1943 (PL113)	Provided federal payment for guidance and placement services, physical rehabilitation, living expenses, and occupational equipment; mentally retarded and psychiatric clients are now eligible for these services
1954	Vocational Rehabilitation Amendments of 1954 (PL565)	Provided assistance to state to educate and train disabled people so that they take a place in the workforce, funds to train health care personnel, and grants for research to aid disabled people
1965	Vocational Rehabilitation Amendments of 1965	Provided grants for the establishment of sheltered workshops
1973	Rehabilitation Act of 1973 (PL112)	Prohibited discrimination against handicapped individuals in any federally assisted program or activity; employability is the eligibility criterion
1974	Rehabilitation Act of 1974 (PL516)	Extended definition of handicap beyond employability
1975	Education for All Handicapped Persons	Provided the appropriate public educational services to all handicapped individuals between 3 and 21 years of age
1976	Educational Amendments of 1976, Title II (PL482)	Mandated that 10% of all federal funding for vocational education be spent on the handicapped and that this amount be matched by state and local funds
1977	Rules and Regulations to Implement (PL516)	Provided guidelines for the implementation of nondiscriminatory hiring practices
1978	Rehabilitation Amendments	Provided for the funding of independent living centers on a demonstration basis; recognized independent living as part of rehabilitation. Also established a National Council on the Handicapped; and called for the establishment of a National Center for Rehabilitation Research
1980	Education Amendments (PL96-374)	Provided for increased access to education
1980	Social Security Disability Amendments (PL96-265)	Extended the initial trial work period under which Social Security benefits would remain to two years
1982	Surface Transportation Assistance Act (PL97-424)	Encouraged transportation industry to identify and remove architectural barriers
1983	Education of Handicapped Act (PL98-199)	Provided for increased access to education for disabled children
1984	Vocational Educational Act (PL98-524)	Mandated state funding to ensure that disabled individuals would have access to vocational education
1984	Rehabilitation Amendments (PL98-221)	Extended the provisions of the rehabilitation Act of 1973. Modified the definition of severely disabled and set 16 years of age as the lower age limit for individuals affected by the 1973 act.
1986	Rehabilitation Amendments (PL99-506)	Provided funding for rehabilitation engineering. Recognized rehabilitation needs of disabled Native Americans. Expanded influence of the National Council on the Handicapped.

Modified from Federal Register 22676-22694, May 4, 1977; and Watson G: Rehabilitation legislation of the 1980's: implications for nurses as health care providers, Rehabilitation Nurs 13:136, 1988.

was defined as the number of cases of a specific condition or impairment during a specific interval. Incidence was defined as the number of cases of a specific condition or impairment having their onset during a specified period. The survey also looked at the impact of certain impairments as measured by limitation of activity, number of bed days and restricted activity days, frequency of visits to the physician, and frequency and degree of bother to the disabled individual. These results, according to the impairments under study, are summarized in Table 25-3. This survey by no

TABLE 25-2 Prevalence and Incidence of Selected Impairments In Noninstitutionalized Individuals in the United States in 1977

Impairment	Prevalence (in thousands)	Incidence* (in thousands)
Visual impairments	11,415	884
Severe visual impairments	1,391	85
Other visual impairments	10,024	798
Hearing impairments (includes tinnitus)	16,219	900
Speech impairments	1,995	113
Paralysis, complete or partial	1,532	22
Upper only	91	
Lower only	264	22
Orthopedic impairments (except paralysis or absence)		
Back or spine	9,365	792
Upper extremity or shoulder	2,500	304
Lower extremity or hip	7,147	684
Other and multiple areas, areas not elsewhere classified, and ill-defined areas of limbs, back, or trunk	1,213	146

Modified from DHHS Pub No (PHS) 81-1562, Hyattsville, 1981, Office of Health, Research, Statistics and Technology.
*Incidence is defined as the estimated number of conditions having their onset in a specified time period, in this case, within 12 months of the week of the interview. Onset of a condition is defined as the time when the condition is first noticed.

TABLE 25-3 Selected Impairments and Their Impact on Non-Institutionalized Individuals in the United States in 1977

	Prevalence			Disability days	
	Number (in thousands)	Number (per 1000 persons)	Conditions that cause limitations of activity (%)	Restricted activity days per condition per year	Work loss days per condition per year*
Visual impairments	11,415	53.8	13.1	6.8	0.3
Severe	1,391	6.6	37.0	23.1	
Other	10,024	47.2	9.8	4.5	0.3
Hearing impairments (includes tinnitus)	16,219	76.4	4.7	0.7	0.1
Speech impairments	1,995	9.4	9.3	3.8	1.3
Paralysis, complete or partial	1,532	7.2	58.4	45.6	9.2
Absence of major extremities	358	1.7	65.9	32.8	4.0†
Upper only	91	0.4	48.4	7.9	4.0†
Lower only	264	1.2	71.2	41.8	4.0†
Orthopedic impairments (except paralysis or absence)					
Back or spine	9,365	44.1	25.5	17.7	3.1
Upper extremity or shoulder	2,500	11.8	21.4	12.6	3.1
Lower extremity or hip	7,147	33.7	26.6	18.8	3.0
Other and multiple, not-elsewhere classified, and ill-defined, impairments of limbs, back, or trunk	1,213	5.7	54.8	46.7	5.7

Modified from DHHS Pub No (PHS) 81-1562, Hyattsville, Md, 1981, Office of Health, Research, Statistics and Technology.
*Work loss days per condition per year were computed for currently employed population only.
†Impact questions were not asked in the case of missing extremities.

means covers the range of physical impairments seen in individuals but is useful as a guide to the prevalence of certain conditions in the community and their impact on the individuals affected.

APPLYING THE NURSING PROCESS TO DISABLED INDIVIDUALS AND THEIR FAMILIES

Critical to the construction of an effective nursing care plan is the systematic collection of a comprehensive data base. (See Chapter 3.)

Assessment

In dealing with disabled individuals, certain portions of the data base assume more relevance. The initial assessment should include a complete history and a physical, environmental, and family assessment of the client.

History and Physical Assessment

The history taken from a disabled individual is essentially the same history as is used for any other client. The physical examination should be comprehensive and cover all the body systems. However, special attention should be paid to the systems involved by the disability, such as the musculoskeletal or neurologic systems. Since one of the main functions of the nurse will be to help the client regain or acquire skills, a sound baseline of the client's sensory functioning and psychosocial functioning should be obtained. In regard to the client's sensory functioning, the nurse should assess the client's auditory, visual, and kinesthetic responses to cue systems by noting verbal responses or body movements. The nurse should note the communication pattern used by the client (verbal or nonverbal), the processing time required for an appropriate response, and whether the client can process 1-2-3 step commands. The appropriateness of motor activities and sequential activities, as well as the client's method of thought integration (abstract vs. concrete), should be observed. As part of the assessment of sensory functioning, the nurse should note the client's orientation, response to pain, and level of interaction with the environment—self, personal belongings, and immediate and larger environment (Syllabus, 1986).

The psychosocial assessment might include the nurse's perception of the clients' developmental stages according to the theories of Erikson, Freud, or Maslow, their relief behaviors, or activities used to relieve anxiety, sexual development and functioning, level of anxiety, classified as mild, moderate, or severe, manner of relating, perception of self, perception of health status, attitude, motivation, insight, affect, and balancing factors in their lives such as material assets and social support (Syllabus, 1986).

Environmental Assessment

The environmental assessment should look at both the individual's immediate environment, that is, the home or living unit, and the larger environment, that is, the area surrounding the home. Figs. 25-2 and 25-3 are examples of environmental assessment tools addressing a general environment and the environment of an individual with low vision, respectively. In general, when assessing the area around a disabled client's residence, the nurse should focus on the type and condition of the residences, architectural barriers, such as narrow doorways and high curbs, that may inhibit mobility, sanitation; safety of the larger environment; availability of transportation; accessibility of schools, churches, and recreational facilities in the area; and accessibility of services such as grocery stores and pharmacies to the disabled individual.

When assessing the immediate living environment of a disabled client, the nurse should look at the overall condition and location of the residence and the client's personal living space. Pa-

Assessment of Immediate Living Environment

Client's Name ______________________

Date ______________________

Parameters	Assessment	Recommendations
Neighborhood	Adequate ___ Inadequate ___	
Amount of Physical Space	Adequate ___ Inadequate ___	
Cleanliness	Adequate ___ Inadequate ___	
Convenient toilet facilities	Adequate ___ Inadequate ___	
Useable and accessible telephone	Adequate ___ Inadequate ___	
Adequate and safe heating	Adequate ___ Inadequate ___	
Stairways and halls	Adequate ___ Inadequate ___	
Cooking facilities	Adequate ___ Inadequate ___	
Tub, shower, hot water	Adequate ___ Inadequate ___	
Laundry facilities	Adequate ___ Inadequate ___	
Physical barriers in home	Present ___ Absent ___	
Physical barriers to exits from home	Present ___ Not present ___	
Physical hazards	Present ___ Not present ___	
Home accessible to care-givers	Yes ___ No ___	
Use of alcohol or drugs by patient or care-giver	Yes ___ No ___	
Client mobility	Adequate ___ Inadequate ___	
Client safety	Adequate ___ Inadequate ___	
Escort necessary	Yes ___ No ___	
Pets	Yes ___ No ___	

Strengths of Physical Environment: ______________________

Areas of Concern: ______________________

Fig. 25-2. Environmental assessment tool for general environments.

STATE UNIVERSITY OF NEW YORK AT BUFFALO
SCHOOL OF NURSING

Low Vision Environmental Assessment Tool*

Client Name ______________________

Date ______________________

AREA	1	2	3	4	INTERVENTIONS RECOMMENDED
I. Activities of Daily Living					
a. Use of stove					
b. Use of oven					
c. Use of washer					
d. Use of dryer					
e. Use of can opener					
f. Reading food labels					
g. Kitchen storage (food, as well as nonedible items)					
h. Dressing hygiene					
i. Ambulation/mobility					
j. Use of cutting utensils					
k. Use of iron					
l. Other ______________					
II. Medications					
a. Storage of medications					
b. Identification of labels					
c. Storage of equipment					
III. Personal (Psychosocial)					
a. Recreational pastimes					
b. Transportation/Travel					
c. Social contacts					
IV. Physical Environment					
A. Lighting					
1. General environment					
2. Stairways					
3. Glare					
B. Clutter/organization					
C. Presence of architectural barriers					
D. Thermostat					
V. General Safety					
Match/lighter use					
Smoking					
Use of telephone					
Plan for emergency assistance (fire; MD)					

*Key to assessment. 1 = Fully independent, adequate; no problem noted. 2 = Requires assistance, requires some remediation or intervention. 3 = Inadequate; safety concern; problem noted. 4 = N/A

Fig. 25-3. Environmental assessment tool for individuals with low vision.

rameters to be assessed include aroma, noise level, lighting, privacy, heat and ventilation, condition of railings, stairs, and stairways, and presence of vermin. The kitchen and bathroom should be assessed for such things as wheelchair and bathtub accessibility, sanitation, medication storage, and lighting. Safety is a primary concern for disabled individuals and should be assessed in both the immediate and broader environments. In the home the nurse, bearing in mind the nature of the disability and its effect on the individual, should assess the arrangement of the furniture, adequacy of available space, presence of potential obstacles such as scatter rugs and low footstools, location and accessibility of electric outlets, and emergency exits. Based on these observations, it should be possible to determine whether adaptive equipment is needed (Syllabus, 1986).

Family Assessment

Physically disabled individuals who live in the community often do so in a family setting, either traditional or nontraditional. Families and significant others can offer support, provide motivation and encouragement, and provide physical care to disabled individuals. These same individuals can foster dependency, noncompliance, and rejection of health services. The impact of disability or the diagnosis of a chronic illness can upset the equilibrium of a family and create new stress on members' health. Crucial to the formation of a client-centered nursing care plan is an assessment of disabled individuals' families or living groups, assessment of their significant others, or, in the absence of an identifiable family or significant other, a careful appraisal of how individuals' social and emotional needs are being met.

Family assessment includes basic demographic data, environmental data, and data related to the health status of the family and their interactions with the health care delivery system. The demographic data to be collected include the age and sex of each family member, family financial resources, roles of the different family members, the cultural and religious orientation of each member, and the occupation and educational background of family members. The family's recreational or leisure activities should be noted, as well as their pattern of communication. It is optimal to obtain a developmental history of the family noting the family's social class status and social mobility.

Looking at the environment of the family, as opposed to the environment of the client, the nurse assesses the family's associations and networking within the community to determine the amount and type of social support available to them. Is the family mobile geographically? What are the unique characteristics of the family's home? What are the unique characteristics of the family's neighborhood?

The health status of family members, the interactions with the health care delivery system, their definitions of health and illness and their level of knowledge should be assessed. Of equal importance is how each family member perceives the health status of the disabled family member and the implications of the disability for themselves. The family's self-care practices, preventive health measures, patterns of usage of health services, and logistic problems to receiving care should be identified.

For disabled individuals who do not have an identifiable family but who do have a significant other, the interaction between the significant other and client should be assessed and the significant other's perception of the health status of the disabled individual should be noted. For those individuals who do not have an identifiable family or a significant other, the nurse should assess how the client's emotional and social needs are being met and identify any available support systems.

Nursing Diagnosis

Based on careful review of the data base collected, the nurse can compile a prioritized list of actual and potential problems for a client. Using the problem list as a guide, the nurse can formulate a nursing diagnosis for each problem identified. Examples of nursing diagnoses applicable to clinical situations involving disabled individuals are shown in the following box.

Planning

The nursing care plan for a disabled individual should be jointly established by the nurse and client. Objectives should be formulated to help direct nursing interventions. The best objectives are behaviorally stated, since those can be most readily measured. Since physical disabilities often require long-term treatment, it is often beneficial to establish both short-term and long-term objectives with a specified time frame for attainment of the objectives.

Implementation

A knowledge of teaching and learning principles is extremely important in the implementation phase, as well as in the planning phase, of the nursing process. Health teaching in a community-based setting is discussed in Chapter 5. A multidisciplinary team approach is often used to deliver care to a disabled individual in the community. The disciplines involved most frequently include medicine (pediatrics, neurology, orthopedics, and ophthalmology), occupational therapy, physical therapy, speech and hearing therapy, special education, rehabilitation, and nursing. In working with this multidisciplinary team, the nurse often assumes the role of case manager who coordinates the different disciplines while maintaining a holistic view of clients as members of their families. Nursing "brings it all together" so that clients receive services based on their individual needs and the "total person" is not lost.

Involving the Family

Often the family becomes the primary means of therapy for a disabled client. In this situation the nurse needs to be especially sensitive to the

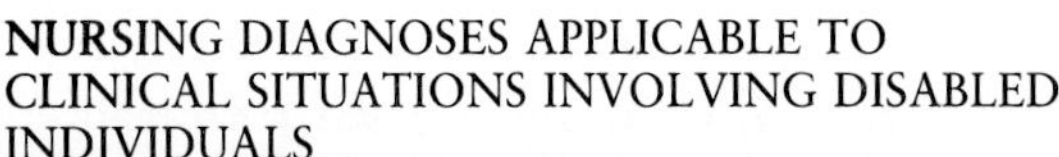

NURSING DIAGNOSES APPLICABLE TO CLINICAL SITUATIONS INVOLVING DISABLED INDIVIDUALS

Activity intolerance
Ineffective airway clearance
Anxiety
Potential for aspiration
Constipation
Diarrhea
Bowel incontinence
Pain
Impaired verbal communication
Ineffective individual coping
Ineffective family coping: Compromised
Ineffective family coping: Disabling
Family coping: potential for growth
Decisional conflict (specify)
Defensive coping
Potential for disuse syndrome
Diversional activity deficit
Dysreflexia
Fatigue
Fear
Fluid volume deficit
Potential fluid volume deficit
Impaired gas exchange
Anticipatory grieving
Dysfunctional grieving
Altered health maintenance
Health-seeking behaviors (specify)
Impaired home maintenance management
Ineffective denial
Potential for injury
Knowledge deficit (specify)
Impaired physical mobility
Noncompliance (specify)
Altered nutrition: less than body requirements
Altered nutrition: more than body requirements
Parental role conflict
Powerlessness
Body image disturbance
Personal identity disturbance
Self-esteem disturbance
  Chronic low self-esteem
  Situational low self-esteem
Sensory/perceptual alterations (specify)
Sexual dysfunction
Impaired skin integrity
Potential impaired skin integrity
Sleep pattern disturbance
Social isolation
Spiritual distress (distress of the human spirit)
Altered thought processes
Altered patterns of urinary elimination

Modified from: Campbell C: Nursing diagnosis and interventions in nursing practice, New York, 1978, John Wiley & Sons Inc.

additional burdens placed on family members. In planning for this family role, opportunities should be provided for both the client and family members to ask questions and discuss their feelings. Families should not be bombarded with suggestions, since this may make them feel their abilities to deal with disabled family members are inadequate. Praise should be provided for innovations and adherence to prescribed regimens. Families involved in these functions require reliable sources of information, support in coping with the emotional burdens of caring for disabled individuals, and access to community resources. It is in these areas that the nurse can make important contributions.

Community Resources Referral

Because of their extensive knowledge of the community, community nurses working with disabled individuals and their families are in an excellent position to make referrals to community resources that might provide services to the client. Referrals may also be made for more extensive assessment of the client's condition or treatment and for testing for placement in specialized education or vocational training situations. A listing of possible community resources may be obtained by contacting the local United Fund or by looking in the local telephone directory. Beginning nurses working in community-based settings should be encouraged to develop their own directory of local agencies including telephone numbers, contacts within the agency, and brief descriptions of services provided. If the client has a fairly common disorder such as cerebral palsy, the first step would be to contact the national organization associated with that disorder, in this case the United Cerebral Palsy Association.

Evaluation

Instead of being a final step, evaluation is often an ongoing activity in the application of the nursing process. Evaluation should be first directed toward the objectives—were they met? If not, attention should be given to the nursing interventions intended to achieve the objectives. Perhaps new methods to achieve the objectives need to be formulated. Perhaps the interventions need to be more specific or broader. Perhaps the interventions are proper but the client requires more time to meet the objectives. Evaluation should be done mutually by the client and nurse. Often clients or their families can best pinpoint why a specific goal is not achieved. The evaluation conference also provides an excellent opportunity for a joint reappraisal of the nursing care plan and setting of new priorities and client-centered objectives.

PHYSICAL DISORDERS SEEN IN THE COMMUNITY

Cerebral Palsy

Cerebral palsy is the most commonly occurring permanent disability in children. It is estimated that approximately 15,000 infants are born with cerebral palsy annually and that there are 750,000 people in the adult population with cerebral palsy in varying degrees (Stryker, 1977).

Definition

Cerebral palsy is a nonspecific term applied to clinical conditions characterized by impairments of muscular control associated with injury to the cranium, especially the motor cortex of the cerebrum. Cerebral palsy is not a progressive disorder, nor is it fatal. The primary disturbances seen in the child or adult are abnormalities of muscle tone and difficulties with coordination, posture, and balance.

Cause

Cerebral palsy may be congenital or acquired. The exact cause of cerebral palsy is often obscure.

The single most important known causal factor is cerebral anoxia. Other known congenital factors include prenatal irradiation, intrauterine infections from TORCHS (toxoplasmosis, rubella, cytomegalic inclusion disease, herpes, and syphilis), drug ingestion by the mother in the prenatal period, mechanical trauma during the birth process, cardiorespiratory or metabolic problems in the newborn period, hyperbilirubinemia, electrolyte disturbances such as hypoglycemia and hypocalcemia in the newborn, and head trauma, toxic ingestion of such agents as lead and carbon monoxide, and infections such as meningitis postnatally (Whaley, 1987). Acquired types of cerebral palsy are usually seen as a result of infections such as meningitis and encephalitis, vascular abnormalities such as arteriovenous malformations and aneurysms, or trauma.

It is important for the community health nurse to remember that in addition to disorders of muscle tone, movement, and posture, other neurologic abnormalities and associated conditions may be seen in clients with cerebral palsy. These other manifestations are not a result of cerebral palsy but of the underlying central nervous system lesion. However, the concomitant abnormalities combine with the cerebral palsy to contribute to the overall outcome seen in the child. Examples of other disorders seen in individuals with cerebral palsy include speech and hearing disorders, attention deficit disorders, disorders of perception, seizure disorders, and mental retardation. Mental retardation often accompanies cerebral palsy, and its incidence is greater in people with cerebral palsy than in the general population. However, many people with cerebral palsy, especially clients with athetosis, have good mentality and high intelligence quotients.

Assessment

Cerebral palsy can be classified in the five following categories depending on the type of neuromuscular dysfunction involved (Whaley, 1987):

1. Spastic cerebral palsy
2. Dyskinetic cerebral palsy (athetosis)
3. Ataxic cerebral palsy
4. Mixed-type cerebral palsy
5. Rigid, tremor, and atonic types of cerebral palsy

The most common categories are spastic cerebral palsy and dyskinetic cerebral palsy, or athetosis.

The major manifestations of spastic cerebral palsy include increased muscle tone (hypertonicity), which is often seen with muscle weakness, persistence of the primitive reflexes such as asymmetric tonic neck reflex and tonic labyrinthian reflex, which are often increased by any active attempts at motion (Fig. 25-4), poor control of posture, balance, and coordination, impairment of fine and gross motor skills, and contractures. These contractures are due to the continuous state of muscle contraction and cause further limitation of mobility. Facial muscles, including muscles of the oral cavity, are often involved and present difficulties with eating and speech (Finnie, 1975).

Dyskinetic cerebral palsy is most often manifest as athetoid movements involving the extremities, trunk, neck, facial muscles, and tongue. These movements disappear in sleep and are increased by stress and fatigue. This type of cerebral palsy is also known as athetosis. Individuals with dyskinetic cerebral palsy often have difficulties articulating (dysarthria) and controlling drooling because of an inability to accommodate their secretions, and may have high-frequency hearing losses and disorders of the extraocular eye muscles including strabismus and conjugate, upward gaze palsy). Joint deformities are rare because of the continual movements of the extremities.

Ataxic, mixed, and rigid-tremor-atonic types of cerebral palsy are rare and infrequently seen in a community setting.

Case Finding

Early diagnosis of cerebral palsy is essential to promote optimum development of the individual.

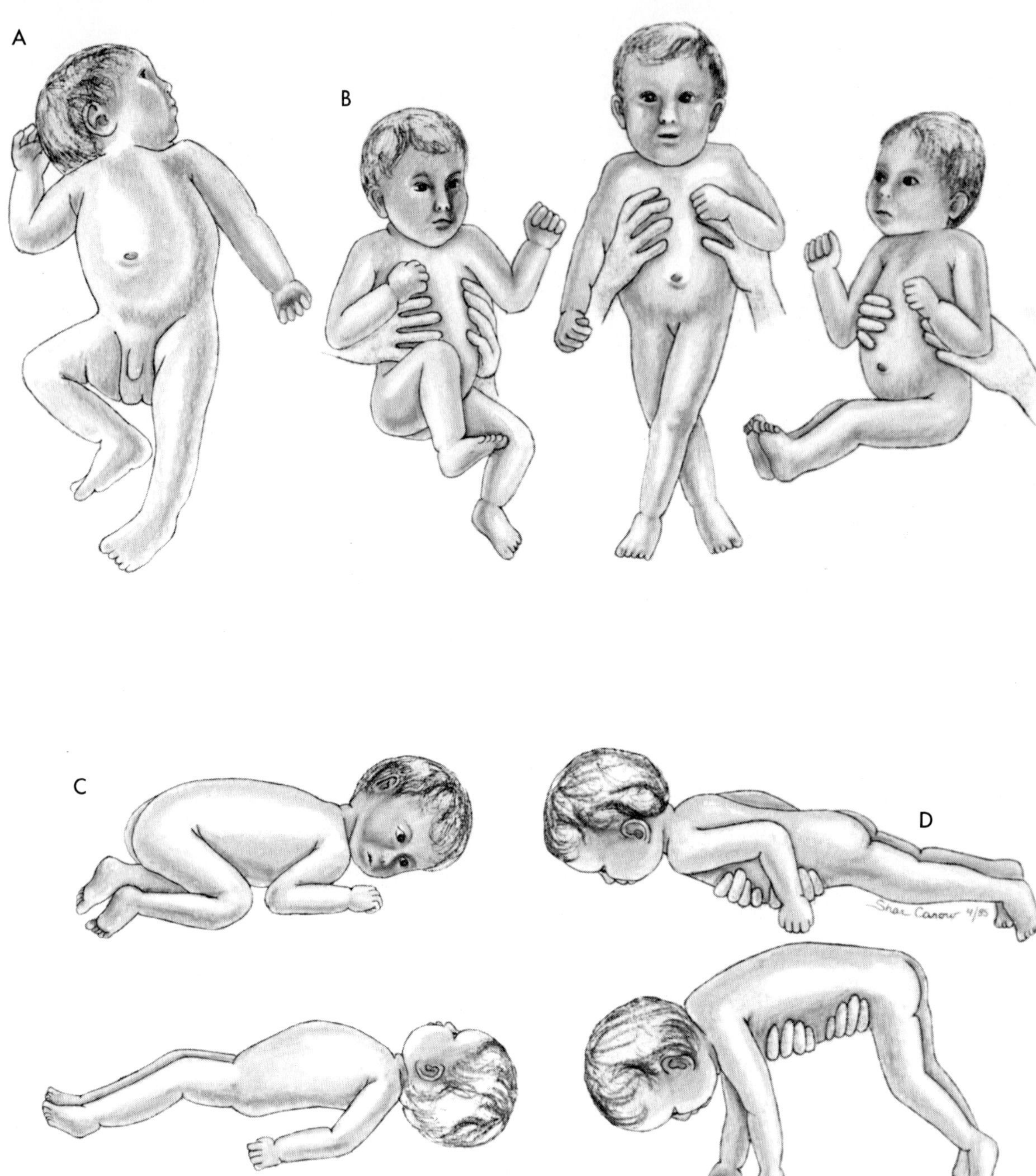

Fig. 25-4. Abnormal positions seen in cerebral palsy. **A,** Asymmetric tonic neck reflex (ATNR). **B,** Extensor spasticity of the legs. **C,** Tonic labyrinthine reflex. **D,** Landau reflex. *Top,* Reaction of normal child (age 3 months to 3 years). *Bottom,* Child with cerebral palsy. From Hellquist J: Cerebral Palsy, Physician's Assistant 80:25, 1985.

This is complicated because, even though it may be suspected at birth that an infant has cerebral palsy, cerebral palsy usually is not diagnosed until after six months of age because of the absence of reliable neonatal neurologic signs and because impairment of voluntary motor control cannot be seen until two to four months of age. Clues that can alert the nurse to the possible existence of cerebral palsy in the young infant are summarized in the following box.

CLUES TO THE PRESENCE OF CEREBRAL PALSY IN INFANTS

1. Is there any history of potential neurologic insult, such as anoxia, hemorrhage, prematurity or metabolic disturbance in the prenatal, perinatal, or postnatal period?
2. Have developmental delays in fine and gross motor achievements, such as delays in raising the head, sitting, and crawling, been noted? This is especially significant if the child's development in other areas is not delayed.
3. Have any abnormalities in the performance of motor activities, such as difficulties with nursing or feeding, including tongue thrust, non–lip closure, inability to suck effectively, and difficulties with swallowing, facial grimacing, writhing movement of the extremities, and lack of movement, been noted?
4. Does the child assume any abnormal postures such as scissoring of extremities, asymmetric tonic neck reflex, and tonic labyrinthine reflex at rest or with movement? (See Fig. 25-4)
5. Have the primitive infantile neurologic reflexes persisted past when you would normally expect to see them be extinguished or are these primitive reflexes weaker or stronger than you would expect to see? Are they asymmetric?
6. Does the child exhibit alterations in muscle tone such as spasticity, hypotonicity, or absence of a Landau reflex, as shown in Fig. 25-4?
7. Do you observe other impairments, such as seizures or sensory impairments, that usually coexist with cerebral palsy?

Modified from Whaley LL and Wong DL: Nursing care of infants and children, ed 3, St Louis, 1987, CV Mosby Co.

Planning

A multidisciplinary team approach is used in the treatment of cerebral palsy. Since the neurologic damage in cerebral palsy is permanent, therapy is aimed at maximizing functional abilities. A family-based treatment program is best. Parental involvement is essential. The treatment team often consists of the physician, rehabilitation nurse, psychologist, physical therapist, occupational therapist, orthopedist, speech therapist, teacher, and social worker. The major goals of therapy include the following (Whaley, 1987):

1. Promotion of locomotion and communication
2. Correction of defects
3. Establishment of self-care
4. Provision of educational opportunities based on a careful assessment of each individual (Whaley, 1987).

To achieve locomotion and self-care, braces and splints may be used. Early referrals to visual and auditory specialists and speech pathologists and therapists facilitate communication.

Orthopedic surgery may be used to decrease muscle imbalances and the stress they cause. The most common surgery done for people with cerebral palsy is tendon-lengthening procedures and osteotomy to realign and stabilize joints. Medications to decrease spasticity have little use in improving overall function but may be used in an attempt to decrease spasticity. Antianxiety agents may be administered to clients with continual motion or excessive tension. Individuals who also have seizures (estimated to be as high as 50% of clients with cerebral palsy) receive antiseizure medications.

Community-Based Nursing Care

Nurses are involved in all aspects of care for children and adults with cerebral palsy and are in the best position to provide guidance and support to the family. Since people with cerebral palsy are essentially "well" people with a chronic disability, most of the nurse's interventions are directed toward home-based care, the overall goal being to help the client capitalize on abilities and minimize or compensate for any disabilities.

Implementation

The diagnosis of cerebral palsy is only the beginning. After the diagnosis the nurse can begin to provide guidance and support to the individual and family that enables maximization of the individual's potential for independence. The major functions of the nurse are to help the individual and family identify specific needs and how they might be met. General features of a home-based nursing care plan categorized by nursing diagnoses for an individual with cerebral palsy include the following:

1. The nursing care plan for individuals in whom alterations in health maintenance is diagnosed includes routine physical examinations; dental care; age-appropriate health screening such as Papanicolaou and glaucoma testing; maintenance of a balanced diet; attention to weight; vigorous, prompt treatment of chronic constipation and other effects of immobility; regular immunizations; a well-regulated daily schedule to prevent fatigue; and adequate sleep and rest.
2. The nursing care plan for individuals in whom impaired verbal communication is diagnosed includes early referral to speech therapists; early referral for hearing evaluation and routine screening; encouraging parents to talk to their child slowly and using articles or pictures to reinforce speech and warning them that responses may be slow in developing; maintaining eye contact while speaking, even if a communicative device or an interpreter is present; allowing sufficient time for the individual to answer; teaching parents feeding techniques that facilitate the development of speech by use of the lips, teeth, and various tongue movements; and employing and teaching augmentative communication methods to dysarthric individuals using Bliss symbol and word boards, signing, optic devices, and electronic voice simulators or microprocessor computers.
3. The nursing care plan for individuals in whom impaired physical mobility is diagnosed includes teaching parents skills in handling disabled children and allowing them an opportunity for supervised practice; employing aids or helping families secure aids to facilitate locomotion and allow families and individuals with cerebral palsy an opportunity to practice with supervision; referring individuals with cerebral palsy to physical or occupational therapy for evaluation as needed; evaluating the disabled individual's environment and assistive devices to prevent injury (individuals may need to wear helmets or may need restraints in their wheelchairs if seizures are not controlled); encouraging sitting, crawling, and walking at appropriate ages; providing for rest before and after exercise; providing motivators for locomotion, especially for children, and incorporating exercises into a play activity; preventing deformity by teaching the family correct usage of braces and splints; and teaching stretching exercises and active and passive range of motion exercises.
4. The nursing care plan for individuals in whom altered growth and development is diagnosed includes screening for additional impairments, such as speech, hearing, and vision impairments and seizure disorders, that might affect the child's cognitive performance; selecting toys and activities that provide both sensory and motor input and encourage both bimanual and unimanual activity; talking to adults or children with

cerebral palsy at their mental level, encouraging attendance at schools that meet the individual's needs; encouraging children to become involved with other children who have similar problems; and encouraging recreational outlets and after-school activities such as handicapped camping, Girl Scouts or Boy Scouts, and special horseback riding programs for disabled individuals.

5. The nursing care plan for individuals in whom self-care deficits and self-concept disturbances are diagnosed includes promoting a positive self-image, capitalizing on individuals' assets and compensating for any liabilities, and praising individuals for work accomplishment and partial accomplishment of a task; encouraging individuals with cerebral palsy to assist in their own care; adapting utensils, food, and clothing to facilitate self-help by padding and weighting utensils, using finger foods and nonslippery, textured foods, and sewing Velcro fasteners in clothing; assisting families in toilet training their children and establishing feeding, bathing, grooming, dressing, and undressing routines; assisting families in setting realistic goals and preventing undue pressures to accomplish goals; and teaching children skills for independent learning and referring children for vocational counseling as they reach adolescence.
6. The nursing care plan for individuals in whom family coping: potential for growth is diagnosed includes encouraging early participation in a treatment program; allowing parents and siblings to discuss their feelings about cerebral palsy and the effect it has had on their lives; evaluating the amount of stress caused by care of the individual and the existence and efficacy of the coping mechanisms being used; helping families work toward a realistic view of the capabilities and outlook for the future of individuals with cerebral palsy; referring families for counseling as needed and encouraging participation in parental groups; and referring families to community organizations providing special services to individuals with cerebral palsy.

Community Resources

There are a variety of community resources that provide services to individuals with cerebral palsy, and often the nurse can advise families of these services and how they might be used. Since other impairments may coexist with cerebral palsy, services for the other impairments should also be contacted.

Nationally the United Cerebral Palsy Association, Inc. promotes education in regard to cerebral palsy, aids cerebral palsy research, and promotes early diagnosis and treatment. Local chapters often provide direct client services such as nursery school for children 3 to 4 years of age, kindergarten classes for children 5 to 6 years of age, educational day-care developmental classes for children 5 to 16 years of age, and social recreation for individuals older than 16 years of age. Appendix 25-1 contains a list of community resources available to help individuals with cerebral palsy and their families.

Visual Impairment

Incidence

It has been estimated that approximately 1 million Americans are blind with 50,000 new cases being added to that total annually (Brunner, 1984). This number is increasing because each year there are more people older than 65 years of age in the United States.

Definition

There are many degrees of visual loss or impairment. Blindness does not necessarily mean total loss of sight. Legal blindness is defined as less than 20 degrees of visual field or a corrected vision of 20/200 or worse in the better eye (Luckmann, 1980). Therefore some "blind" people may be able to distinguish size, shape, and color and in some instances even read large print with corrective lenses. The degree of visual loss has implications for the planning of nursing care, treatment, and rehabilitation, since many individuals with impaired vision are eligible for financial aid, tax deductions, or nonfinancial aids such as talking books, braillewriters, and large print materials.

Cause

There are many different factors that are known to cause visual impairment and blindness; they include infections, trauma, normal changes seen secondary to aging, intrinsic eye diseases, and systemic diseases. However, 40% of all blindness can be attributed to three disorders—cataracts, which are surgically correctable, glaucoma, which usually can be prevented with treatment, and diabetes mellitus, which has an improved prognosis with the newer forms of treatment.

Community-Based Nursing Care

Community health nurses can interact with visually impaired individuals in three areas—prevention, casefinding, and management.

Prevention

Nurses are often in an ideal position to teach individuals and families about care of the eyes and the prevention of blindness. For individuals older than 40 years of age yearly eye examinations with tonometry (measurement of intraocular tension) are as important as regular physical examinations, since findings in the eye are often a reflection of general health. Nurses should encourage eye safety measures such as wearing safety goggles and using protective sports equipment and shatterproof glass in automobiles and eyeglasses. Families should be made aware of the possibility of damage to the eyes from toys or fireworks.

Nurses aid in the prevention of visual impairment by conducting vision screening clinics for preschoolers and seeing that there are routine eye examinations carried out in schools. Parents should be alerted to the importance of the early identification and treatment of strabismus to prevent strabismic amblyopia (cortical suppression of central vision because of disuse). Parents should be taught the importance of early treatment of eye disorders and to avoid the use of home remedies and, more important, eye drops prescribed for another person or another disorder. There are seven danger signals seen in the eye that require immediate medical evaluation. They include the following (Luckmann, 1984):

1. Changes in vision status such as persistent diplopia, floaters, sudden loss of vision, and rainbow halos around lights
2. Redness of the eye
3. Pain in or around the eye
4. Opacities in the transparent portions of the eyes or growths on the eyelids
5. Crossing of the eyes
6. Irregularities of the pupil
7. Persistent discharge from the eyes or crusting or tearing of the eyes

If any of these symptoms are detected, the individual should seek prompt medical treatment.

Assessment

A thorough, comprehensive history should be obtained on any clients who have a complaint involving the eye. Eye pain and loss of vision are always considered important symptoms and should be referred immediately for further evaluation. The nurse should obtain a history of the present illness including any past history of problems with the eyes, trauma to the head or eyes, and systemic diseases, especially those known to cause ocular symptoms, including diabetes, thyroid disease, hypertension, connective tissue disorders, blood dyscrasia, neurologic disease, and renal disease. A family history of eye problems should be obtained, since a strong hereditary component has been associated with certain ocular tumors, various degenerative disorders of the eye, glaucoma, myopia, and strabismus. The client's occupation should be noted with regard to any job hazards and safety precautions used. Hazardous types of recreation, as well as alcohol and drug use and any history of sexually transmitted diseases, should also be noted. The present status of the visual impairment, that is, temporary or permanent, and the length of time the individual has been impaired, as well as the patient's self-care capabilities, should be obtained. Visual loss, whether temporary or permanent, has major psychosocial implications for both affected individuals and their families. During the course of the interview it is important to assess the degree of acceptance of the impairment. That is, does the client exhibit any evidence of body image disturbance, anxiety, powerlessness? It is also important to assess the coping mechanisms being used and their effectiveness and the adequacy of support from family or significant others (Tucker, 1984). Community resources currently used by clients and their families should be noted.

A review of systems for the eye might include asking clients whether they experience any of the following (Luckmann, 1980):

1. Pain
2. Foreign body sensations
3. Retinal or vitreous hemorrhages
4. Scotomas (blind spots)
5. Proptosis (abnormal displacement or "bulging" of the eye)
6. Loss of vision or blurred vision
7. Diplopia
8. Headaches, nausea, or vomiting
9. Photophobia
10. Conjunctival discharge or subconjunctival hemorrhages
11. "Spots" or "floaters" in front of their eyes
12. "Showers of sparks" before their eyes
13. "Halos" or "rainbows around lights"
14. "Curtains passing in front of their eyes"

In young children it may be difficult to obtain a history of visual changes or impairment. However, there are behavioral clues that alert the nurse to the need for an eye examination. Some of these clues include the following (Whaley, 1987):

1. Lack of orientation response to a stimulus such as not following a moving light or lack of eye contact with caregiver
2. Excessive rubbing of the eyes
3. Holding books or toys close to eyes
4. Poor school performance
5. Clumsiness and inaccurate judgments in picking objects up
6. Squinting or frowning
7. Closing one eye or tilting head to side to see

Any of these behaviors seen in a young child should cue the nurse to investigate further. In this situation early identification and treatment may prevent further visual impairment.

Physical signs of eye disorders include redness or swelling of the eye or adnexa oculi, excessive tearing, blepharospasm, corneal haziness or opacities, foreign bodies in the eye, enlargement of the eyeball with or without proptosis, heterophoria (misalignment of the eyes), discharge from the eyes, nystagmus, lesions around the eyes or on the eyelids, ptosis, lacerations or contusions, and loss or defects in peripheral field vision. The nurse who becomes proficient in the use of the ophthalmoscope can also gather further information on the client's visual status by carefully assessing the ocular fundus—the condition of the lens and the retina including the optic disc, retinal background, arterioles and venules, and macula.

Planning

Rehabilitation of visually impaired individuals is directed toward normalizing their lives as much as possible. The nurse can often guide the client

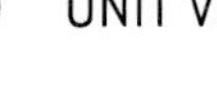

WHAT EVERYBODY SHOULD KNOW ABOUT BLINDNESS

WHEN YOU MEET A BLIND PERSON YOU SHOULD ALWAYS DO THE FOLLOWING:

Identify yourself.
If there are others present, address the person by name so that there is no mistake to whom you are talking.
Remember that an unseen smile can be conveyed by a warm handshake and a friendly tone of voice.
Talk directly to the blind person and not through a companion.
Be sure blind people know when you leave so that they aren't left talking to an empty space.

WHEN YOU ARE TALKING WITH A BLIND PERSON YOU SHOULD ALWAYS DO THE FOLLOWING:

Don't worry about avoiding words such as "look," "see," and "blind"—most blind people are not offended by these words and use them in their own speech.
Use a normal tone of voice—most blind people have normal hearing, so there is no need to shout.

WHEN OFFERING ASSISTANCE TO A BLIND PERSON YOU SHOULD ALWAYS DO THE FOLLOWING:

If you think a blind person needs help, offer assistance but allow the person to decide whether help is needed.
If you escort blind people somewhere, offer your arm and let them hold on just above your elbow—you will find this is the easiest and most comfortable way to walk together.
When seating a blind person, placing the individual's hand on the back of the chair allows the person to be seated independently.
If you must leave blind people alone for a few minutes, leave them in contact with some stationary object.
When giving directions, make them as clear as possible—use *left* and *right* according to the way the blind person is facing.
Remember to be verbal—hand gestures are meaningless to a blind person.

ALSO:

When dining with a blind person, read the menu and the prices; describe the position of food on the plate; if more help is needed, the person will ask.
It is best to leave doors fully opened or closed—a door left ajar can be confusing, especially for a person with partial sight.
Do not rearrange things in a blind person's home or work setting; if something must be moved for safety reasons, be sure to inform the person of the change.
Do not pet or otherwise distract a guide dog because blind persons' safety depends on their dogs' attention—do not touch or offer food without the master's permission.

Courtesy Blind Association of Western New York.

into a beginning rehabilitation program. The basic philosophy of this program should be similar to that of the nursing care plan in that both should be focused on clients' assets and not their disabilities.

When working with visually impaired individuals, especially a blind client, the community health nurse should be aware of some helpful guidelines. These guidelines are summarized in the preceding box. Nursing interventions in a community setting are mainly involved with assistance in learning self-care activities and client and family education.

Implementation

General features of a community-based home nursing care plan categorized by nursing diagnoses for an individual with visual impairment include the following:

1. The nursing care plan for individuals in whom impaired home maintenance management is diagnosed includes assessing the arrangement of furniture, clutter, and rugs on floor; making sure the client and family understand the importance of leaving furniture and commonly used articles in the same place; encouraging clients not to smoke when they are alone or in bed; encouraging regular rest and exercise; and stressing the importance of ongoing visual care.
2. The nursing care plan for individuals in whom impaired physical mobility is diagnosed includes helping clients explore their environments, including location of commonly used utensils, doors, and windows; using clients' sense of touch in familiarizing them to new environments; always identifying yourself when approaching clients and explaining the purpose of visits; and never touching clients without first identifying yourself.
3. The nursing care plan for individuals in whom self-care deficits are diagnosed in-

cludes assessing what clients can do for themselves, helping them learn self-care activities, and withdrawing assistance gradually; helping clients find clothing without a lot of buttons and shoes without laces; using clock orientation for describing food placement and location of bath equipment; explaining events before they happen; providing outlets for client frustration and verbalization of anxiety; helping clients use their senses of touch, smell, and hearing to the fullest potential; and using assistive devices when appropriate.

4. The nursing care plan for clients and families in whom knowledge deficits are diagnosed includes making sure the client and family understand the nature of the disability, its prognosis and treatment, and the goals of both the medical and nursing care plans; advising clients to wear sunglasses if they are photophobic or using mydriatric eye drops; advising clients to use extra lighting if they are experiencing difficulty with night vision or using miotic eye drops; making sure the client and family are familiar with any eye medications prescribed, including the medications' generic and trade names, purpose, dosage, side effects, and method and time of administration (even if the client is independent in this area of self-care, a family member should also be familiar with the procedure in case the client becomes incapacitated), advising the client to have an extra bottle of eye medications available, especially when traveling; making sure the client and family are aware of the signs and symptoms that should be reported to the eye physician immediately (these include headache, fever, eye pain, changes in visual acuity, discharge from the eyes, or any changes in the appearance of the eyes); counseling clients not to use other individuals' eye medications or over-the-counter medications without checking with a physician.
5. The nursing care plan for individuals in whom social isolation, disturbances in self-concept, and ineffective individual and family coping are diagnosed includes involving the client in care as much as possible to enhance self-esteem; providing for recreational activities and participation in groups with similar disabilities; encouraging independence; avoiding overprotectiveness and excessive sympathy; being aware that the client may still have a body image disturbance or may still be in the stage of denial or grieving over the loss of sight; assessing whether clients have ways of venting their feelings and whether they have a significant other to talk to; referring client and family to community organizations providing services to visually impaired individuals.

Home-Based Care of Clients with Diabetes

Since diabetes is one of the major factors causing visual impairment, the nurse should be familiar with the resources available to help clients be independent in their self-care. Table 25-4 identifies five major self-care tasks necessary for clients with diabetes and possible interventions that might be implemented to assist in these tasks. Although this list is by no means exhaustive, it does show how simple items such as magnifiers, lights, and highlighters can help keep clients independent. Most of these resources are fairly inexpensive and can be purchased at local drugstores or discount department stores. Literature is also available to the nurse in working with the blind diabetic in the areas of meal preparation, self-care, and activities of daily living (Van Son, 1982). A variety of self-help aids are also available for use with the blind person with diabetes.

Hearing Impairment

In their daily practice community health nurses often encounter individuals with a variety of degrees of hearing impairments. Hearing impair-

TABLE 25-4 Guide to Low-Vision Interventions—Diabetes Self-Care

Task	Interventions	Task	Intervention
Indicating units on a U-100 insulin syringe	Handheld magnifiers Magnifying glasses Stapelet Insulin needle guide C-Better magnifiers for syringe Low-dose syringe 100 watt lighting Use of gooseneck lamp	Identifying and interpreting Keto-diastix values	Use of Megadiastix Magnifying glasses Magnifiers 100 watt lighting Use of interpretation charts with large color areas (reagent areas) Enlargement of test strip (color area and stem) Labeling with large letters Interpretation of chart colors Talking blood analyzer Talking urine analyzer
Reading an insulin label	Magnifiers Magnifying glasses Large printed labels from pharmacy 100 watt lighting Use of highlighter for identification Use of rubber band for identification Hand-lettered large print labels in black ink against a white background	Inspection of skin for changes secondary to diabetes such as erythema (infection), presence of skin lesions (insulin allergy), lipodystrophy	Palpating areas of insulin injection for heat; nodules; tenderness; hypertrophy; atrophy Use of magnifiers (especially over insulin injection sites) Magnifying glasses 100 watt lighting Gooseneck lamps Repositioning extremities for better inspection Use of magnification mirrors for areas that cannot be seen directly
Reading oral hypoglycemic agent label	As above		

Modified from Skelly A and Van Son-Martinez A: 1985.

ments are the most prevalent type of disability seen in the United States, with more individuals being affected than those with heart disease, impairments of vision, or other types of chronic disabilities (You and Your Deaf Patient, 1978).

Definition

Individuals can be said to be hearing impaired, deaf, or hard of hearing. Hearing-impaired individuals are those whose hearing deficits have prevented them from developing proper language, participating in conversation, or living a productive life. A hard-of-hearing individual is one who has a hearing impairment but sufficient ability to understand speech, often with a hearing aid. A deaf individual has total lack of hearing or hearing impairment so severe that everyday auditory communication is impossible or nearly impossible (Davis and Silverman, 1978).

Incidence

There are approximately 14 million people in the United States who are hearing impaired, and 6.5 million of these people have a significant bilateral impairment that makes it difficult to both hear and understand speech. In the United States 1 million people are deaf (You and Your Deaf Patient, 1978). It has been estimated that 5% of schoolchildren in the United States have some type of hearing impairment and that almost half of these children have impairments severe enough to require special educational and speech services.

Cause

A number of causes of hearing impairment have been identified. In adults, primary ear disorders, such as otitis media, otosclerosis, Ménière's disease, mastoiditis, labyrinthitis, acoustic nerve tumors, and presbyacusis, systemic disorders, such as onset of anemia, neurologic disorders, renal disease, diabetes mellitus, hypertension, and syphilis, trauma, such as head injuries, and drugs are all factors that have been implicated in hearing loss.

In children, the causes of hearing impairment can be classified according to when the damage occurred—prenatally, natally, or postnatally. Prenatal causes of hearing impairment include congenital malformations of the ear, hereditary factors, and rubella. Natal causes include prematurity, hypoxia, and trauma caused by delivery. Postnatal causes of hearing impairment in children include rubeola, rubella, scarlet fever, pertussis, meningitis, severe jaundice in the newborn, or Rh incompatibility. Prolonged use of certain ototoxic medications can also cause a permanent type of sensorineural hearing loss in both adults and children. Otitis media is the major cause of a reversible type of conductive hearing loss in childhood. Prompt treatment of otitis media during childhood can prevent permanent disability.

Community-Based Nursing Care

Community nurses can interact with hearing-impaired individuals in three areas—prevention, casefinding, and management.

Prevention

Prevention of hearing loss in the community involves attention to the amount and type of environmental noise, use of safety precautions in loud situations, community education about the relationship of medications and hearing loss, and the prompt treatment of ear infections.

The amount of environmental noise present in the work, home, and social settings, as well as the provision and use of protective devices in loud situations, should be assessed. Although research is still being conducted on the overall effect of noise on the human body, it has been found that exposure to noise of 90 dB or greater has distinct physiologic effects including contraction of the stomach muscles, flushing of the skin, and increased emotional outbursts. Loud persistent noise can cause constriction of peripheral blood vessels and difficulty with equilibrium (Brunner, 1984). The length of exposure to extensive noise also affects the risk of hearing impairment.

Clients and families should be knowledgeable about the relationship of medications and hearing loss. Certain drugs and chemicals are known to be ototoxic. Certain cytotoxic and diuretic drugs are also known to cause hearing impairment. A brief list of these agents is shown in the following box. When nurses take a medication history, they should remember that certain drugs and chemicals are ototoxic and should find out to what extent the individual has used these agents. Clients with a history of renal disease are especially sensitive to the effects of these medications.

Middle ear problems, such as dysfunction of the eustachian tube leading to otitis media, can cause hearing impairment if treatment is delayed or inadequate. Parents should be told of the importance of prompt treatment of these disorders.

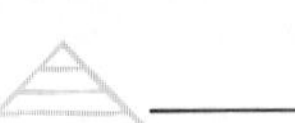

KNOWN OTOTOXIC AGENTS

Acetylsalicylic acid
Chloramphenicol
Chloroquine
Ethacrynic acid
Furosemide
Gentamicin
Kanamycin
Neomycin
Nitrofurantoin
Polymyxin B
Quinidine
Quinine
Streptomycin
Tobramycin
Vancomycin
Viomycin

Community nurses further aid in the prevention of hearing impairment by conducting hearing acuity screening clinics for preschoolers and making sure there is a routine program of audiometry examinations carried out in the schools. Children who have impaired hearing should be referred to a member of the health care team for immediate evaluation and treatment.

Thompson and Bowers (1980) list six risk factors for the potential development of hearing deficiencies. The risk factors include the following:

1. History of a long exposure to loud noise
2. History of medication sensitivity
3. History of chronic nasal allergies
4. Long history of cigarette smoking
5. History of systemic disease associated with hearing impairment, including diabetes mellitus, renal disease, and hypertension
6. Generalized physical or emotional disability (which is correlated with diminished acuity of hearing)

Identifying any of these risk factors promptly could prevent permanent loss of hearing.

Assessment

A thorough, comprehensive history should be obtained on any client with a complaint involving the ear. A history of the current illness should be taken using the analysis of symptoms format. Nurses should assess the degree of onset of the problem, that is, gradual or acute, the specific type of sounds that the individual has difficulting hearing, such as the doorbell or stove timer, the type of treatment or assistive devices the client has tried and their result, and the degree to which the hearing problem interferes with the client's life. Nurses should also note any history of trauma or injury to the ears, including foreign bodies in the ears, harsh wax removal, and exposure to environmental noise, and any history of the systemic diseases that are associated with loss of hearing. A history of recent problems with the mouth, throat, nose or paranasal sinuses, as well as any dental work, should be taken. In addition, the nurse should take history of childhood ear problems or infections, their frequency and treatment, and any residual problems. A family history of ear disorders or loss of hearing should be obtained. The nurse should take a careful history of exposure to ototoxic agents, as well as exposure to environmental or employment noise. If the client reports a positive history of such exposure, the extent of the exposure and any safety precautions used should be noted. Finally, a history of sexually transmitted diseases, recreational hazards such as swimming in polluted waters, and the use of alcohol and tobacco should be obtained. As with visual loss, the present status of the hearing impairment, that is, temporary or permanent, and the length of time the individual has been impaired should be noted.

Hearing loss has major psychosocial implications for both affected individuals and their families. Impairment in hearing may affect not only the way individuals communicate, but also their basic personality, awareness of surroundings, and safety. During the course of the interview it is important for nurses to assess the degree of acceptance of the impairment. They must note any evidence of disruption of body image such as loss, grief, or shame, anxiety, powerlessness, as well as coping mechanisms being used, their effectiveness, and the adequacy of support from family and significant others. Community resources the client is using should also be noted.

A review of systems for the ear and hearing loss might include asking clients whether they have any of the following signs or symptoms:

1. Pain or discomfort in the ear
2. Active discharge from the ear noting color, consistency, amount, odor, duration, and associated symptoms
3. Decreased or absent hearing noting whether it is unilateral or bilateral
4. Any trauma to the ear
5. Excessive cerumen
6. Congenital deformities of the ears
7. Foreign bodies in the ear
8. Vertigo (a sense of whirling or rotation)
9. Dizziness (lightheadedness)
10. Tinnitus (ringing or buzzing in the ears)
11. Nausea or vomiting
12. Headache
13. Changes in speech such as slurring of words, dropped endings of words or excessive nasality
14. Feeling of fullness in ear or own voice echoing
15. "Popping" sensation in ear when swallowing
16. Use of cotton swabs or hairpins to clean ears
17. Use of a hearing aid or another type of assistive device
18. Ability to read lips or use sign language

If a client's parent states that the client is using a hearing aid, the nurse might wish to question the client further about the functioning of the device and find out whether the client hears any whistling noises or has static interference or pain from the mold.

In young children it may be difficult to obtain a history of hearing impairment. However, there are certain behavioral clues that should alert the nurse to the need for a hearing examination (Your Child's Hearing, 1977).

Clues Suggesting Hearing Impairment

In the newborn the absence of the startle reflex to a handclap at three to six feet suggests hearing impairment. In children eight to 12 months of age hearing impairment should be suspected if they do not turn their heads toward familiar sounds or vocalize in response to their mothers. Children 18 months of age should be able to use a few single words if their hearing is not impaired. Children 2 years of age who are unable to follow a simple command without a visual clue, children 3 years of age who are unable to localize the source of a sound, children 4 years of age who are unable to give a cohesive account of a recent experience or follow a two-step command, and children 5 years of age whose speech is difficult to understand or who are unable to carry on a simple conversion may be hearing impaired. Finally, school-age children who have lack of attention or concentration and whose school performance is poor may be hearing impaired. Children exhibiting any of these behaviors should be assessed further. Early identification and treatment of hearing problems can prevent further hearing impairment.

Physical signs of disorders of the ears include an abnormal configuration of the ears, low-set or unequal positioning of the auricle, redness, tenderness, swelling, lesions or nodules of the auricle, and bleeding or discharge from the external auditory meatus. The nurse who has become proficient in the use of the otoscope can also gather further information on the client's tympanic membrane and condition of the external auditory canal including swelling, inflammation, growths, presence of cerumen, discharge, or presence of foreign bodies. Abnormalities of the tympanic membrane include perforation, bulging or retraction, lack of movement when the Valsalva maneuver is applied or when swallowing, obliteration of the classic landmarks, hyperemia (increased vascularization), and color changes. Normally the tympanic membrane is pearly gray and reflects the light from the otoscope. When infected the tympanic membrane is red or pink. A yellow-amber tympanic membrane indicates the collection of serous fluid behind the eardrum; a bluish tympanic membrane indicates the presence of blood. A tuning fork helps distinguish between sensorineural and conductive types of hearing loss.

Planning

Rehabilitation of hearing-impaired individuals is directed toward normalizing their lives as much as possible. The nurse can often guide the client into a beginning rehabilitation program. The basic philosophy of a rehabilitation program should be similar to that of a nursing care plan in that both should be focused on a client's assets, not disabilities.

When working with hearing-impaired individuals, nurses should be aware of some helpful guidelines, which are summarized in the following box. Nursing interventions in a community setting mainly involve establishing a means of communication, maintaining a safe environment, and educating the client and family.

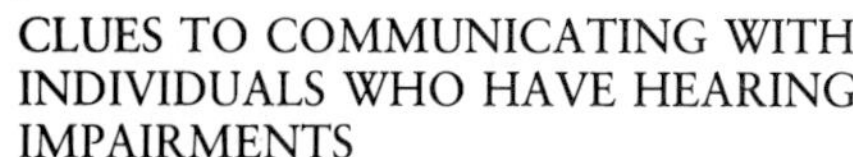

CLUES TO COMMUNICATING WITH INDIVIDUALS WHO HAVE HEARING IMPAIRMENTS

Face the individual directly on the same level within 4 feet.
Never stand with your back to a window.
Speak slowly; do not exaggerate your lip movements.
Avoid talking with your mouth full.
Avoid having more than one person speak to the client at once.
Give full attention to the individual.
Try to anticipate replies.
Speak in simple phrases and rephrase as necessary.
Do not obscure the client's view of your mouth.
Indicate the subject of the conversation by pointing.
Pause more frequently than you would in normal conversation.
If you are unsure whether the client understands the communication, write the message to prevent misunderstandings.

IF THE CLIENTS' SPEECH IS DIFFICULT TO UNDERSTAND NURSES SHOULD ALWAYS DO THE FOLLOWING:

Engage clients in conversation frequently so that you are familiar with their speech patterns.
Allow clients time to answer.
Try to catch the essential meaning of what is being said.
Do *not* indicate that you understand the client if you do not.
If you cannot understand what clients are saying, have them write it down. Having clients read their written messages aloud helps you become more familiar with speech patterns.

IF THE CLIENT IS USING A HEARING AID NURSES SHOULD ALWAYS DO THE FOLLOWING:

Make sure the hearing aid is turned on.
Make sure the pitch is adjusted to a comfortable level for the client.
Follow the same guidelines as for other hearing-impaired individuals.

Implementation

The general features of a community, home-based nursing care plan categorized by nursing diagnoses for hearing-impaired individuals include the following:

1. The nursing care plan for individuals in whom impaired home maintenance management is diagnosed includes locating clients' beds so that they can see the door; orienting clients to surroundings, since hearing impaired individuals use sight and touch extensively and are sensitive to movement and light changes; employing a call bell for summoning assistance; installing flashing lights and amplifiers to augment doorbells, telephones, timers, and alarm clocks; and making sure lighting is adequate,

since it is critical for visibility when communicating with other individuals.

2. The nursing care plan for individuals in whom alterations in communication is diagnosed includes making sure clients have a pad and pencil available; allowing clients time to answer; and writing messages simply, using short phrases.
   a. If clients *can read lips* (speechreaders), avoid having more than one person talk to the client at one time; speak slowly, be natural, and do not exaggerate sounds; position yourself within four feet of clients, facing them; stay on the same visual plane as the client; never talk with your back to a window, since light should be on your face; speak in simple phrases and rephrase if clients have difficulty understanding; indicate the subject of conversation by printing if possible; consider use of hearing guide dogs to assist impaired masters.
   b. If *clients* use sign language, determine whether they use American Sign Language (ASL)—the nurse can use a pad and pencil for this; locate an interpreter—a family member may fill this role; and talk directly to them—stand or sit next to the interpreter so that the client can see both of you.
   c. If the client has a hearing aid, make sure it is in place and turned on; and establish a comfortable pitch while standing where the client can see you (Tucker, 1984).
3. The nursing plan for individuals in whom social isolation, disturbances in self-concept, and ineffectiveness individual and family coping are diagnosed includes providing for adequate rest, since many deaf individuals are fatigued by the energy expended in communication; encouraging communication with significant others; maintaining a quiet, nonstressful environment; encouraging verbalizations and being aware of body language; waking clients by placing the hand gently on one arm if their eyes are closed; avoiding overprotectiveness and excessive sympathy; letting clients actively participate in their own care; trying to involve clients with groups of individuals who have similar disabilities; and providing for diversional activities, hobbies, and travel.
4. The nursing care plan for individuals in whom client and family knowledge deficits are diagnosed includes making sure the client and family understand the nature of the disability, its prognosis and treatment, and the goals of both the medical and nursing care plan; making sure the client and family are familiar with ear medications prescribed, including the medications generic and trade names, purpose, dosage, side effects, and method and time of administration; making sure the client and family are aware of the signs and symptoms that should be reported to a physician immediately, including changes in hearing acuity, ear pain, discharge, persistent tinnitus, vertigo, and lightheadedness; advising the client to have duplicate prescriptions for ear medications available when traveling; advising clients not to use other people's medications or over-the-counter medications without checking with their physician first; and referring clients and families to community organizations that provide services to hearing-impaired individuals.

SUMMARY

Community-based nurses play an active role in the lives of physically handicapped people and people needing rehabilitation through prevention of disability, casefinding, which enables earlier interventions and better prognoses, and management, a joint client-nurse approach to normalization of the client's life with maximization of optimum levels of functioning.

It is important that nurses be aware of the signs and symptoms of various disabilities they may encounter in the community and knowledgeable about nursing interventions that would benefit the clients and their families. Knowledge of community resources that may provide services to the disabled client is also essential to the total team rehabilitation effort.

Above all it is important for nurses to remember that the disabled person is a unique individual who is worthy of respect and often admiration. Disabled clients should remain active participants in their own care and help make decisions about the objectives the nursing care plan addresses. Through recognition of these facts and modeling of a humanistic attitude toward the disabled, the nurse may also be instrumental in changing some of the age-old stereotypes about the physically handicapped.

QUESTIONS FOR DISCUSSION

1. When clients and their families are faced with a new disability, they often go through a period of crisis. How might the nurse be helpful in this situation?
2. What kinds of barriers are faced by disabled persons?
3. Describe the nursing process as it relates to a client with cerebral palsy.
4. What suggestions can the nurse make to help a partially blind diabetic client better cope with the home environment?
5. List five age-appropriate clues that might suggest a hearing impairment at various points in the life span.

REFERENCES

American Nurses Association: Standards of community health nursing practice, Kansas City, Mo, 1973, The Association.

Barrell LM: Crisis intervention—partnership in problem solving, Nurs Clin North Am 9:9, 1974.

Bowe F: Handicapping America—barriers to disabled people, New York, 1978, Harper & Row, Publishers Inc.

Brunner LS and Suddarth D: Textbook of medical-surgical nursing, ed 5, Philadelphia, 1984, JB Lippincott Co.

Davis H and Silverman SR: Hearing and deafness, ed 4, New York, 1978, Holt, Reinhardt & Winston Inc.

Diamond M and Jones SL: Chronic illness across the life span, New York, 1983, Appleton & Lange.

Finnie NR: Handling the young cerebral palsied child, ed 2, New York, 1975, EP Dutton.

Haber L and Smith RJ: Disability and deviance, Soc Secur Bull 30:17, 1967.

Janken JK: The nurse in crisis, Nurs Clin North Am 9:18, 1974.

Jarvis LL: Community health nursing: keeping the public healthy, ed 2, Philadelphia, 1985. FA Davis Co.

Luckmann J and Sorensen K: Medical-surgical nursing, ed 2, Philadelphia, 1955, WB Saunders Co.

Nagi S: Some conceptual issues in disability and rehabilitation. In Sussman M, editor: Sociology and rehabilitation, Washington, DC, 1966, US Department of Health, Education and Welfare.

Prevalence of Selected Impairments—United States—1977, DHHS Pub No 81-1562, Hyattsville, Md, 1981, Office of Health Research, Statistics and Technology.

Safilios-Rothschild C: The sociology and social psychology of disability and rehabilitation, New York, 1970, Random House Inc.

Spradley BW: Community health nursing concepts and practices, ed 2, Boston, 1985, Little, Brown & Co Inc.

Stryker R: Rehabilitative aspects of acute and chronic nursing care, ed 2, Philadelphia, 1977, WB Saunders Co.

Syllabus for continuity of care for individuals with chronic illness, Buffalo, 1986, State University of New York at Buffalo, School of Nursing.

Thompson JM and Bowers AC: Clinical manual of health assessment, ed 3, St Louis, 1988, CV Mosby Co.

Tucker SM and others: Patient care standards, ed 4, St Louis, 1988, CV Mosby Co.

Van Son A: Diabetes and patient education: a daily nursing challenge, New York, 1982, Appleton & Lange.

Watson PG: Rehabilitation legislation of the 1980's: implications for nurses as healthcare providers, Rehabilitation Nurs 13:136, 1988.

Whaley LF and Wong DL: Nursing care of infants and children, ed 3, St Louis, 1987, CV Mosby Co.

You and your deaf patients, Washington, DC, 1978, Gallandet University Press.

Your child's hearing, Buffalo, NY, 1977, St Mary's School for the Deaf.

APPENDIX 25-1

Agencies That Provide Information and Services to Disabled Individuals and Their Families

Although this list is by no means exhaustive, it should provide a beginning source for referrals.

General/Cerebral Palsy

American Academy of Pediatrics
1801 Hinman Ave.
Evanston, Il 60204

Association for Children with Learning Disabilities
2200 Brownsville Rd.
Pittsburgh, PA 15210

Bureau of Education for the Handicapped
U.S. Office of Education
U.S. Dept. of Health and Human Services
Seventh and D Streets SW
Washington, DC 20036

Child Welfare League of America
67 Irving Place
New York, NY 10003

Council for Exceptional Children
900 Jefferson Plaza
1499 Jefferson Davis Highway
Arlington, VA 22202

Day Care and Child Development Council of America, Inc.
1426 H St. NW
Washington, DC 20005

Epilepsy Foundation of America
733 15th St. NW, Suite 1116
Washington, DC 20005

Muscular Dystrophy Association of America, Inc.
1790 Broadway
New York, NY 10019

National Association for Mental Health
10 Columbus Circle
New York, NY 10019

National Association for Retarded Citizens
2709 Ave. E East
Arlington, TX 76011

National Association for the Education of Young Children
1834 Connecticut Ave. NW
Washington, DC 20009

National Association of Coordinators of State Programs for the Mentally Retarded, Inc.
c/o Mr. Robert Gettings, Executive Director
National Easter Seal Society for Crippled Children and Adults
2123 West Ogden Ave.
Chicago, IL 60612

National Foundation–The March of Dimes
1275 Mamaroneck Ave., PO Box 2000
White Plains, NY 10602

National Multiple Sclerosis Society
257 Park Ave. S
New York, NY 10010

National Society for Autistic Children
621 Central Ave.
Albany, NY 12206

National Society for Autistic Children
169 Tampa Ave.
Albany, NY 12208

Office of Child Development
U.S. Department of Health and Human Services
PO Box 1182
Washington, DC 20013

United Cerebral Palsy Association, Inc.
66 E 34th St.
New York, NY 10016

Visual Impairment/Blindness

American Foundation for the Blind
15 W 16th St.
New York, NY 10011

American Printing House for the Blind
1839 Frankfort Ave.
Louisville, KY 40206

Association for the Education of the Visually Handicapped
711 14th St. NW
Washington, DC 10005

National Society for the Prevention of Blindness
16 E 40th St.
New York, NY 10019

Hearing Impairment

American Deafness and Rehabilitation Association
814 Thayer Ave.
Silver Spring, MD 20910

Convention of American Instructors of the Deaf
5034 Wisconsin Ave. NW
Washington, DC 20016

National Theatre of the Deaf
305 Great Neck Road
Waterford, CT 06385

Registry of Interpreters for the Deaf
PO Box 1339
Washington, DC 20013

Alexander Graham Bell Association for the Deaf
Headquarters: The Volta Bureau
1537 35th St. NW
Washington, DC 20007

The American Speech-Language-Hearing Association
10801 Rockville Pike
Rockville, MD 20852

The John Tracy Clinic
806 West Adams Blvd.
Los Angeles, CA 90007

The National Association of Hearing and Speech Agencies
919 18th St. NW
Washington, DC 20006

The National Association of the Deaf
2025 I Street
Washington, DC 20006

Parents' Groups

International Association of Parents of the Deaf
814 Thayer Ave.
Silver Springs, MD 20910

International Parents Organization
Alexander Graham Bell Association of the Deaf
3417 Volta Place NW
Washington, DC 20007

CHAPTER

26

Sexuality and Community Nursing

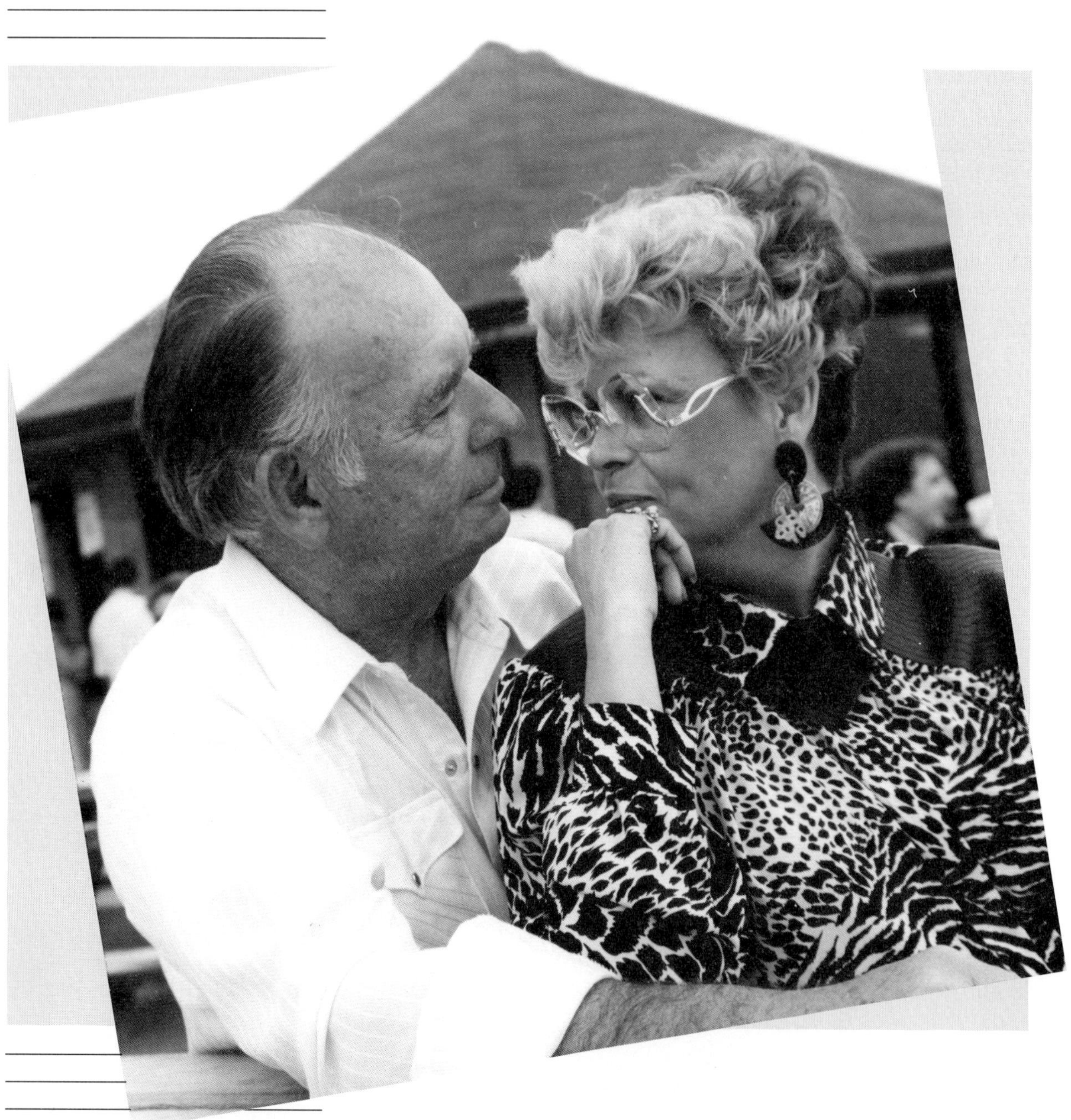

CHAPTER OUTLINE

OBJECTIVES

After completing this chapter, the reader should be able to:

1. Distinguish between the various forms of sexually transmitted diseases (STDs) and explain their causal agents.
2. Explain some of the unique problems facing clients with STDs.
3. Understand the background of the acquired immunodeficiency syndrome crisis and the challenge it presents to the nurse.
4. Explain the importance of taking a sexual case history.
5. Understand the extent of sexual diversity in the United States.
6. Realize the importance to nurses of understanding their clients' sexuality.

HISTORICAL PERSPECTIVE

Sexuality was once a subject that was seldom mentioned or officially discussed among nurses. In fact, women as a group in the nineteenth century were supposed to pretend they knew little or nothing about sex, and "proper" ladies did not talk about it at all. Instead, sexuality was something people (particularly women) tried to ignore; sex was only for having children. These attitudes, sometimes labeled Victorian because they were associated with the reign of Queen Victoria in England, both preceded her reign and continued after her death at the turn of the century. A medical misunderstanding of sex contributed to conservative attitudes.

The origin of these erroneous assumptions can be traced to the seventeenth century when there was vast confusion over the effects of tertiary syphilis, which were confused with the effects of sexual activity itself. This confusion was compounded by some of the medical theories of the day that were concerned with saving energy and body fluids and establishing an equilibrium. The person most responsible for popularizing the mishmash of theories about sexuality that had such great influence on future generations was the Swiss physician, S.A.D. Tissot who wrote a book called *Onanism,* which was translated into many different languages.

Tissot believed that the key to health was a balance of body fluids. Death, he theorized, was caused by loss of body fluids that could not be replaced. He recognized that such things as perspiration and urination were necessary bodily functions and believed that these fluids normally were replaced by fluid intake. Loss of blood, even in menstruation, as well as loss of fluid through diarrhea, excessive perspiration, great discharges of mucus, and of course the loss of semen and a female equivalent that Tissot never really described, caused problems according to his theories. Since many fluid losses could not be controlled by the individual, nature had to run its course, but certain losses, such as those resulting from sexual activity, could be controlled. Tissot thought sexual activity should be restricted to preserve health. Tissot supported his theory by documenting that mentally ill or feebleminded individuals often masturbated. Tissot also diagnosed what is now called tertiary syphilis and thought this was caused by an overactive sex life. Weakening caused by loss of blood was also documented.

With this evidence Tissot condemned all nonprocreative sex, which he termed "onanistic sex" from the Biblical story of the punishment of Onan. His ideas had particular influence in the United States, perhaps because of their adoption by Benjamin Rush, a physician who signed the Declaration of Independence and one of the most influential medical practitioners in America (Bullough, 1980). Other writers, including Sylvester Graham, after whom the Graham cracker is named, and John Harvey Kellogg, who began manufacturing corn flakes and other breakfast cereals with his brother, popularized these ideas in their books designed to raise the levels of health consciousness. Inevitably this misinformation worked its way into the nineteenth century nursing texts (Bullough and Seidl, 1987).

The sequelae of tertiary syphilis were not fully recognized until almost the end of the nineteenth century. It was then realized that the effects of tertiary syphilis include aortic insufficiency, aneurysms, tabes dorsalis, and a number of other manifestations depending on where the spirochete lodged (Brandt, 1985). The discovery that *Spirochaeta pallida* and not sex was the cause of syphilis, however, did not immediately change attitudes about the dangers of sex, since syphilis was incurable and abstinence was regarded as the best protection. Nurses found themselves at a loss, since it was clear to them that a significant percentage of clients in long-term care institutions were there because of the sequelae of syphilis and yet official U.S. censorship of sexual discussion prevented them from talking about prophylactic devices that might cut the spread of syphilis.

Margaret Sanger, one of the most famous of

American nurses, was arrested for writing and trying to distribute a pamphlet titled, *What Every Girl Should Know,* because among other things it included references to syphilis and gonorrhea (Gordon, 1976). As late as 1924 when the Venereal Disease Division of the U.S. Public Health Service polled state officials on their positions regarding prophylaxis and venereal disease, Pennsylvania was the only state with any kind of program, and even their program was soon dropped because of public pressure (Brandt, 1985).

Gradually several factors came together that lessened censorship and changed public attitudes. These factors included the work of Sigmund Freud and his association of sexual repression with neurosis, a better understanding of the physiology of sex, the development of effective contraceptives and prophylactics, and discovery of cures, or at least better treatments, for some sexually transmitted diseases (STDs). Not until the 1930s did official discussion take place in public health circles. The leader in bringing about change was Thomas Parran, surgeon general of the United States under Franklin D. Roosevelt. Parran mounted the first government campaign against STDs. Still no overnight changes in public attitudes took place and prohibitions against the use of condoms, which were considered contraceptives, as well as prophylactics, existed in many states.

It was not until the 1950s and 1960s that the major barriers preventing discussion of human sexuality were either eliminated or lessened for most nurses in a community health setting. Since one of the jobs of the community health nurse is to screen groups at risk to detect and begin treatment as early as possible, a knowledge of STDs is critical (see box). Nurses are often invited or required to carry out education programs, give information about prophylactic measures and devices, and supervise clients who have STDs. Nurses must also pay attention to sexual issues when taking a health history, since this can often lead to the diagnosis of an unsuspected STD. With the appearance of the acquired immunodeficiency syndrome (AIDS) epidemic nurses have had to learn to take precautions to prevent the spread of AIDS to themselves and others.

SEXUALITY AND THE NURSE

Because sexuality has been such a forbidden topic, the nurse must be particularly aware of the social interaction involved in dealing with clients in whom an STD has been diagnosed. With few exceptions, and these are mentioned in the text, the only way a person can contract an STD is to have genital contact with an infected person. Individuals who have sexual contact with a single partner throughout their lives or who abstain from sex are unlikely to contract an STD. The overwhelming majority of people with STDs are intimate with more than one person or are involved with a partner who is not monogamous.

When one person in a relationship contracts an STD, the implication is that one partner has been unfaithful to the other, something the unfaithful person would prefer to keep secret. Initially an unfaithful person may surreptitiously try to discover whether the faithful partner has already contracted the disease. If the faithful partner is still disease free, the infected partner will probably heave a sigh of relief and undergo treatment with the hope that the faithful partner will never find out. Unfortunately, the absence of easily recognizable symptoms does not mean that the disease has not been passed on to the partner. Many people with STDs are asymptomatic, although the infection might pass the placental barrier or ultimately have other consequences. Individuals in whom an STD is diagnosed should be made aware of this problem and encouraged to share information with their sexual partners, but in many cases they refuse to do so.

SEXUALLY TRANSMITTED DISEASES

Although old nursing texts use the term "venereal disease" for all diseases that can be spread by sexual contact, the current term for these diseases is "sexually transmitted diseases" (STD). In the late 1950s and the 1960s the number of cases of STDs dropped to a record low and there was a widespread belief that the problem had been controlled by the use of penicillin and other antimicrobial agents. Unfortunately, the allocation of federal funds for controlling STDs dropped 83% between 1948 and 1955 (Webster, 1972). Current statistics suggest that the belief that STDs were declining as a serious health problem was overly optimistic. Gonorrhea is now the most common infection reported to public health authorities and has been diagnosed in more than 1 million Americans every year since 1975. Nongonococcal urethritis may affect an equally large number of people, and it is estimated that more than 20 million Americans now have recurrent genital herpes infections. AIDS is of course epidemic.

Perhaps the best way to describe the various forms of STDs is by their causal agents—bacteria, viruses, and genital parasites.

Bacterial Infections

Today STDs caused by bacteria are relatively easy to cure. Included in this group are gonorrhea, chlamydial infections, syphilis, chancroid, granuloma inguinale, lymphogranuloma venereum, and shigellosis.

Gonorrhea

Gonorrhea is widespread. There are over 1 million cases recorded annually by the Centers for Disease Control, and it is estimated the number of actual cases is probably twice as high. Those at greatest risk are in the age group 20 to 24, and usually about a third of the reported cases comes from that group. The next largest age group is those between 15 to 19. Any age group that has sexual contact, however, is susceptible, and in 1979, for example, 300 cases of gonorrhea in children younger than 10 years of age were reported; most of these children were victims of abuse.

Gonorrhea is caused by *Neisseria gonorrhoeae,* a gram-negative diplococcus that thrives on the mucous membranes of the mouth, urethra, vagina, and anus. This means that it can be transmitted by kissing (if the locus of infection is in the mouth) and oral, anal, or vaginal sex. The incubation period ranges from two to 14 days, and the onset of the disease is marked by copious mucopurulent discharges created by phagocytosis. Discharge is vaginal in the female, and urethral in the male, or pharyngeal if contracted from oral sex and anal if contracted from anal sex.

Of the women who have contracted gonorrhea, 80% have mild symptoms or are asymptomatic. In most other women, in addition to the vaginal discharge, they have some pain during urination, mild pelvic discomfort, or abnormal menstruation. A few women have concomitant pelvic inflammatory disease (PID). Some men are asymptomatic, although not in as large a proportion as women, and the most noticeable symptom in males is painful urination.

Diagnosis is confirmed by a culture of the vaginal or urethral discharge using a Thayer-Martin medium. The normal treatment is by procaine penicillin G or ampicillin with probenecid, but this is no longer foolproof because some penicillin-resistant strains, such as penicillinase-producing *N. gonorrhoeae* (PPNG), first reported in 1975, have developed (Culliton, 1976). Both the increase in the number of cases of gonorrhea and the appearance of penicillin-resistant strain correlated with the war in Vietnam, and since then the number of resistant cases has been increasing. In 1979 836 such cases were reported in the United States and in 1981 more than 2000 U.S. cases were reported. Other antibiotics, such as tetracycline, still work against gonorrhea, but there is growing concern over resistant strains.

In a sense people with gonorrhea who are symptomatic are more fortunate than those who are not, since thousands of men and women become infertile each year from the scar tissue in their fallopian tubes or vas deferens that is often a sequela of untreated cases. The most serious complication of gonorrhea is PID, of which perhaps as many as 200,000 cases are reported each year

(Curran, 1979 and 1980). Gonorrheal PID is marked by intense lower abdominal pain, tenderness, and fever as the infection invades the uterine cavity and produces inflammation and abscesses of the fallopian tubes and occasionally the ovaries. The cause of PID may be determined with a culture of the cervical mucosa. Most clients with acute PID respond to treatment with penicillin, ampicillin, or tetracycline, and recovery is usually rapid once PID is diagnosed. Women who use an intrauterine device (IUD) are more likely to have PID develop from gonorrhea or other genital infections than are women who do not use an IUD (Scott, 1978).

Ectopic pregnancy is a serious complication of untreated gonorrhea or PID. The increase in the incidence of gonorrhea is one reason it is estimated that the rate of ectopic pregnancy tripled between 1967 and 1977. Occasionally gonorrhea is marked by salpingitis, cervicitis, peritonitis, and abscesses of the Skene's or Bartholin's glands in the female and the epididymis and prostate in the male. Although no one is immune to gonorrhea, there has been some recent success with a vaccine developed at the University of Pittsburgh by C.C. Brinton and his colleagues (Brinton and others, 1982). The vaccine stimulates the body to develop antibodies that coat the hairlike projections of the gonococcus, making it more difficult for the bacterium to attach to the mucous membrane. One of the reasons newborn infants are treated with penicillin (or in the past why 1% aqueous silver nitrate was instilled in the eyes of infants) is to prevent gonococcal infection of the conjunctiva or ophthalmia neonatorum, which can cause blindness.

Chlamydial Infections

Chlamydial infections are caused by the microorganism, *Chlamydia trachomatis,* a species of bacteria that are surrounded by a thick sheath or capsule. It is estimated that there are somewhere between 3 million and 5 million people with chlamydia in the United States; the incidence must be estimated, since unlike other epidemic diseases, chlamydial infections do not have to be reported. Chlamydial infections are responsible for more than 40% of the nonspecific urethritis in men and a high percentage of PID in women. Chlamydial infections are known to cause infertility, as well as a greater likelihood of ectopic pregnancy, in women, which makes them life-threatening infections. Some researchers estimate that 30% of sexually active teenagers carry *C. trachomatis.* Babies born to women with chlamydial infections are susceptible to eye infections and chlamydial pneumonia if they are not delivered by caesarian section.

Like many other STDs chlamydial infections can be carried and transmitted without producing any symptoms at all. This has led it to be called the silent epidemic, since as many as 80% of the women who are infected with *C. trachomatis* do not know it until and unless complications develop. Symptoms of chlamydial infections in the female include break-through bleeding, lower abdominal pain and cramping, frequency and burning on urination not attributable to obvious urinary tract infection, cervicitis, vaginal discharge, and painful intercourse.

Symptoms of the disease in the male are not often present, but if they are, they are marked by a urethral discharge that is usually thin and whitish, burning and frequency on urination not attributable to obvious urinary tract infection, and pain in the testicles or rectum (epididymitis or proctitis).

Chlamydial infections are diagnosed in women by using a culture, and if results are negative for gonorrhea but signs of inflammation are present, then a chlamydial infection is usually suspected, although diagnosis of a chlamydial infection must always be confirmed with a laboratory test. The prescribed treatment is 500 mg of tetracycline four times a day for one week to 10 days or 100 mg of doxycycline two times a day for one week to 10 days. Pregnant women are advised to use erythromycin, and tetracycline eye ointment should be used in the newborn's eyes. Penicillin is not effective. A good preventive is the use of a condom or spermicide.

Lymphogranuloma Venereum

Chlamydia trachomatis also sometimes causes lymphogranuloma venereum (LGV). This is not common in the United States (fewer than 500 cases a year), but many cases might go unreported. It is a disease of the lymphatic system, and it appears as a small lesion on the genitals or perineum. The lesion is painless and usually disappears quickly, although it might be accompanied by fevers, chills, abdominal pain, loss of appetite, and backache. To diagnose LGV, the lymphogranuloma venereum complement fixation (LGV-CV) test is used. The prescribed treatment of LGV is sulfisoxazole or tetracycline for three weeks or longer if the infection is not treated early. If treatment is delayed, in severe cases of LGV the inguinal lymph nodes swell, forming buboes, and secondary ulcers appear on the genitals. Ultimately the penis in the male and the labia or clitoris in the female may swell, and a painful elephantiasis develops.

In older texts the term *nongonococcal urethritis* (NGU) is used as a synonym for chlamydial infections. In addition to *C. trachomatis,* other organisms cause NGU, including *Ureaplasma urealyticum* (T-mycoplasma), another strain of bacteria that is also transmitted through sexual contact. Symptoms in the male are similar to those of chlamydial infections, and NGU causes urethritis in females. NGU can be treated with tetracycline or in the same way as chlamydial infections, with which it is often grouped. Like chlamydial infections, NGU appears one to three weeks after contact.

Syphilis

The origins of syphilis have been subject to much debate. In the sixteenth century it was believed to be a new disease; at that time it was epidemic. Scholars today are not certain whether syphilis was a new disease at that time, but there is almost general agreement that it was not imported from the New World by Columbus as some argued a generation ago. It is caused by a corkscrewlike organism called *Treponema pallidum.* Syphilis is transmitted through sexual contact and goes through several phases. The primary stage is marked by the appearance of a more or less painless ulcer called a chancre, which varies with the type of sexual contact; it can be in the mouth, vagina, urethra, or anus or on external genitals. This primary phase lasts from 10 to 90 days and is infective. The chancre then disappears almost spontaneously, leaving syphilis victims with the false impression that they have no infection, although they are still highly contagious. Since there is little pain associated with the chancre, a woman might not notice it if it appears on her cervix; the same is true of men if a chancre appears in the urethra or anus.

If syphilis is untreated, it enters into a secondary stage anywhere from two weeks to one month after the chancre has healed. Secondary syphilis is characterized by a generalized body rash that is sometimes accompanied by headache, fever, indigestion, sore throat, and pains in the joints or muscles. It is highly contagious. The disease process then enters another latent phase that might last anywhere from one to 40 years. Some authorities break the latent phase into an early and a late latent phase, but infected people have no physical symptoms in any part of the latent phase. After the early latent period the person is no longer infectious. During the second latent phase the bacteria lodge in internal body parts such as the brain, spinal cord, bones, and bodily tissues, and eventually a third-stage, or tertiary syphilis develops in roughly one half of all untreated clients. This third stage of syphilis takes various forms, depending on where the bacteria concentrated, and might be marked with gummas, or rubbery tumors on the skin, bones, liver, or stomach, a central nervous system involvement with optic atrophy, deafness and general paresis, aortic insufficiency or aneurysms, endarteritis, or insanity.

In the early stage, syphilis is usually diagnosed through an examination of the blood sample for antibodies, although sometimes a false positive can be given because the antibodies were there from a related or past infection or exposure. Syphilis is treated with benzathine penicillin G, although in 1981 there was some indication that some strains of *T. pallidum* might be developing resistance to benzathine penicillin G; there are now attempts to find alternative treatments (Norgard and Miller, 1981). Natural immunities to syphilis do not develop, and thus a person who has had syphilis can be reinfected.

Since the bacteria can cross the placental barrier, a woman with untreated syphilis can infect the fetus. This makes it critical that the nurse be alert to symptoms of syphilis when taking a history of a pregnant woman. In most cases when *T. pallidum* crosses the placental barrier, which occurs in perhaps as many as 90% of pregnant women with syphilis, the result is a spontaneous abortion or a stillbirth. The newborn who survives can be treated to prevent further damage, but treatment does not undo the damage that has already occurred, which might include blindness, deafness, and deformities of the bones and teeth.

Chancroid

Chancroid is caused by a *Haemophilus ducrevi,* a bacterium that is usually, at least in the United States, transmitted by sexual intercourse. In some areas of the world, notably the tropics, *H. ducreyi* might be spread by physical contact. Those individuals who wash their genitals regularly are not as susceptible to the disease, and in the United States it is not widespread (not many more than 1000 cases per year). Small bumps appear at the site of chancroid infection, usually the genitals, three to five days after physical contact with an infected person. These eventually rupture to form irregular soft sores or craterlike ulcers. Chancroid chancres are soft and painful in contrast to the hard and usually painless syphilis ulcers. Lymph nodes on the infected side of the groin often become infected, inflamed, and swollen, forming a bubo that might eventually rupture. This is more likely to happen in men than women. Diagnosis of chancroid is made by visual inspection of the lesions and buboes and microscopic examinations of the smears from the ulcer. Chancroid is treated with sulfa drugs or tetracycline. Sometimes a chancroid heals on its own.

Granuloma Inguinale

Granuloma inguinale is now rare; fewer than 100 cases are reported annually. It is caused by the bacterium *Donovania granulomatis,* but it is not particularly contagious. It can be transmitted either sexually or nonsexually, and infection is marked by the appearance of a pimple on the genitals or thighs. Eventually the pimple begins to ulcerate, produces a strong odor, and spreads to adjacent areas until it is treated. If the pimples ulcerate, the infected tissue is permanently destroyed. Granuloma inguinate is diagnosed by microscopic examination of a smear from the lesions, which contain the bacteria, and is treated with tetracycline or gentamicin, neither of which can reverse the damage already done. If granuloma inguinale is not treated, continued spreading can lead to death (Morton, 1976).

Shigellosis

Shigellosis is caused by bacteria of the genus *Shigella* and may be transmitted through feces or sexual contact. Oral stimulation of the anus of someone with shigellosis exposes the stimulator to the disease, and perhaps for this reason some 30% of the reported cases occur among homosexual men (Bader, 1978). Pain, fever, diarrhea, and inflammation of the mucous membranes of the large intestines are among the symptoms. Some also experience a burning rectal sensation and vomiting. Shigellosis is diagnosed using a culture of a stool specimen and is treated with ampicillin or tetracycline, although *Shigella* bacteria rapidly develop resistance to antibiotics.

Viral Infections

Although bacteria that cause STDs traditionally have been regarded as the most serious agents of disease associated with sexual activity, the diseases they cause can now be treated relatively easily if they are diagnosed early enough. This is not true of another category of STDs, namely those transmitted by viruses, which at the time of this writing are approaching epidemic proportions.

Acquired Immunodeficiency Syndrome (AIDS)

The most serious of the virally transmitted diseases is acquired immunodeficiency syndrome (AIDS), which was not described until the period between 1980 and 1981. In those years Michael S. Gottlieb, a University of California at Los Angeles physician, identified several men with *Pneumocystis carinii* pneumonia (PCP), a rare type of pneumonia that was usually seen only in people whose immune system had become depressed, such as kidney transplantation clients who took drugs to prevent rejection of the transplant. At about the same time Alvina Friedman-Kien of New York University saw a young gay man with Kaposi's sarcoma, an uncommon, slow-growing cancer usually found only among elderly men of Mediterranean lineage. In the New York man the disease took a more deadly form similar to those cases prevalent in equatorial Africa. Friedman-Kein found that other physicians in New York and San Francisco had come across homosexual clients with this form of Kaposi's sarcoma as early as 1979. Both physicians informed the Centers for Disease Control of their unusual findings, and it was quickly realized that a new STD had been found. Further research identified the causal factor as a virus that specifically attacks the T_4 lymphocytes, a subgroup of white blood cells that plays a major role in defending the body against infections and some cancers. The virus, called the type 1 human immunodeficiency virus (HIV) (as of this writing researchers believe a type 2 virus will be found), is an RNA retrovirus that has a selective tropism for the T_4 lymphocyte cell, the critical cell in most immunologic functions. The HIV incorporates itself into the genetic materials, or DNA, in the T_4 lymphocyte cell nucleus, and when the T-cells are activated, as they are in the presence of an infection, the virus reproduces itself and kills the T-cell. When the T-cell dies, new viruses are released and invade and kill other T_4 cells. As a result of losing many T_4 cells HIV-infected people have difficulty fighting infections, particularly some of the rarer ones to which AIDS clients seem particularly susceptible. The boxed material describes some of the diseases commonly associated with AIDS. One of the difficulties in writing about AIDS is that the disease is so new and breakthroughs in information are so frequent that data become outdated quickly.

Epidemiologists are fairly certain that the HIV originally came from Central Africa, where it was picked up by homosexual men who transmitted it to the United States and Europe. Before the disease was recognized and the virus was identified, some people contracted the disease through blood transfusions. When it was realized that AIDS could be contracted through blood transfusions, stored blood samples were checked. Researchers found that as early as 1978 some 1% of the blood samples taken in a San Francisco STD clinic showed HIV antibodies. By 1984, 65% of the samples taken in the same clinic had HIV antibodies. As of this writing it is assumed that all people who test positive for HIV antibodies will develop the symptoms of AIDS. Between 1 million and 2 million people have been exposed to the AIDS virus in the United States, and by 1991 there will be 270,000 cumulative cases of AIDS (Fauci, 1988). The virus may live in humans for years before actual symptoms appear, and the U.S. Public Health Service

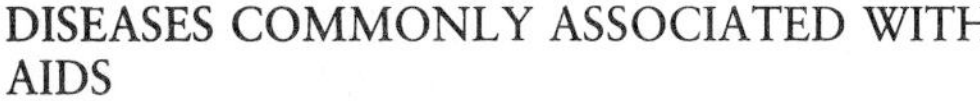

DISEASES COMMONLY ASSOCIATED WITH AIDS

Cytomegalovirus (CMV's) one of a group of herpes viruses causing cell enlargement of various internal organs.

Kaposi's sarcoma is a rare form of cancer of the skin and connective tissue that formerly was confined to older men.

Pneumocystis carinii pneumonia is a form of pneumonia resulting from infection with *P. carinii* and previously observed only in cancer or transplant clients who received immune suppression drugs to prevent rejection of a transplant or treatment.

estimated (and so far its estimates have been accurate) that the number of new AIDS cases in the United States would increase approximately 75,000 a year by 1991, 50% more than all cases reported up to the end of 1987. At that time AIDS had been diagnosed in 49,793 people, 27,909 of whom are dead (Curran and others, 1988). By the middle of 1989, 102,621 cases of AIDS had been reported in the United States; 59,391 people in whom AIDS was diagnosed had died, and 944 of the cases were reported in children younger than 13 years of age (Centers for Disease Control, 1989). Although AIDS was first diagnosed in gay men, the disease is not a homosexual disease even though it is spread more easily through anal intercourse than through penile-vaginal intercourse. As of 1989, 20,619 of the cases of AIDS that were reported occurred among people with a history of intravenous drug use. In addition, there were 7173 AIDS cases reported in intravenous drug users who had a history of homosexual activity (Centers for Disease Control, 1989).

Since AIDS leads to a diminished capacity to combat any infection or malignancy, the symptoms of AIDS are not always the same; the symptoms of the disease that AIDS prevents the body from combating become the symptoms of AIDS. There can be a broad range of symptoms depending on the type and location of the infection. Symptoms include swollen lymph glands, fatigue, general malaise, fever, night sweats, diarrhea and gradual weight loss, mental and neurologic problems, impaired speech, tremors and seizures progressing to dementia, as well as particular susceptibility to certain diseases mentioned previously. When AZT is given to people with AIDS, the drug has strong toxic side effects, especially to bone marrow, and it tends to lose effectiveness if it is taken for a long period. It is more effective when given to people wio have only recently been infected with HIC. Other drugs, such as DDI, look promising. As of this writing, however, there is no cure for AIDS, even though there is a worldwide effort to find a vaccine or treatment; the immediate solution is to lessen the chance for infection and to overcome the hysteria and panic the disease has caused (Koff and Hoth, 1988). The nurse is on the front line of the AIDS battle, since both the diagnosis of AIDS and the care of AIDS clients are often done by nurses. In addition, nurses must disseminate information about AIDS to clients under their care.

In fact, disseminating information on AIDS is so important that in 1988 Surgeon General C. Everett Koop sent a pamphlet titled *Understanding AIDS* to every address in the United States.

The pamphlet emphasized that AIDS is one of the most serious health problems ever to face the American public. Certain behaviors put individuals at risk, and nurses must alert people to the risky behaviors listed in the first box on the following page.

Since home care is the preferred and least expensive treatment option for AIDS clients at this time, nurses who care for AIDS clients must make certain that appropriate isolation precautions are used, although these depend on the type of contact caregivers have with clients (see box in the second column on p. 642) (O'Brien, Oerlemans-Bun, Blanchfield, 1987; Smith, 1987).

Contaminated equipment such as linen is disinfected with bleach and water in a 1:10 concentration. Nurses who care for clients who require

WHAT BEHAVIOR PUTS YOU AT RISK

You are at risk of being infected with the AIDS virus if you have sex with someone who is infected or if you share needles and syringes with someone who is infected.

Since you cannot be sure who is infected, your chances of coming into contact with the virus increase with the number of sex partners you have. Any exchanges of infected blood, semen, or vaginal fluids can spread the virus and place you at great risk.

The following behaviors are risky when performed with an infected person. You cannot tell by looking whether a person is infected.

RISKY BEHAVIOR

Sharing needles and syringes
Anal sex, with or without a condom
Vaginal or oral sex with someone who shoots drugs or engages in anal sex
Sex with someone you do not know well (a pickup or prostitute) or with someone you know has several sex partners
Unprotected sex (without a condom) with an infected person

SAFE BEHAVIOR

Not having sex
Sex with one faithful, uninfected partner
Not shooting drugs

TO THESE WE ADD

When having sex with a new partner, make sure a latex condom is used, preferably with a spermicide and a lubricant.

SPECIAL PRECAUTIONS FOR NURSES WHO CARE FOR AIDS CLIENTS

Gloves must be worn when coming in contact with clients' blood, body fluids, or secretions, as well as when handling soiled items and surfaces, and materials contaminated with blood or body fluids.

Gowns are required only if soilage of clothing with clients' blood or body fluids may occur.

Masks are not required except when tuberculosis is suspected or present or when performing procedures, such as suctioning, that may cause blood or body fluids to splash directly onto the face.

Hands and other skin surfaces should be washed immediately and thoroughly if they are contaminated with blood or other body fluids from clients.

injections should be supplied with puncture-proof containers for used needles and syringes. These should be returned to the hospital for disposal. Many AIDS clients are also drug users; additional precautions need to be taken with them.

The average age for a person with AIDS is in the thirties, and dealing with such a debilitating, life-threatening illness is difficult for clients, significant others, and caregivers (Schoen, 1986). The nurse is one of the key support persons with whom the AIDS client comes in contact. The ability of society to deal with an epidemic such as AIDS basically depends on how nurses perform as information givers, diagnosticians, and caregivers. The boxed material on p. 643 lists nursing diagnoses commonly associated with the care of AIDS clients.

Herpes

The most widespread of the viral STDs is herpes simplex 2, or genital herpes, the incidence of which increased thirteenfold between 1966 and 1979. The incidence of herpes continued to increase in the early 1980s, but as of this writing the incidence of new cases seems to be declining. Still, more than 20 million people in the United States have been infected with the virus, and even with the leveling off of new herpes cases, there are more than 500,000 new cases reported every year. Like the "cold sore" or "fever blister" that many people with herpes simplex 1 have on their lip, a painful vesicle is present in people with herpes simplex 2. Neither of the herpes simplex viruses is curable. Even though the herpes simplex viruses are dormant most of the time, they often erupt during times of physiologic or psychologic

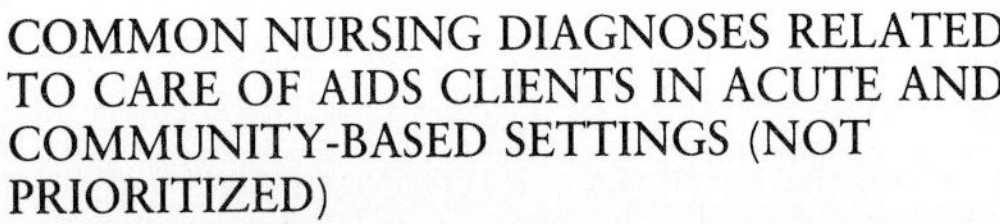

COMMON NURSING DIAGNOSES RELATED TO CARE OF AIDS CLIENTS IN ACUTE AND COMMUNITY-BASED SETTINGS (NOT PRIORITIZED)

1. Knowledge deficiency of client, family, and significant others regarding the disease process and its transmission and regarding legal, moral and ethical rights and responsibilities, such as rights to treatment and humanistic care and responsibilities of communication with partners
2. Alterations in functioning of the immune system, including compromise of respiratory status manifested as cough, fever, and dyspnea and potential for the development of infection in self and others
3. Alterations in functioning of the gastrointestinal system manifest as weight loss, anorexia, diarrhea, dehydration (fluid and electrolyte balance), and oral lesions
4. Potential for the development of pain and potential for the development of skin lesions, edema, and other symptoms related to the disease process
5. Activity intolerance manifest as fatigue and weakness, dyspnea, and general malaise
6. Social isolation and fear of rejection manifest as loss of self-esteem and control, fear of transmitting AIDS to others accompanied by intensified needs for physical contact and emotional intimacy and dependency, potential for loss of income, and occupation, guilt regarding life-style, and loss of social support
7. Alterations in functioning of the neurologic system manifest as impairments in cognitive functions, disorders of gait and balance, seizures, central nervous system infections, paralysis, and coma
8. Powerlessness and depression manifest as anger, hostility, withdrawal, fear, and guilt related to variability in access to participation in decision-making process and treatment
9. Fear of death and fear of the unknown

stress. There is a difference between the two types of herpes simplex. Although herpes simplex 1 is irritating and disfiguring for brief periods, herpes simplex 2 has more serious sequelae. It should also be emphasized that herpes simplex 1 may be spread to the genitals and herpes simplex 2 can be spread to the lips by oral contact. Genital herpes is normally transmitted by sexual contact, and there is an incubation period of three to seven days. The onset of the disease is marked by minor itching or an extensive rash of the genital region, and this is followed by a cluster of bullae that ruptures and ulcerates and that is pruritic and painful especially during intercourse. In women the bullae break out on the labia minora and labia majora, vagina, clitoral hood, and cervix. In men the bullae tend to form on the glans or foreskin of the penis. When the vesicles break out, the infection can spread to other parts of the body and the open wounds are also susceptible to other infections. Usually the bullae disappear from two to six weeks after the first infection; when they reappear, they usually last less than two weeks. People with herpes simplex are highly infectious during the active period when there are sores, although infection is still possible during the dormant phase.

Some cases of herpes simplex 2 are asymptomatic, particularly those where infection is on the cervix, which has relatively few nerve endings. Herpes simplex can be diagnosed by direct observation of the blisters, by microscopic examination of the ulcerous tissues, and by a variety of tests using cultures of the virus for positive identification. Although herpes simplex has no cure, acyclovir in ointment form (Z ovirax) may reduce contagion. The drug reduces pain for men but not for women.

Hot baths and exposure of sores to air and warm heat help reduce the discomfort of outbreaks. Clothing that reduces air circulation, such as nylon panties, pantyhose, close-fitting shorts, or jock straps, should be avoided.

Two major dangers are associated with herpes simplex—its threat to the fetus and its link with cancer. The herpes simplex 2 virus can pass through the placenta in pregnant women, and if the fetus is not infected before birth, it may become infected when it passes through the cervix and vagina if the virus is in the active stage. Infection of the fetus is often fatal, but if the fetus survives, it is probable that in at least 25% of cases the infant will have some birth defect, including brain damage. If herpes simplex 2 is active when the woman is in labor, a caesarian section should be performed. Herpes simplex 2 may also cause cervical cancer. Cervical cancer develops in about 6% of women with herpes simplex 2, and more than 80% of women in whom cervical cancer is diagnosed have herpes simplex 2. This correlation may not be significant, and other factors might be involved. Whenever nurses or clients apply acyclovir, they should wear gloves to prevent reinfection or transmission to other areas.

Genital warts, sometimes called venereal warts or more technically condyloma acuminatum, are caused by a human papovavirus, are soft, pink, and painless, and occur in single or multiple growths resembling cauliflower as warts do on other parts of the body. Genital warts are transmitted through direct contact with the warts during vaginal, oral, or anal intercourse, but they may also be contracted through nonsexual contact. The warts are highly contagious, but if they are on the penis or in the vagina, the likelihood of spreading the infection can be greatly lessened by use of a condom. The warts usually appear from one to three months after contact and can be diagnosed visually. They may be removed by freezing (cryotherapy), burning (usually with the chemical podophyllin), or dehydration with an electric needle. Sometimes genital warts regress without treatment, but they may spread, sometimes to the extent that they block the vaginal or rectal opening. The virus has also been linked to cervical cancer and can be transmitted to the baby as it moves through the birth canal.

Hepatitis B

Hepatitis B is another viral disease that can be sexually transmitted. Hepatitis B was formerly known as serum hepatitis, and it is quite different from infectious hepatitis or hepatitis A. It is believed that as many as 40% of all hepatitis B cases may be sexually transmitted. Approximately 65% of homosexual men in the United States have antibodies for hepatitis B, suggesting previous infection. About 10% of those infected with hepatitis B become chronic carriers of the virus, although most show no symptoms. Hepatitis B can be transmitted by exposures to semen, saliva, and blood of infectious carriers, whereas hepatitis A is spread by direct or indirect contact with feces contaminated with the hepatitis A virus.

Symptoms of hepatitis B appear within 30 to 120 days after exposure and include mild fever, fatigue, sore muscles, headache, upset stomach, skin rash, joint pains, and dark urine. The sclera becomes yellow, and the skin is jaundiced. Diagnosis is made using the hepatitis B surface antigen test. Those who have had hepatitis B are at increased risk for developing cancer of the liver and about 1% of those hospitalized for hepatitis B die. Although there is no cure, there is a safe and effective vaccine (Heptavax-B) now available, although it is still expensive. It is the first vaccine successfully developed to prevent an STD. Health professionals may, however, contract the disease without sexual contact. Dentists are particularly at risk because of saliva spread by high-speed drills.

Parasites

Community health nurses should know about a number of parasitic infections that result from sexual contact. Perhaps the most serious and life-threatening parasitic infection is amebic dysentery, or intestinal amebiasis, caused by the one-celled *Entamoeba histolytica.* It can be transmitted through exposure to contaminated water and food, as well as sexual contact. The most likely sexual transmission of amebic dysentery is oral contact with the anus. Many cases occur among homosexual men, but heterosexual couples who engage in anal intercourse may also contract the disease (Felman and William, 1978).

Pinworm, or *Enterobius vermicularis,* is spread by contact with the eggs of the pinworm. Cunnilingus or manual foreplay with the anus of a person having pinworm can transmit the parasite, which has been spreading among homosexual men (Waugh, 1976). Pinworm can be diagnosed by visual inspection of the worms in a stool sample or microscopic identification of pinworm eggs. It is treated with pyrvinium pamoate tablets or similar drugs.

Scabies is a highly contagious infestation of eight-legged parasitic mites, *Sarcoptes scabiei,* and can be transmitted both sexually and nonsexually. When the eggs of the mites hatch, they cause red, itchy, pimplelike bumps on the skin. Victims often appear with irritated scratch marks of the pubis. Diagnosis is through microscopic inspection of infected skin. Treatment is with gamma benzene hexachloride (Kwell) shampoo, which is applied from the neck down. Bedding and clothing must also be washed to get rid of the eggs, which can be spread by sleeping in an infected bed.

Crabs, or more technically *Pthirus pubis,* are six-legged creatures the size of a pinhead. They inhabit the hairy areas of the pubic region, anus, and underarms, as well as the eyelashes. The nits, or eggs, are laid by the female lice and mature in two or three weeks, whereupon they begin feeding on blood, producing inflammation of the skin and pruritus. Diagnosis is by identification of the nits or insects with a low-power microscope. As with scabies, crabs can be transmitted sexually or nonsexually through contact with infected bedding, towels, or clothing. Treatment is with gamma benzene hexachloride shampoo, although crabs can be eliminated with piperonyl butoxide (RID), which unlike gamma benzene hexachloride can be purchased without a prescription in most states.

Other Sexually Transmitted Diseases

Both men and women are susceptible to other infections through sexual activity. In women many of these infections go under the general heading of vaginitis and are usually marked by pruritus, and leukorrhea. Infections in women are mostly caused by a flagellated protozoan from the genus *Trichomonas,* or the yeastlike fungus *Candida albicans,* although not all causes of vaginitis have been identified.

Candidiasis is not normally sexually transmitted. *Candida albicans* is part of humans' normal gastrointestinal flora and is usually in balance with the human flora. When there is a disturbance in the balance of flora, *C. albicans* can become pathogenic in the vagina. Irritation, itching, and a white cheesy discharge resembling the curd of cottage cheese mixed with egg white tend to appear in the vagina, particularly during pregnancy or following antibiotic therapy or at other times when the pH of the vaginal flora is altered. Sometimes this can happen when women douche too frequently. Candidiasis often results in inflammation of the vaginal wall; the labia sometimes swell, and intercourse can be painful. Diabetic and postmenopausal women are more likely to become infected than other women. Candidiasis can be diagnosed by microscopic examination of a fresh specimen of discharge or by growing the fungus in a culture. Women with candidiasis can be treated with antifungal vaginal preparations, including nystatin (Mycostatin) or clotrimazole (Gyne-Lotrimin). During treatment the male partner should wear a condom to avoid infecting or reinfecting his partner.

Trichomoniasis vaginitis, caused by the protozoan *Trichomonas vaginalis,* can be transmitted through sexual contact, but infection can also result from using washcloths or towels that contain *T. vaginalis* or contact with perianal discharge. It is estimated that nearly 1 million women a year are infected with *T. vaginalis* in the United States. Incubation periods range from four days to one month. Many but not all women who contract trichomoniasis vaginitis have a foamy, yellow-green (or sometimes whitish yellow), foul-smelling vaginal discharge. Many women, however, are asymptomatic, and some authorities believe that the protozoa are part of the normal vaginal flora. Diagnosis of the trichomoniasis vaginitis is made by dropping a sample of the discharge on a prepared slide and looking for trichomonads. Women with trichomoniasis vaginitis are treated with metronidazole (Flagyl), and the infected woman, as well as her partner, should be treated, since some men can be carriers. Metronidazole should not be taken in combination with alcohol because it reacts in a way similar to disulfiram (Antabuse) and poses risks for people with peptic ulcers, blood disease, and central nervous system disorders. Metronidazole also poses a danger to the fetus, so it should not be prescribed for pregnant women (Boston, 1984).

Haemophilus vaginalis is a bacterium associated, possibly causally, with vaginitis and is most prevalent among women of childbearing age. Usually this type of vaginitis is asymptomatic, but symptoms include leukorrhea and a discharge with an unpleasant odor. Ampicillin is given to both the woman and her partner to prevent reinfection (Kaufman, 1976). In men the infection is usually asymptomatic.

Cystitis is inflammation of the urinary bladder caused by infection and involves both men and women, although it is more common in women. It is sometimes called the honeymoon disease because it is often preceded by frequent intercourse. Cystitis is caused by a variety of bacteria including *Escherichia coli,* which can be transmitted either sexually or nonsexually. Women wiping from the anus toward the uretha may bring *E. coli* from the rectum into the urethral opening. Vigorous intercourse may have the same effect. The onset of the disease is marked by frequency, urgency, burning during urination, and pain in the lower back or abdomen. It is often treated with sulfisoxazole (Gantrisin) or a combination of trimethoprim and sulfamethoxazole (Bactrim). Treatment also includes drinking large quantities of fluids, since this helps eliminate the infection.

Prostatitis, inflammation of the prostate, is confined to males. It is an infection of the prostate gland that primarily afflicts men between 20 and 40 years of age. Perhaps as many as 40% of males have had such an infection. Like cystitis it can be caused by *E. coli.* In this case it is called infectious prostatis. Congestive prostatitis is different and may result from either infrequent ejaculation or abstinence from sexual activity. Infectious prostatitis often is contracted during sexual contact; congestive prostatitis afflicts priests and other celibates, although many are asymptomatic. Symptoms include groin and lower back pain, fever, and a burning sensation during and following ejaculation. In some men there is a thin, watery discharge from the urethra before urination. The bacterial infection can be treated with antibiotics, whereas inflammation of the prostate may be reduced by palpating or manipulating the penis (Masters and Johnson, 1970).

OTHER SEXUAL PROBLEMS

After reading this chapter so far, nurses may think the reason they need information about sexuality is to deal with STDs. This, however, is only part of the sex information needed. Since sex is important in society, the nurse must be cognizant of developments in the whole field. In some cases the nurse must act as detective, ferreting out incidents of sexual assault, either of children or, as in the case of rape, of adults. This topic is discussed in Chapter 27 as part of the topic of abuse in a family setting. Incest is also included there.

In other cases the nurse must act as supporter and consoler in cases such as breast cancer, cancer of the cervix, cancer of the prostate, or similar cancers in which clients worry about their body image and their ability to function as sexual partners. These topics are also discussed in Chapter 18. Chapter 18 also discusses contraceptives and abortion, which are two topics about which the nurse is called on to give information.

Information giving, in fact, whether formally or informally, is one of the major tasks of the nurse in sexual matters. This, as has been indicated earlier, implies a willingness to frankly and openly discuss sexual problems with clients. Sometimes this comes when taking a client history or when preparing a nursing plan for convalescent clients in their homes. Since sex is often such a forbidden topic, it takes a special awareness by the nurse to recognize a client's problems. The best way for nurses to deal with sexual matters when taking a history is for them to ask the simple question, "Do you have any sexual problems?" The same is true when preparing a nursing plan. Many physicians and even a few nurses skirt the sexual issue by asking clients at the end of history taking whether there is anything else bothering them. Be open with clients and include questions about STDs when other questions about communicable diseases are asked. Questions about sexual dysfunction and contraception should be part of the review of reproductive and genitourinary systems. In cases where the client initiates a discussion on a sexual topic without prompting, the nurse should listen with sensitivity and in as nonjudgmental a way as possible. In responding the nurse also must be careful to use unambiguous terms the client can understand. No other area of human behavior is so full of euphemisms, and since the euphemisms vary among social class and cultural groupings, it is easy for an unwary counselor to offend a client or cause misunderstanding. If the nurse somehow manages to project a sincere interest in the client's problems and indicates a willingness to enter into open sexual discussions, it is likely that "almost any individual's sexual history will be reported with sufficient accuracy and adequate detail for treatment purposes" (Masters and Johnson, 1970). This was the advice of William Masters and Virginia Johnson to sexual and family therapists and it applies equally well to nurses, although community nurses do not ask the number and variety of questions that a sex therapist would.

Neurologic impairment is a major physiologic cause of sexual dysfunction. Although sexual dysfunction may have a variety of causes, the major cause is diabetes mellitus. Diabetic neuropathy is caused by the impairment of the autonomic nervous system; it is usually manifest in male clients as a failure to achieve tumescence. However, recent research also indicates that in many cases sexual dysfunction might be psychologic, since the association of diabetes with impotence is widely known and believed. Diabetic women are less likely to achieve orgasm than nondiabetic women, but in a practice setting this is not usually mentioned as a problem by the client (Kolodny, 1971; Pieper and others, 1983; Whitley and Berke, 1983). It might be that diabetic women are more ashamed to mention this or are less aware of their loss than men.

Other endocrine disorders, including anterior pituary deficiency and Addison's disease, are occasionally the cause of a loss of libido. Leriche's syndrome, a localized atherosclerosis, and thrombosis of the bifurcation of the aorta can also cause a loss of tumescence because of the diminished blood supply. Sexual dysfunction can also result from psychologic reaction to an illness, either through misinformation or misunderstanding. Nurses can serve a particularly valuable function in being able to deal with client problems in this area. Myocardial infarction, in particular, has proved sexually frustrating to many clients. Clients, as well as partners of clients, who have had a myocardial infarction often want to resume a sexually active life but fear the exertion will kill them. Research indicates that most clients can resume coitus six to eight weeks after an acute myocardial infarction, providing there is no anginal pain. Specifically, when clients can perform exercises at levels of 6 to 8 calories per minute without accompanying symptoms of abnormal pulse rate and blood pressure or electrocardiogram changes, they can resume sexual activity (Hellerstine and Friedman, 1969). When clients can climb 20 stairs briskly without any of the above signs, as a rule they can also engage in intercourse. Some cautions should be observed, however. Namely sexual activity should be consistent with past patterns, if only because too radical a change from past patterns has been known to cause anxiety in the spouse or partner of the client. The nurse might have to initiate discussion about sexual activity in cardiac clients. Failure to do so can lead not only to client anxiety and possible sexual dysfunction, but also to a slow recovery rate.

Drugs themselves often affect both libido and sexual performance, and nurses should be on the alert to explain the consequences. There are four large groupings of drugs that might affect sexual behavior. Clients might not know the sexual consequences of receiving these drugs. The first group comprises sedatives, including alcohol, barbiturates, and narcotics. Alcohol in small amounts may act to overcome inhibitions, but in larger quantities alcohol acts as an anaphrodisiac, repressing or destroying sexual desire. Methadone, a common substance used in stabilizing drug addicts, also acts as an impairment to sexual function. All sedatives can suppress sexual interest and response.

The antiandrogens, a family of drugs that counter the stimulating effect that androgen has on the brain, also diminish sexual response. Medications in this group are used to treat some allergic reactions, reduce swelling in tissues, and minimize the body's fluids in certain illnesses. Estrogen, a hormone used commonly in menopausal women to minimize the effects of the loss of the body's natural production of estrogen, falls into this antiandrogenic category when given to men for cancer of the prostrate or similar diseases.

The anticholinergic and antiadrenergic drugs used to treat hypertension, circulatory problems, and diseases of the eye also block the blood vessels and nerves connected to the genitals. Reserpine and methyldopa, two drugs sometimes used to treat hypertension, can cause loss of sexual interest, erectile incompetence, and depression.

Psychotropic drugs, including tranquilizers and muscle relaxants, cause ejaculatory and erectile difficulties. Haloperidol and thioridazine can both cause retarded ejaculation.

Nurses must be on the alert to explain the consequences of these drugs to prevent noncompliance with the drug regimen. Spouses or other significant persons in the client's life should also be alerted so that pressure from them will not encourage noncompliance.

VARIANT LIFE-STYLES AND SEXUAL PATTERNS

Nurses also serve as information givers about a variety of sexual orientations, since they are often in a position to participate in educational forums or talk to the relatives of clients. One of the more difficult emotional problems that many parents and relatives have is accepting that their son, daughter, or loved one is homosexual. Part of the difficulty here is that society is not in agreement about what constitutes sexual health, and instead people have been influenced by punitive and arbitrary standards of "normalcy" promulgated by various moral regulators of society. These standards have little to do with what we know about such behaviors. Health professionals as a group have not been any less condemnatory of variant sexual behaviors in the past than society at large; they incorporated into their own definitions of normality what society said and labeled as pathologic what religion had once defined as sinful or what the law labeled criminal. In the not-too-distant past, the only form of sexual behavior generally accepted as "healthy" was heterosexual intercourse within marriage. Even this was qualified by the stipulation that coitus be engaged in only to procreate. In fact, until the past two decades or so, most states outlawed any sexual activity other than penile-vaginal intercourse between legally married people. Although other sexual activities took place, they were technically illegal (Bullough, 1975).

Complicating the problem for the community health nurse is that many clients and many parents or loved ones of clients think they have a sexual "perversion," since they have often read outdated medical literature. Outdated literature often convinces them that something is wrong with either them or their loved one. The medical professional must deal with variant sexual life-styles with great caution, since much that was written and accepted by the medical community before 1980, as well as some that is still believed, is inaccurate if not actually harmful. It was only in 1974 that the American Psychiatric Association removed homosexuality from the category of illness, although not all psychiatrists accepted the decision. A homosexual person could be regarded as ill in 1973 (American Psychiatric Association, 1968) and not ill in 1975 without any change in life-style (American Psychiatric Association, 1980). One cynic stated that more people became well in 1973 than any year before or since.

The action of the American Psychiatric Association emphasizes just how our concepts of illness and disease change. It also emphasizes the necessity for community health nurses to be aware of societal and cultural norms in dealing with clients and to put aside personal prejudices. This brief synopsis of the past history of medical views of homosexuality is also important because many people hold strongly to some of the ideas advanced by earlier generations of researchers, and parents and loved ones of people who proclaim their homosexuality often feel they have failed somehow. This is because in the past homosexuality was attributed to a weak father figure, an overly assertive mother, or an unstable childhood environment, and the parents of homosexual people often suffer untold remorse because they think they have failed. One of the functions that effective nurses can serve when they find themselves dealing with such parents or loved ones is to try to assuage the guilt and hurt.

Nurses might also run into homosexual couples in the course of a home visit or in a clinic. Although such individuals are unlikely to disclose their sexual preference to a community health nurse, when nurses run across couples of the same sex living together, they should be prepared to deal with them in the same way they deal with a heterosexual couple. However, nurses must also be alert to some of the special medical problems of STDs to which homosexual people are susceptible.

A person does not become a homosexual by having one homosexual experience, and one of the counseling tasks that a community nurse often encounters is to assure a young man or young woman of this. Many individuals experiment both heterosexually and homosexually before they proclaim their identity, and some continue to do so for long periods. If a client proclaims himself or herself a homosexual, the decision should be accepted by the nurse. Adults who do seek a nurse's help about their homosexuality are usually more concerned about making a better adjustment to their homosexuality than in altering their sexual orientation. Although some individuals can change from homosexuality to heterosexuality and vice versa, such changes are highly unlikely, and some would argue they are impossible.

Separate from homosexuality is transvestism, a rather complex behavior with many variations. Simply defined it is the desire to wear the clothes of the opposite sex, but the desire to live the role of the oppostie sex and even to be identified with the opposite sex at least part-time is often associated with transvestism. The phenomenon is more commonly found among men than women, since on this issue at least, women have more freedom. The spouse of a transvestite may bring the situation to the nurse's attention, or the nurse may notice transvestite behavior in the client. Many, if not most, transvestites are heterosexual and married. Transvestism is not uncommon. There are no valid estimates of the incidence of transvestism. It does pose a psychologic strain on the spouses of transvestites. Because discovery by children or exposure to the public is feared by many transvestites, transvestism also poses psychologic difficulties for the transvestite that might manifest themselves as organic illnesses or sexual dysfunction in one of the partners.

Transvestism is a behavior dealing with gender identity; transsexualism is a problem with sexual identity, since a transsexual person is not so concerned about dressing or acting out the role of the opposite sex as in having the sexual organs of the opposite sex. Although the phenomenon was reported in the medical literature of the nineteenth century, it was not labeled as transsexualism until 1950 (Bullough, 1975). Transsexualism achieved widespread publicity in 1952 when Christine Jorgensen, a former American soldier, had her sex surgically changed from male to female in Denmark. Even then Dr. Christian Hamburger, the surgeon in charge, identified Jorgensen as a transvestite. He also indicated that when news of the sex change became public he was flooded with communications requesting sex change (Hamburger, 1954). Since then the number of surgical sex changes has increased, but most reputable surgeons require the person to live the role of the opposite sex for at least one year before surgery is performed. A psychiatric examination is also required. Surgically it is easier to transform a male into a female than it is to change a female into a male, although both are now done in approximately equal ratios. Again, the nurse can serve as information giver and as a referral person.

A number of other variant sexual behaviors that community nurses run across exist; some psychiatric-oriented specialists call them "paraphilias," a term we do not use because of its implication of mental illness. The list of variant sexual behaviors is too long to discuss every behavior in detail. Perhaps the most troublesome behaviors are sadomasochistic practices for sexual pleasure. In these cases both partners consent to the behavior, and sometimes the injuries are visible to the nurse. Such behavior becomes problematic when one of the partners does not consent. When these individuals are unwilling to bring charges, the nurse should move with caution. Spouse beating is a serious offense (of which wives often are the victims) as the chapters on women and the family indicate, but sometimes the behavior is mutually agreeable.

SEXUAL CHROMOSOMAL ABNORMALITES

Observing clients, particularly infants and children, closely is one of the most valuable tasks the nurse can perform. Nurses should look for cases of possible chromosomal abnormality. Although the vast majority of individuals have a sexual chromosomal arrangement of XX or XY, a number of viable genetic possibilities exist, including X, XXX, XXY, XYY, and perhaps others. A single X chromosome results in a condition known as Turner's syndrome, which occurs in about one infant in 5000 and results in a female phenotype of short stature with sexual infantilism caused by rudimentary "streak" ovaries and somatic manifestations such as distinctive facies and webbing of the neck. Since the ovaries are nonfunctional or have degenerated entirely, the child does not develop normally at puberty. Usually Turner's syndrome also has a growth-hindering effect; affected individuals seldom grow as tall as 5 feet. Girls who show signs of inadequate growth, even when they do not have the other characteristic stigmata, should be subjected to a chromosomal test; such a test should always be given if the girl fails to develop secondary sex characteristics or exhibits primary amenorrhea. Once the condition is diagnosed, estrogen therapy induces development of the breasts and secondary characteristics, as well as some growth in the genital tract, usually enough to permit normal sex activity.

Much more common is Klinefelter's syndrome (XXY), which is believed to exist in about one case in 500. Clients are phenotypic males with small firm testes, and, like those suffering from Turner's syndrome, they are sterile. During puberty gynecomastia and signs of androgen deficiency occur in about one half of these clients.

Other sex chromosome abnormalities do not necessarily appear through any gonadal defects but are nonetheless associated with a high incidence of mental retardation. Treatment for people in whom chromosomal abnormalities are diagnosed is not yet agreed on.

Even when normal chromosomal patterns develop, other factors can also serve to confuse sexual identity of the child. Since embryologically the external organs are the last stage of sexual development to be completed, it is not uncommon for the external genitalia to be left unfinished, neither fully masculinized nor fully feminized. Because the unfinished state of either sex looks remarkably similar, unfinished external genitalia have caused great traumas over sexual identification in the past. Nurses dealing with newborns are urged to examine them closely and in doubtful cases to recommend holding off conferring a sexual identity until chromosome and other tests can be done.

The professional should also be observant of the developing child, since there are strong psychologic factors involved in sex behavior and most sexual behavior and orientation does not have an innate, instinctive base. Even children deliberately reared in a sex different from the one to which they anatomically should have been assigned seem to accept their sex of rearing (Money and Erhard, 1972). Probably the greatest problem the nurse might face with feminized boys or masculinized girls is in dealing with the parents; in many cases counseling should be recommended for the parents.

SUMMARY

It is extremely important for the community health nurse to be aware of the importance of sexuality, to ask about sexual problems, to be able to recognize venereal disease, and to be acquainted with sexual behaviors that might cause anxieties to the individual or the family. To do this nurses must accept their own sexualities, including the peculiarities of their sexuality, to be as nonjudgmental as possible about a client with sexual problems. Clients who tell about sexual problems should be listened to, organic causes of dysfunction should be recognized and dealt with, and all clients with sex problems should be advised or referred. The nurse must be aware of the diversity of sexual activity and the traumas that result from a hasty generalization or a misunderstanding. No matter how old a client is, sex is one of the motivating factors in life, and a happy, well-adjusted sex life can contribute to clients' well-being throughout their lives.

QUESTIONS FOR DISCUSSION

1. List the major bacterial STDs and identify the causative organism for each.
2. Why is tertiary syphilis seldom seen today?
3. Define the term AIDS.
4. What are the major clinical manifestations of infection with HIV?
5. Is homosexuality an illness?

REFERENCES

American Psychiatric Association: Diagnostic and statistical manual—II, Washington, DC, 1968, The Association. (This manual was revised later to include the 1974 statement.)

American Psychiatric Association: Diagnostic and statistical manual—III, Washington, DC, 1980, The Association.

Bader M: Sexual transmission of shigellosis, Med Aspects Hum Sexuality 12:75, 1978.

Boland MG and Klug RM: AIDS: implications for home care, Am J Maternal/Child Nurs 11:404, 1986.

Boston Women's Health Book Collective: The new our bodies, ourselves, ed 2, New York, 1984, Simon & Schuster.

Brandt AM: No magic bullet: a social history of venereal disease in the United States since 1880, New York, 1985, Oxford University Press.

Brinton CC and others: The development of a neisserial pilus vaccine for gonorrhea and meningococcal meningitis. In Westein L and Fields BN, editors: Seminars in infectious diseases, Vol 4, New York, 1982, Thieme Medical Publishers Inc.

Bullough VL: Transsexualism in history, Arch Sex Behav 4:561, 1975a.

Bullough V: Sex and the medical model, J Sex Res 11:291, 1975b.

Bullough VL: Sexual variance in society and history, Chicago, 1980, University of Chicago Press.

Bullough VL and Seidl A: Sexuality in nursing texts, Holistic Nurs Practice 1:84, 1987.

Centers for Disease Control: Recommendations for prevention of transmission in health care settings, MMWR 36:55, 1987.

Centers for Disease Control, HIV/AIDS: Centers for Disease Control, National AIDS Clearing House, HIV/AIDS surveillance hot line, 800-458-5231, statistics compiled monthly.

Culliton BJ: Penicillin-resistant gonorrhea: new strain spreading worldwide, Science 194:1395, 1976.

Curran JW: Economic consequences of pelvic inflammatory disease in the United States, Am J Obstet Gynecol 138:848, 1979.

Curran JW: Management of gonococcal pelvic inflammatory disease, Sex Transm Dis 6:174, 1980.

Curran JW and others: Epidemiology of HIV infection and AIDS in the United States, Science 239:610, 1988.

Fauci AS: Human immunodeficiency virus: infectivity and mechanisms of pathogenesis, Science 239:617, 1988.

Felman YM and William DC: Sexually transmitted amebiasis, Med Aspects Human Sexuality 12:155, 1978.

Gordon L: Woman's body, woman's right: a social history of birth control in America, New York, 1976, Grossman.

Hamburger C: Desire for change of sex as shown by personal letters from men and women, Acta Endocrinol 8:231, 1954.

Hellerstine HK and Friedman EH: Sexual activity and the post-coronary patient, Med Aspects Human Sexuality 3:70, 1969.

Kaufman RH: Sexual transmission of *Haemophilus vaginalis,* Med Aspects Human Sexuality 10:133, 1976.

Koff WC and Hoth DF: Development and testing of AIDS and vaccines, Science 241:426, 1988.

Kolodny RC: Sexual dysfunction in diabetic females, Diabetes 20:557, 1971.

Masters WH and Johnson VE: Counseling with sexually incompatible marriage partners. In Klemer RH, editor: Counseling in marital and sexual problems, Baltimore, 1965, Williams & Wilkins.

Masters WH and Johnson V: Human sexual inadequacy, Boston, 1970, Little, Brown & Co Inc.

Money J and Erhard A: Man & woman/boy & girl, Baltimore, 1972, John Hopkins University Press.

Morton BM: VD: a guide for nurses and counselors, Boston, 1976, Little, Brown & Co Inc.

Norgard MV and Miller JN: Plasmid DNA in *Treponema pallidum* (Nichols): potential for antibiotic resistance by syphilis bacteria, Science 213:553, 1981.

O'Brien AM, Oerlemans-Bun M, and Blanchfield JC: Nursing the AIDS patient, AIDS Patient Care 1:21, 1987.

Pieper BA and others: Perceived effect of diabetes on relationship to spouse and sexual function, J Sex Ed Ther 9:46, 1983.

Schoen K: Psychosocial aspect of hospice care for AIDS patients, Am J Hospice Care 3:22, 1986.

Scott WC: Pelvic abscess in association with intrauterine contraceptive devices, Am J Obstet Gynecol 131:149, 1978.

Smith AM: Alternatives in AIDS home care, AIDS Patient Care 00:28, 1987.

Smith AM: Understanding Aids, Washington, DC, 1988, US Department of Health and Human Services.

Waugh M: A sexually transmitted disease: *Enterobius vermicularis,* Med Aspects Human Sexuality 10:119, 1976.

Webster B: Report of the National Commission on Venereal Disease, Rockport Md, 1972, HEW Pub No (HSM) 72-8125 Department of Health, Education and Welfare.

Whitley MP and Berke PA: Sexual response in diabetic women, J Sex Ed Ther 9:51, 1983.

CHAPTER 27

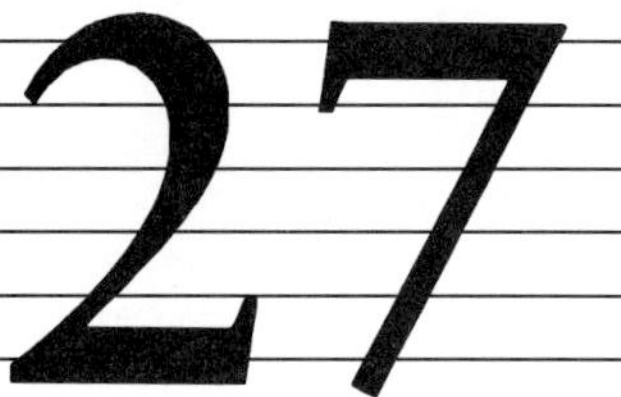

Abuse in a Family Setting

Vern Bullough
Richard Seibert

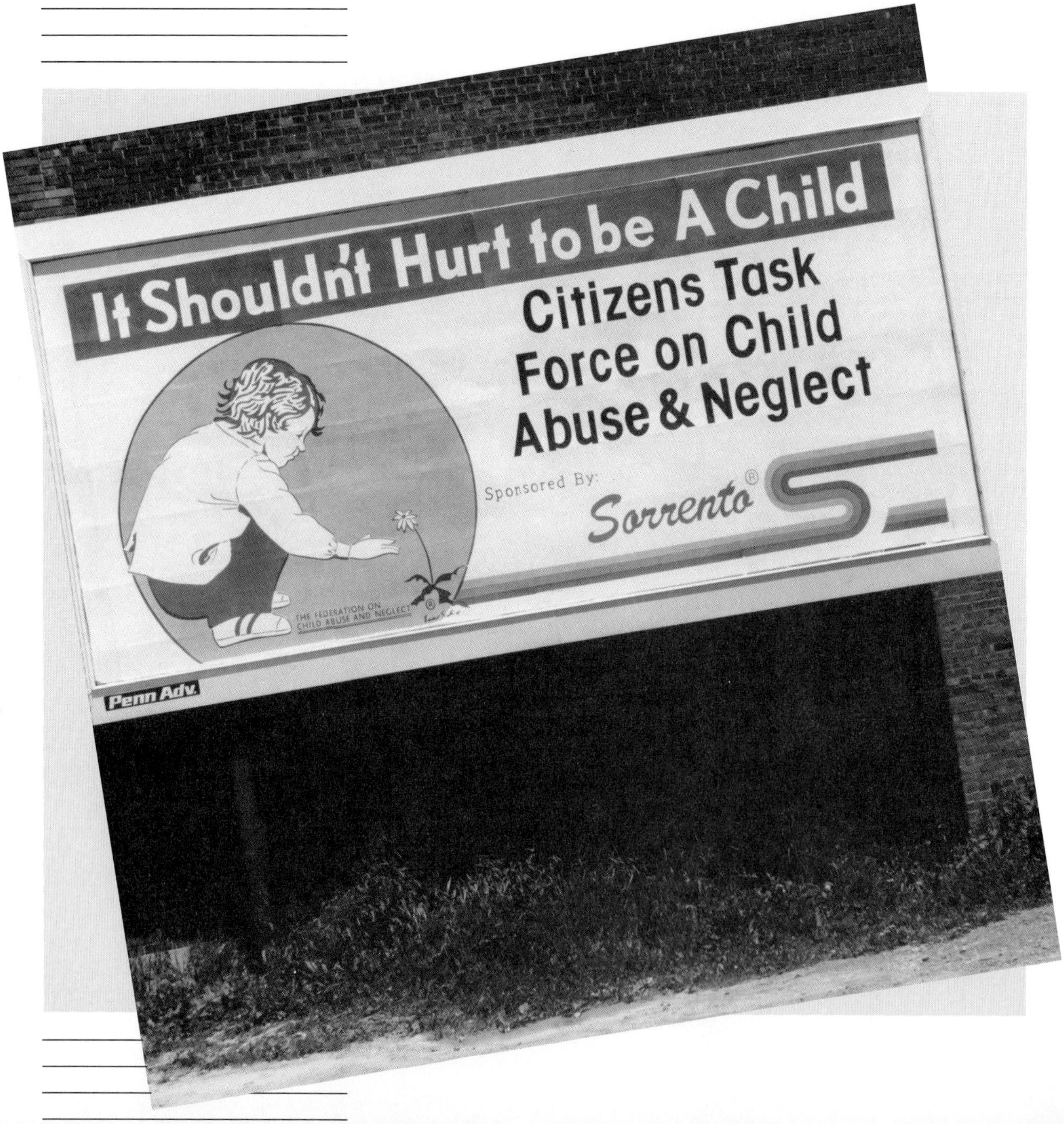

CHAPTER OUTLINE

OBJECTIVES

After completing this chapter, the reader should be able to:

1. Explain why cultural factors are important in understanding and defining abuse.
2. Define child abuse.
3. Distinguish between normative and situational child abuse.
4. List physical indicators of child abuse, as well as indicators of neglect.
5. Describe characteristics of abused children.
6. Explain why the number of battered wives is disproportionate to the number of battered husbands.
7. Explain why the increase in home care might lead to greater client abuse.

COMMUNITY NURSES see abused children, battered wives, and neglected family members; often nurses can help these people. Some words of caution, however, are in order. The terms abused, battered, and neglected have different meanings for different people. They are also terms the media have adopted, often without any discrimination as to their use and with little understanding of what constitutes an abused child, a battered wife, or a neglected person. Each of the terms must be put into a social setting and a cultural perspective. Madeleine Leininger, the nurse anthropologist, popularized the term "transcultural nursing" to emphasize those cultural variables that are crucial but often overlooked aspects of client care (Leininger, 1970 and 1977). Nurses with a sociologic or historical background would call the same thing cultural variables or social factors in nursing care. At least three crucial elements need to be considered in transcultural nursing—basic knowledge about the culture of the client, the necessity for assessing the client from the standpoint of the nurse's own belief system, and an ability to apply a broad knowledge base and an individual assessment to the health care problem at hand. Treatment strategies that are compatible with the client's own beliefs have a better chance of success. Treatments that violate a nurse's strong beliefs, even if the nurse is convinced the treatments are proper, should not be carried out unless the nurse comes to terms with those beliefs. This is particularly true in trying to deal with the issues discussed in this chapter.

CHILD ABUSE AND NEGLECT

Problems in Identification

The definition of child abuse and neglect varies according to social and economic class, as well as ethnic or cultural origins. Ultimate reaction of nurses to an abused or neglected child, a battered wife, or other neglected family members, however, is determined to a large extent by the nurse's own bias. Recognition of this individual orientation, although difficult, is essential in proper intervention techniques and delivery of appropriate services to clients.

Specifically it can probably be assumed that the typical health care professional either comes from or has adopted a middle-class life-style. On the other hand, a disproportionate number of the clientele served by community nurses are likely to be from the lower class. This raises several different kinds of questions. Can the middle-class nurse identify with and empathize with the person from the lower class? Do such simple things as the presence of roaches in the kitchen constitute neglect? When several children are found sharing a single mattress in a cramped room, should the nurse take steps to rectify the situation? Is a sharp slap on the face of a two-year-old child excessive force or a reasonable disciplinary technique?

Potential subjectivity is an issue in other areas as well. What is the proper attitude toward the roles of husband and wife? Does a husband have the right to strike his wife under certain circumstances? What about the sanctity of the home? Does anyone have the right to intervene in the privacy traditionally granted to spouses, parents, and family members?

Although it is easy to ask these questions, there is often no right answer. The discretion and judgment of nurses are severely tested when they deal with the issues raised in this chapter. Acceptable behavior varies widely among social classes and cultural groups. In modern day Sweden, parents who spank their children are guilty of a criminal offense punishable by imprisonment. Yet in many parts of the United States spanking a child is considered a normal part of parenting. Such spankings today usually are less violent and less frequent than they once were because American attitudes are changing. When the razor strap used for honing and sharpening a razor was a standard part of household equipment 50 years ago, beating a child with a strap was the norm in many parts of the country. One of the authors, as a child, lived next door to a child who was beaten every morning on the grounds that he would probably get into trouble sometime during the day and he might as well get spanked early. Many senior citizens have recalled for the authors how as children their hand or fingers were deliberately burned so that they would know to avoid the stove. Young boys who wet the bed were often put into girl's clothing for days at a time and called "sissies" in front of their peer groups, whereas young girls who had difficulty controlling their bladder were required to wear visible diapers or signs proclaiming their inadequacies. A standard expression that was often repeated was, "spare the rod and spoil the child." Many practices that are now considered abuse were considered normal in the not-too-distant past.

These kinds of historical details are important because there is a widespread popular belief, undoubtedly encouraged by media sensationalism, that the incidence of child abuse is rising or that battered wives did not exist in the past and that everyone had a loving place in the family. Nothing could be further from historical reality. Instead in the past few decades we have had a growing sensibility to the dangers of abuse and violence.

Another problem is that domestic violence of all kinds is an invisible phenomenon. Because domestic violence takes place for the most part within the private confines of a home, it is difficult to determine the actual incidence. In 1984, for example, 1,726,649 children were reported as either abused or neglected children by various child protection agencies throughout the United States. That reflected an increase of 185% since 1978. There is disagreement about what such figures mean. Some argue that the numbers reflect an increase in actual incidence, whereas others, such as us, believe that the increased reports are a reflection of increased awareness. This last view is more hopeful than the former because it implies that society is finally recognizing that child abuse and neglect are real and that something should be done about them (NCPCA, 1986).

The health care community, teachers, and even the general public are aware of the existence of child abuse. Feminist sensibilities have been raised enough to emphasize that a wife need not take a beating by her husband, and as women have become somewhat better able to survive economically without a husband, they have asserted their right to be free of abuse. Although elderly people, one of the groups most subject to abuse in the past, still face some forms of discrimination, increasing proportions of them are able to live independently of their children. In fact Social Security, Medicare, and pensions in general have given elderly people the kind of independence that was an almost impossible dream for them in the past. Laws have been and are being changed to conform to these changing societal standards. Institutions have also been established, although not in sufficient quantity or quality, to help deal with some of the problems the nurse might encounter.

Anyone who has read historical reports of public health or community health nurses realizes the difficulty their predecessors faced in finding solutions to the problems they saw among their clients. Often the only solution available for neglected or battered children was to pull them from the family setting and put them into large-scale institutions, where there were often hundreds of other children. Although this removed abused children from the home and freed them from parental battering, such children were not likely to receive loving support in such institutions. As one reads the court records of the past, it becomes apparent why there was such great reluctance to remove children from family settings even though they might have continued to be abused. The same was true of battered wives. If they fled the family, they had to worry about their children, and if a wife took her children with her, the support network of services enabling her to function independently of a husband was almost totally lacking. Invariably professionals advised a battered wife to resign herself to her situation, or she herself decided that with her limited options sticking it out was the best alternative until her children were grown.

Widowed or ill mothers or fathers who were forced to move in with their adult children often produced a tense situation for both the parents and the adult children. Unfortunately, the only alternative was a county old folks' home, the less desirable forerunner of today's nursing home. Often elderly people who found themselves in such situations retreated to their rooms and tried to be as inconspicuous as possible. Conditions undoubtedly varied according to economic level, but the community health nurse usually saw the cases at the lower social and economic levels. Individuals such as Lillian Wald tried to deal with some of these problems by establishing settlement houses in communities to give the poor options and to air their difficulties to the public, but there were never enough settlement houses to deal with all those who needed this kind of support.

Nurses who saw battered children often found little support when they reported the abuse. One nurse of the authors' acquaintance remembers visiting a household and observing a toddler sitting on a potty chair in a closet. While investigating she found that the mother forced her daughter to sit on the chair during all waking hours to toilet train her. If the child did not produce any results or had a bowel movement in her diaper during the night, she was beaten. Eventually, regardless of what the child did, the mother closed the door on the closet and left the child there all day. Ultimately the child was taken from her mother but only after the nurse made many frantic reports to the authorities.

The situation has changed considerably since that time, in large part because of the willingness of professionals to intervene and the development of specialized agencies to help. There are, however, still problems. The most important legislation in terms of child abuse was the Child Abuse Prevention and Treatment Act of 1974. This law established the National Center on Child Abuse and Neglect and provided funds to gather statistics, do research on the causes of child abuse, prevent child abuse, and treat abused children. It also provided for the establishment of regional child-abuse centers. One result was the bring the issue of child abuse to the forefront of public consciousness.

The distinction between child abuse and child neglect is often blurred, especially in the popular media. An appropriate operational definition distinguishing between the two was developed by New York State (1980). In the guidelines issued by the state's department of social services, an abused child was defined as

> a child less than 18 years of age whose parents or other persons legally responsible for their care inflict or allow to be inflicted serious physical injury by other than accidental means; create or allow to be created the risk of such injury; and commit or allow to be committed a sexual offense against the child.

On the other hand, a neglected child may be defined as

> a child less than 18 years of age whose physical, mental, or emotional condition has been impaired or is in danger of being impaired due to parents' failure to provide: adequate food, clothing, shelter, medical care, education, supervision, and guardianship. The infliction of excessive corporal punishment and abandonment of the child is also included in this category.

Child Abuse

Although the types of child abuse and neglect vary somewhat with social and economic condition, child maltreatment takes place at all levels of society. It is, however, more frequent in certain situations of which the nurse should be particularly aware. One such situation results in what might be called normative child abuse, that is, the parents believe severe punishment is part of "good parenting." Often cited in this connection is the belief that to spare the rod is to spoil the child. The nurse must be particularly wary in such situations, remembering the social and cultural variables involved. Some cautious questioning might elicit the belief patterns responsible for punishment, and perhaps if the ongoing punishment is mild enough, the nurse should not intervene. If it is serious, the nursing intervention might be to indicate some of the dangers. Sometimes the nurse can work through institutions such as churches to which the parents belong or suggest some alternatives to physical punishment. Sometimes the only thing the nurse can do is report child abuse to the proper agencies.

Another kind of child abuse, however, is situational child abuse. The key to this is the theory of frustration/aggression, which explains aggressive behavior as a response to frustration. Children tend to become targets of violence by one of two routes. Children may be a real target for parental violence because they are the source of the parent's frustration. Unwanted children may be a target of violence because they are unwanted, but even children who were once wanted might no longer be wanted if they are handicapped, hyperactive, or perceived in other ways as infringing on the social, economic, and emotional goals of their parents. In short, any child who for whatever reason is or becomes unwanted is a potential target for violence (Gelles, 1973).

In addition, children can become targets for parental violence when the real source of anger on the part of the mother or father lies somewhere else. That is, although the real problem for the parent may be an employer, for example, children become the victims because they are weaker than the employer and more accessible to the parent (O'Brien, 1971).

Media attention to some of the more bizarre cases of abuse and neglect leaves the impression that abusive parental behavior is a manifestation of pathologic personalities. This is rarely the case. The majority of abusive and neglectful parents are, by most standards, normal. Their behavior reflects a response to conditions over which they have little or no control or their own cultural upbringing (Straus, 1980).

With prevention and constructive intervention of utmost importance, it is helpful for the nurse to know what kind of families have potentially abusive parents in terms of the aggression/frustration theory. Such families include impoverished families, families experiencing crises such as unemployment or prolonged illness of a spouse, families in which one or both parents are substance abusers, families that are physically or socially isolated, one-parent families, and families in which one or both parents have a history of deviant activity or pathologic behavior or were themselves abused as children.

Failure to thrive may be diagnosed in an abused child at an early stage (approximately one third of these are likely to be infants or toddlers younger than 3 years of age). These children have been physically and emotionally damaged by an adult or sometimes an older child or relative to the extent that someone in the helping professions, often a nurse, becomes aware of a problem. Child abuse can occur not only in a family setting, but also in institutional settings such as day-care centers, schools, and childcare agencies (Kempe, Cutler, and Dean, 1980).

The physical indicators of abuse in the boxed material based on the definitions of the New York State Department of Social Services) do not necessarily indicate that child abuse has occurred. The nurse must consider such injuries in light of inconsistent medical history, the developmental ability of children to injure themselves, or other possible indicators of abuse. These indicators do, however, raise an alert sign and cue the nurse to look further. The questions the nurse should seek to answer include the following:

1. Are bruises bilateral or are they found on only one surface (plane) of the body?
2. Are bruises extensive? Do they cover a large area of the body?
3. Can the broken bones be explained by individual activity?
4. Are there bruises in various stages of healing indicating that injuries occurred at different times?

PHYSICAL INDICATORS OF ABUSE

1. Bruises and welts that may indicate abuse include bruises on any infant, especial facial bruises; bruises on the posterior side of a child's body; bruises in unusual patterns that might reflect the pattern of an instrument or human bite marks; clustered bruises indicating repeated contact with a hand or instrument; and bruises in various stages of healing
2. Broken bones that may indicate abuse most often include multiple breaks in arms or legs that are inconsistent with a child's age or activity
3. Burns that may indicate abuse include immersion burns indicating dunking in a hot liquid ("stocking" burns on the arms or legs or doughnut-shaped burns on the buttocks and genitalia); rope burns that indicate confinement; and dry burns indicating that a child has been forced to sit on a hot surface or has had a hot implement applied to the skin
4. Lacerations and abrasions that may indicate abuse include lacerations of the lip, eye, or any portion of an infant's face including tears in the gum tissue that may have been caused by force feeding; and any laceration or abrasion to external genitalia
5. Head injuries that may indicate abuse include absence of hair or hemorrhaging beneath the scalp caused by vigorous hair pulling; subdural hematomas (hemorrhaging beneath the dura) caused by shaking or hitting; and peritonitis, or inflammation of the peritoneum, caused by a ruptured organ

5. Are there patterns caused by particular instruments such as a belt buckle, a wire, a straight-edge razor, or a coat hanger?
6. Are injuries inconsistent with the explanation offered?
7. Are the patterns of injuries consistent with abuse? (A good example is the shattered eggshell pattern of skull fractures commonly found in children who have had their heads thrown against walls.)
8. Are the patterns of burns consistent with forced immersion in a hot liquid? Is there a distinct boundary line where the burn stops ("stocking burn") or a doughnut pattern caused by forcibly holding a child's buttocks in a tub of hot liquid?
9. Are the patterns of burns consistent with a spattering of hot liquids?
10. Are the patterns of burns consistent with the explanation offered?
11. Are the burns caused by a particular kind of implement such as an electric iron or the grate of an electric heater or are they circular cigarette burns?

Obviously the nurse must exercise judgment in deciding whether a case of child abuse has occurred. It is better, however, to erroneously suspect child abuse than to rationalize that child abuse has not occurred and then find on another visit that the child is in critical condition or even dead from additional incidents.

Often the parent or parents involved in child abuse contradict themselves when they describe the injury, become irritated when questioned about it, are angry with the child about the injury, and give no indications of feeling guilty about their lack of care or concern for the child (see box on opposite page).

If the child is admitted to the hospital, the parents often tend to disappear after the child has been admitted and fail to visit the child during the hospitalization. Surprisingly many children, out of love and loyalty to the parent or fear of losing the parent, may distort the truth in an attempt to protect the responsible parent.

Observers find, however, that the behavior patterns of abused and neglected children are not all the same. In general there seem to be four different categories, although as in any list these categories can be extended to five or six or reduced to two or three depending on how a person wants to include them. The box in the second column of the following page shows one such list.

Child Neglect

Nurses must be alert for indicators of neglect (see box on p. 662). Unfortunately, many of the preceding issues have a high correlation with poverty, and it is important to separate poverty from

Jack Burt, 3 years old, was dead on arrival and had welts around both arms and across his back, a large swelling on his head, and old burn scars from chest to lower abdomen. As his stepfather carried him in, a nurses' aide heard the man say, "I don't want any more of this; I won't take any more of this. No more." Depositing the boy's body on an examining table, he walked across the room, saying in casual social tones to the aide, "Don't I know you from somewhere? I'm sure I've met you somewhere before."

When the physician asked what happened, Jack's stepfather replied, "I just hit him like I always do when he pees the bed. This time he went and fell on his head. . . ."

Although both Jack's mother and grandmother knew he was being "punished" by being placed on a hot gas burner, neither woman had asked for protective placement. Legal charges against the stepfather came after Jack's death (Costin and Rapp, 1984).

SUMMARY OF BEHAVIORS THAT CHARACTERIZE ABUSED CHILDREN

1. Overly compliant, passive, undemanding behaviors aimed at maintaining a low profile and avoiding any possible confrontation with a parent that could lead to abuse; in cases of severe abuse, this could mean avoiding any situation in which the abusive parent even notices the child; often the child is wary of adult contact, apprehensive when other children cry, and intolerant of physical contact or touch
2. Extremely aggressive, demanding, and rageful behaviors caused by the child's repeated frustrations at not getting basic needs met; these behaviors are more common in a child who is mildly or inconsistently abused, since such a child has learned to have some expectations of love and support
3. Overly adaptive behavior in response to unresolved need of the parent; certain abusive parents, unable to satisfy their own needs appropriately, turn to children for fulfillment. If parents need parenting themselves, the child may be expected to assume this task and become inappropriately adult and responsible; other parents, with a need to keep their child dependent, produce clinging, babyish behavior in the child long after a child in a healthy family would have become more self-reliant
4. Lags in development; children who are forced to siphon off energy normally channeled into growth because of a need to protect themselves often fall behind the norms for their age in toilet training, motor skills, socialization, language development, and emotional development

genuine neglect. There are also differing cultural expectations, values, and childrearing practices. It is important to emphasize that sometimes the symptoms of neglect can occur through conditions over which the parent has no control. This is best illustrated by the frustrations experienced by an editor of this text in the 1950s (Bullough, 1953).

In 1953, rats mutilated and killed an infant in an area next to the district in which I was working. In my own district, they chewed the hand of a small black newborn infant named William Henry. William's mother and four siblings lived in a dugout basement under a dilapidated row house. Mrs. Henry had been awakened in the middle of the night by the cries of her baby and found two huge gray rats on top of him. When she snatched him up, his hand was a bleeding mass of mangled flesh. She took her baby to Cook County Hospital for emergency care.

Cook County, however, was more than an hour away by bus, and in order to get there, she borrowed money from her neighbors to take a taxi. Because she was afraid to leave her other four children alone at home, she took all of them with her and she spent the night in the emergency room, waiting for the baby to be treated and admitted. Most of William's hand could be saved, although he lost the distal portion of three fingers. When William was discharged from the hospital, the Health Department was notified. I was sent to visit the family. I found them living in a basement that had probably never been meant to be used as a residence.

Most of the houses in this particular area had been built in the 1870s and 1880s, long before electrical outlets were a standard feature in a home and when food storage posed serious problems. The basements in many of these houses had been designed to store food and coal, and the

INDICATORS OF NEGLECT

1. Abandonment. Children are abandoned totally or for long periods.
2. Lack of supervision. Children are observed engaging in dangerous activities or are inadequately supervised for long periods, for example, children are left in the care of children too young to protect them.
3. Lack of adequate clothing and good hygiene. Children are dressed inadequately for the weather or suffer persistent illnesses such as pneumonia, frostbite, or sunburn that are associated with excessive exposure; children have severe diaper rash or other persistent skin disorders resulting from improper hygiene; children are chronically dirty and unbathed.
4. Lack of medical or dental care. Children's needs for medical or dental care or medication and health aids are unmet.
5. Lack of adequate education. Children are chronically absent from school.
6. Malnutrition (a particularly important clue). Children lack sufficient quantity or quality of food; children consistently complain of hunger or rummage for food; sometimes a key to malnutrition is severe developmental lag.
7. Lack of adequate shelter. Children live in housing that is structurally unsafe or unsanitary or has exposed wiring or inadequate heating.

original owners probably never thought of these dugouts as possible residences. It obviously was not a suitable place for five children to live.

I felt the rats would attack the infant again unless something was done. I called the office of the city housing inspector, met with officials in the urban renewal office, and had long discussions with my own supervisor. In spite of all my efforts, some of which became quite frantic, no public official would be talked into doing anything about the rats, and there seemed to be no other housing available at the level the Henry family could afford. . . . Mrs. Henry . . . was on welfare, but her welfare checks were smaller than those families of comparable size because she had tried to keep the arrival of her new baby a secret. She was convinced that her social workers would cut off her aid entirely if it became known that she had conceived again without finding a stable male breadwinner for the family.

The house above the Henrys' basement was scheduled to be torn down as part of a large urban renewal project. The official at the Office of Urban Renewal whom I contacted explained that his department might eventually use its influence to place the Henrys in public housing, since finding other kinds of replacement housing on the open market for such a large family, at a price they could afford, was next to impossible. However, the official refused to speed up the process or even let Mrs. Henry know that she had a chance to obtain public housing, because he felt it would be "bad for neighborhood morale." He explained to me that the only way to get "those old mamas off their cans was to frighten them with the bulldozer."

Unfortunately, the slum clearance itself was a major factor in creating the rat problem in the first place. The large luxury buildings being built on the cleared land were largely ratproof, and the displaced rats, like the displaced people, made their way to nearby slum areas. Because of increased concentration, the appetites of the rats soon outstripped the available uncollected garbage supplies and they turned to attacking infants in their cribs.

Several families in the area had built heavy screen cages over their children's beds and, sometimes at night, they would hear rats gnawing on the screens. Mrs. Henry, however, lacked money to buy screens and apparently had little talent as a carpenter. After the baby came home from the hospital, she tried to keep herself awake at night to guard him, but soon the state of chronic exhaustion made this difficult. In a desperate attempt to do something constructive to help her, I begged two half-grown cats from another family I knew and took them to her. Before a week was past, the rats had eaten the cats.

William Henry was a neglected infant, but the neglect was at that point beyond the mother's control. In part because of such cases, the federal government in the 1960s and 1970s made concerted efforts to enact legislation prohibiting this kind of societal neglect. Some of this legislation no longer exists. Even when it was in effect, if a person was poor and had no supporting relatives, society still did not cope well with this kind of neglect except to remove the child from the parent, which in cases like William Henry's is really no solution.

Role of the Nurse in Working With Abused and Neglected Children

The problem of detecting and dealing with abused and neglected children is not only a nursing problem. It crosses many disciplines and involves many different groups. Nurses are obviously a key factor, but law enforcement officers, many persons in the legal system, the staff in medical care facilities, social workers, teachers, ministers, priests, rabbis, self-help groups, and counseling and family therapy groups are also important in dealing with abused and neglected children. Often laypeople, family, friends, and fellow church members are important in helping deal with the problem; at other times, groups such as Parents Anonymous or Alcoholics Anonymous may be called in (see box).

The goal of any intervention is to reduce the stress that encourages abusive behavior, as well as to protect the abused or threatened persons. In extreme cases criminal prosecution might be a result of intervention, although this is usually reserved for those cases in which there seems to be no hope of change. Often it is necessary to remove a child from a dangerous situation, although there are still societal problems on where to place such children, particularly in the long run.

The best treatment for abuse is preventive treatment, and it is in this area that the nurse can be most effective. Nurses need to be alert not only to actual child abuse, but also to those conditions that are breeding grounds for abuse and neglect. Often parents are aware of the potential for abuse in themselves and are willing to discuss the issue with an empathetic nurse. If nurses become aware of potential danger, they should try to identify support systems for both the person who is doing the abusing and the person likely to be abused.

SELECTED NATIONAL GROUPS DEALING WITH ABUSED CHILDREN

American Humane Association, Children's Division, 5351 Roslyn St., Englewood, CO, 80110

National Center for the Prevention and Treatment of Child Abuse and Neglect, University of Colorado Medical Center, 1205 Oneida St., Denver, CO, 80229

Parents Anonymous, 22330 Hawthorne Blvd., Torrace, CA, 90505

National Center on Child Abuse and Neglect, PO Box 1182, Washington, D.C., 20113

Alcoholics Anonymous. Local chapters or hot lines can be found in local telephone books

Many communities have hot lines that can be called; in other instances, it is important to turn to families or various shelters for support. The nurse must also be alert to situations where abuse exists only as a potential, such as the case of a handicapped child where the parents seem unable to cope or where nurses find uncomplaining acceptance of intolerable conditions.

Nurses must report suspected child abuse in many jurisdictions. Persons who report suspected child abuse, even if they do so without much evidence, are immune from any civil or criminal liability that might result from such action. If prosecution of child abusers results from such a report, however, the nurse might be called on to testify. It is probably best to take a sympathetic yet objective attitude in such cases. Even though society has made considerable progress in the past few decades, there is still no easy answer to the problem of child abuse by parents. Often the abused child is placed in a foster home for protective reasons, but the child is often re-placed several times, which can lead to serious problems in the child. This is why most agencies still strive to involve the family in therapy programs. The abusing parent is most often viewed as a potentially good parent who has gone wrong and not as one who is deficient. If experience demonstrates that a parent is deficient, removal of the child from the family still remains the only answer.

BATTERED SPOUSES

Although battered husbands exist, women are more often battered perhaps because men traditionally have had greater opportunities to escape the house and live lives more independent of the family. Men, as a group, are also physically stronger than women. Like child abuse, the battered-wife phenomenon is both a new and an old problem. The extent of the problem is unknown and in part depends on definition. In a survey of 2143 couples, Murray Straus (1980) reports that 28% of the respondents reported incidents of violence in their marriage. For various reasons, such as the victim's shame, much violence goes unreported. Straus estimates that violence might occur in as many as 50% to 60% of all American marriages.

In large part because of the feminist concerns expressed in the 1960s and 1970s, wife battering became an issue of national concern. The first widely publicized shelter for battered women, the Chiswick Women's Aid, was established in England in 1971. One of its founders, Erin Pizzey, furthered awareness of the problem through speaking tours and a book titled, *Scream Quietly or the Neighbors Will Hear* (1974). Because of successful lobbying by Pizzey and others, two British parliamentary committees investigated wife beating. The result was the passage of a 1976 law in the United Kingdom giving broader protection to battered women (Tierney, 1982).

In the United States the first organized response to wife beating was the opening of the Rainbow Retreat in Phoenix, Arizona, in 1973, and other shelters quickly followed. Haven House in Pasadena, California, began sheltering battered women in 1974, although it was originally restricted to helping women beaten by alcoholic husbands. La Casa de las Madres in San Francisco and Transition House in Cambridge, Massachusetts, two other early shelters, were models of feminist grass-roots shelters followed by others.

Even before the shelters appeared, Women's Advocates, Inc., of St. Paul, Minnesota, established a hot line in 1972 to provide telephone crisis counseling to battered women. Group members later took to sheltering victims informally in their own homes. A hot line began in New York City in 1975 (Abused Women's Aid in Crisis), and after that hot lines and shelters began springing up across the United States.

The impulse behind these concerns was the growth of the feminist movement, and what started on a local level soon became a project for national groups. The National Organization for Women formed the National Task Force on Battered Women/Household Violence at its eighth annual conference in October 1975 to raise consciousness and promote shelters. Del Martin, coordinator of the task force, wrote *Battered Wives* (1977), which proved as influential in raising American consciousness as Pizzy's book did in raising British public opinion. Between 1975 and 1978 some 170 shelters opened in the United States (Battered Families, 1979).

The growing movement concerned with battered wives quickly moved into the legislative arena, and public policy was established. The initial legislation was designed to broaden protection for battered wives by increasing the criminal penalties for battering, strengthening civil protection, and making it easier for women to file charges against their husbands. By 1980 most states, as well as the District of Columbia, had enacted special legislation for cases of wife beating (Kalmuss and Straus, 1981), and although law enforcement agencies initially were reluctant to intervene, they have become increasingly active in the field. So far no federal legislation has been enacted, although bills have been introduced. Instead various government agencies have either established new programs or extended old programs to address the issue. The Law Enforcement Assistance Administration, for example, put several million dollars into combating family violence. The Department of Labor instructed regional administrators to direct local governments to fund programs, and the Department of Health and Human Services in 1979 created the Office on Domestic Violence.

During this same time the National Institute of Mental Health began funding research into the field of family violence. The United State Commission on Civil Rights (Tierney, 1982) also moved into the field by sponsoring a national conference on policy issues regarding wife beating. The list of agencies and projects could be continued, but the point is that a new awareness of an old problem has occurred. Much of the recent research that has taken place emphasizes that it is more often an economic dependency than a psychologic dependency that keeps women in severely abusive marriages (Kalmuss and Straus, 1981). Abused women are often in a catch-22—beaten if they stay in a marriage and economically lost if they quit the marriage. In many ways the battered wife finds her relationship with her husband similar to the relationship between a child and a parent. She is physically weaker than her husband, and she is an easily accessible target for her husband's anger. Although roles are changing in this society, a battered wife is still quite likely to perceive herself as inferior to her husband. A significant section of society still believes women are inferior to men. Finally, as is also the case with children, the role of the wife has historically been defined as one the husband needs to control. Traditionally, husbands not only had the right to beat their wives, they could also beat them anytime and for any or no reason (Hotaling and Straus, 1980).

Changing this situation requires fundamental changes in the male-female relationships, some of which are now taking place, as well as the kind of institutional support necessary to give women greater independence. These support services include childcare services, reduced occupational discrimination against women, and an end to sex-based wage differentials. Therapeutic education and support services designed to build a woman's self-confidence, independence, and belief that she can survive outside of marriage can help individual cases, but as long as the basic inequalities between marriage partners continue to be a part of society, wife abuse, despite reforms by the feminist movement, is not going to be eradicated easily (Gelles and Straus, 1988; Dutton, 1988; Shupe and Stacey, 1987).

The nurse must deal with wife abuse somewhat differently than child abuse, since the law assumes that women, as adults, have greater freedom of action. It is probably wise for the nurse who believes there is evidence of wife abuse to try to seek confirmation from the victim before she reports it, since abused wives often are either unwilling or unable to speak out publicly against their husbands. Police have also generally been reluctant to intervene in domestic disputes, even those involving violence, since in some cases after dealing with the abusive husband, they find that the woman is not willing to press charges after the incident. Often, in fact, the abused wives join their husbands in attacking the police (Baro, 1980).

Police, however, have increasingly come to realize the seriousness of domestic violence, since it can and does lead to murder, sometimes the wife killing the husband, other times the husband beating the wife to death. Bernadette Powell (Jones, 1985) gained national attention when she shot and killed her ex-husband who had continued to harass and physically abuse her even after the two were divorced. Police had apparently not taken his violent actions so seriously as they should have, and Powell's case added impetus to the movement to educate police more effectively about how to intervene in cases of domestic violence. Laws have also changed, and in many jurisdictions police now have the right to arrest and detain husbands overnight if they batter their wives. Husbands can be held overnight even if the wife does not file a complaint. If the police have difficulty intervening in domestic struggles, the problem for the nurses is compounded. The best thing the nurse can do is give a referral to a battered women's shelter or hot line and extend a sympathetic ear.

OTHER CASES OF FAMILY ABUSE

Although anyone living in a family situation is a potential target of abuse, next to children and wives, elderly people constitute the group most likely to be the subject of growing tension and therefore possible abuse. Elderly people are often brought back into the family home because of illness or frailty. Often in today's world elderly parents who are unable to take care of themselves must be brought into their adult children's home, but sometimes adult children must be brought back into the parents' home for the same reason (Quinn and Tomita, 1986).

A good example is Stanley Aiken,* a widower with Alzheimer's disease who had lived alone for several years after his wife's death but who, because of the increasing severity of his disease, was brought to the home of his daughter and son-in-law who had teenage children. Although the daughter, Althea Lowman,* loved her father, his conduct grew more and more erratic. Stanley could not remember what he had said and sometimes forgot where he was. Although Stanley loved to walk, he became lost and disoriented when he took walks alone. He became incontinent at night, and Althea began waking Stanley in the middle of the night to take him to the bathroom as if he were a small child. One day Stanley went into the backyard with Althea's eldest son's target pistol and began shooting in the air to frighten away people whom he thought were sent to attack him. This necessitated police intervention and temporary commitment. The discharge nurse investigated the home before Stanley was sent there again, and although the nurse felt the father should be institutionalized, Althea was so insistent she could handle the situation that Stanley was sent back to her home. The nurse alerted the outpatient department to keep a close watch on the situation. When a nurse visited the home about two weeks later she found Stanley with a deep scratch on his face. After the nurse inspected further, she found that Stanley had bruise marks on his back. When questioned, Mrs. Lowman said her father had fallen over a bicycle in the garage, but since the bruises on the back did not support such a story, the nurse gently probed deeper. Althea immediately burst into tears and said that her father had put on his hat to go for a walk at a time when she was not free to go with him. Stanley had insisted on going, and Althea had tried to stop him by hitting him on the face. Althea's ring scratched him. Stanley still insisted on leaving, and Althea Lowman had literally tackled him to hold him down. Once Stanley was down Althea lost control of herself and pummeled him on the back. She was ashamed of her actions. After some further conversation Althea began to vent her frustrations to the nurse, who listened patiently and nonjudgmentally. Ultimately Stanley was institutionalized. The daughter, however, went to the institution every day for a couple of hours. Althea found that she could oversee the care of her father better than if he had stayed at her home. Cases such as this are complicated because of the guilt that children often feel about "neglecting" their parents. In this case a solution was found, but each situation is different.

Cases like Stanley Aiken's are likely to increase rather than decrease because of changes in the health care system related to deinstitutionalization (Pillemer, 1985). This is true not only of elderly clients, but also of family members with long-term illnesses or who are otherwise bedridden but not in need of enough nursing care to justify hospitalization. Although many family members are receptive to taking care of their loved

*Names have been changed to protect the clients' identity.

ones at home, if they have to do so for long periods, the chances for possible abuse increase. The kinds of cases a nurse might run into during home visits, either as a discharge nurse or while doing a nursing assessment, are exemplified by the case of Donald Knorr.*

Donald Knorr was 37 years of age, single, and used to living by himself or with various women friends. He worked in steel mills from the time he was 18 years of age until the mills in his city closed. To save money while he went to a community college for retraining, Donald moved back into the home of his widowed 77-year-old mother. Donald fell asleep at the wheel of his car, went off the road at a high speed, and suffered severe neck injuries three days after he graduated and started working (for the first time in two years). Donald found himself a quadriplegic after surgery, but there is some hope that he will recover at least partially. By the time Donald was removed from the intensive care unit he had exhausted his insurance and was sent home to his mother. Medicaid and a private nursing service took over much of the care, but the aged mother still had to take on heavy burdens, particularly since the private duty aides and licensed practical nurses did not always show up, and she became frazzled. Donald, even though he tried not to be overbearing, demanded service and attention. When the nurse supervisor visited the family, she realized quickly the emotional state of the mother and the need to give greater support service to her. In fact, the mother confessed that she had stood crying by her sleeping son's bed the day before. She was angry and frustrated with the way life had treated her. She was fearful that she might do something drastic unless she could get away for a while. The mother also felt guilty.

In such situations abuse is likely to occur, and the nurse must be alert for the possibility. In the case of Mrs. Knorr, the nurse contacted Mrs. Knorr's sister who sent her college-age son to stay with Donald for a week while Mrs. Knorr visited an old friend in another city. She came back somewhat refreshed, albeit still not anxious to resume the burden thrust on her.

Community-based nurses, if current trends in client care continue, will be called on to use their nurturing skills to help not only the client, but also members of the client's family. The burden of an elderly parent, a severely handicapped or bedridden adult child, or a dying spouse who has been sent home from the hospital are all situations calling for sophisticated nursing intervention. Unfortunately, much of the care is given by the least skilled members of the nursing team, and the registered nurse is only called in occasionally. The nurse then must make rapid assessments and quick investigations, but the skilled and knowing nurse can prevent untold tragedies of abuse. In fact, one of the selling points for skilled nursing is not only client care, but also the ability to perceive growing family crises and do something about them.

*Names have been changed to protect the clients' identity.

SUMMARY

Although the incidence of abuse of vulnerable family members has probably lessened in recent years, it is still a significant problem that nurses need to be able to recognize and report. Briefly defined, child abuse is inflicting a serious physical injury on or committing a sexual offense against a child. Child neglect is causing a serious physical, mental, or emotional problem by failure on the part of caregivers to provide adequate food, clothing, shelter, medical care, education, or supervision. These same problems can occur with other vulnerable family members including wives, mentally retarded or sick adults, or elderly people. The causes of abuse and neglect by family members are multiple, but often abusers were themselves victims of abuse, or they are people who are under great stress and have not developed positive coping strategies.

Nurses who work in the community or emergency rooms need to be particularly aware of the physical indicators of abuse including multiple bruises, broken bones, and burns and the signs of neglect including poor hygiene, lags in development, overcompliance, or extreme aggressiveness. Suspected abuse or neglect should be thoroughly investigated and reported to the authorities when appropriate.

Family members who abuse or neglect others can sometimes be helped with group therapy or temporary respite services, which may defuse what seems like a hopeless situation to them. With the support of career counseling or assertiveness training battered wives can sometimes help themselves.

QUESTIONS FOR DISCUSSION

1. What is the difference between child abuse and child neglect?
2. List at least four clues that might suggest child abuse.
3. List at least four clues that might suggest child neglect.
4. In what types of situations might elder abuse occur?
5. Speculate as to why an abused wife might stay with her husband.

REFERENCES

Baro M: Functions of the police and the justice system in family violence. In Green M, editor: Violence and the family, Boulder, Colo, 1980, Westview Press Inc.

Battered families: a growing nightmare, US News and World Report, p 60, January 15, 1979

Bullough B: Unpublished case notes, 1953.

Costin LB and Rapp CA: Child welfare policies and practices, New York, 1984, McGraw-Hill Inc.

deYoung M: The sexual victimization of children, Jefferson, NC, 1982, McFarland & Co Inc, Publishers.

Dutton D: The domestic assualt of women, Boston, 1988, Allyn & Bacon Inc.

Fotjik K: Wife beating: how to develop a wife assault task force and project, Pamphlet, Ann Arbor, Mich, 1976, Ann Arbor-Washtenau County National Organization for Women.

Garbarino J and Gwen W: Understanding abusive families, Lexington, Mass, 1980, DC Health.

Gelles R: Child abuse as psychopathology: a sociological critique and reformulation, Am J Orthopsychiatry 43:11, 1973.

Gelles R and Straus M: Intimate violence, New York, 1988, Simon & Schuster Inc.

Green M: Violence and the family, Boulder, Colo, 1980, Westview Press Inc.

Hotaling G and Straus MA: Culture, social urbanization, and irony in the study of family violence. In Straus MA and Hotaling GT, editors: The social causes of husband-wife violence, Minneapolis, 1980, University of Minnesota Press.

Hymovich D, Hymovich B, and Underwood M: Family health care, New York, 1973, McGraw-Hill Inc.

Jones A: Everyday death: the case of Bernadette Powell, New York, 1985, Holt, Rinehart & Winston Inc.

Kalmus D and Straus MA: Ideological and social organizational factors associated with state and local response to domestic violence, Unpublished paper presented at the meeting of the Academy of Criminal Justice Sciences, Philadelphia, March 11, 1981.

Kempe S, Cutler C, and Dean J: The infant with failure to survive. In Kempe C and Helfer RE, editors: The battered child, ed 3, Chicago, 1980, University of Chicago Press.

Leininger MM: Nursing and anthropology: two worlds to blend, New York, 1970, John Wiley & Sons Inc.

Leininger MM: Transcultural nursing, St. Paul, Minn 1979, Masson Publishing.

Martin D: Battered wives, San Francisco, 1977, Glide Publications.

Mayhall PD and Norgard KE: Child abuse and neglect, New York, 1983, John Wiley & Sons Inc.

National Committee for the Prevention of Child Abuse, NCPCA Memorandum, Feb 1986.

New York State Department of Social Services: Guidelines for Detecting Child Abuse, New York, 1980, The Department.

O'Brien J: Violence in divorce-prone families, J Marriage Fam 33:92, 1971.

Pillemer K: The dangers of dependency: new findings on domestic violence against the elderly, Soc Problems 133:146, 1985.

Pizzey E: Scream quietly or the neighbors will hear, Short Hills, NJ, 1974, Ridley Enslow Publishers.

Quinn MJ and Tomita SK: Elder abuse and neglect: causes, diagnosis and intervention strategies, New York, 1986, Springer Publishing Co Inc.

Sgroi M: Handbook of Clinical Intervention in Child Sexual Abuse, Lexington, Mass, 1982, DC Heath.

Shupe A, Stacey W, and Hazelwood L: Violent men, violent couples, Lexington, Mass, 1987, DC Health & Co.

Straus MA and Hotaling GT, editors: The social causes of husband-wife violence, Minneapolis, 1980, University of Minnesota Press.

Straus MA: A sociological perspective on the causes of family violence. In Green MR, editor: Violence and the family, Boulder, Colo, 1980, Westview Press Inc.

Straus MA: Wife beating: how common and why? In Straus M and Hotaling G, editors: The social causes of husband-wife violence, Minneapolis, 1980, University of Minnesota.

Steinmetz S and Straus M: Violence in the family, New York, 1974, Dodd, Mead & Co Inc.

Tierney KJ: The battered women: issues of public policy. Proceedings of a Consultation Sponsored by the US Commission on Civil Rights, Washington, DC, 1982, US Commission on Civil Rights.

CHAPTER

28

Substance Abuse

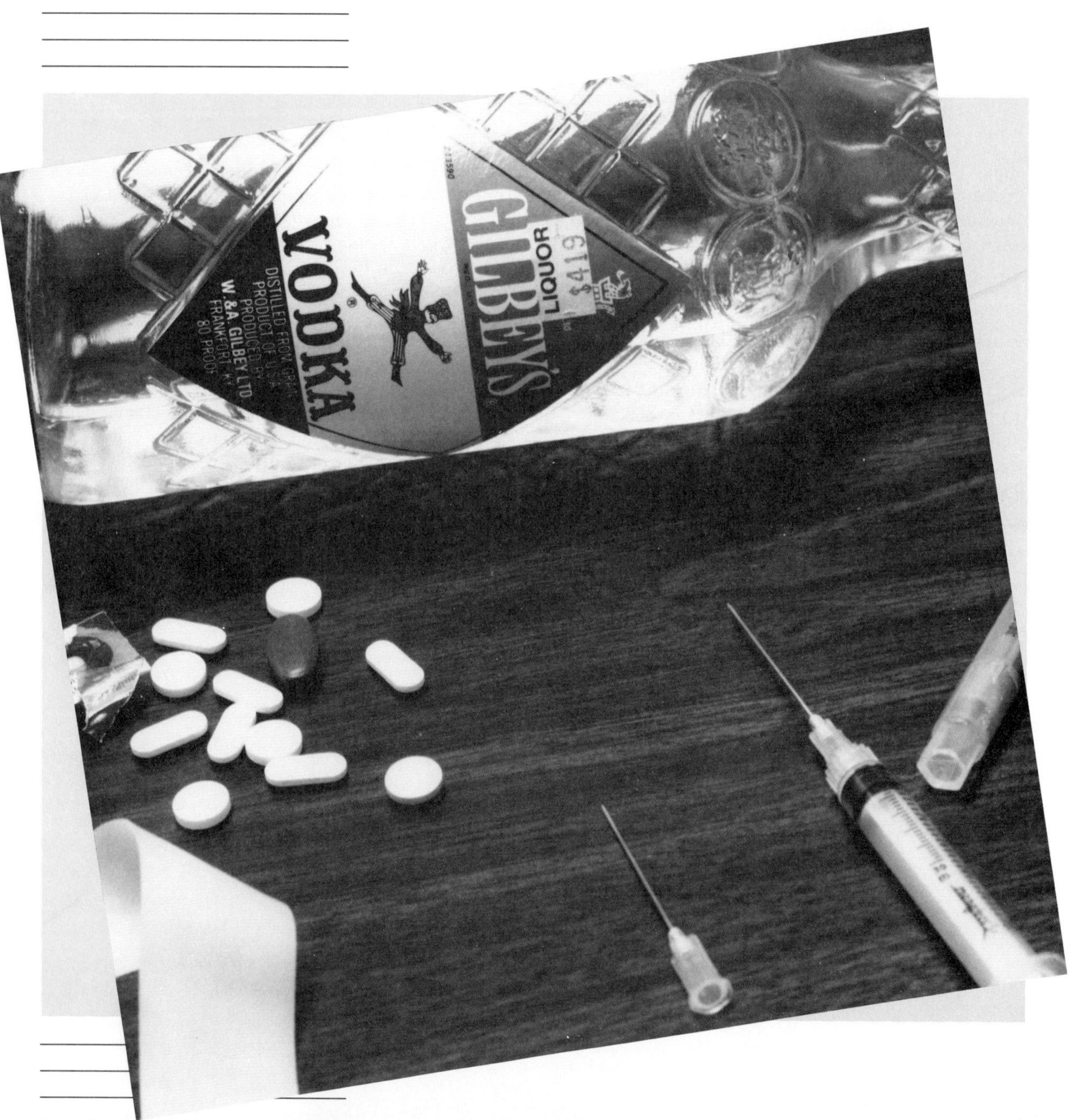

CHAPTER OUTLINE

Historical perspectives

Current perspectives

Types of commonly abused substances

- Xanthines
- Tobacco
- Central nervous system depressants
- Stimulants
- Cocaine
- Opiates and other analgesics
- Cannabis
- Hallucinogens and other drugs
- Glues, solvents, and aerosols

Using the nursing process to treat substance abuse

- The nursing process: assessment
- Nursing diagnosis
- Planning
- Implementation: primary prevention
- Implementation: secondary and tertiary prevention
- Evaluation

Substance abuse and populations at risk

- Drug abuse and AIDS
- Drug-exposed infants
- Nurses who abuse substances

Summary

OBJECTIVES

After completing this chapter, the reader should be able to:

1. Identify the major types of substances that are abused.
2. Understand the actions of these substances, the symptoms of their use, and, as appropriate, the symptoms of withdrawal.
3. Understand the five-step nursing process as it relates to substance abuse.
4. Discuss the special problems of selected at-risk populations, including intravenous drug users, pregnant women, and nurses.

HISTORICAL PERSPECTIVES

Florence Nightingale, under whose image modern nursing developed, would probably have considered substance abuse a major nursing problem—but for quite different reasons than we do today. What we now call substance abuse was in her day seen as a moral rather than a medical illness, and thus a vice and not a disease. Since Nightingale believed that one of the tasks of nurses was to impart moral training to their clients, she probably would have urged nurses to help their clients overcome their failings by emphasizing moral values. The debate over whether "addiction," as it was then termed, was a moral or medical problem lasted well into the twentieth century, and as late as 1968, when Terry and Pellens (1970) surveyed health officials across the United States, 425 health officials stated that most physicians in communities under their jurisdiction considered addiction a disease, whereas 542 reported that most physicians in communities under their jurisdiction regarded addiction as a vice.

It was not only the debate about whether addiction was a vice or an illness that made the nursing problems of an earlier generation different from ours, but also the definition of what was a harmful drug. Opiates were widely used in the nineteenth century without any consideration of consequences. Teething babies had their gums rubbed with drugs such as paregoric or morphine, and laudanum was put into formulas to soothe infants. The original formula for Coca-Cola included cocaine. Physicians regularly prescribed drugs for various client ills. In fact until the Harrison Narcotic Act was approved in 1914, American physicians were responsible for a significant portion of what we would now call substance abuse. Even after the act was passed, those addicted to drugs could get them by prescription from their physician, although in 1919 the U.S. Treasury Department issued regulations that prohibited prescribing narcotics to maintain addicts on their customary usage. Although it took some years before the U.S. Supreme Court finally ruled favorably on the legality of these regulations, most physicians ceased providing drugs for addicts and all clinics providing stabilizing doses were closed by 1923.

Deprived of their legal source of drugs, addicts had to either stop using illegal drugs or use illegal sources to obtain them. Many addicts turned to illegal sources, and when they were caught, they were arrested; if convicted, they were sent to federal prison. By 1928 narcotic drug law violators constituted about one third of the populations of major federal penitentiaries at Atlanta, Leavenworth, and McNeil Island (Bennett, 1958). This crackdown on narcotic addiction coincided with Prohibition in the United States. If those arrested and convicted of alcohol-related crimes were also included in the prison population count, it is clear that the majority of inmates in federal prisons were there for their connection with some form of drug use.

The inevitable result of criminalizing drugs was an escalation of inmates and a growing crisis of prison congestion. Superintendent of Prisons James W. Bennett proposed that special federal institutions be established for treatment and rehabilitation of addicts. This was the first major indication that attitudes toward substance abuse were changing from regarding it as a vice and crime to regarding it as an illness. Although the U.S. Public Health Services did not want to take responsibility for such institutions, they were forced to. Legislation providing for two rehabilitation centers was passed in 1929, but the first center, built near Lexington, Kentucky, did not open until 1935. It was designed to serve 1200 persons. Although it was originally called the U.S. Narcotics Farm (inmates worked on a farm while recovering), its name was soon changed to the U.S. Public Health Service Hospital. A second center was opened in 1938 near Fort Worth, Texas, and was always known as a U.S. Public Health Service Hospital. Individuals either were committed to the hospitals by the courts or signed themselves in voluntarily, but one of the early findings from this procedure was that approximately 70% of the clients who entered voluntarily left before treatment was complete. Both centers originally dealt only with men, and it was not until 1941 that women were admitted, first at Lexington and later for a brief time at Fort Worth. The Fort Worth center closed in 1971 and the Lexington center closed in 1974 as new views of substance abuse, as well as different treatment modalities, developed. As this happened, community-oriented substance abuse centers became the dominant treatment modality (Maddux, 1978).

CURRENT PERSPECTIVES

As attitudes toward substance abuse changed, so did the definition of what constituted substance abuse. The current definition is twofold including a list of substances that can be abused and a description of what happens when substance abuse occurs. In general terms substance abuse involves taking through any route of administration any substance that alters mood, level of perception, or brain function. Such a broad definition allows the inclusion of substances ranging from prescribed medications to alcohol or even solvents. More narrowly, substance abuse is defined as use of mind-altering substances in ways that differ from generally approved medical or social practices. The use of the term "social practices" means that definitions can change as social practices change. Usually substance abuse involves dependence or habituation and compulsive use that implies a psychologic or physical need for the drug. The following box defines terms commonly associated with substance abuse.

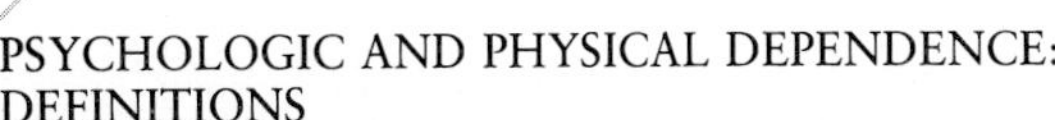

PSYCHOLOGIC AND PHYSICAL DEPENDENCE: DEFINITIONS

1. Psychologic dependence is an attribute of all definitions of substance abuse and derives from the user's perceived need for the substance to reach a maximum level of functioning and to avoid negative effects associated with its absence.
2. Physical dependence is a state of physiologic adaptation to chronic use of the substance to the point that symptoms of withdrawal develop when drug intake is stopped. Physical symptoms, however, are also interrelated with behavior conditions and psychologic factors. Physical dependence usually encompasses two important aspects—tolerance and withdrawal.
A. Tolerance is the need to have larger and larger doses of a substance to achieve the same effects as were achieved the first time the drug was taken. This phenomenon occurs both through alterations in the drug metabolism such as the liver destroying the substance more quickly *(metabolic tolerance)* and through alterations in the target cells' (usually in the nervous system) functioning in the presence of the drug such as the tissue reaction to the drug being diminished *(pharmacodynamic tolerance)*. This is a general statement and is not applicable to each individual, since there are variations in individuals. One person may develop tolerance to one aspect of a drug's action and not another. Usually the development of tolerance to one drug of a class indicates *cross-tolerance* to other drugs of the same class (see following box).
B. Withdrawal is the appearance of physiologic symptoms when the intake of a substance is stopped too quickly. This phenomenon was first and most completely described for drugs like opiates that tend to depress the action of the central nervous system. Today we know that when drugs with different actions than opiates, such as stimulants, are stopped withdrawal signs occur. Withdrawal, it should be noted, is not an all-or-none phenomenon and usually consists of a syndrome or mixture of a variety of possible symptoms.

Modified from Schuckit MA: Drug and alcohol abuse: a clinical guide to diagnosis and treatment, ed 2, New York, 1984, Plenum Publishing Corp.

TYPES OF COMMONLY ABUSED SUBSTANCES

Some substances of potential abuse are more widely used than others. Alcohol, nicotine, and caffeine, for example, are probably the most widely used drugs in Western culture. Of the three, nicotine in the form of smoking tobacco is the most potent and destructive, although alcohol is a close second. The potential abuse of these three substances emphasizes another important distinction in any discussion of substance abuse, that is, the distinction between the substance and

SUBSTANCE ABUSE TERMINOLOGY: SELECTED TERMS

Abstinence. Cessation of use of a psychoactive substance previously abused or on which the user has developed drug dependence.
(Drug) Addiction. A chronic disorder characterized by the compulsive use of a substance resulting in physical, psychologic, or social harm to the user and continued use despite that harm.
Alcoholism. A chronic, progressive, and potentially fatal biogenetic and psychosocial disease characterized by tolerance and physical dependence on alcohol manifested as a loss of control, as well as diverse personality change and social consequences.
Blackout. Acute anterograde amnesia with no formation of long-term memory, that is, a period of memory loss during which there is no recall of activities, resulting from the ingestion of alcohol or other drugs.
Cannabis dependence. The psychologic need for a routine pattern of cannabis use to the point where social-occupational functioning is impaired to some degree.
Cross-tolerance. Tolerance, originally produced by long-term administration of one drug, that is accompanied by tolerance of a second drug that has not been administered previously. (For example, tolerance to alcohol is accompanied by cross-tolerance to volatile anesthetics or barbiturates.)
(Drug) Dependence. A generic term that relates to physical dependence, psychologic dependence, or both. It is characteristic for each pharmacologic class of psychoactive drugs. Impaired control over drug taking is implied.
Detoxification. A process of withdrawing a person from an addictive substance in a safe and effective manner.
Disease concept. Recognition that chemical dependency is a chronic, progressive, and potentially fatal biogenetic and psychosocial disease characterized by tolerance of and physical dependence on a drug manifest as a loss of control, as well as diverse personality changes and social consequences.
Drug abuse. Any use of drugs that causes physical, psychologic, economic, legal, or social harm to the user or to others affected by the drug user's behavior.
Drug free. Ongoing disassociation from the use of any psychoactive substance.
Loss of control. The inability to limit the use of substances via an internal locus of control.
Maintenance. A form of therapeutic intervention applied to opiate addicts and consisting of the oral administration of a substitute opiate drug to minimize the reinforcement of drug taking and prevent a withdrawal reaction while rehabilitation is achieved.
Overdose. The inadvertent or deliberate consumption of a much larger dose than that habitually used by the individual in question and resulting in serious toxic reactions or death.
Polydrug abuse. Concomitant use of two or more psychoactive substances in quantities and with frequencies that cause the individual significant physiologic, psychologic, or sociologic distress or impairment.
Prevention. Social, economic, legal, or individual psychologic measures aimed at minimizing the use of potentially addicting substances or lowering the dependence risk in susceptible individuals.
Primary prevention. Attempts to reduce the incidence of new cases of drug abuse (or drug problems) in a general population.
Rehabilitation. The restoration of an optimum state of health by medical, psychologic, social, and peer group support for chemically dependent people and their significant others.
Relapse. Recurrence of alcohol- or drug-dependent behavior in an individual who has previously achieved and maintained abstinence for a significant time beyond detoxification.
Sobriety. Generally the state of complete abstinence from alcohol and other drugs of abuse in conjunction with a satisfactory quality of life.
Substance abuse. The use of a psychoactive substance in a manner detrimental to the individual or society but not meeting criteria for substance or drug dependence.
Tolerance. Physiologic adaption to the effect of drugs such that effects are diminished with constant doses or the intensity and duration of effects are maintained through increased doses.
Treatment. Application of planned procedures to identify and change patterns of behavior that are maladaptive, destructive, or unhealthful or to restore appropriate levels of physical, psychologic, or social functioning.
Withdrawal. Cessation of drug or alcohol use by an individual in whom dependence is established.
Withdrawal syndrome. The onset of a predictable constellation of signs and symptoms involving altered activity of the central nervous system after the abrupt discontinuation of, or rapid decrease in dosage of, a drug.

Modified from Rinaldi RC and others: Clarification and standardization of substance terminology, JAMA 259:555, 1989.

TABLE 28-1 Xanthine Content in Selected Beverages, Foods, and Drugs

Item	Caffeine (mg)	Theobromine (mg)	Theophylline (mg)
DRINKS (6 OZ CUP)			
Percolated coffee (Maxwell House)	94	—	—
Instant coffee (Nescafe)	81	—	—
Instant coffee (Tasters' Choice)	68	—	—
Decaffeinated coffee, percolated or instant Sanka or Brim	4	—	—
Lipton tea	52	6	8
Constant Comment tea	29	14	—
Rose Hip Herbal tea	—	—	—
Pepsi Cola	46	—	—
Mountain Dew	57	—	—
Carnation hot cocoa	—	32	—
CANDY (1 OZ)			
Ghiradelli dark chocolate	24	40	—
Hershey's milk chocolate	4	13	—
DRUGS (USUAL MG DOSE)			
Aqua-Ban tablets	100	—	—
Cafergot tablets	100-200	—	—
Dietac capsules	200	—	—
Fiorinal	40	—	—
Extra Strength Excedrin	65	—	—
Theophylline (Theolar, Theophyl, Bronkodyl)	—	—	100-250

Modified from Minton JP: To whom it may concern, Unpublished letter, 1981; Bullough B, Hindi-Alexander M, and Fetouh S: Methylxanthines and fibrocystic breast disease, Nurse Pract, 1989 (in press); Ratings: chocolate bars, Consumer Rep 51:61, 1986.

its potential abuse—in the case of alcohol, between drinking alcoholic beverages and alcoholism. The vast majority of Americans drink alcohol occasionally, and a substantial number, perhaps as many as one third, drink to the point of getting into temporary interpersonal or legal difficulties. Not all drinkers who get into temporary difficulty, however, are alcoholics. Similar statements might be made about other substances including nicotine and caffeine, which can also be abused.

To fine-tune the handling of problems of substance abuse, researchers have had a tendency in recent years to add still another element to the definition of substance abuse, namely, the potential occurrence of serious social and health problems resulting from ingesting the substance. This definition has particular value in dealing with substances such as tobacco or caffeine in which only epidemiologic studies demonstrate the serious dangers involved in addiction to smoking or caffeine. The preceding box shows a list of additional definitions to clarify the language used by experts in the field of substance abuse.

Xanthines

The xanthines (methylxanthines) are the most culturally accepted legal drugs in our society. Table 28-1 shows the xanthine content of selected beverages, foods, and drugs. They are relatively mild in normal dosages and are highly attractive psychoactive substances that are widely used in our society. They are found in coffee, tea, colas, chocolate, and a large number of prescription and over-the-counter drugs. A key xanthine is caffeine, but also included in the xanthines is theobromine, found in tea and chocolate, and theophylline, a drug used in the treatment of asthma and found in small amounts in some teas. Most beverages containing xanthines also have significant amounts of oils, which may cause gastric irritability, and tannin, which is somewhat constipating. The effects of the xanthines are dose related with more mild results from low doses and more troublesome effects from higher doses. All are stimulants and bronchodilators with their other effects varying with dosages. Most individuals who consume more than 500 to 600 mg of xanthines a day have withdrawal symptoms when they begin to cut down, which indicates the addictive nature of xanthines. High intake levels are associated with gastrointestinal distress, overstimulation of the central nervous system, and tachycardia (Schuckit, 1984). Xanthines are not linked to breast cancer, but xanthines tend to exacerbate the pain associated with fibrocystic breast disease (Bullough and others, in press; Hindi-Alexander and others, 1985; Minton, 1981).

Tobacco

Nicotine, along with the tars and other substances present in tobacco, is regarded as the major cause of lung cancer, laryngeal cancer, chronic bronchitis, and cardiovascular disease. The percentage of cigarette smokers in the United States reached its height in the mid-1960s when 52% of American males and 32% of American females were classified as regular smokers. Total U.S. consumption was 600 billion cigarettes per year. Since 1964 when the Advisory Commission to the Surgeon General of the United States reported that tobacco intake was a major health hazard, tobacco consumption has dropped. This achievement has not been easy, and most of the success has been in convincing people who are already smoking to stop, rather than in keeping young people from starting to smoke. Smoking in both men and women has fallen to approximately 30%. It is estimated this change will have prevented approximately 3 million smoking-related deaths between 1964 and the year 2000 (Warner, 1989a). There is, however, still much to be done. The American Cancer Society calculated that in 1985 alone, 390,000 persons died as a result of smoking. This estimate is based on the assumption that 30% of all cancer deaths, 21% of deaths from coronary artery disease, 18% of stroke deaths, and 82% of deaths from chronic obstructive lung disease are attributable to smoking. The correlation between smoking and cancer is most noticeable in women, who early in this century smoked rarely. At that time their lung cancer death rate tended to be similar to the rate of nonsmokers (12 deaths per 100,000 women). In 1960 women smokers had a lung cancer death rate of 23.9 deaths per 100,000 women, and by the mid-1980s, when large numbers of women had been smoking for many years, the rate for women smokers had escalated to 130.4 deaths per 100,000 women (Warner, 1989b). These data suggest that smoking is still the major substance abuse problem in the United States. The smoking issue is further complicated by the growing realization that some of the harmful sequelae of smoking tobacco can result from simply being around people who smoke (Sandler, 1989).

Central Nervous System Depressants

Just as alcohol and caffeine can be classified as abused substances when they are taken in excessive doses, other drugs that have clinical usefulness can also be classified as abused substances. This is particularly true of the central nervous system (CNS) depressant drugs such as hypnotics and antianxiety drugs (see Table 28-2). The CNS

TABLE 28-2 Commonly Used Central Nervous System Depressants

Type	Generic name	Trade name
HYPNOTICS		
Barbiturates		
Long acting	Phenobarbital	Luminal
Short acting	Thiopental	Pentothal
	Methohexital	Brevital
Intermediate acting	Pentobarbital	Nembutal
	Secobarbital	Seconal
	Amobarbital	Amytal
	Butabarbital	Butisol
Barbiturate-like	Methaqualone	Quaalude
	Ethchlorvynol	Placidyl
	Methyprylon	Noludar
	Glutethimide	Doriden
Others	Temazepam	Restoril
	Flurazepam	Dalmane
	Chloral hydrate	Noctec
ANTIANXIETY DRUGS		
Carbamates	Meprobamate	Miltown
		Equanil
	Tybamate	Solacen
		Tybatran

Modified from Schuckit MA: Drug and alcohol abuse: a clinical guide to diagnosis and treatment, ed 2, New York, 1984, Plenum Publishing Corp.

depressants all have clinical usefulness, as well as abuse potential. When used alone CNS depressants can cause a high, but some people use the depressants with other drugs. The specific pharmacologic mechanisms for most of these drugs are not completely known, but the depressants bring about a reversible depression of the activity of all excitable tissues—especially those of the CNS, where the greatest effect occurs on the synapse. The resulting sequelae range from a slight lethargy or sleepiness, through various levels of anesthesia, to death from depressed respiration and heart depression. Paradoxically the hypnotics and the antianxiety drugs sometimes cause extreme excitement when given to children and elderly clients. Since alcohol is also a depressant, if barbiturates are taken with alcohol, the effect can be lethal. All CNS depressants produce a withdrawal state when stopped abruptly after relatively continual administration.

TABLE 28-3 Commonly Used Stimulants

Generic name	Trade name
Amphetamine	Benzedrine
Benzphetamine	Didrex
Caffeine	
Chlorphentermine	Pre-Sate
Cocaine	
Dextroamphetamine	Dexedrine
Diethylpropion	Tenuate, Tepanil
Fenfluramine	Pondimin
Methamphetamine	Desoxyn
Methylphenidate	Ritalin
Phenmetrazine	Preludin
Phentermine	Ionamin

Stimulants

Stimulants encompass a wide variety of drugs that share the ability to stimulate the nervous system at multiple levels. As a group they work, at least in part, by causing the release or blocking the reuptake of neurotransmitters such as norepinephrine from nerve cells. Some, in addition, mimic the functions of transmitters like norepinephrine through a direct effect on the nerve cells themselves (see Table 28-3). Clinically the drugs cause euphoria and decrease fatigue and the need for sleep; they may increase feelings of sexuality, interfere with normal sleep patterns, decrease appetite, increase energy, and tend to decrease the level of distractibility in children with a hyperkinetic syndrome.

Cocaine

The most widely abused stimulant as of this writing is cocaine, which is a local anesthetic harvested from a shrub that grows wild in Peru and Bolivia but is grown in many other countries as well. Pharmacologically it is classified as a tropane alkaloid (somewhat related to atropine and scopolamine). It acts at the level of the neurotransmitters to block their reuptake, which produces a norepinephrine and epinephrine effect, as well as at the CNS level to produce dopamine and serotonin effects (Loveys, 1978). Cocaine is sold on the street as an impure powder and is frequently expanded with procaine or amphetamines. It can be taken through many modes of administration, but it is most often taken intravenously or snorted (inhaled through a straw or rolled paper into the nose). Although the drug is smoked in tobacco, this is not efficient, since cocaine sulfate has a melting point of almost 200° C and little of it enters the system when it is smoked. To get around that problem cocaine suppliers developed a freebase cocaine with a melting point of 98° C. Freebase cocaine is produced by adding acid to a strong base, such as buffered ammonia, and to an aqueous solution of cocaine. From this the alkaline freebase precipitate is extracted. In this form it can be sprinkled over tobacco or smoked in special pipes. In 1985 a new method of preparing street cocaine was developed. The product, called crack, is cheaper, and it can be smoked or used intravenously. This has made cocaine accessible to poor people, and it has sparked an increase in cocaine use.

The physiologic response to cocaine is often biphasic. Intranasal ingestion produces an initial bradycardia because low doses of the drug stimulate the vagus nerve. Eventually with low doses or with higher plasma concentrations, cocaine produces an increased heart rate, an elevated blood pressure, euphoria, garrulousness, and a decrease in fatigue. Additional effects may include nausea, vomiting, and an increased body temperature. The sequelae could be arrhythmias probably brought about both by the effects of the drug and through catecholamine release. Tolerance to the drug develops rapidly. For example, doses of cocaine that would be lethal to a first-time user are needed by an experienced user to get a high. The half-life of the drug also decreases as the metabolic tolerance is increased.

Withdrawal symptoms such as nausea or pain ordinarily do not occur, yet cocaine is highly addictive because as the drug wears off there is a profound sense of depression. This feeling can be so negative that an obsessive desire for cocaine follows. The chronic abuser may focus total attention on obtaining the drug and neglect personal hygiene, food, and other life activities (Loveys, 1978). Death from cocaine toxicity is caused by a fatal arrhythmia, respiratory arrest, myocardial ischemia, or stroke. Other cocaine-related causes of death include septicemia, hepatitis, or acquired immunodeficiency syndrome from contaminated intravenous equipment.

Opiates and Other Analgesics

Both natural substances and semisynthetic drugs make up a category of pain-killing drugs that includes opiates and other analgesics shown in Table 28-4. Although opiates and other analgesics undergo similar metabolism in the body, they differ from other drugs in their degree of oral absorption. Detoxification occurs primarily in the liver, and the resulting metabolites are excreted through the urine and bile. All opiates and other analgesics produce analgesia, drowsiness, changes in mood, and, when administered in large doses, a clouding of mental functioning through the depression of CNS and cardiac activity. Tolerance develops rapidly to most opiates, particularly to the potent analgesics. The substances are addicting, since they produce euphoria and quickly produce tolerance and dependence. Physical dependence develops after relatively short-term use. Recent research has produced the discovery of opiate receptors in specific areas of the brain that have some function in mediating or regulating the perception of pain. (These receptor sites are the same ones to which endorphin and enkephalin bind.)

TABLE 28-4 Opiate Analgesics

Generic name	Trade name
Paregoric	—
Heroin	—
Morphine	—
Codeine	—
Hydromorphone	Dilaudid
Oxycodone	Percodan
Methadone	Dolophine
Propoxyphene	Darvon
Meperidine	Demerol
Pentazocine	Talwin, Fortral

The number of individuals addicted to opiates is unknown, but addicts are divided into two categories—the prescription abusers and the street abusers. Prescription abusers tend to be elderly and middle class, whereas street abusers tend to be young and lower class. But that is too simplistic a definition, and significant overlap exists. Unlike most other drugs, opiates are not known to produce any type of temporary psychosis. The major negative symptom produced by opiate administration is depression. Two major problems exist for the opiate abuser, namely, overdose and the discomfort of withdrawal. Overdose is marked by blue lips, a pale blue tinge to the body, pinpoint pupils, recent needle marks, pulmonary edema, bradycardia, depressed respiration, cardiac dysrhythmia, and convulsions. Death results from a combination of respiratory depression and pulmonary edema, cerebral edema, or both.

Withdrawal, which usually occurs within 12 hours of an addict's last dose, is marked first by physical discomfort including tearing of the eyes, running of the nose, sweating, and yawning. Other symptoms of withdrawl include dilated pupils, loss of appetite, gooseflesh, back pain, and tremors. This gives way to insomnia, incessant yawning, a flu-like feeling of weakness, nausea, vomiting, chills, flushing, muscle spasms, ejaculation, and abdominal pain. In the acute phases of withdrawal the syndrome decreases in intensity. By the fifth day of withdrawal the symptoms are reduced, and the symptoms disappear in a week to 10 days.

Cannabis

"Cannabis," the term for the hemp plant, is sold as marijuana or hashish. It is among the most widely used drugs in the United States. The most active ingredient is δ-9-tetrahydrocannabinol (THC). It produces fewer physiologic and psychologic alterations than do most other classes of drugs, including alcohol. Cannabis, however, does affect the brain, the cardiovascular system, and the lungs, although most changes appear to be reversible. Although THC is sometimes called a hallucinogen, its effects at the doses usually taken are euphoric and result in a change in the level of consciousness without hallucinations. The drug can be ingested through smoking, eating, and (rarely) intravenous injection. Only about half the potency is absorbed through smoking, although the potency depends on the quality of the marijuana and the amount of time elapsed since the plant was harvested. Potency decreases over time, and the stems and leaves of marijuana plants are less potent than the flowering tops. Peak THC plasma levels are reached within 10 to 30 minutes of ingestion, and intoxication usually lasts between two and eight hours depending on the dose. When the plant is eaten, a greater percentage of the drug is absorbed, resulting in a long and less predictable high. Once peak THC plasma levels are reached, the drug tends to disappear from the plasma rapidly and is absorbed in tissues, especially in tissues with high levels of fat such as the brain and testes.

Physical changes are dependent on the amount of cannabis ingested. Usually changes include euphoria, relaxation, sleepiness, and heightened sexual arousal. The user is unable to keep track of time, experiences hunger, and exhibits decreased social interaction. Large doses of cannabis may produce hallucinations that are often accompanied by paranoid delusions. Moderate intoxication brings about shakes or tremors, a decrease in body temperature, a decrease in muscle strength and balance, decreased motor coordination, a dry mouth, and bloodshot eyes. Some individuals also experience nausea, headache, nystagmus, and lowered blood pressure. Neither tolerance nor physical dependence is a major clinical problem. Toleration of increasing doses of the drug does develop through both metabolic and pharmacodynamic mechanisms, and there is a mild level of cross-tolerance to alcohol. There is a debate about whether withdrawal occurs. If it does occur, the intensity probably parallels the length and amount of exposure to the drug and consists of nausea, poor appetite, mild anxiety, and insomnia. More severe symptoms might result from those accustomed to high doses.

TABLE 28-5 Hallucinogenic Drugs

Type	Drug name
Indolealkylamines	Lysergic acid diethylamide (LSD) Psilocybin Psilocin Dimethyltryptamine (DMT) Diethyltryptamine (DET)
Methoxy-amphetamine	MDA
Phenethylamines	Mescaline (peyote)
Phenylisopropylamines	2,5-dimethoxy-4-methylamphetamine (DOM or STP)
Related drugs	Phencyclidine (PCP) Nutmeg Morning glory seeds Catnip Nitrous oxide Amyl nitrate or *n*-butyl nitrite

Hallucinogens and Other Drugs

Although marijuana can produce hallucinations, its effect is usually to alter the "feeling state" without producing hallucinations. However, a wide variety of substances do produce hallucinations. These substances can be synthetic products such as lysergic acid diethylamide (LSD), plant products such as peyote or mescaline, or fungi such as psilocybin. Structurally they resemble amphetamines, and many have been used at religious ceremonies and social gatherings for centuries. Table 28-5 lists some of the common hallucinogenic drugs.

Sometimes hallucinogenic drugs are called psychedelic drugs. The effects of hallucinogenic drugs are an increased awareness of sensory input, a subjective feeling of enhanced mental activity, a perception of normal environmental stimuli as novel events, altered body images, a turning inward of thoughts, and a decreased ability to tell the difference between oneself and one's surroundings. In addition to hallucinations, hallucinogenic drugs tend to produce adrenergic effects such as dilated pupils, a flushed face, a fine tremor, increased blood pressure, elevations in blood sugar, and an increase in body temperature.

Tolerance of larger and larger doses of hallucinogenic drugs develops rapidly after as little as three or four days of ingesting one dose per day but disappears within four days to a week after everyday ingestion is stopped. Cross-tolerance exists between hallucinogenic drugs and most other drugs, but this does not extend to marijuana. There is no clinically significant withdrawal syndrome in users of hallucinogenic drugs. The most common difficulties former users have are panic reactions, flashbacks, and toxic reactions including temporary psychoses.

Note that some substances in Table 28-5 are traditional ones that may produce some hallucinogenic reactions, since they contain atropine-like substances.

Nutmeg plants can be ground and either inhaled or ingested in large amounts to produce a change of consciousness. Nutmeg in such quantities has unpleasant side effects such as vomiting, and chronic use apparently causes constipation. The side effects of nutmeg ingestion prevent its more widespread use except among those desperate to obtain drugs such as the prison population. Similarly morning glory seeds, if ingested in large amounts, can produce a mild hallucinatory state. Morning glory seeds taken intravenously are dangerous and can produce a lethal, shocklike state. Catnip can be smoked and produces an intoxication similar to that of marijuana, but the intoxication is usually also associated with headaches. In the western United States a similar reaction comes from locoweed (genera *Astragalus* and *Oxytropis)*, which causes locoism in horses, cattle, and sheep. Locoweed apparently can produce hallucinations in humans, but it also causes uncoordination, depression, difficulty in eating, and an exaggerated reaction to stress. Nitrous oxide (N_2O) is a relatively weak anesthetic that was used in the nineteenth century to produce hallucinations. Continued use of the drug can cause a paranoid psychotic state, but this ceases when nitrous oxide ingestion is stopped. Amyl nitrate and *n*-butyl nitrate are vasodilators that are believed by the street culture to cause a slight euphoria, flushing, and a slowing of time perception. They are also said to enhance orgasm, and for this reason they are often sold in adult bookstores.

Of these hallucinatory drugs, the most widely used is phencyclidine (PCP). PCP was first introduced as a general anesthetic under the names of Sernyl, Sernylan, Ketamine, Ketalar, Ketaject, and Ketavet. PCP had the benefit of allowing anesthesia through a dissociative state in which the subject was not in a deep coma, and thus there was little depression of blood pressure, respiration, and other vital signs. Its use in humans, however, was severely restricted after it was found that approximately 20% of the individuals to whom PCP was administered developed agitation and even hallucinations during the immediate postoperative period. PCP affects the basic brain centers, probably through interference with the synaptic transmission between cells. It is readily absorbed by mouth or intravenously, as well as by smoking or snorting. Metabolism occurs primarily in the liver. PCP penetrates easily into fat stores, and thus it can have a half-life as long as three days. PCP has a relatively complex interaction with a number of different systems. It is sympathomimetic, increases CNS catecholamines, and produces a subsequent increase in blood pressure, heart rate, respiratory rate, and reflexes. PCP also has cholinergic effects that increase CNS acetylcholine and results in sweating, flushing, drooling, and pupillary constriction. CNS serotonin systems might be affected by ingestion of PCP, and effects on the cerebellum are fairly prominent with resulting dizziness, uncoordination, slurred speech, and nystagmus. Behavioral toxicity is dose related. Low doses of PCP give a feeling of floating, euphoria, and heightened emotionality along with mild increases in heart rate, sweating, and lacrimation. A 10 mg dose results in a drunken state. Theoretically there could be withdrawal symptoms in PCP users, but there is little evidence of this other than a rebound effect, which can be expected after abrupt discontinuation of any drug.

Glues, Solvents, and Aerosols

Glues, solvents, and aerosols constitute a heterogenous group of inhalants that produce generalized CNS depression. Use of these products was first noted in the early 1960s when teenagers began to inhale model airplane glue. Since then the list of inhalants has grown to include toluene (glues and paint thinners), the hydrocarbons (solvents and Freon), and other household or industrial substances. They are popular because they induce euphoria and are readily available, cheap, legal, and easy to conceal. Onset of mental change occurs rapidly after these products are inhaled and disappears fairly quickly. With the exception of headaches, serious hangovers are usually not observed.

The danger with inhalant drugs is that they are often part of a fad adopted by adolescents in their early teens. Usually the drugs are harmless, but they sometimes result in toxic reactions including organic brain syndromes and various other medical complications. A life-threatening toxic reaction is characterized by respiratory depression and cardiac dysrhythmias followed by a rapid loss of consciousness. There is no clinically relevant withdrawal syndrome described in users of these drugs. Most of the disorders are transient and disappear with supportive care, but severe liver or kidney damage can result in some instances (Bailey, 1989; Bennett, Vourakis, and Woolf, 1983). Table 28-6 lists some commonly used inhalants.

Almost any over-the-counter drug can be abused, including antihistamines, analgesics, decongestants, expectorants, bromides, laxatives, and weight-control products, as can almost any prescription drug. As indicated earlier, many of the first addicts in this country became addicted to prescription drugs; this is still possible. Nurses should know this and with prescription drugs should be alert to possible multidrug misuse.

TABLE 28-6 Commonly Used Inhalants

Type	Drug Name
Glues	Toluene, naphtha, acetates, hexane, benzene, xylene, chloroform
Cleaning solutions	Trichloroethylene, petroleum products, carbon tetrachloride
Nail polish removers	Acetone
Lighter fluids	Naphtha, aliphatic hydrocarbons
Paints and paint thinners	Toluene, *n*-butyl acetate, acetone, naphtha, methanol
Aerosols	Fluorinated hydrocarbons, nitrous oxide
Other petroleum products	Gasoline, benzene, toluene, petroleum ether
Propellants	Nitrous oxide

USING THE NURSING PROCESS TO TREAT SUBSTANCE ABUSE

The Nursing Process: Assessment

The five-step nursing process can be used for working with many problems related to substance abuse, although the assessment process varies with the nursing role. The community health nurse starts with a broad picture of community needs. Although past experience and knowledge of the literature are important for this assessment, periodic reassessment of the community is important because patterns of drug abuse change. Because marijuana was used heavily by members of the youth culture, it was the major public concern 20 years ago, even though alcohol, cigarettes, and heroin were causing the most serious problems. The hallucinogens, including LSD, were also worrisome because even one dose can occasionally trigger a psychosis. Cocaine was snorted, but for the most part only affluent people dabbled in its use, and few became seriously addicted.

Currently community health nurses who are assessing their communities are indicating that cocaine in the form of crack is the most serious problem. Many cocaine users now are poor people, and cocaine is now more often taken intravenously or smoked than it is snorted. Marijuana, tobacco, and heroin use has decreased in most communities, although it is distressing to find that many young people still start to smoke. These observations are documented in a poll of substance abuse done by the Department of Health and Human Services. It was estimated that 23 million people used illicit drugs in 1985. This estimate dropped dramatically in 1988 to 14.5 million users of illicit drugs. The change was primarily due to fewer marijuana and casual cocaine users. However, the number of regular crack users has increased substantially (Amons, 1989).

Community-wide assessment is important to help structure planning and the use of resources. It also helps shape nursing education to keep it up to date. Being up to date is particularly important for the school nurse. The assessment process in the school should include gathering data

TABLE 28-7 Street Names for Commonly Used Drugs

Drug	Street name	Drug	Street name
DEPRESSANTS		HALLUCINOGENS	
Amobarbitol	Blue birds, blue devils, blue heaven, blues, and bullets	Dimethyltryptamine	AMT, Businessman's Lunch, and DMT
Amobarbitol and secobarbitol	Down trouble, downs, goofballs, green and white librium, greenies, reds and blues, rainbows, and tooies	Lysergic acid (LSD)	Acid, barrels, battery acid, berkeley blood, blotter acid, blue acid, blue, blue dots, blue microdots, cube, HCP, owselys, pearly gates, morning glory, seeds, sugar, sunshine, window pane, and zen
Chloral hydrate	Peter and librium-tranqs		
Methaqualone	Ludes, quads, sopors, and T-bird		
Pentobarbital	Nembies, peanuts, yellows, and yellow jackets	Mescaline	Bad seed, big chief, cactus, chief, mescal, peyote, pink wedge, and white light
Secobarbital	Red birds, red devils, seccy, and seggy	Psilocybin	Exotic mushroom and God's flesh
Nonspecific drug	Doll		
STIMULANTS		OTHERS	
Amphetamines	Bennies, blue angels, black beauties, chris, christine, christmas trees, coast to coast, peaches, pep pills, pinks, roses, truck driver, uppers, ups, and wake ups	Heroin	Horse, brown, scat, junk, shit, skag, and smack
		Cannabis	Acapulco gold, ace, ashes, baby, bhang, grass, hay, hash, hemp, jive, joint, lid, locoweed, Mary Jane, pot, reefer, roach, rope, stick, and sweet Lucy
Cocaine	Coke, copilot, crack, criss-cross, crossroads, dope, double cross, flake, footballs, gold dust, and green and clears	Phencyclidine (PCP)	Angel dust, busy bee, criptal, dummy mist, flying saucers, goon, green, hair, horse, tranquilizer, shermans, sherms, and whack
Dextroamphetamine	Dexies, hearts, lip poppers, and oranges		
Methamphetamine	Crystal, dexies, meth, speed, and whites		

Modified from Bennett G, Vourakis C, and Woolf DS: Substance abuse, pharmacologic, developmental, and clinical perspectives, ed 2, New York, 1983, John Wiley & Sons.

about the ages and educational levels of users, the patterns of use, and the social support systems that encourage use. Alternative social support systems need to be surveyed to identify possible allies in the difficult struggle against substance abuse. A particularly important tool in this analysis is the anthropologic approach, which allows one to be an observer by listening, avoiding being judgmental, and hearing not only what is being said, but also what is not being said.

The listening task in the school setting is complicated because adolescents use an informal patois that is ever changing, so the slang of 10 years ago is out of date. The drug culture has slang terms that change over time. Table 28-7 shows some street names for commonly used drugs.

TABLE 28-8 Clues of Possible Substance Abuse

Substances	Paraphernalia	Symptoms	Withdrawal symptoms	Other clues
Marijuana	Cigarette paper and roaches (smoked ends of marijuana cigarettes)	Animated behavior followed by stuporous behavior		Smell of burnt rope
Cigarettes	Packs of cigarettes	Cough and pharyngitis	Agitation and hunger	Finger stains
Alcohol	Bottles and cans	Depression and intoxication	Thirst and hallucinations	Absenteeism
Cocaine	Eyedroppers, needles, syringes, white powder or flakes, and rolled paper	Excessive activity and garrulousness	Depression	Irritated nasal septum and scars on arms
Heroin	Bent spoons, needles, syringes, and eyedroppers	Constricted pupils and euphoria	Nausea, vomiting, and agitation	Scars on arms
Glue	Bags or rags with glue on them	Watering eyes, running nose, and drowsiness		

The assessment done by the home health care nurse or the nurse practitioner is more narrowly focused on the individual or the family as it affects the individual. Questions about substance abuse should be included in all health histories. These questions can follow the items on prescription drugs. The best place to start is probably with smoking and alcohol because they are less stigmatized. Questions about marijuana and other drugs can then follow easily. The tone of voice and body language of the questioner should be relaxed and matter of fact so that barriers to communication are not created. It is interesting how people are often willing to report their drug usage when they are not threatened. A recent study of the reliability of survey data on cigarette smoking compared survey totals with excise tax records of cigarette sales collected by the U.S. Department of Agriculture and found that 72% of the cigarette consumption was reported. Although this suggests considerable underreporting, it also indicates that people reported nearly three quarters of their consumption (Hatziandreu, 1989).

In addition to the openly revealed substance use, the nurse may want to look for more subtle clues of abuse such as frequent absence from work, which tends to accompany any serious addiction, child abuse, which may suggest alcoholism, and tracks, or scars (and abscesses) along the arm, which frequently mark an intravenous drug user. A single observation may not mean drug abuse, but it can certainly alert the nurse to the need for further questions and observations. Table 28-8 classifies clues that suggest common types of substance abuse.

Nursing Diagnosis

The nursing diagnosis as it relates to substance abuse is a summary statement of the problem or problems to be addressed. When the community is the client, the diagnosis could be one of the escalating abuse of cocaine in the community. If single clients are the focus of the nursing process, the diagnoses would focus on those clients and the problems they are ready to deal with, such as alcoholism. For the pregnant woman the concern should broaden to include the fetus, as well as the woman. When the community health nurse's client is a child, the diagnostic statement might well focus on the problematic behavior of an adult whose problems are affecting the child.

Planning

Although planning and implementation are often intertwined, it is important to carry out both processes. The formal reason for planning is to set goals of intervention and decide on a methodology for reaching those goals. Planning also has some less obvious functions. It notifies people that an intervention is being considered and thus helps enlist their cooperation. Consequently a fairly public planning process can often help the intervention strategy succeed.

Implementation: Primary Prevention

Most implementation activities carried out by nurses in the community are aimed at either primary prevention of substance abuse or treatment combined with secondary and tertiary preventive measures. Although there has been significant media attention about substance abuse for the last two decades, the United States has not been particularly effective in developing preventive campaigns. Although it is true that the antismoking campaign, which started in 1964 with the surgeon general's report, has yielded some good results, the United States still has a long way to go. It is important to realize that the campaign has been hampered by the vigorous efforts of the tobacco industry (Warner, 1989a), which issues counter reports and blocks antismoking campaigns and laws whenever possible. Over the years the tobacco industry has successfully lobbied Congress and convinced members to defeat efforts to repeal the subsidies paid to tobacco farmers. These subsidies motivate farmers to continue to grow tobacco instead of switching to food or fiber crops with social usefulness. At the executive level the industry has most recently pressured President Bush to threaten Japan, South Korea, and Taiwan with trade sanctions if they do not open their markets to American cigarettes (Health Groups, 1989). Similar observations can be made about the alcohol industry, which spends huge amounts of money on lobbying and media campaigns.

The efforts of these two major industries to push their cause pale beside the illicit drug industry. One of the problems is that the illicit drug industry's activities are more difficult to track because the industry operates outside the law. This means that it has the additional advantage of being tax exempt. Instead of paying taxes, the illicit drug industry spends a significant amount of its capital on the bribery and corruption of public officials at all levels of government. The public power of the industry was dramatically demonstrated in the 1987 Iran-Contra hearings when Oliver North calmly testified that there were connections between South American drug dealers and U.S. government officials, including himself. The power of the illicit drug industry does not mean the United States is helpless in efforts to curtail substance abuse, but it does put the problem in perspective. On the positive side, recent public opinion polls have indicated that the American people see substance abuse as the No. 1 problem facing the country, and media coverage is reflecting this concern (Drug Crisis, 1989). A "drug czar," William Bennett, has been appointed by President Bush, so there is hope that some effective strategies will be worked out.

It should be emphasized, however, that any effective strategy to cut down illicit drug use will be costly. Joseph Westermeyer (1989) did a comprehensive review of the efforts that have been made to suppress various illicit drugs on both the national and international level. From this review he argued that international efforts to suppress production, particularly of opium, have not been effective in the long run. Although the efforts have succeeded in cutting down opium production in one part of the world, the result has been increased opium production in other areas. The poverty in developing countries and the huge profits to be made in illicit drug trade make drug trade too attractive to be easily controlled at the source. Westermeyer therefore argues that the most effective campaigns are at the national level. Unfortunately, the only totally effective national campaign he could cite was the one carried out in the People's Republic of China. The campaign involved strict anticorruption policies at all levels, total government control of the media, long prison sentences for addicts, death penalties for drug dealers and corrupt public officials, and involuntary drug screening. In addition, block groups or work groups were organized to cut down the social isolation of individuals and to monitor their behavior. The social cost of this approach seems too great; it would in effect be the end of the American way of life.

There may, however, be some aspects of the program that can be useful. In summarizing his observations of the international scene, Westermeyer proposes the following four steps for an American national drug policy:

1. Eliminate illicit drug production within our boundaries. This would involve increased police work and heavy penalties for not only drug manufacturers, but also those who finance drug production and public officials who furnish protection.
2. Enforce laws against those who engage in drug commerce including all those who buy, sell, exchange, give, share, carry, and ship drugs.
3. Treat drug abusers. Westermeyer argues that as the supply of drugs disappears, abusers will be willing to seek early and more effective treatment. Treatment facilities are already in short supply, and if the supply of drugs disappears, the treatment facilities would have to be significantly expanded.
4. Stop illicit drug trade at our borders. The current law enforcement officials can stop only 1% to 3% of the drug shipments. Westermeyer argues that this is ineffective, but if 10% of drug shipments could be stopped, much of the profit of the industry would be cut (Westermeyer, 1989).

The four-step program outlined above is probably significantly more costly than the program that will be proposed by the drug czar. The political climate probably does not support such expensive measures. The cost would escalate even more if the root of despair that leads many inner-city residents to take drugs was tackled. The big picture does not look hopeful, but nurses who work in the front lines can help develop more rational policies if they participate in the public debate, as well as work with their individual clients.

At the community level preventive efforts to date have been focused primarily on schoolchildren. Outcome studies of antidrug educational programs suggest that ordinary teaching about drugs is not particularly useful in changing attitudes and behaviors about substance abuse. In fact some of the courses seem to have had the opposite effect, stimulating an interest in trying selected substances (Kinder, Pape, and Walfish, 1980). Programs that combine educational efforts with strategies to strengthen peer pressure against drug use and lessen some of the negative pressures by dealing with homelessness, unemployment, and boredom are more successful (Bailey, 1989; Burpo, 1988; Kinder, Pape, and Walfish, 1980).

Other approaches to preventive programs use social learning theory combined with a problem-solving approach. These programs teach problem-solving and decision-making skills, cognitive skills for resisting social pressure, enhancement of self-esteem, nondrug alternatives for coping, and assertiveness. These skills and attitudes are taught using demonstrations, reinforcements, role playing, behavioral rehearsals, and homework assignments (Bailey, 1989).

Timing of any of these programs is important. A study of the readiness of children to experiment with alcohol suggests that this developmental stage tends to occur at about 14 or 15 years of age, so programs instituted when the pressure for experimentation occurs are most effective (Castiglia and others, 1989). There is a body of research that suggests that some children move from alcohol, to cigarettes, to illicit drugs. This implies that dealing with early addictive behavior is a useful strategy (Fleming and others, 1989; Kandel, 1975).

Implementation: Secondary and Tertiary Prevention

When the nursing diagnosis is focused on an individual who is already a substance abuser, treatment and secondary prevention of further psychologic and physiologic damage is the focus of nursing intervention. Most of the time a referral to a community facility is needed, so knowledge of community resources for treatment is important. The box lists national organizations that deal with substance abuse; these sources may be helpful in locating local facilities. But a local list of agencies for referral should be developed.

In selecting the agency for referral it is important to know something about the range of services offered, whether the facility is an inpatient or an outpatient facility, the cost, the availability of treatment slots, the entry requirements, and the treatment philosophy of the facility. All of these characteristics should be discussed with the client as the planning process is carried out.

The treatment philosophy of the agency depends partly on the view of its staff in regard to the causality of substance abuse. As was indicated earlier there are two major views of addiction; it is often viewed as either a moral problem or an illness. However, the illness model is further divided into a focus on a genetic or biologic cause, a psychologic origin, or cultural and social causality.

In a review of the theoretic models of addiction, Hughes points out that the support for the genetic or biologic model developed after the discovery of the endorphins, endogenous substances produced by the pituitary gland that tend to mimic the opiates. The genetic or biologic model was further supported with a study done by Goodwin and his colleagues in the early 1970s. They studied 5483 adopted sons of alcoholics in Denmark and found that the sons whose biologic fathers were alcoholics were more than three times as likely to become alcoholics as were the adopted sons of nonalcoholic fathers (Hughes, 1989).

The psychologic approach posits that addiction is due to a disorder in the psychologic development of the individual. It views the client as having an addictive personality, which can span a variety of substances. Those who favor cultural and social causative factors posit that there is an addictive behavior pattern similar to the addictive personality type used by the psychologists, but they emphasize a multivariate causality.

These models suggest different treatment modalities. Treatment plans that view alcoholism as an illness, such as the one developed by Jellenick, view alcoholism as based on predisposing factors that are inborn, although the alcoholic still can make choices. The condition is progressive, and the client must abstain absolutely to be successfully treated. According to Hughes, the need for total abstinence as the only approach to treatment has been refuted in several studies (Hughes, 1989).

The biochemical model could also suggest an alternative drug regimen such as the methadone treatment plan for heroin addiction. Clients are taken off heroin and put on oral methadone, which produces an alternative addiction. Methadone does not produce the same euphoria that is seen with heroin, so people are less likely to escalate use of the drug, and some can turn their attention from a complete absorption with drugs to other concerns including work, care of their children, and activities of daily living. Although there is a high attrition rate (up to one half over four years) and occasional cheating, methadone treatment is a useful therapy.

The psychologic approach suggests psychotherapy as the treatment modality. A social and cultural causality suggests dealing with problems such as underemployment by providing job training, day care, and social support systems.

Alcoholics Anonymous (AA) is probably the most well-known treatment option. It has suc-

RESOURCES FOR PREVENTION AND TREATMENT OF SUBSTANCE ABUSE

Addiction Research Foundation
33 Russell St.
Toronto, Canada M5S2S1

Al-Anon Family Group Headquarters
PO Box 182
Madison Square Station
New York, NY 10010

Alcoholics Anonymous
World Services
PO Box 459
New York, NY 10017

American Cancer Society
777 Third Ave.
New York, NY 10017

American Lung Association
1740 Broadway
New York, NY 10019

Delancey Street Foundation
2563 Divisadero St.
San Francisco, CA 94115

DO IT NOW Foundation
PO Box 5115
Phoenix, AZ 85010

Families Anonymous
PO Box 344
Torrance, CA 90501

Food and Drug Administration
Room 15B32, Parklawn Building
5600 Fishers Lane
Rockville, MD 20857

Narcotics Anonymous
World Service Office
PO Box 622
Sun Valley, CA 91352

National Association of Gay Alcoholism Professionals (NAGAP)
204 W 20th St.
New York, NY 10011

National Association of Recovered Alcoholics in the Profession
PO Box 95
Stanton Island, NY 10305

National Cancer Institute
Room 10A18, Building 31
National Institutes of Health
Bethesda, MD 20205

National Council on Alcoholism
733 Third Ave.
New York, NY 10017

National Clearinghouse for Alcohol Information
PO Box 2345
Rockville, MD 20852

National Clearinghouse for Drug Abuse Information
PO Box 416
10325 Kensington Pkwy
Kensington, MD 20759

March of Dimes Birth Defects Foundation
1275 Mamaroneck Ave.
White Plains, NY 10605

National Institute on Alcohol Abuse and Alcoholism
U.S. Department of Health and Human Services
5600 Fishers Lane
Rockville, MD 20857

National Institute on Drug Abuse
U.S. Department of Health and Human Services
5600 Fishers Lane
Rockville, MD 20857

National Nurses Society on Alcoholism
Suite 1405
733 Third Ave.
New York, NY 10017

National Self-Help Clearing House
33 W 42nd St.
New York, NY 10036

Office on Smoking and Health
U.S. Department of Health and Human Services
Park Building, Room 116
5600 Fishers Lane
Rockville, MD 20857

Palmer Drug Abuse Program
PO Box 223581
Dallas, TX 75222

Pills Anonymous
814 E 76th St.
New York, NY 10021

Potsmokers Anonymous
316 E Third St.
New York, NY 10009

Renaissance Project
2 Hamilton Ave.
New Rochelle, NY 10801

Schick Laboratories
1901 Avenue of the Stars
Suite 1530
Los Angeles, CA 90067

Secular Organization for Sobriety (SOS)
Box 15781
North Hollywood, CA 91615-5781

SMOKENDERS
525 Prospect St. at Memorial Pkwy.
Phillipsburg, NJ 08865

Synanon
PO Box 786
Marshall, CA 95940

Vista Hill Foundation
Drug Abuse and Alcoholism Newsletter
Suite 100
3420 Camino del Rio N
San Diego, CA 92108

Women for Sobriety, Inc.
Box 618
Quakertown, PA 18951

Modified from Bennett G, Vourakis C, and Woolf RDS: Substance abuse, pharmacologic, developmental, and clinical perspectives, New York, 1983, John Wiley & Sons Inc.

cessfully helped thousands of alcoholics over the years. It uses a combination of models viewing alcoholism as a moral problem that stems from a physiologic predisposition and psychologic factors. Because it is viewed as a moral problem, public confession and contrition are called for. Peer support and total surrender of self to the support of a higher power are the psychologic support mechanisms. AA is probably least effective with people who are not religious and those who want to feel more in control of themselves instead of surrendering to the higher power.

A recent alternative to AA is the Secular Organization for Sobriety (S.O.S.), which now claims chapters in 90 localities. It uses some of the same approaches as AA including confessions and group support at meetings, but there is no mention of a higher power. Rather individuals are urged to take control of their own lives (SOS, 1988).

Evaluation

Periodic evaluation of the intervention strategy that is used is important. Sometimes a different referral or a rethinking and a new approach are needed. At the community level the evaluation component uses a research process. Research is still much needed in the field of substance abuse because all of the answers are not yet in.

SUBSTANCE ABUSE AND POPULATIONS AT RISK

There are some populations that present special problems relative to substance abuse including those at risk for acquired immunodeficiency syndrome (AIDS), pregnant women, teenagers, and nurses. Teenagers are covered in Chapter 16. The others are briefly discussed here.

Drug Abuse and AIDS

During the early years of the AIDS epidemic in America the victims were primarily gay white males from the East Coast. The distribution of the disease, however, quickly broadened to include all 50 states and a widening circle of populations. The number of AIDS cases has continued to increase each year. In 1987 the rate of increase, which had been declining, increased, but only because the definition of AIDS was revised to include more cases. The definition now includes anyone with human immunodeficiency virus (HIV) antibodies and one of the following secondary conditions—*Pneumocystitis carinii* pneumonia, Kaposi's sarcoma, esophogeal candidiasis, extrapulmonary tuberculosis, or HIV dementia. Women constituted 10% of the new cases of AIDS in 1988 and children constituted 1.8%. The ethnic mix has changed with a rapidly growing minority contingent from the inner-city poverty areas. Most of the children who have AIDS are younger than 5 years of age, and most contracted AIDS in utero. Few will survive to adulthood.

The reason for the shift in infection source from gay white males to the broader group is mainly attributed to intravenous drug use. Nearly 70% of the women with AIDS were infected when either they or their sexual partners used drugs (Leads from MMWR, 1989). Intravenous drug use is more of a risk factor in the United States than in European countries such as England or the Netherlands where sterile syringes and needles are easily obtainable. In United States, a prescription is required to purchase these supplies, a practice originally instituted to discourage illicit drug use. Although requiring a prescription for needles and syringes does not seem to have been particularly effective in accomplishing this goal, it has encouraged the sharing of needles and syringes. Sometimes a supply of needles and syringes is owned by a drug pusher who establishes a "shooting gallery" for drug clients where a single needle and syringe can be used by dozens of people in a day or evening. Since blood-to-blood contact is the most efficient mode of transmission of the HIV, sharing a needle is a more certain way of spreading the disease than sexual contact. It is crucial that we as community-oriented nurses use every available opportunity to prevent further spread of AIDS by addicts who use intravenous drugs.

Even with the most successful preventive efforts, intravenous drug users who test positive for the HIV will turn up in the client loads of community health nurses, home health care nurses, nurse practitioners, and even school nurses. An assessment of the client's needs and strengths is the first step in the nursing process. The planning that follows should involve the client as much as possible.

The stigma of AIDS adds to the depression, anger, and loneliness the intravenous drug user may already feel. This makes it difficult to de-escalate the drug habit. In fact de-escalation may not, at this time, be the primary goal of the nursing intervention. Instead, the initial goal is to stop the spread of AIDS. A first step for heroin users could be to get them on a methadone maintenance program to bypass the needle and syringe as a source of contamination for others. In addition, the client needs to be taught other protective measures. That a client's route of infection was intravenous drug use does not mean that this is the only route for spreading the disease. Blood and other body fluids can also transmit AIDS, so condoms should be urged for all sexual encounters.

Female clients of childbearing age who are HIV positive and intravenous drug abusers should try at all costs to avoid getting pregnant. Not only should they be urged to insist that all male partners use condoms, but also they should use an additional method of contraception such as oral contraceptives or an intrauterine device. This is because condoms are only 85% effective. A baby born to a woman with AIDS will almost certainly test positive for the HIV, and the infant will have a 50% chance of developing AIDS. If the AIDS victim is pregnant, nurses should not force the client to have an abortion but an abortion should certainly be seriously considered. Babies and children with AIDS need expert home or hospital nursing and loving supportive care.

All intravenous drug users should be made aware of the danger of AIDS and hepatitis B. A 1987 study found that there were an estimated 1.1 million people injecting illicit drugs intravenously; up to 80% of this group sometimes shared needles. One positive finding was that approximately 20% of this group were willing to stop injecting heroin if they could get into a methadone maintenance program. Unfortunately, not enough programs were available.

This again suggests the importance of the role of the nurse as an advocate and a participant in the political process. More methadone clinics are needed, and since they are not profitable, public funds will have to be used to establish and maintain them. This can be achieved only through the political process. Nurses may also want to debate and perhaps advocate free needles and syringes for all addicts of intravenous drugs and free condoms for all sexually active clients who are not strictly monogamous.

Drug-Exposed Infants

AIDS is not the only danger faced by an infant whose mother abuses drugs. The drugs themselves can cause serious damage to the developing fetus. The following three types of damage to the fetus are reported depending on the type of drug the mother uses (Weston and others, 1989):

1. The infant is born with a drug addiction and consequently faces withdrawal symptoms.
2. The neonate is sick because of the toxicity of the drug.
3. The neonate has brain damage or other congenital anomalies because of the teratogenic characteristics of the drug.

The number of infants facing one or all these types of damage is increasing rapidly. A hospital survey done in 1988 indicated that in a sample of 36 hospitals, 11% of the newborns were affected by substance abuse (Weston, 1989). Since it has been the practice to remove these infants from the care of their mothers, foster care facilities are being overwhelmed and many infants are being left in the hospitals as border babies.

Intervention in the problem is complex, but it is a problem on which society needs to start working immediately. A major issue is that there is a severe shortage of treatment facilities for drug-addicted pregnant women. Congressional hearings have documented that most women who seek treatment for their substance abuse cannot get it. The second problem is a shortage of programs to follow and treat the damaged infants in homes with their mothers, in the hospital, or in foster homes.

If the mother is too drug damaged to keep the infant, hospital and foster care are not the only alternatives. There are some loving people who will adopt if they understand the infant's situation and if the paperwork can be cleared. A recent best selling novel, *The Broken Cord* tells the story of an unmarried man, Michael Dorris, who adopted an Indian boy with fetal alcohol syndrome that had caused mental retardation (Dorris, 1989). Dorris did not understand the full impact of the problem and only came to do so as his son grew older. It is a sad and beautiful book that makes a plea for dealing with the problem before it develops.

Nurses Who Abuse Substances

Substance abuse is the major cause for discipline by state medical boards. This is also true for the members of the other health professions. In addition to all the other factors faced by the ordinary individual who becomes a substance abuser, health professionals have the additional problem of having access to drugs. Until recently the profession, as distinct from the licensing boards, has not been concerned about nurses who become involved with alcohol or drugs. Fortunately there is now a growing realization that this problem is our professional responsibility. One result has been the establishment of rehabilitative programs for impaired nurses.

Peer support in identifying the impaired nurse is also important, although it may not be appreciated at the time. It is difficult to think of reporting the suspicious activity of a colleague as a helpful act, but it is. Early treatment of substance abuse is usually more successful than later interventions; impaired nurses can also do serious damage to clients unless they are detected and treated (Green, 1989).

One of the authors of this book served as a member of a state board of nursing. Nurses, in an effort to gain access to drugs, sometimes acted without consideration of their clients. The most distressing situations were those in which nurses abused narcotics by removing a narcotic from a bottle and then filling it with normal saline or water so that clients in pain were given an injection that contained little narcotic. Clients in such situations often cry out begging for more medication. Other nurses, who responded to the care and observed the chart indicating narcotic had been given, fearful of addicting clients (even terminal cancer clients), would force the clients to wait as long as four hours before giving them more diluted narcotic. Although nurses often suspected a colleague of substance abuse, they would usually say nothing unless they were certain. Sometimes if they did have courage enough to report the problem, the hospital simply discharged the nurse without reporting it to the Board. This allowed the nurse to move to another hospital and repeat the process. One of our responsibilities as nurses is to report impaired nurses as soon as possible so that they can be removed from a job where clients can be harmed and can be given help to recover. Ignoring the problem makes the situation worse.

SUMMARY

From the Nightingale era until the present nurses have been concerned about substance abuse, although the definition of the problem has changed to regard substance abuse as a moral problem to an illness. Substance abuse can be defined as the intake of a mind-altering substance when it is not approved by medical or social practice. The major categories of substance abuse include smoking, intemperate use of alcohol or caffeine, and the use of cannabis, hallucinogens, or inhalants such as glue and solvents. In addition, the abuse of drugs that are not prescribed, including the central nervous system depressants, stimulants, and opiates and other analgesics, can be problematic.

Substance abuse patterns change over time, and the most recent problem is the epidemic of abuse of cocaine in the form of crack. The use of intravenous cocaine and heroin is particularly dangerous when taken by pregnant women because of the dangers to the developing fetus.

The five-step nursing process can be used to structure the role of the nurse as it relates to substance abuse. The intervention phase of the nursing process tends to focus primarily on two types of activity—primary prevention and treatment, which is often aimed at preventing further damage.

QUESTIONS FOR DISCUSSION

1. If you planned a community assessment for your own community, what do you think would be the major substance abuse problem?
2. How would you proceed with the assessment process?
3. What factors have lead to the upsurge in the use of cocaine?
4. What are the major sources for referral for clients with substance abuse problems in your community?
5. Why is intravenous drug use more dangerous now than it was a few years ago?

REFERENCES

Amons M: Illegal drug use drops but crack addiction soars, Los Angeles Times, p 15, August 1, 1989.

Bailey GW: Current perspectives on substance abuse in youth, J Am Acad Child Adolesc Psychiatry 28:151, 1989.

Becker MH and Joseph JC: AIDS and behavioral change to reduce risk: a review, Am J Public Health 78:394, 1988.

Bennett G, Vourakis C, and Woolf CS, editors: Substance abuse: pharmacologic, developmental, and clinical perspectives, New York, 1983, John Wiley & Sons Inc.

Bennett JVA: A prison administrator views today's narcotic problem. In Livingston RB, editor: Narcotic drug problems, Washington, DC, 1958, US Government Printing Office.

Bullough B, Hindi-Alexander M, and Fetouh S: Methylxanthines and fibrocystic breast disease, Nurse Pract, 1989 (in press).

Burpo RH: A step beyond "just say no," MCN 13:428, 1988.

Castiglia PT and others: Influence on children's attitude toward alcohol consumption, Pediatr Nurs 15:263, 1989.

Dorris M: The broken cord, New York, 1989, Harper & Row, Publishers Inc.

The drug crisis: hour by hour; Crack, Newsweek, p 64, November 28, 1988.

Fleming R and others: The role of cigarettes in the initiation and progression of substance abuse, Addict Behav 14:261, 1989.

Fortin ML: Community health nursing. In Bennett G, Vourakis C, and Woolf DS, editors: Substance abuse: pharmacologic, developmental, and clinical perspectives, New York, 1983, John Wiley & Sons Inc.

Gebbie K: The president's commission on AIDS: What did it do? Am J Public Health 79:868, 1989.

Green P: The chemically dependent nurse, Nurs Clin North Am 24:81, 1989.

Hatziandreu EJ and others: The reliability of self-reported cigarette consumption in the United States, Am J Public Health 79:1020, 1989.

Health groups condemn threats by United States on tobacco trade, The Nation's Health 19:1, 1989.

Hindi-Alexander M and others: Theophylline and fibrocystic breast disease, J Allergy Clin Immunol 75:709, 1985.

Hughes TL: Models and perspectives of addiction, Nurs Clin North Am 24:1, 1989.

Jellinek EM: The disease concept of alcoholism, New Haven, Conn, 1960, Hillhouse.

Kandel DB: Stages in adolescent involvement in drug use, Science 190:912, 1975.

Kastrup ER: Facts and comparisons, 1980 Edition, St Louis, 1979, Facts and Comparisons.

Kinder VN, Pape NE, and Walfish S: Drug and alcohol education programs: a review of outcome studies, Int J Addict 15:1035, 1980.

Leads from MMWR update, acquired immunodeficiency syndrome—United States, 1981-1988, JAMA 261: 2609, 1989.

Loveys BJ: Drug abuse in critical care: physiologic effects of cocaine with particular reference to the cardiovascular system, Heart Lung 16:175, 1978.

Maddux JF: History of the hospital treatment programs, 1935-74. In Martin E and Isbell H, editors: Drug addiction and the US Public Health Service, DHEW Publication No (ADM) 77-434, Washington, DC, 1978, US Government Printing Office.

Minton JP: To whom it may concern, Unpublished letter, February 1981.

Minton JP and others: Caffeine, cyclic nucleotides and breast disease, Surgery 86:105, 1979.

Ratings: chocolate bars, Consumer Rep 51:61, 1986.

Sandler DP and others: Deaths from all causes in nonsmokers who lived with smokers, Am J Public Health 79:163, 1989.

Schuckit MA: Drug and alcohol abuse: a clinical guide to diagnosis and treatment, ed 2, New York, 1984, Plenum Publishing Corp.

SOS Meetings: collective suggestions from readers SOS: Save ourselves, SOS Newsletter 1:1, 1988.

Terry CE and Pellens M: The opium problem, Montclair, NJ, 1970, Patterson Smith.

United States Public Health Service: Smoking and health report of the advisory committee to the Surgeon General of the Public Health Service, Department of Health, Education and Welfare, Public Health Service (PHS Pub No 1103), Washington, DC, 1964, US Government Printing Office.

Warner KE: Effects of the antismoking campaign: an update, Am J Public Health 79:144, 1989a.

Warner KE: Smoking and health: a 25-year perspective, Am J Public Health 79:141, 1989b.

Westermeyer J: National and international strategies to control drug abuse, Adv Alcohol and Subst Abuse 8:1, 1989.

Weston DR and others: Drug exposed babies: research and clinical issues; zero to three, Bull Nat Center Clin Infant Programs 9:1, 1989.

BIBLIOGRAPHY

Nuckols CG and Greeson J: Cocaine addiction: assessment and intervention, Nurs Clin North Am 24:33, 1989.

Smith J: The dangers of prenatal cocaine, MCN 13:174, 1988.

Index

Page numbers in *italics* indicate illustrations and boxed material.
Page numbers followed by *t* indicate tables.

X

Y

Photography Credits

pp. 22, 53, 54, 86, 128, 171, 172, 188, 206, 224, 242, 296, 372, 404, 438, 470, 519, 520, 598, 632, and 654—Ruth E. Heintz.

pp. 104, 223, 274, and 492—courtesy Hospital Home Health Care Agency of California.

pp. 343 and 558—Harry A. Sparks. p. 558—courtesy also Kids in the Middle.

p. 344—courtesy Constance D. Blair.

p. 2—from Duffus RL: Lillian Wald: neighbor and crusader, New York, 1938, Macmillan Publishing Co.

The photographer thanks the following agencies and their representatives for their assistance in providing opportunities for photographing their clients and facilities: Allentown Industries of Buffalo, NY; Buffalo VA Medical Center Hospital Based Home Care Department (HBHC); City Mission of Buffalo; Erie County Health Department; James Liederhouse, P.T.; Seneca Nation Health Center on the Cattaraugus Indian Reservation; The Sheehan Memorial Hospital Family Care Center in the Buffalo Perry housing project; and the WNY AIDS Program.

Ruth E. Heintz